MASTER TECHNIQUES IN ORTHOPAEDIC SURGERY™
■
FRACTURES

MASTER TECHNIQUES IN ORTHOPAEDIC SURGERY™

■

Series Editor
Roby C. Thompson, Jr., M.D.

Volume Editors

THE FOOT AND ANKLE
Kenneth A. Johnson, M.D.

RECONSTRUCTIVE KNEE SURGERY
Douglas W. Jackson, M.D.

KNEE ARTHROPLASTY
Paul A. Lotke, M.D.

THE HIP
Clement B. Sledge, M.D.

THE SPINE
David S. Bradford, M.D.

THE SHOULDER
Edward V. Craig, M.D.

THE ELBOW
Bernard F. Morrey, M.D.

THE WRIST
Richard H. Gelberman, M.D.

THE HAND
James W. Strickland, M.D.

FRACTURES
Donald A. Wiss, M.D.

FRACTURES

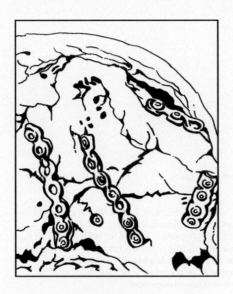

Editor

DONALD A. WISS, M.D.
**Southern California Orthopedic Institute
Van Nuys, California**

Illustrator

Christopher Blake Williams, M.A.

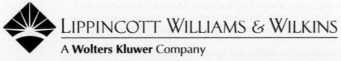

LIPPINCOTT WILLIAMS & WILKINS
A **Wolters Kluwer** Company

Philadelphia · Baltimore · New York · London
Buenos Aires · Hong Kong · Sydney · Tokyo

Acquisitions Editor: Kathey Alexander
Developmental Editor: Juleann Dob
Manufacturing Manager: Tim Reynolds
Production Manager: Jodi Borgenicht
Production Editor: Raeann Touhey
Cover Designer: Patricia Gast
Indexer: Lynne Mahan
Compositor: Maryland Composition
Color Separator/Prepress: Chroma Graphics (overseas), Pte Ltd.
Printer: Toppan Printers, Pte Ltd., Singapore

Printed and bound in **Japan**

9 8 7 6 5 4 3 2

Library of Congress Cataloging-in-Publication Data
Fractures / editor, Donald A. Wiss ; illustrator, Christopher Blake Williams.
    p.   cm. — (Master techniques in orthopaedic surgery™ [v. 10])
    Includes bibliographical references and index.
    ISBN 0-397-51703-3
    1. Fracture fixation—Atlases.   I. Wiss, Donald A.   II. Series.
    [DNLM: 1. Fractures—surgery.   WE 168 M423 1994 v.10]
  RD103F58F73   1998
  617.1'5—dc21
  DNLM/DLC   98-15918
  for Library of Congress   CIP

To my wife, Deborah,
my sons, Jeremy and David,
and my parents, Dorothy and William,
whose guidance, love, and support made this book a reality

∎

CONTENTS

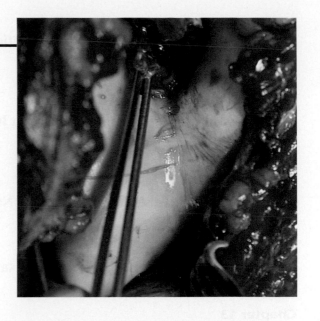

PART III   PELVIS AND ACETABULUM

CONTRIBUTORS

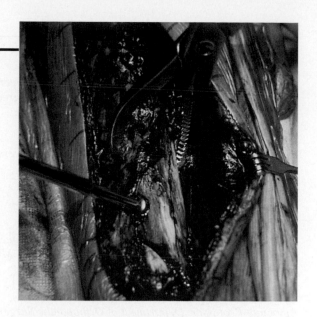

Craig S. Bartlett, M.D.
Clinical Assistant Professor, Department of Orthopaedic Surgery and Rehabilitation, University of Vermont, McClure Musculoskeletal Research Center, Robert T. Stafford Hall, Burlington, Vermont 05405-0084

Fred F. Behrens, M.D.
Professor and Chairman, Department of Orthopaedics, New Jersey Medical School, Doctors Office Center, Suite 5200, 90 Bergen Street, Newark, New Jersey 07103-2499

Stephen K. Benirschke, M.D.
Associate Professor, Department of Orthopaedics, Harborview Medical Center, 325 Ninth Avenue, Seattle, Washington 98104

Louis U. Bigliani, M.D.
The Shoulder Service, New York Orthopaedic Hospital, Columbia-Presbyterian Medical Center, 161 Forth Washington Avenue, New York, New York 10032

Piotr A. Blachut, M.D., F.R.C.S.C.
Clinical Associate Professor, Department of Orthopaedics, Division of Orthopaedic Trauma, University of British Columbia, Vancouver Hospital and Health Sciences Center, 910 West 10th Avenue, Vancouver, British Columbia, V5Z 4E3, Canada

Brett R. Bolhofner, M.D.
All Florida Orthopedic Associates, St. Petersburg, Florida 33702

Michael J. Bosse, M.D.
Department of Orthopaedic Surgery, Carolinas Medical Center, 1000 Blythe Boulevard, P.O. Box 32861, Charlotte, North Carolina 28232

Timothy J. Bray, M.D.
Associate Clinical Professor, Department of Orthopaedic Surgery, University of California, Davis Medical Center, Sacramento, California; and Associate, Reno Orthopaedic Clinic, 555 North Arlington Avenue, Reno, Nevada 89503

Bruce D. Browner, M.D.
Gray-Gossling Professor and Chairman, Department of Orthopaedic Surgery, University of Connecticut Health Center, John Dempsey Hospital, 10 Talcott Notch Road, Farmington, Connecticut 06034-4037

Andrew E. Caputo, M.D.
Department of Orthopaedics, University of Connecticut Health Center, 10 Talcott Notch, Farmington, Connecticut 06034-4037

Peter A. Cole, M.D.
Assistant Professor, Department of Orthopaedic Surgery, University of Mississippi Medical Center, 2500 North State Street, Jackson, Mississippi 39216

Charles N. Cornell, M.D.
Associate Professor, Department of Surgery, Cornell University Medical College, Hospital for Special Surgery, 535 East 70th Street, New York, New York 10021

Christopher W. DiGiovanni, M.D.
Clinical Instructor, Department of Orthopaedics, Brown University, 14 Balmoral Avenue, Providence, Rhode Island 02908

Alan E. Freeland, M.D.
Director, Hand Surgery and Professor, Department of Orthopaedic Surgery and Rehabilitation, University of Mississippi Medical Center, 2500 North State Street, Jackson, Mississippi 39216

William B. Geissler, M.D.
Associate Professor, Department of Orthopaedic Surgery and Rehabilitation, University of Mississippi Medical Center, 2500 North State Street, Jackson, Mississippi 39216

Thomas P. Goss, M.D.
Professor, Department of Orthopaedic Surgery, University of Massachusetts Medical Center, 55 Lake Avenue North, Worcester, Massachusetts 01655

James A. Goulet, M.D.
Associate Professor, Department of Orthopaedic Surgery, University of Michigan Hospitals and Health Center, Taubman Center 2914, 1500 E. Medical Center Drive, Ann Arbor, Michigan 48109-0328

Pierre Guy, M.D., F.R.C.S.C.
Assistant Professor, Department of Orthopaedic Surgery, McGill University Health Center, 1650 Cedar Avenue, D10-160, Montreal, Quebec H3G 1A4, Canada

David L. Helfet, M.B., Ch.B.
Associate Professor, Department of Orthopaedic Surgery,
Cornell University Medical College, 535 East 70th Street,
New York, New York 10021

Eric E. Johnson, M.D.
Professor, Department of Orthopaedic Surgery, University
of California at Los Angeles Medical Center, 10833
LeConte Avenue, Room 62-266CH, Los Angeles,
California 90095-6902

Kenneth D. Johnson, M.D.
Professor, Department of Orthopaedic Surgery, Vanderbilt
University Medical Center, 2100 Pierce Avenue, 131 MCS,
Nashville, Tennessee 37212

Jessie B. Jupiter, M.D.
Associate Professor, Department of Orthopaedic Surgery,
Massachusetts General Hospital, Wang Ambulatory Care
Building, 15 Parkman Street, Boston, Massachusetts 02114

James F. Kellam, M.D., B.Sc.
Director of Orthopaedic Trauma, Department of
Orthopaedic Surgery, Carolinas Medical Center,
1000 Blythe Boulevard, P.O. Box 32861, Charlotte,
North Carolina 28203

Kenneth J. Koval, M.D.
Chief, Fracture Service, Department of Orthopaedic
Surgery, Hospital for Joint Diseases, 301 East 17th Street,
New York, New York 10003

Mark D. MacLeod, M.D., F.R.C.S.C.
Clinical Assistant Professor, Department of Surgery,
Division of Orthopaedics, University of Western Ontario,
345 Westminster Avenue, London, Ontario N6C 4V3,
Canada

Arthur L. Malkani, M.D.
Chief, Adult Reconstruction, and Assistant Professor,
Department of Orthopaedic Surgery, The University of
Louisville, 530 South Jackson Street, ACB Third Floor
Bridge, Louisville, Kentucky 40292

Joel M. Matta, M.D.
Clinical Professor, Department of Orthopaedic Surgery,
University of Southern California, 637 South Lucas
Avenue, Suite 605, Los Angeles, California 90017

Augustus D. Mazzocca, M.D.
Department of Orthopaedics, University of Connecticut
Health Center, 10 Talcott Notch, Farmington,
Connecticut 06034-4037

Dana C. Mears, B.M., B.Ch., Ph.D.
Professor, Department of Orthopaedic Surgery, Albany
Medical College, 47 New Scotland Avenue, Mail Code:
61OR, Albany, New York 12208

Berton R. Moed, M.D.
Professor, Department of Orthopaedic Surgery, Wayne
State University, University Health Center, Suite 7C, 4201
St. Antoine Boulevard, Detroit, Michigan 48201

Bernard F. Morrey, M.D.
Department of Orthopaedics, Mayo Medical School; and
Department of Orthopaedics, The Mayo Clinic and Mayo
Foundation, 200 First Street, Southwest, Rochester,
Minnesota 55905

Brent L. Norris, M.D.
Department of Orthopaedic Surgery, Carolinas Medical
Center, 1000 Blythe Boulevard, P.O. Box 32861, Charlotte,
North Carolina 28232

Peter J. O'Brien, M.D., F.R.C.S.C.
Assistant Professor, Department of Orthopaedics,
University of British Columbia, Vancouver Hospital and
Health Sciences Center, 910 West 10th Avenue, Vancouver,
British Columbia V5Z 4E3, Canada

Brendan M. Patterson, M.D.
Assistant Professor, Department of Orthopaedic Surgery,
MetroHealth Medical Center, Case Western Reserve
University School of Medicine, 2500 MetroHealth Drive,
Cleveland, Ohio 44109

Mark C. Reilly, M.D.
Clinical Instructor, Department of Orthopaedic Surgery,
Harbor—University of California at Los Angeles Medical
Center, Torrance, California 90509

Barry L. Riemer, M.D.
Professor, Department of Orthopaedic Surgery, and
Director, Orthopaedic Trauma Division, Allegheny
University of The Health Sciences, 420 East North Avenue,
Suite 401, Pittsburgh, Pennsylvania 15212-4734

M. L. Chip Routt, Jr., M.D.
Associate Professor, Department of Orthopaedics,
University of Washington, Harborview Medical Center,
325 Ninth Avenue, Seattle, Washington 98104

Thomas A. Russell, M.D.
Associate Professor, Department of Orthopaedic Surgery,
University of Tennessee, and Memphis Orthopaedic Group,
Inc., 1325 East Moreland Street, Suite 260, Memphis,
Tennessee 38104

Roy W. Sanders, M.D.
Professor, Department of Orthopaedics, University of
South Florida, 12901 B. B. Downs Boulevard, Tampa,
Florida 33612

Bruce J. Sangeorzan, M.D.
Professor of Orthopaedic Surgery, Department of
Orthopaedics, University of Washington, Harborview
Medical Center, 325 Ninth Avenue, Box 359798, Seattle,
Washington 98104

Gregory J. Schmeling, M.D.
Director, Division of Orthopaedic Trauma, Associate
Professor, Department of Orthopaedic Surgery, MCW
Clinics at Froedtert East, 9200 West Wisconsin Avenue,
Milwaukee, Wisconsin 53226

Andrew H. Schmidt, M.D.
Clinical Assistant Professor, Department of Orthopaedic Surgery, University of Minnesota, Hennepin County Medical Center, 701 Park Avenue, Minneapolis, Minnesota 55415

David Seligson, M.D.
Professor, Department of Orthopaedics, University of Louisville, Louisville, Kentucky 40202; and Ortho Trauma Associates, Louisville, Kentucky 40207

Randy Sherman, M.D.
Chairman, Division of Plastic and Reconstructive Surgery, University of Southern California—University Plastic Surgeons, 1450 San Pablo Street, Ground Floor, South Entrance, Suite 1900, Los Angeles, California 90033-4680

John M. Siliski, M.D.
Assistant Professor, Department of Orthopaedic Surgery, Massachusetts General Hospital, Harvard Medical School, Wang ACC, Suite 525,15 Parkman Street, Boston, Massachusetts 02114

Peter T. Simonian, M.D.
Associate Professor, Department of Orthopaedic Surgery, University of Washington; and Chief, Sports Medicine Clinic, Department of Orthopaedic Surgery, University of Washington Medical Center, Box 356500, Seattle, Washington 98195

Stephen H. Sims, M.D.
Department of Orthopaedic Surgery, Carolinas Medical Center, 1000 Blythe Boulevard, P.O. Box 32861, Charlotte, North Carolina 28232

Marc F. Swiontkowski, M.D.
Professor and Chair, Department of Orthopaedic Surgery, University of Minnesota Medical School, 420 Delaware Street Southeast, Box 492, Minneapolis, Minnesota 55455

David C. Templeman, M.D.
Wayzata Orthopaedics, 2805 Campus Drive, Plymouth, Minnesota 55441

Paul Tornetta III, M.D.
Department of Orthopaedic Surgery, Boston University Medical Center, 88 East Newton Street, Boston, Massachusetts 02118

Peter G. Trafton, M.D.
Professor and Vice Chairman, Department of Orthopaedic Surgery, Brown University, Providence, Rhode Island 02903

Thomas F. Varecka, M.D.
Assistant Professor, Department of Orthopaedic Surgery, University of Minnesota, Hennepin County Medical Center, 701 Park Avenue, 862B, Minneapolis, Minnesota 55415

Mark S. Vrahas, M.D.
Associate Professor, Department of Orthopaedic Surgery, Louisiana State University, 2025 Gravier, New Orleans, Louisiana 70112

J. Tracy Watson, M.D.
Senior Staff Surgeon, Division of Orthopaedic Trauma, Wayne State University, 2799 West Grand Boulevard, Detroit, Michigan 48201

Lon S. Weiner, M.D.
Section Chief, Department of Orthopaedic Trauma, Lenox Hill Hospital; and Assistant Clinical Professor, Department of Orthopaedics, Mt. Sinai Hospital, 130 East 77th Street, New York, New York 10021

Raymond R. White, M.D.
Trauma and Fracture Surgery, Orthopaedic Associates of Portland, P.A., 33 Sewall Street, Portland, Maine 04102

John H. Wilber, M.D.
Associate Professor, Department of Orthopaedic Surgery, Case Western Reserve University, University Orthopaedic Associates, 11100 Euclid Avenue, Cleveland, Ohio 44106

Robert A. Winquist, M.D.
Orthopaedic Physician Associates, 1229 Madison Street, #16, Seattle, Washington 98104

Donald A. Wiss, M.D.
Southern California Orthopedic Institute, 6815 Noble Avenue, Van Nuys, California 91405-3730

Daniel M. Zinar, M.D.
Associate Clinical Professor and Chair, Department of Orthopaedic Surgery, Los Angeles County-Harbor—University of California at Los Angeles Medical Center, 1000 West Carson Street, Box 422, Torrance, California 90509

ACKNOWLEDGMENTS

Master Techniques in Orthopaedic Surgery: Fractures was edited in Los Angeles and Van Nuys, California between 1994 and 1997, while I was practicing at the Southern California Orthopedic Institute (SCOI). It reflects nearly twenty years of study and treatment of fractures and their sequelae. Anyone undertaking such a work will incur debts of gratitude to a number of people who worked on this project with considerable commitment and little public recognition.

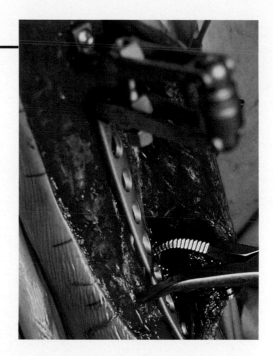

I am particularly grateful to Christopher Blake Williams, the medical illustrator of this text, for his magnificent artwork depicting fractures and their fixation. Abandoning the traditional methods of illustration, all of the artwork in the text is computer-generated, permitting more typographical detail and improved three-dimensional reality.

I would like to acknowledge and extend my gratitude to Eleanor O'Brien who typed and retyped virtually all of the manuscripts during the inevitable revision process. This book would have been enormously more difficult without her editorial and organizational talents, as well as her cheerful and patient attitude. Pam Swan, my medical secretary, also handled many of the details with the authors, and their staffs, as well as the publishing team at Lippincott–Raven. Thanks are due to Kathey Alexander and her staff at Lippincott–Raven for editorial assistance, support, and patience while completing this final volume of the *Master Techniques in Orthopaedic Surgery* series.

Finally, my heartfelt thanks and appreciation to each of the contributing authors who answered the "bell" once again with yet another academic request for their precious time. Their willingness to share their considerable expertise, explaining the details and nuances of fracture cases will unequivocally benefit orthopaedic surgeons everywhere who care for patients with musculoskeletal trauma.

SERIES PREFACE

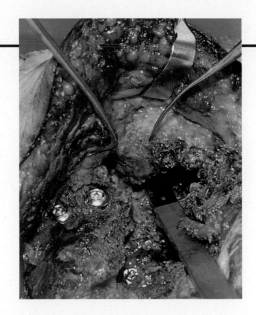

Master Techniques in Orthopaedic Surgery is a ten-volume series of operative atlases designed to provide in-depth descriptions of surgical techniques that are preferred by surgeons recognized by their peers a master surgeons in their area of specialization.

The ten volume editors, all recognized leaders based on their research and educational contributions, have advanced the surgical state of the art in our field. The chapter authors were selected for their experience and skills, and were asked to present their material in a personal manner, highlighting their unique perspectives and observations for the reader.

These atlases are designed to help the practitioner deal with the difficult but common problems encountered in daily practice. Surgical procedures that are in the developmental phase, such as vascularized fibular grafting for osteonecrosis, or procedures largely restricted to referral centers, such as reconstruction for limb salvage following tumor resection, have not been covered since procedures such as these are rarely performed by the orthopaedic practitioner. Likewise, the common, straightforward procedures that offer few complications and little difficulty have also been avoided.

These book take you into the operating room and let you peer over the shoulder of the surgeon at work. The color photographs and accompanying drawings guides the orthopaedist step-by-step through a procedure. The commentary, organized in a standard format throughout the series, offers one specific technical advice, as well as tips and pearls gained through the surgeon's years of experience.

The shared knowledge and expertise found in these pages are presented to enable the surgeon to undertake surgical procedures with greater confidence and improved proficiency.

Roby C. Thompson, Jr., M.D.
Series Editor

PREFACE

American medicine is in the midst of a profound and wrenching transformation. Government, Wall Street, and third party payers have demanded improved medical care at lower cost. Better medicine (orthopaedics) occurs when doctors practice medicine consistently on the basis of the best scientific evidence available, set up systems to measure performance, analyze results and outcomes, and make this information widely available to patients and the public. Reduced costs have been achieved partially through a wholesale shift to health maintenance organization, capitation, and managed care.

Trauma is a complex problem where initial decisions often dramatically determine the ultimate outcome. Death, deformity, and medicolegal entanglements may follow vacillation and error. When treatment is approached with confidence, logic, and technical skill, the associated mortality rate, preventable complications, permanent damage, and economic loss may be significantly reduced. Uncertainty, inactivity, and inappropriate investigation by the physician are all detrimental to the patient. Certain traditional concepts need to be abandoned and new approaches learned.

This text attempts to address society's mandate to our profession: better orthopaedics at reduced cost. It provides residents and practitioners with surgical approaches to 42 com-

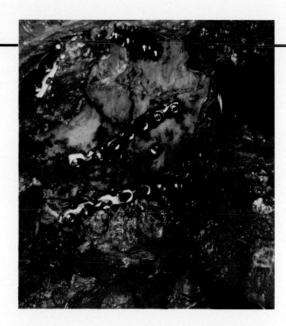

mon but often problematic fractures that, when correctly done, have proven to be safe and effective. It is my hope that this volume becomes a valuable fixture in the catalog of literature on fractures.

Donald A. Wiss, M.D.

MASTER TECHNIQUES IN ORTHOPAEDIC SURGERY™

■

FRACTURES

PART I

Upper Extremity

Master Techniques in Orthopaedic Surgery,
FRACTURES, edited by D. A. Wiss,
Lippincott–Raven Publishers, Philadelphia © 1998.

1

Glenoid Fractures: Open Reduction Internal Fixation

Thomas P. Goss

INDICATIONS/CONTRAINDICATIONS

Fractures of the scapula comprise approximately 1% of all fractures. Because direct high-energy trauma is generally involved, there is a high incidence (80% to 95%) of associated osseous and soft-tissue injuries, which may be multiple, major, and threaten limb or life. Fractures of the glenoid process account for approximately one third of scapular fractures and include disruptions of the glenoid cavity (the glenoid rim and the glenoid fossa; Fig. 1) and disruptions of the glenoid neck (Fig. 2). Although more than 90% of glenoid fractures are minimally displaced and can be treated nonoperatively, approximately 10% are significantly displaced and require surgical reconstruction. Fractures of the glenoid rim are managed surgically if the injury causes persistent subluxation of the humeral head or if the reduction is unstable. Instability can be anticipated if the fracture is displaced 10 mm or more and one fourth or more of the glenoid cavity anteriorly or one third or more of the glenoid cavity posteriorly is involved. Surgical indications for glenoid fossa fractures include (a) an articular step-off of 5 mm or more, (b) such severe separation of the fragments that a nonunion is likely, and (c) a fracture pattern that allows displacement of the humeral head out of the center of the glenoid cavity. Surgical treatment of glenoid neck fractures is considered if there is translational displacement of the glenoid fragment 1 cm or more or angular displacement of the fragment 40 degrees or more in either the coronal or sagittal plane (Type II fractures) or both. Contraindications include severely comminuted fractures of the glenoid cavity and glenoid fractures in which comminution of the surrounding osseous structures precludes satisfactory fixation.

T. P. GOSS, M.D.: Department of Orthopedic Surgery, University of Massachusetts Medical Center, Worcester, Massachusetts 01655.

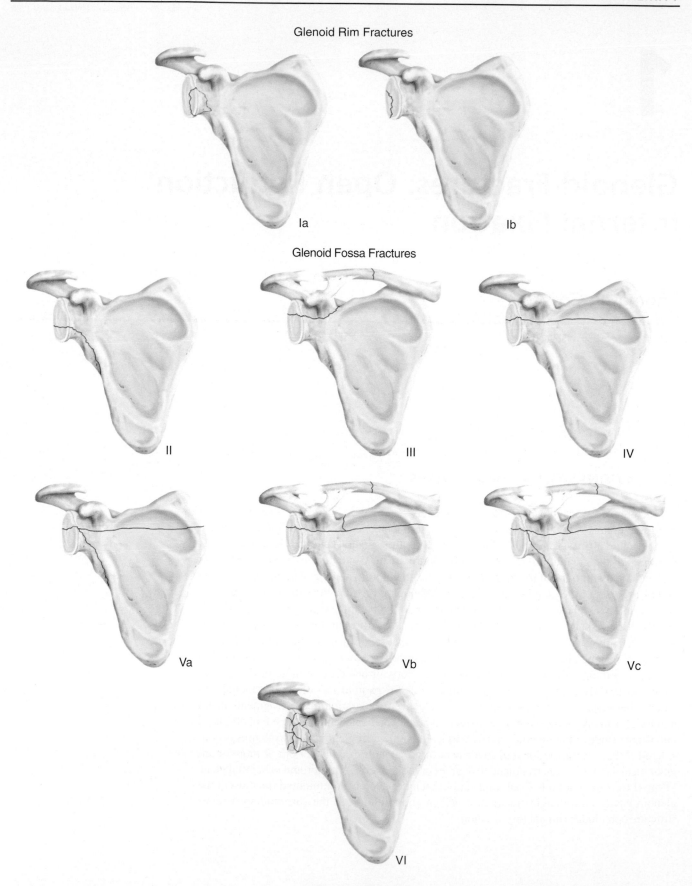

Figure 1. Classification for fractures of the glenoid cavity.

Type I Fractures

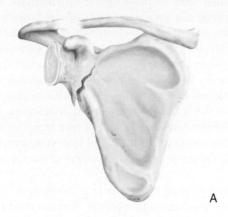

A

Type II Fractures

Translational Displacement

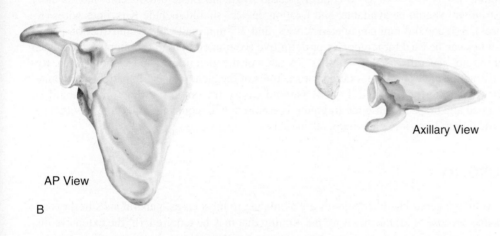

Axillary View

AP View

B   C

Angulatory Displacement

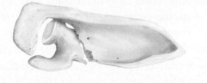

D

Axillary View

Figure 2. A–D: Classification for fractures of the glenoid neck.

PREOPERATIVE PLANNING

Diagnosis is radiologic and begins with a "scapula trauma series," composed of true anteroposterior (AP) and lateral views of the scapula and an axillary projection of the glenohumeral joint. Because of the complex bony anatomy in the area, however, a computed tomography (CT) scan is often required to accurately define these injuries and to allow optimal preoperative planning. These radiographs should also be reviewed carefully to identify associated fractures of the shoulder girdle including the remainder of the scapula, the clavicle, and the proximal humerus, as well as disruptions of the acromioclavicular, glenohumeral, sternoclavicular, and scapulothoracic articulations. Abrasions and open wounds involving the superficial soft tissues must be inspected carefully, and surgery may need to be delayed until they are adequately clean. Although vascular injury is quite uncommon, distal pulses should be palpated and if absent or questionable, arteriography should be performed. Injury to the brachial plexus also is uncommon, but a thorough neurologic examination is necessary to document function of the axillary, musculocutaneous, median, radial, and ulnar nerves. Electromyographic (EMG) testing can be performed 3 weeks after injury if a deficit is found or suspected. Scapulothoracic dissociation is a distinct clinical entity that should be considered. It has a very high incidence of neurovascular involvement and is characterized by (a) a history of violent trauma, (b) massive swelling of the shoulder girdle, and (c) posterolateral displacement of the scapula relative to the rib cage.

Should it be determined that surgical management of the glenoid fracture is necessary, a thorough knowledge of shoulder anatomy is essential. Anterior rim (Type Ia) fractures are approached anteriorly with the patient in the beach-chair position. Posterior rim (Type Ib) fractures, all glenoid fossa disruptions, and glenoid neck fractures are approached at least in part posteriorly. A superior approach may be added if a large displaced superior glenoid fragment (Type III) or glenoscapular fragment (Type IV) is present or if a glenoid neck disruption results in a difficult-to-control glenoid fragment. Basic orthopaedic and shoulder instruments should be available, and fixation devices should include Kirschner wires (K-wires), 3.5- and 4.0-mm cannulated screws, and 3.5-mm malleable reconstruction plates. K-wires can be used for temporary or definitive fixation of glenoid fragments. Cannulated screws are generally used to stabilize fractures of the glenoid rim and glenoid fossa. Reconstruction plates provide fixation for fractures of the glenoid neck. In patients with anterior rim, posterior rim, and Type II glenoid cavity fractures, the iliac crest should be prepped and draped in case the fragment is comminuted, requiring replacement with a tricortical graft to restore glenohumeral stability.

SURGERY

Although nerve-block techniques are available, in most cases, general anesthesia is advisable because of (a) the awkward positioning that may be required, (b) the extensive dissection and manipulation that may be necessary, (c) the prolonged operative time that frequently occurs, and (d) the proximity of the patient's head to the work being done. A regional block before the administration of general anesthesia, however, may be used for postoperative pain control. With the exception of Type Ia fractures of the glenoid cavity (anterior rim injuries), which require an anterior exposure, the primary surgical approach for these fractures is posterior. The patient is placed on the operating room table in the lateral decubitus position—nonoperative side down (a towel roll placed in the axilla), operative side up, and the torso stabilized with a beanbag (Fig. 3). The upper extremity and shoulder complex are prepped and draped free; the elbow, forearm, and wrist/hand are encased in a sterile wrap; and a well-padded sterilely draped Mayo stand is prepared to serve as a mobile adjustable arm rest. Bony landmarks are outlined with a marking pen (Fig. 4).

An incision is made over the lateral spine of the scapula, along the posterior aspect of the acromion to its lateral tip, and extended distally in the midlateral line for a distance of 2.5 cm (Fig. 5). Via sharp and blunt dissection deep to the subcutaneous layer, soft-tissue flaps are developed and retracted, exposing the posterior deltoid muscle (Fig. 6). The posterior deltoid is dissected sharply off the scapular spine and acromion and then split in the line of its fibers for approximately 2.5 cm, starting at the lateral tip of the acromion. The posterior deltoid is bluntly separated from the underlying infraspinatus and teres minor musculotendinous units and retracted down to, but not below, the inferior margin of the teres minor (Fig. 7). The inferior half of the infraspinatus tendon is incised vertically 2.5 cm posterior to the greater tuberosity, and the infraspinatus/teres minor interval is opened.

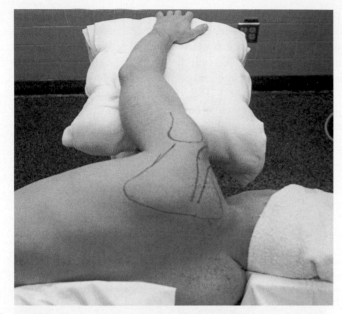

Figure 3. The lateral decubitus position used for posterior and posterosuperior approaches to the glenoid process.

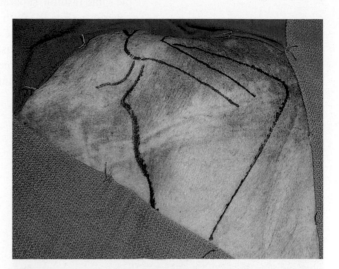

Figure 4. The posterior shoulder complex bony landmarks.

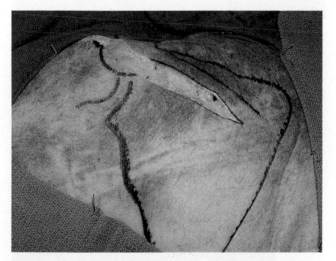

Figure 5. The standard posterior incision extending along the inferior margin of the scapular spine and the acromion. At the lateral tip of the acromion, the incision continues in the midlateral line for 2.5 cm..

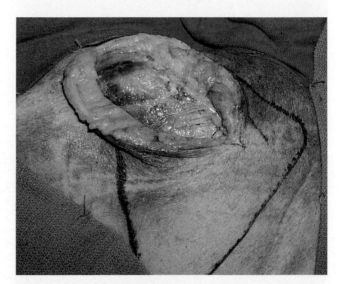

Figure 6. Elevation of superficial soft-tissue flaps to expose the origin of the posterior and middle heads of the deltoid muscle.

The infraspinatus can then be dissected off the underlying posterior glenohumeral joint capsule and retracted superiorly (Fig. 8). The posterior glenohumeral capsule is incised in the same fashion, separated subperiosteally off the posterior glenoid process, and retracted superiorly (Fig. 9). With a Fukuda retractor inserted into the joint and holding the humeral head out of the way, the entire glenoid cavity can be inspected, and the surgeon has ready access to the posterior aspect of the glenoid process (Fig. 10). The entire infraspinatus tendon/posterior glenohumeral capsule can be detached laterally and superiorly and turned back medially for maximal exposure. The interval between the infraspinatus and teres mi-

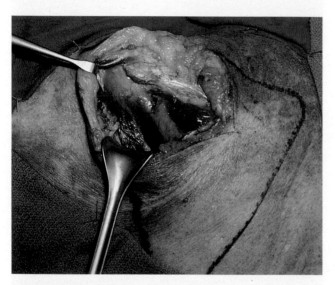

Figure 7. The posterior and middle heads of the deltoid muscle have been detached from the scapular spine/posterior acromial process and retracted distally to expose the infraspinatus musculotendinous unit.

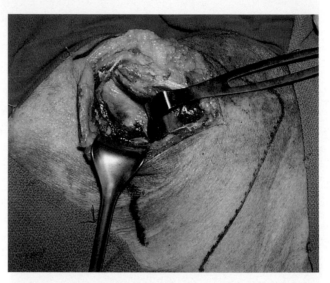

Figure 8. The infraspinatus/teres minor interval has been developed, with the infraspinatus retracted superiorly and the teres minor retracted inferiorly to expose the posterior glenohumeral joint capsule (the inferior portion of the infraspinatus insertion has been released).

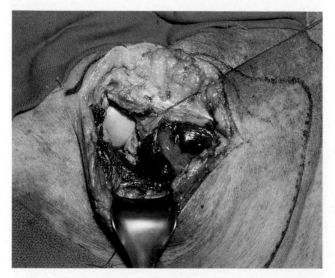

Figure 9. The inferior portion of the posterior glenohumeral joint capsule has been incised and reflected medially to expose the humeral head and glenohumeral joint space.

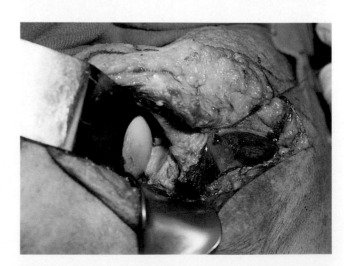

Figure 10. With the posterior glenohumeral joint capsule reflected medially and a humeral head retractor in place, ready access is available to the glenoid fossa and the posterior glenoid rim.

nor muscles can be further developed and the underlying soft tissues elevated subperiosteally to gain access to the inferior aspect of the glenoid process and the lateral border of the scapula (Fig. 11).

Thick solid bone for internal fixation is at a premium because much of the scapula is paper-thin. Four regions of substantial bone are available: the glenoid neck, the coracoid process, the base of the scapular spine, and the lateral border of the scapular body (Fig. 12). A variety of fixation devices are available, but the most useful are (a) easily contoured 3.5-mm reconstruction plates, (b) 3.5- or 4.0-mm cannulated interfragmentary compression screws, and (c) K-wires (Figs. 13–15). These devices may be used alone or in combination. The final choice depends on the available bone stock and the surgeon's preference. Obviously, stable internal fixation is the goal, but often lesser fixation is either all that can be provided or all that is needed. The posterior exposure should be sufficient for Type Ib (posterior rim) and Type II glenoid cavity fractures, as well as for most fractures of the glenoid neck. For Type Ib fractures, the posterior fragment is reduced anatomically and fixed in position with two 2.0-mm guide wires. These wires are then used to drill, tap, and finally insert two 4.0-mm cannulated compression screws (the second screw is placed to control rotation). If the posterior rim fragment is comminuted, a tricortical bone graft harvested from the iliac crest is used to reconstruct the posterior rim. For Type II (inferior glenoid fossa) fractures, similar fixation is provided; however, the inferior fragment must be well mobilized by dissecting subperiosteally inferiorly and anteriorly, and the cannulated screws are placed posteroinferiorly to anterosuperiorly. For fractures of the glenoid neck, the infraspinatus/teres minor interval must be developed, exposing the lateral scapular border. The glenoid fragment is then reduced as anatomically as possible relative to the scapular body (a supplemental superior approach may be useful to place a K-wire into the glenoid fragment to aid in reduction) and fixed in position with a contoured 3.5-mm reconstruction plate applied along the posterior aspect of the glenoid fragment and the lateral scapular border. Glenoid cavity fractures with a significantly displaced superior fragment (Types III and IV injuries) generally require a supplemental superior approach (Figs. 16–18). A 2.0-mm guide wire can then be placed into the superior fragment and used to manipulate it into position while visualizing the reduction via the posterior exposure. The

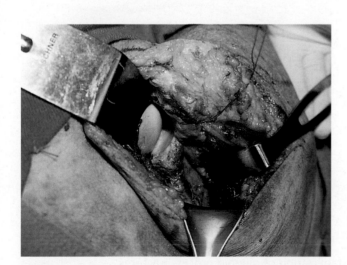

Figure 11. With the infraspinatus/teres minor interval developed further, the two musculotendinous units retracted, and the long head of the triceps muscle released, access to the inferior aspect of the glenoid process and the lateral scapular border is available.

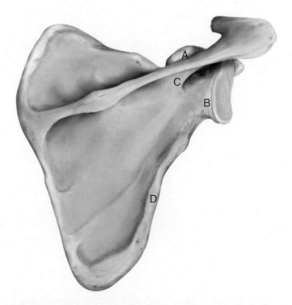

Figure 12. Areas of adequate bone stock for internal fixation in the glenoid region of the scapula. A, Coracoid process; B, glenoid neck; C, base of the scapular spine; D, lateral border of the scapula.

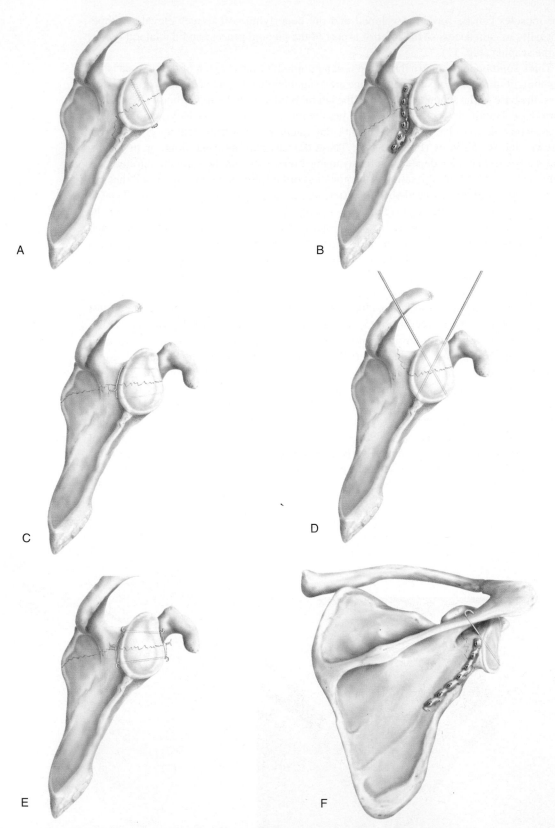

Figure 13. Internal-fixation techniques for stabilization of glenoid process fractures.
A: Interfragmentary compression screw. **B:** Reconstruction plate. **C:** Cerclage wire/suture. **D:** K-wires. **E:** Two K-wire–cerclage wire/suture technique. **F:** Reconstruction plate plus K-wire (used for temporary or permanent fixation).

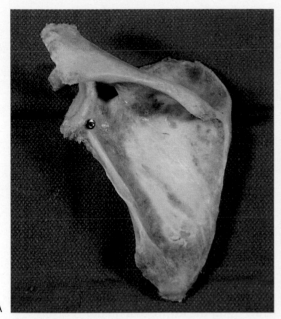
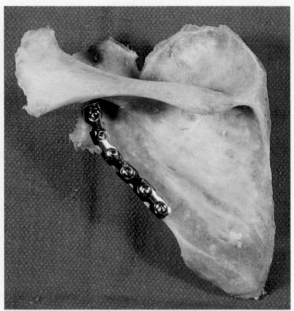

Figure 14. The two most useful devices for internal fixation of glenoid process fractures. **A:** A cannulated interfragmentary compression screw. **B:** A 3.5-mm malleable reconstruction plate.

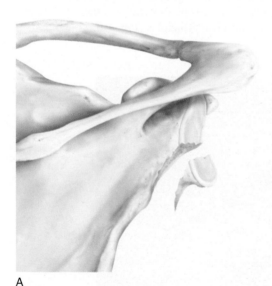
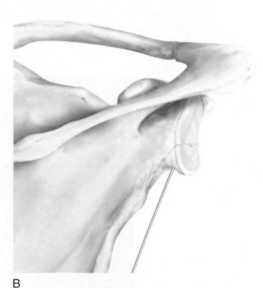

Figure 15. Reduction and internal fixation of a glenoid fracture by using an interfragmentary cannulated compression screw. **A:** Displaced Type II glenoid cavity fracture. **B:** Temporary reduction and fixation of fragment by using a K-wire. (*figure continues*)

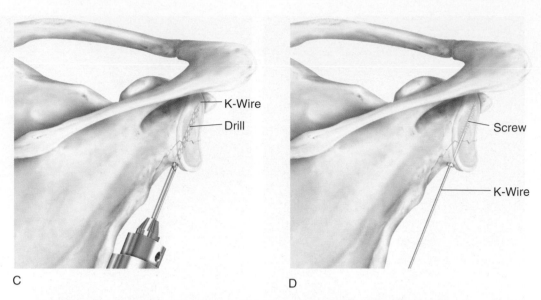

Figure 15. *(continued)* **C:** Passage of a cannulated drill using the K-wire as a guide. **D:** Passage of a cannulated compression screw using the K-wire as a guide.

guide wire is then passed across the fracture site into the inferior aspect of the glenoid process and used to drill, tap, and finally place a cannulated compression screw. Type V fractures of the glenoid cavity are combinations of the Type II, III, and IV disruptions and therefore follow the same management principles. If bleeding is a concern, medium hemovac drains are placed in the wound—one deep and one superficial to the infraspinatus muscle. Closure of the wound follows routine surgical principles (Fig. 19).

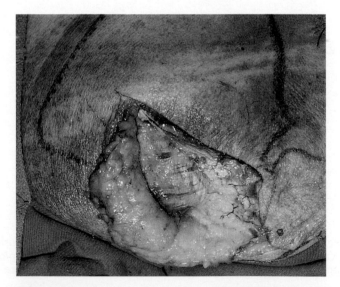

Figure 16. This and the next two figures show the superior approach to the glenoid process. The inferior aspect of the scapular body is at the top, the superior angle of the scapula is to the left, and the glenohumeral joint is to the right. The incision is the same as that in Figure 5; however, in this case, the superior soft-tissue flap has been developed and reflected, exposing the trapezius muscle (in the center of the figure), which is inserting along the scapular spine and acromial process.

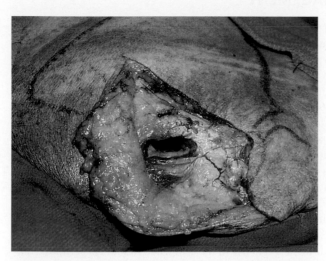

Figure 17. In the interval between the clavicle and the scapular spine/acromial process, the trapezius has been split in the line of its fibers to expose the underlying supraspinatus muscle.

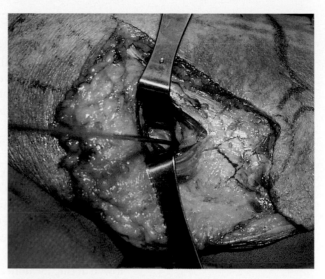

Figure 18. In the interval between the clavicle and scapular spine/acromial process, the trapezius muscle and the supraspinatus musculotendinous unit have been split in the line of their fibers and retracted to expose the superior aspect of the glenoid process lateral to the coracoid process. A K-wire has been placed into the glenoid process. If this were a separate fracture fragment, the K-wire could be used to manipulate the fragment into position relative to the remainder of the glenoid process (a posterior exposure is necessary to make sure articular congruity has been restored). The K-wire could then be used to place a cannulated interfragmentary compression screw.

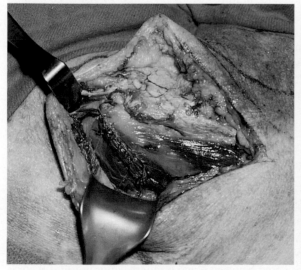

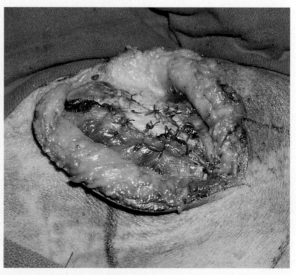

A   B

Figure 19. A: Closure of the infraspinatus/teres minor interval and repair of the infraspinatus insertion. **B:** Closure of the split in the trapezius muscle by using a running 2-0 absorbable suture, and reattachment of the origin of the deltoid muscle by using no. 1 nonabsorbable sutures placed through drill holes in the scapular spine/acromial process.

POSTOPERATIVE MANAGEMENT

Most patients are discharged to home with their arms immobilized in a sling and swathe bandage. Early care after operative treatment of glenoid fractures is dependent on the degree of stability achieved. With stable internal fixation, patients are begun on a program of simple passive range-of-motion exercises, which include dependent circular and pendulum movements and external rotation to but not past neutral during the first 2 weeks after surgery. Between weeks 3 and 6, further passive stretching exercises in all ranges are initiated. The goal is to achieve 90 degrees of forward flexion by postoperative day 14, 120 degrees by postoperative day 28, and 150 degrees by postoperative day 42; internal rotation to the small of the back by postoperative day 28, and to the high part of the lower back by postoperative day 42; 0 degrees of external rotation by postoperative day 14, 30 degrees of external rotation by postoperative day 28, and 60 degrees of external rotation by postoperative day 42. The patient sees a therapist 2 to 3 times a week and performs a self-directed home exercise program 3 to 4 times a day. During the first 2 weeks, the patient's arm is totally immobilized between physiotherapy sessions. Light use of the arm while sitting is allowed during the third and fourth week. Light use of the arm when indoors is permitted during weeks 5 and 6. The patient is seen by his physician at 2-week intervals between weeks 1 and 6. AP radiographs in neutral rotation and axillary views of the shoulder are obtained on each occasion to ensure maintenance of the reduction and hardware and correct positioning of the humeral head within the glenoid cavity. Range of motion of the shoulder is documented, and updated physiotherapy instructions are generated accordingly. If fixation is with K-wires, cerclage wires, or isolated screws, the shoulder may need to be immobilized in a sling and swathe dressing, an abduction brace, or even overhead olecranon-pin traction for 7 to 14 days to allow early healing to occur before beginning any physiotherapy. At 6 weeks, healing is usually advanced, protection is discontinued, and functional use of the shoulder is encouraged. As range of motion improves, progressive strengthening exercises are added. The rehabilitation program continues until range of motion and strength are maximized. The patient should limit the use of the arm to light activities through week 12, and heavy, physical athletic activities are prohibited for 4–6 months after surgery.

Unfortunately, because scapular fractures are uncommon, there are few personal series, and no well-controlled multicenter studies. Hardegger et al. (11) reported 79% good-to-excellent results associated with five displaced glenoid neck fractures treated surgically (6.5-year follow-up). Kavanaugh et al. (13) at Mayo Clinic reviewed 10 displaced glenoid cavity fractures treated with open reduction and internal fixation and found it to be a "useful and safe technique which can restore excellent function of the shoulder." Until more data are available, it is reasonable to predict a good-to-excellent functional result if (a) surgical management restores normal or near-normal glenoid anatomy/articular congruity/glenohumeral stability, (b) the fixation is secure, and (c) there is a well-structured and intensive rehabilitation program.

COMPLICATIONS

Complications associated with fractures of the glenoid are in four categories.

1. Complications associated with injuries to bony and soft tissue structures in the zone of injury due to the severe traumatic forces involved.

   Examples: although uncommon, injuries to the axillary nerve do occur but usually represent a neurapraxia and have a good prognosis for recovery. EMG testing may be performed 3 weeks after injury or as needed thereafter to monitor recovery. Exploration and repair should be considered between 3 and 6 months after injury if there is no sign of function or if improvement is not satisfactory. Exploration and repair should be performed by 12 months at the latest. Glenohumeral arthrodesis should be considered if the patient fails to recover functional arm elevation.

   On occasion, fractures of the glenoid neck may be associated with a fracture of the clavicle. This combination of injuries has been called a "floating shoulder" and represents a double disruption of the superior shoulder suspensory complex. Because of instability, the glenoid neck or clavicle fracture can be severely displaced. Regardless of how the glenoid neck fracture is managed, if unacceptable displacement persists at the clavicular fracture site, open reduction and internal fixation (ORIF) is indicated.

2. Complications associated with the scapular fracture.

If ORIF of a glenoid fossa fracture fails to restore satisfactory articular congruity, resulting in symptomatic posttraumatic glenohumeral arthritis, a shoulder arthroplasty may be indicated. In older individuals, a total replacement is the procedure of choice. In younger individuals, a hemiarthroplasty with or without reshaping of the glenoid and biologic resurfacing (with the option to convert to a total shoulder replacement at a later date) may be considered. Arthrodesis is an option in those who must use their shoulders for heavy, manual, physical work.

3. Complications associated with the surgical management.

Superficial infections are managed with local irrigation and debridement, closure over drains, and a short course of appropriate antibiotic therapy. Deep infections must be recognized as early as possible and treated aggressively. The wound is opened surgically, thoroughly debrided and irrigated, and closed over drains. Hardware is maintained if at all possible and certainly if fixation is firm. Six weeks of appropriate intravenous antibiotic therapy is frequently indicated.

4. Complications associated with the postoperative management.

A poorly supervised physiotherapy program may lead to postoperative shoulder stiffness. Close follow-up by the physician, dedication on the part of the therapist, and maximal effort by the patient should result in functional shoulder range of motion. Most patients will lose some range of motion; however, 135 degrees or more of forward flexion, internal rotation to the small of the back, and 30 degrees of external rotation should be achieved. If postoperative loss of motion occurs, closed manipulation under anesthesia is generally unsuccessful because this type of shoulder stiffness is caused by dense posttraumatic and postoperative scarring. An open surgical release can result in even more scarring and loss of motion. Treatment therefore consists of a long-term aggressive stretching program, hoping that the contracted soft tissues will gradually stretch out over time.

ILLUSTRATIVE CASES FOR TECHNIQUE

Fracture of the posterior glenoid rim is shown in Figure 20. Fracture of the glenoid cavity is shown in Figure 21. Figure 22 shows a fracture of the glenoid neck.

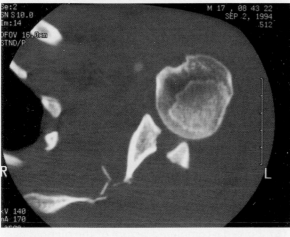
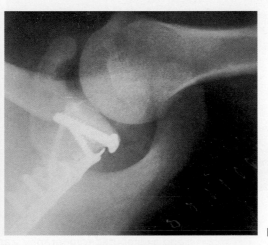

A   B

Figure 20. A 17-year-old boy had multiple blunt trauma including a left shoulder injury after a motor vehicle accident. Plain radiographs and a computed tomography scan **(A)** showed a severely displaced posterior glenoid rim fragment with a significant articular step-off and posterior subluxation of the humeral head (a Type Ib fracture of the glenoid cavity). Five days after injury, he underwent an open reduction and internal fixation via a posterior approach. Fixation was achieved with two interfragmentary cannulated screws and a buttress plate. Articular congruity and glenohumeral stability were restored **(B)**.

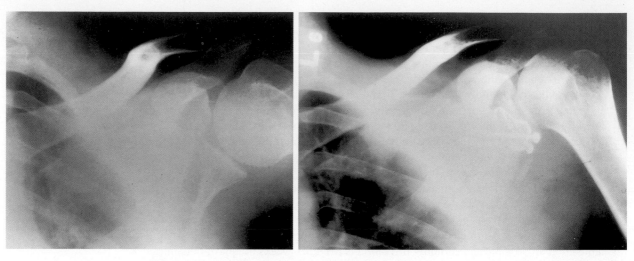

A   B

Figure 21. A 37-year-old man had blunt trauma to his left shoulder caused by a fall down a flight of stairs. Plain radiographs **(A)** showed a severely displaced inferior glenoid cavity fragment (Type II fracture) with a significant articular step-off and inferior subluxation of the humeral head. Two days after the injury, he underwent an open reduction and internal fixation via a posterior approach. Fixation was achieved with two interfragmentary compression screws and a cerclage wire. Articular congruity and glenohumeral stability were restored **(B)**.

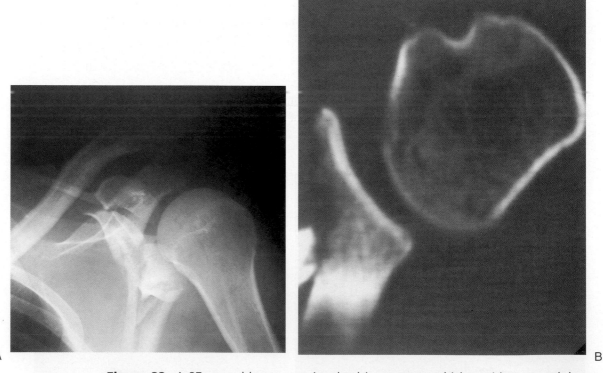

A   B

Figure 22. A 27-year-old man was involved in a motor vehicle accident, sustaining multiple blunt trauma, including an injury to his left shoulder. Plain radiographs **(A)** and a computed tomography scan **(B)** showed a complete fracture of the glenoid neck and a fracture of the coracoid process, resulting in severe angulatory displacement of the glenoid fragment (a Type II glenoid neck fracture). (*figure continues*)

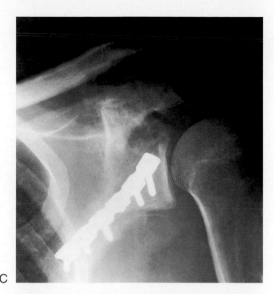

C

Figure 22. *(continued)* Two days after the injury, he underwent an open reduction and internal fixation via a combined posterior/superior approach. Fixation was achieved with a 3.5-mm reconstruction plate. Anatomic position and stabilization of the glenoid fragment were achieved **(C)**.

RECOMMENDED READING

 1. Ada, J.R., and Miller, M.E.: Scapular fractures: analysis of 113 cases. *Clin. Orthop.*, 269:174–180, 1991.
 2. Butters, K.P.: The scapula. In Rockwood, C.A., Jr., Matsen, F.A., II, (eds.): *The Shoulder.* W.B. Saunders, Philadelphia, 1990, vol. 1, pp. 335–366.
 3. DePalma, A.F.: *Surgery of the Shoulder,* 3rd ed. J.B. Lippincott, Philadelphia, 1983.
 4. Goss, T.P.: Double disruptions of the superior shoulder suspensory complex. *J. Orthop. Trauma,* 7:99–106, 1993.
 5. Goss, T.P.: Fractures of the glenoid cavity. *J. Bone Joint Surg. [Am],* 74:299–305, 1992.
 6. Goss, T.P.: Fractures of the glenoid cavity: operative principles and techniques. *Techniques Orthop.,* 8:199–204, 1994.
 7. Goss, T.P.: Fractures of the glenoid cavity [videotape]. American Academy of Orthopaedic Surgeons Physician videotape library, 1994.
 8. Goss, T.P.: Fractures of the glenoid neck. *J. Shoulder Elbow Surg.,* 3:42–52, 1994.
 9. Goss, T.P.: Scapular fractures and dislocations: diagnosis and treatment. *J. Am. Acad. Orthop. Surg.,* 3(1):22–33, 1995.
10. Goss, T.P.: The scapula: coracoid, acromial and avulsion fractures. *Am. J. Orthop.,* 25(2):106–115, 1996.
11. Hardegger, F.H., Simpson, L.A., and Weber, B.G.: The operative treatment of scapular fractures. *J. Bone Joint Surg. [Br],* 66:725–731, 1984.
12. Ideberg, R.: Unusual glenoid fractures: a report on 92 cases [Abstract]. *Acta. Orthop. Scand.,* 58:191–192, 1987.
13. Kavanaugh, B.F., Bradway, J.K., and Cofield, R.H.: Open reduction and internal fixation of displaced intra-articular fractures of the glenoid fossa. *J. Bone Joint Surg. [Am],* 75:479–484, 1993.
14. Miller, M.E., and Ada, J.R.: Fractures of the scapula, clavicle, and glenoid. In Browner, B.D., Jupiter, J.B., Levine, A.M., et al. (eds.): *Skeletal Trauma: Fractures, Dislocations, Ligamentous Injuries.* W.B. Saunders, Philadelphia, 1992, Vol. 2, pp. 1291–1310.
15. Nordqvist, A., and Petersson, C.: Fracture of the body, neck or spine of the scapula: a long-term follow-up study. *Clin. Orthop.* 283:139–144, 1992.

Master Techniques in Orthopaedic Surgery,
FRACTURES, edited by D. A. Wiss,
Lippincott–Raven Publishers, Philadelphia © 1998.

2

Proximal Humeral Fractures: Percutaneous Fixation

Raymond R. White

INDICATIONS/CONTRAINDICATIONS

Percutaneous fixation of proximal humeral fractures is an excellent example of indirect reduction and minimal stable fixation. This procedure allows rapid healing and return to a normal function. The Neer classification accounts for displacement and angulation and is used to classify proximal humerus fractures (Fig. 1). Percutaneous fixation is most commonly used to treat two-part fractures or those involving the surgical neck and the isolated greater tuberosity fracture. However, this technique is also optimal for three-part fractures because it preserves the tenuous blood supply to the head fragment. This technique, therefore, should be considered for physiologically young patients who wish to save their own humeral head and avoid prosthetic replacement. Occasionally percutaneous fixation can be used on four-part fractures. The risk of avascular necrosis associated with this procedure precludes its use in circumstances other than for young patients who want to save the humeral head.

Contraindications for percutaneous fixation are head-splitting fractures, four-part fractures in the elderly, uncooperative patients, pathologic bone, and metaphyseal extension. This technique is not a substitute for prosthetic replacement in the elderly with four-part fractures or fractures in which the humeral head is split and not able to be reconstructed. Patients must be cooperative and not confused. Postoperative patient confusion may lead to loss of fixation and poor results. If adequate fixation is not possible because of osteopenia or pathologic (tumor) bone, another technique should be used. This technique cannot be used in fractures with metaphyseal comminution. These fractures, in which length is an important issue, should be stabilized with plate fixation.

R. R. White, M.D.: Trauma and Fracture Surgery, Orthopaedic Associates of Portland, P.A., Portland, Maine 04102.

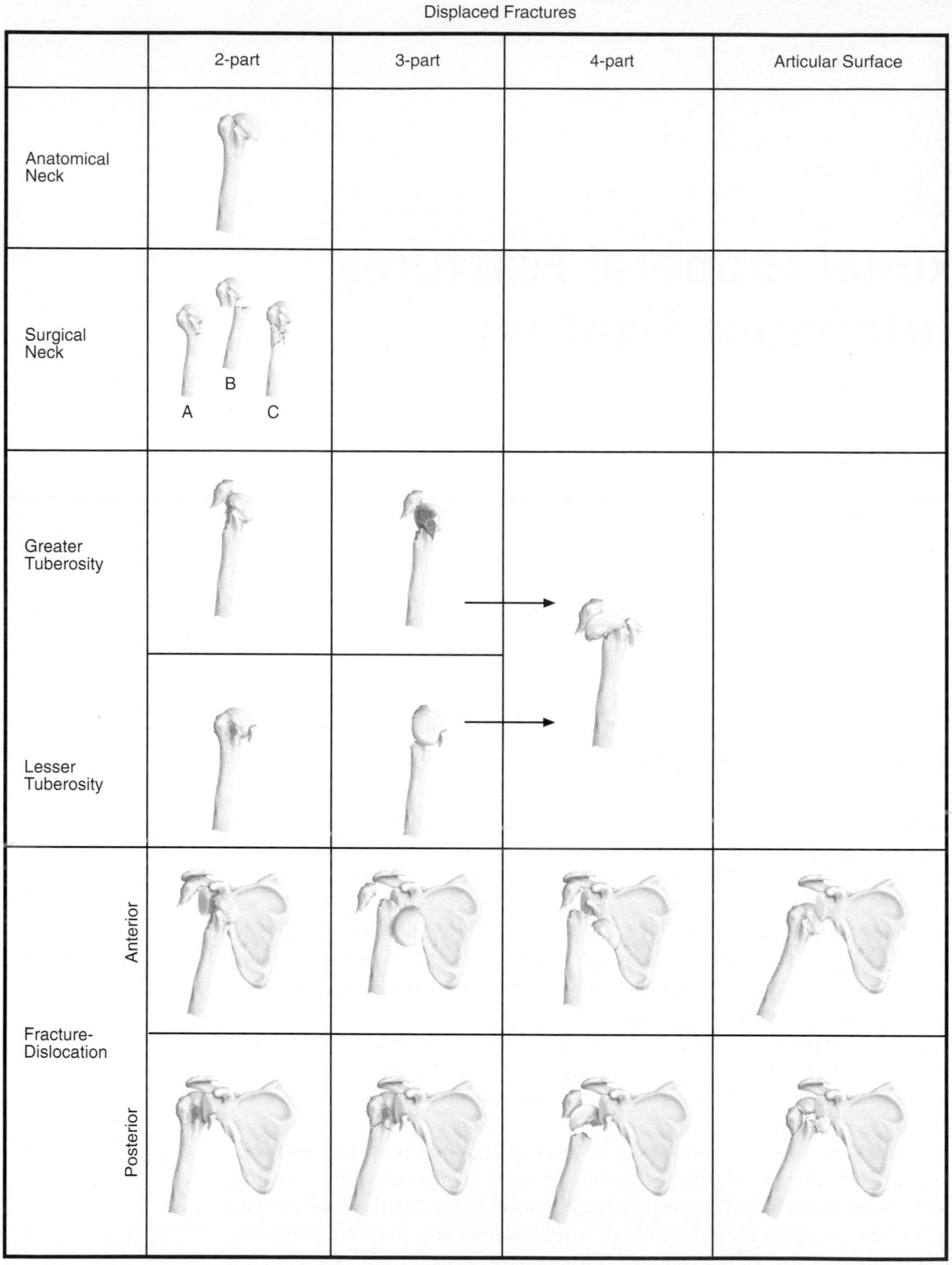

Displaced Fractures

	2-part	3-part	4-part	Articular Surface
Anatomical Neck				
Surgical Neck	A B C			
Greater Tuberosity				
Lesser Tuberosity				
Fracture-Dislocation — Anterior				
Fracture-Dislocation — Posterior				

Figure 1. Neer classification of proximal humerus fractures

PREOPERATIVE PLANNING

Initially, the patient's limb is evaluated for neurovascular compromise, especially the axillary nerve. Considerable shoulder swelling is not unusual, and ecchymosis often extends into the forearm and chest wall.

Radiographic views include an anteroposterior (AP), scapular Y, and axillary lateral view of the shoulder (Fig. 2A–C). A true AP view of the humerus (with the arm in a neutral position) may be useful to determine head impaction. The axillary view is helpful in determining anteroposterior angulation and lesser tuberosity displacement (Fig. 2C). A computed tomography (CT) scan is rarely necessary, and magnetic resonance imaging (MRI) is not helpful in determining head vascularity in the acute phase.

Timing of the surgery is critical only if the head is dislocated. A dislocated humeral head must be relocated as an emergency. Occasionally it is possible to reduce the head dislocation by closed methods, but an open approach is usually required. If the head is not dislocated, surgery can be done on an elective basis, usually 3 to 7 days after injury. If there are no associated medical problems, surgery can be done in an outpatient setting. The patient is placed in a sling-and-swathe shoulder immobilizer until surgery. Pre- and postoperative pain management are the same: the patients are given scheduled acetaminophen (1,000 mg, q. 6 h) and ibuprofen (400 mg, q. 6 h), with oxycodone (5 to 10 mg, q. 2 h) for breakthrough pain.

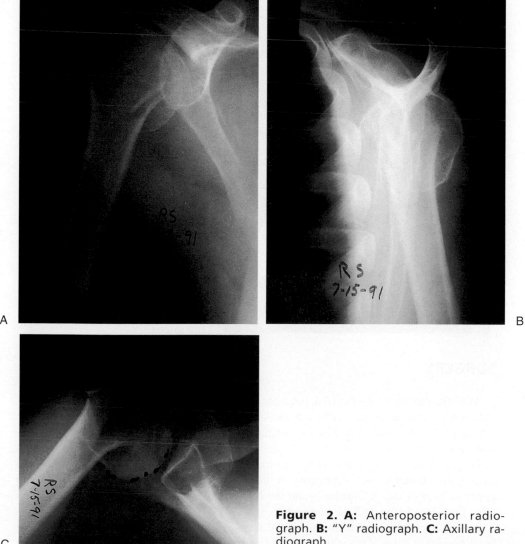

A

B

C

Figure 2. A: Anteroposterior radiograph. **B:** "Y" radiograph. **C:** Axillary radiograph.

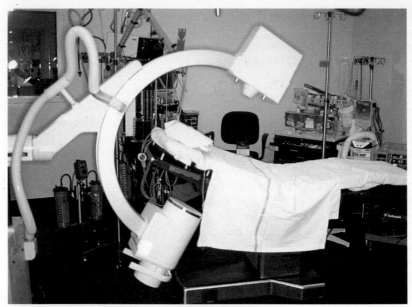

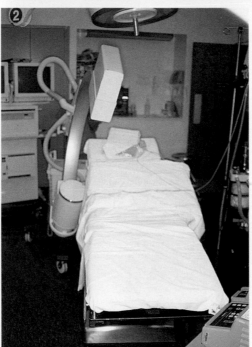

Figure 3. A: The position of the operating room equipment. The table is turned 90 degrees, with the anesthetist and equipment on the unaffected side and the image intensifier at the head of the table. **B:** The C-arm position as seen from the end of the table. Note that the C is tilted to avoid the table's interfering with the image.

SURGERY

After the patient is anesthetized, the table is turned 90 degrees, with the anesthesia staff and their equipment on the unaffected side, allowing sufficient room for the surgeon on the affected side. The image intensifier is positioned at the head of the table with the TV monitors near the base unit on the affected side (Fig. 3A). The C-arm is positioned so the machine can swing 90 degrees to obtain an axillary view. The "C" should be positioned to swing either under or over, depending on the position of the patient. It is helpful to tilt the upper portion of the "C" medially and the lower portion of the "C" laterally to keep the table from interfering with the image (Fig. 3B).

Patients can be positioned in one of two ways. The first is to place the patient flat on a level operating room (OR) table with the head at the foot of the table (backward on the table), so the table cranks are not in the way of the x-ray machine (Fig. 4A). The patient is then moved laterally on a radiolucent board so the shoulder is over the edge of the table. The advantage of this position is threefold: two-part fractures tend to stay reduced; the image-intensifier sending unit is below the table and farther from the surgeon; and the image swings under the drapes, facilitating an axillary view (Fig. 4B).

In the second position, the patient is placed in a "beach-chair" position (Fig. 5A) with the shoulder over the edge of the table. The image intensifier is turned so the sending unit is up and can be swung over the top for the axillary view. This position provides an easy table set-up, and if open reduction is necessary, the position is a familiar one. Unfortunately, the C arm must be swung over the top to obtain an axillary view, and the x-ray sending unit is closer to the surgeon's head, increasing exposure to the surgeon (Fig. 5B).

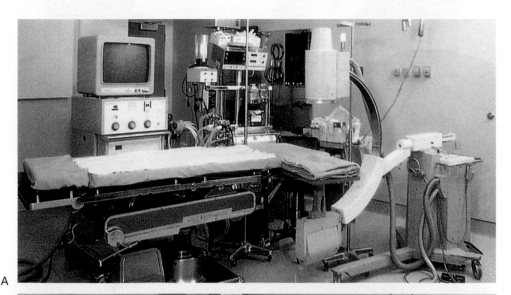

A

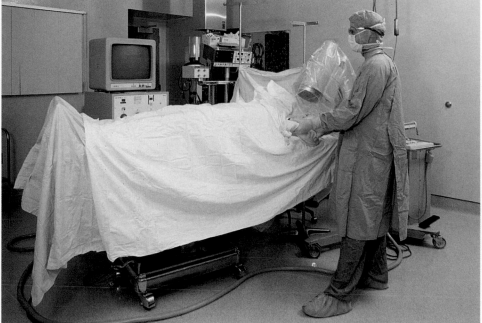

B

Figure 4. A: The patient is positioned flat on the operating room table. The patient's head is at the foot of the table. This keeps the table cranks from interfering with the image intensifier. **B:** The axillary view is easy to obtain in this position by swinging the image under the shoulder.

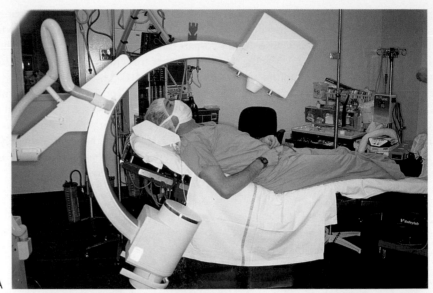

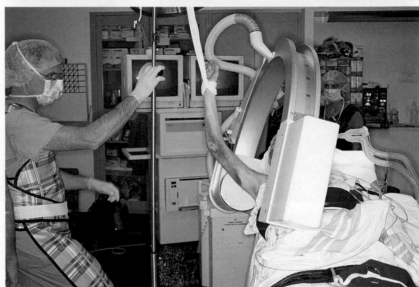

Figure 5. **A:** The "beach-chair" position is shown. **B:** The image must be swung over the top for the axillary view.

Reduction

Head-Shaft Reduction. It is imperative that the head be properly reduced onto the shaft. The pectoralis major pulls the shaft medially, anteriorly, and into internal rotation, exerting a deforming force. The supraspinatus, the other major deforming force, abducts the head fragment. Reduction can usually be accomplished by reversing the deforming forces. The reduction maneuver is longitudinal traction, abduction, posterior displacement, and slight external rotation of the shaft fragment relative to the proximal fragment (Fig. 6A). When impaction is a major component of the fracture, the shaft fragment may need to be moved posteriorly and outward (while longitudinal traction is applied; Fig. 6B). This movement can be aided by placing a rolled towel in the axilla to act as a fulcrum. Reduction must be confirmed in both AP and axillary planes by using the image intensifier before fixation.

Once reduction is obtained, it can usually be maintained by holding the arm suspended while prepping and draping is carried out (Fig. 7). After draping, the assistant holds the reduction while the surgeon places the fixation.

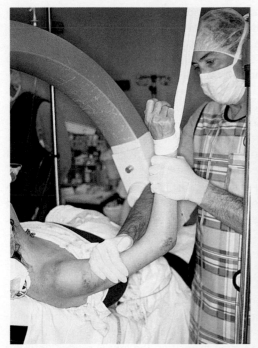
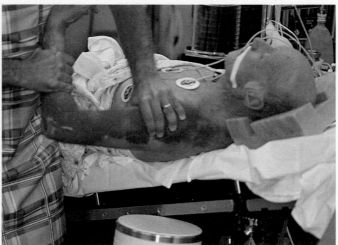

A   B

Figure 6. A, B: The maneuver used to reduce two- and three-part fractures. The shaft is distracted and mobilized posteriorly relative to the head fragment.

If an acceptable reduction cannot be obtained or maintained, a small-diameter Schanz pin inserted into the head acts as a joystick. The pin should be placed via the greater tuberosity to control the head fragment so the shaft fragment can be reduced to it.

Occasionally the fracture cannot be reduced closed because of biceps tendon interposition. A limited deltopectoral approach can be used to remove the tendon, permitting fracture reduction. Formal open reduction is occasionally necessary when there is a significant displacement or irreducible impaction. In these cases, fixation can be either percutaneous or internal.

Greater Tuberosity Reduction. Greater tuberosity fractures can be reduced percutaneously. First, rotate the shoulder until the displaced fragment is seen in its greatest profile and displacement. The fragment is usually a little posterior; some internal rotation of

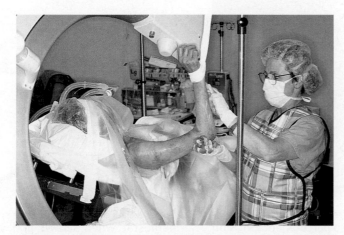

Figure 7. The arm is held suspended for prepping and draping. This position usually holds the reduction.

the arm will give the best view of displacement. A cannulated screw guide pin is placed via a 1.5-cm deltoid splitting into the center of the fragment. If the displacement is lateral only, the pin can be directed into the humeral head. If the displacement is superior and lateral, the pin should be directed more inferiorly. The cannulated screw (usually with a washer) will push the fragment either medially, or medially and distally when tightened, thereby reducing the fracture.

Three-Part Fractures. Three-part fractures in which the head is impacted and the greater tuberosity laterally displaced can also be reduced percutaneously. A 2.0-cm deltoid-splitting incision is made at the level of the fracture (this is localized with the image intensifier). A lamina spreader is introduced into the fracture site, and the head is disimpacted by opening the jaws of the spreader (Fig. 8); this tilts the head fragment into position by rotating it around the intact medial soft-tissue structures. The head is then held in place with pins (as described subsequently). The greater tuberosity can then key into place if the head has been tilted into the correct position. It is reduced as described previously, and fixed as noted subsequently (see Internal Fixation).

Fixation

Greater Tuberosity Fractures. In minimally displaced or comminuted tuberosity fractures, a large cannulated cancellous screw (7.0 or 7.3 mm) can be used to obtain both the reduction and the fixation. By using the image intensifier, the arm is rotated until the tuberosity is in greatest profile and displacement. Next, the cannulated screw guide pin is placed through a 1.5-cm incision into the center of the fragment and into the opposite cortex. A screw with a washer is then placed in the standard fashion. As the screw is tightened, the reduction is accomplished. A washer must be used to distribute the force of this powerful screw over a large area to avoid fragmenting the tuberosity. Care must be taken not to entrap the deltoid muscle beneath the washer. A curved hemostat or similar instrument is used to mobilize the muscle as the screw and washer pass through the deltoid (Fig. 9).

Two-Part Fractures. For fixation of a two-part proximal humeral fracture, we use 2.5 × 150-mm terminally threaded pins (Fig. 10) to decrease the chance of pin migration. If

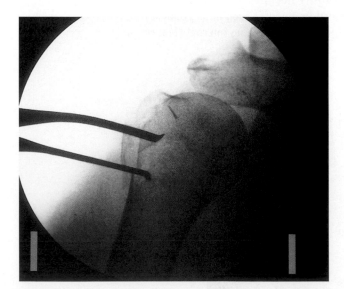

Figure 8. The impacted head fragment of this three-part fracture is reduced through a percutaneous incision with a lamina spreader.

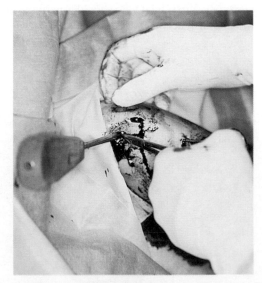

Figure 9. The soft tissues are spread with a hemostat when screws and washers are passed through them.

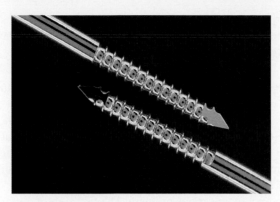

Figure 10. Terminally threaded pins used for percutaneous fixation.

these are not available, the terminally threaded guide pins can be used with a compression hip screw.

By using the image intensifier, position a pin on the anterior shoulder along the ideal line for placement, and mark the line with a skin marker. This line functions as the anteversion guide pin does in pinning femoral neck or intertrochanteric fractures. Ideally, it should be placed just above the deltoid insertion, but it is usually placed a little higher. Care must be taken to avoid damaging the axillary nerve. Four pins should be placed; they need not be parallel. An attempt should be made to spread the pins in the humeral head. Pin placement should be checked on both views with the image intensifier to be certain that they are contained within the humeral head. After the pins have been placed properly, they are cut off beneath the skin.

Another method of fixation uses cannulated screws. With this method, it is possible to use only one or two cannulated screws because of the limiting factor of the size of the starting point, the lateral humeral shaft. The fixation used most often is two 7.0-mm cannulated cancellous screws oriented vertically along the shaft and into the head.

Three- and Four-Part Fractures. In three- and four-part fractures, the head fragment is stabilized in the same way as in two-part fractures. The greater tuberosity fragment is stabilized with a single large cannulated cancellous screw. This screw is directed either into the humeral head or into the proximal metaphysis, depending on which way will best reduce the fragment (see the previous section on fixation of greater tuberosity fractures). The lesser tuberosity is not usually stabilized in four-part fractures.

POSTOPERATIVE MANAGEMENT

The strength of the fixation and the reliability of the patient determine whether the arm is placed in a sling or sling-and-swathe. If the patient is cooperative and excellent fixation was obtained, only a sling is used. If there are any concerns, the swathe also is used. Physical therapy (PT) is started 5 to 7 days after surgery. Initial PT consists of gentle pendulum exercises. Active and active-assisted range of motion is started 3 to 4 weeks after surgery, depending on the fixation quality and the healing. The sling protection is discontinued 4 to 6 weeks after surgery, depending on healing. Strengthening begins at this time. Unrestricted activity begins when healing is complete, usually within 6 to 10 weeks.

The pins are removed at 4 to 6 weeks, depending on healing. This is generally done in the office with local anesthesia. Sometimes sedation is necessary; extremely squeamish patients require a light general anesthetic.

COMPLICATIONS

Pin Protrusion/Migration

The most common causes of pin protrusion through the skin are reduction of swelling in the upper area and outward migration of the pins.

In the first type, the surgeon has two choices: (a) remove the pin if healing has progressed, and the remainder of the fixation is adequate to the point that removal of the pin will not jeopardize the fixation; or (b) leave the protruding pin in place, and treat the pin site as if it were an external fixator pin site. I generally choose the latter approach and have done so without further problems.

Migrating pins pose a more serious problem. The first sign of a migrating pin may be a sudden increase in pain, in either the shoulder or the soft tissues. If the pin has migrated outward and still provides fixation, it can be treated as a protruding pin, as noted previously. If it is no longer providing fixation, protruding through the skin, and causing enough irritation to hamper rehabilitation, it is best removed. If a pin should migrate inward and penetrate the humeral head, it must be removed immediately. These pins are not repositioned because enough healing has taken place that replacement is not necessary.

Loss of Reduction

Loss of reduction is usually associated with fixation failure, either pin or bone failure. Because many patients with proximal humerus fractures are elderly, the problem of poor bone quality is of great concern. Also, many elderly patients become confused and may be more active than they should be. When a patient becomes confused and requires restraints, the arm should be placed in a sling-and-swathe. A fiberglass cast may be used for the swathe so it cannot be removed by the patient.

ILLUSTRATIVE CASES FOR TECHNIQUE

Case 1: Greater Tuberosity Fracture

A 40-year-old man had a displaced greater tuberosity fracture. Operative intervention was chosen because of the displaced nature of this fracture. At surgery the arm was internally and externally rotated until the tuberosity fragment was seen to be maximally displaced (this is shown in Fig. 11A). With the arm in this position, a cannulated screw guide pin was placed into the center of the fragment with the use of the image intensifier. When the pin was in the appropriate position in the fragment, as seen on both the AP and axillary views, it was passed to the opposite cortex or into the humeral head. In this case, the opposite cortex was used (Fig. 11B). The cortical bone below the head is preferred because the bone is stronger and will allow the screw to reduce the fragment as it is tightened. If the screw is placed into the humeral head, it must be short enough so that when the fragment is driven home and the fragment is reduced, the screw does not penetrate the humeral head.

A washer was used to distribute the force over a larger area and to prevent fragmentation of the tuberosity. The screw reduced the fracture as it was tightened. Figure 11C shows the final reduction and screw position.

Postoperatively the shoulder was treated with a sling. The patient was started on immediate pendulum exercises. The sling was discontinued at 4 weeks when active exercises were begun. By 8 weeks, the patient had nearly normal range of motion. The result is shown in Figure 11D.

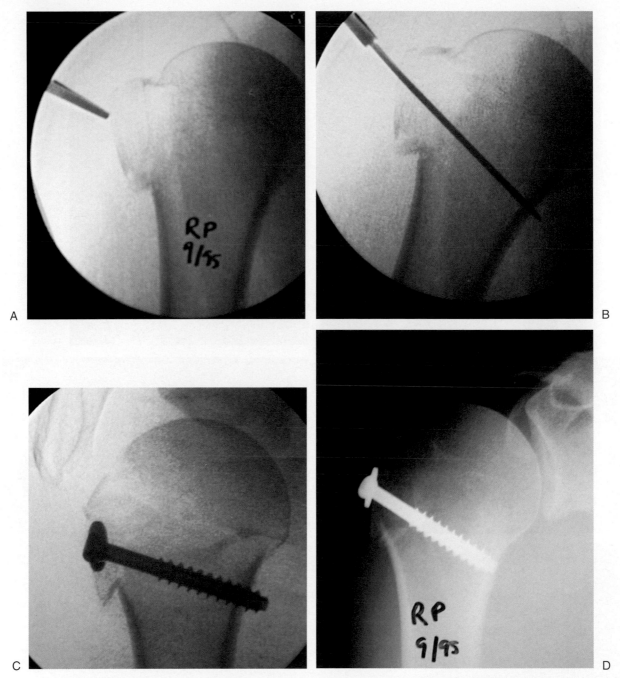

Figure 11. A: The greater tuberosity is seen on greatest profile, and the starting point is identified with a straight hemostat. **B:** A cannulated screw guide pin is passed through the greater tuberosity and into the medial cortex. **C:** The cannulated screw is placed, and the fracture is reduced by the screw and washer. **D:** Result at follow-up.

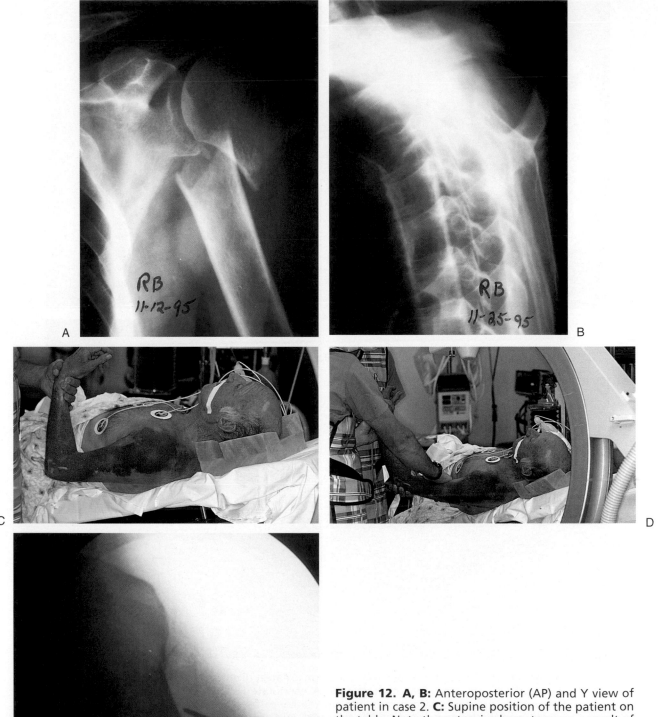

Figure 12. A, B: Anteroposterior (AP) and Y view of patient in case 2. **C:** Supine position of the patient on the table. Note the extensive hematoma as a result of this fracture. **D:** The reduction maneuver. The shaft is mobilized distal, posterior, and lateral relative to the head fragment. **E:** The position of the fragments after reduction and before pinning. This shows a pin placed outside the skin to localize the skin incision.

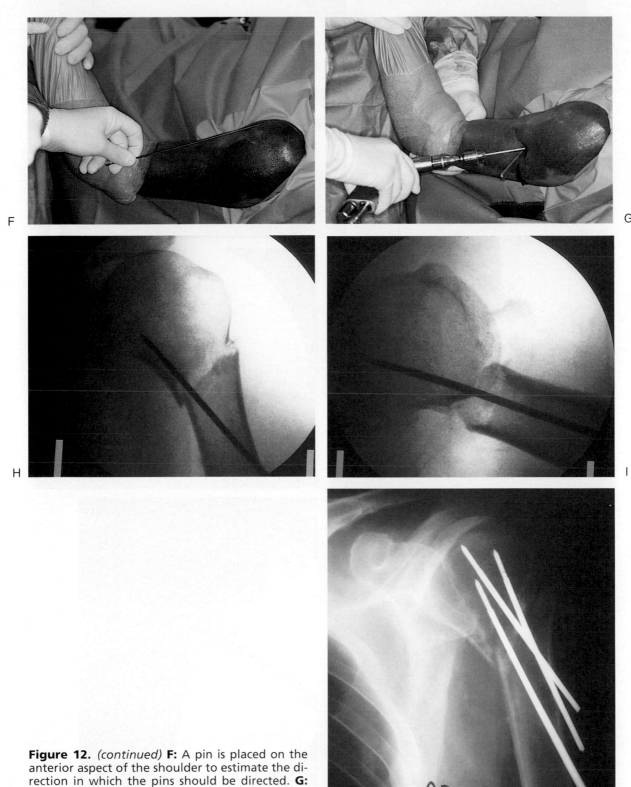

Figure 12. *(continued)* **F:** A pin is placed on the anterior aspect of the shoulder to estimate the direction in which the pins should be directed. **G:** The first pin is drilled. Note the pin is directed in line with the shaft. This will place the pin in the head fragment. **H, I:** The intraoperative placement of the first pin in the AP and axillary views. **J:** The radiograph at 3 weeks shows the final position, and one pin has slightly backed out.

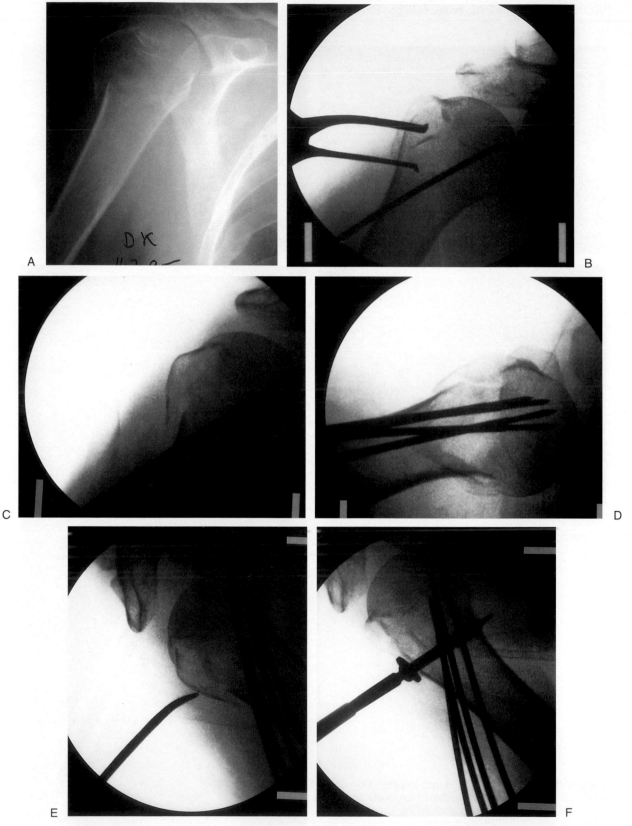

Figure 13. A: Impacted three-part fracture. The head fragment is impacted into a valgus position, and the tuberosity fragment is laterally displaced. **B:** The lamina spreader is shown in position. The head has been elevated and the first K-wire is in place. **C, D:** The position of the pins in the anteroposterior (AP) and axillary views. The tuberosity is still displaced. **E:** An instrument is shown localizing the appropriate starting point for the screw. **F:** The final position after the cannulated screw is placed. The tuberosity is reduced.

Case 2: Two-Part Fracture

A 62-year-old man had a displaced two-part fracture of the proximal humerus, as shown in Figures 12A and B. He was brought to surgery for reduction and fixation. Figure 12C shows his position on the OR table. Also note the extensive hematoma often seen with this fracture. Reduction was accomplished by moving the shaft fragment posteriorly and laterally relative to the proximal fragment. This is shown in Figure 12D. Figure 12E shows the reduction before pinning.

A pin was placed on the anterior aspect of the shoulder to act as a guide for the skin incision (Fig. 12F). Once the appropriate position is determined, a line can be marked on the skin. Pins were placed percutaneously through stab incisions, as shown in Figure 12G. Note how the pin is directed in line with the shaft to the humeral head. Figures 12H and I show the intraoperative placement of the first pin in the AP and axillary views.

Figure 12J shows the fracture at 3 weeks after surgery. One of the pins is backing out.

Case 3: Three-Part Fracture

A 38-year-old woman had a displaced three-part fracture, as shown in Figure 13A. Her fracture is one in which the head is impacted into a valgus position, and the greater tuberosity is laterally displaced. At surgery, the head fragment was disimpacted percutaneously with a lamina spreader. The lamina spreader is placed through a small incision and gradually opened to accomplish the reduction. The lamina spreader is shown in Figure 13B (after one pin was placed). Three additional pins were placed, as shown in Figures 13C and D. The tuberosity fragment is still displaced. Figure 13E shows an instrument localizing the starting point for the cannulated screw. The screw is tightened, and the tuberosity fragment is shown reduced in Figure 13F.

RECOMMENDED READING

1. Cornell, C.N., Levine, D., and Pagnani, M.J.: Internal fixation of proximal humerus fractures using the screw-tension band technique. *J Orthrop. Trauma,* 8:23–27, 1994.
2. Flatow, E.L., Cuomo, F., Maday, M.G., et al.: Open reduction and internal fixation of two-part displaced fractures of the greater tuberosity of the proximal part of the humerus. *J. Bone Joint Surg. [Am],* 73:1213–1218, 1991.
3. Jaberg, H., Warner, J.J., and Jakob, R.P.: Percutaneous stabilization of unstable fractures of the humerus. *J. Bone Joint Surg. [Am],* 74:508–515, 1992.
4. Kocialkowski, A., and Wallace, W.A.: Closed percutaneous K-wire stabilization for displaced fractures of the surgical neck of the humerus. *Br. J. Accident Surg.,* 21:209–212, 1990.
5. Koval, K.J., Sanders, R., Zuckerman, J.D., et al.: Modified-tension band wiring of displaced surgical neck fractures of the humerus. *J. Shoulder Elbow Surg.,* 2:85–92, 1993.
6. Ruedi, T., and Schweiberer.: Fractures of the proximal humerus. In Allgöwer, M. (ed.): *Manual of Internal Fixation,* 3rd ed. Springer-Verlag: Berlin, 1992, pp. 438–441.

Master Techniques in Orthopaedic Surgery,
FRACTURES, edited by D. A. Wiss,
Lippincott–Raven Publishers, Philadelphia © 1998.

3

Proximal Humeral Fractures: Open Reduction Internal Fixation

Charles N. Cornell

INDICATIONS/CONTRAINDICATIONS

The majority of proximal humeral fractures occur in the elderly, are minimally displaced, and are stable, allowing nonoperative management. However, 15% to 20% of proximal humeral fractures have significant displacement, angulation, malrotation, or tuberosity involvement. Fractures that have 1 cm of displacement or have more than 45 degrees of angulation of the humeral head with respect to the shaft or more than 10 mm of displacement of the tuberosities from their anatomic positions may be candidates for open reduction and internal fixation.

The classification system described by Neer (6) is commonly used and is effective in relating both the severity of the injury and appropriate surgical management. In this system, the four anatomic regions of the proximal humerus are identified, and the involvement of these structures by the fracture is described as one-, two-, three-, or four-part fractures. One-part fractures are essentially nondisplaced and are amenable to closed treatment. In this classification system, displacement implies that a fragment is shifted by 10 mm or more or is angulated by more than 45 degrees from its normal alignment. Two-part fractures are those with the head and tuberosities intact but separated from the shaft. In three-part fractures, one of the tuberosities, usually the greater, is split off from the head, which is significantly displaced from the shaft. Four-part fractures involve separation of both tuberosities from the head, as well as significant displacement of the head from the shaft. The classification also describes those injuries associated with dislocation of the head from the glenoid, in addition to the fracture, and identifies these as having a significantly worse prognosis. The greater the number of fragments in a fracture, the greater the risk of avascular necro-

C. N. Cornell, M.D.: Department of Surgery, Cornell University Medical College, Hospital for Special Surgery, New York, New York 10021.

sis, with four-part fractures having the highest risk of this complication. For this reason, it is widely accepted that most two- and three-part fractures are candidates for internal fixation, whereas most four-part fractures should be treated with prosthetic replacement. Exceptions to this rule are young patients with good bone stock and valgus-impacted four-part fractures in which surgical repair of the fracture has been followed by predictable success (7).

Most unstable two-, three-, and four-part fractures require surgical management to restore useful shoulder function. Few patients, regardless of age or associated medical conditions, will not benefit from surgical treatment of an unstable proximal humerus fracture. Specific indications for open reduction and internal fixation include open fractures, those that cannot be closed reduced, and fractures in the elderly with poor bone stock not amenable to closed reduction and percutaneous fixation. Young patients with good bone stock, especially those with multiple injuries, are excellent candidates for closed reduction and percutaneous fixation. Specific contraindications to surgery occur in patients with little hope of functional recovery, such as debilitated elderly patients or those with neurologic lesions that preclude useful muscle function. The presence of severe rotator cuff arthropathy is a relative contraindication to repair and an indication for prosthetic replacement with a large head prosthesis. Four-part fractures with dislocation of the humeral head are associated with nearly a 100% incidence of osteonecrosis and should be selected for hemiarthroplasty.

The majority of proximal humeral fractures occur in elderly women after slips and falls. The bone of the proximal humerus is osteoporotic and provides for poor fixation when plates or screws are used (4,5). Hawkins et al. (4,5) pointed out that the soft-tissue attachments of the rotator-cuff tendons are usually strong in spite of poor adjacent bone quality. They demonstrated that these soft tissues provide excellent sites of fracture fixation when tension-band wiring techniques are used. Furthermore, tension-band wiring does not violate the subacromial space or lead to postoperative impingement and minimizes the stripping and interference with blood supply associated with plates. In younger patients, bone quality is usually superior, allowing excellent fixation with plates and screws. In many cases, fractures in young individuals are the result of high-energy trauma and as such can be severely comminuted in the metaphyseal region. This comminution creates instability that precludes the use of the tension-band technique, as it leads to excessive shortening with loss of deltoid power and inferior subluxation of the humeral head. In such cases, a buttress plate is needed to restore and maintain length. Nonetheless, two-, three-, and four-part fractures in young patients without significant comminution can be ideally managed with the screw–tension-band technique.

PREOPERATIVE PLANNING

In patients with injuries to the shoulder, a careful history should be taken to document the mechanism of injury as well as the presence of associated injuries. The physical examination should assess the degree of swelling, with a careful search for neurovascular injury. Although vascular injury is rare, axillary artery disruption does occur and is most commonly associated with numbness and paresthesia in the limb and an expanding axillary hematoma. Because the collateral circulation of the upper limb is extensive, the presence of pulses at the wrist does not preclude a significant proximal vascular injury. The axillary and musculocutaneous nerves are the most commonly injured nerves, and their function at the time of presentation must be carefully documented. Radiographs should include a true anteroposterior (AP) and transthoracic lateral of the scapula, and an axillary lateral of the glenohumeral joint. If significant comminution exists, full-length views of the humerus may be necessary. If there is a question of comminution of humeral articular fragment, a computed tomography (CT) scan maybe helpful. The surgeon may wish to obtain a view of the opposite shoulder to act as a guide for restoration of the injured side.

The surgeon should develop a careful preoperative plan and create a surgical tactic. Preoperative planning in these cases consists of a careful analysis of the injury radiographs to determine the number and location of the fracture fragments (Fig. 1). A surgical drawing can trace the preoperative location of the humeral head, shaft, and greater and lesser tuberosities. A second drawing is prepared to locate the position of the fragments after open reduction is performed. The position of the screw and tension-band wires is included in this second drawing (Fig. 2). The surgical approach to a proximal humeral fracture can be difficult. Swelling, hematoma, and the disruption of the normal soft-tissue and bony landmarks can frustrate even experienced surgeons. I have found that careful preoperative planning helps predict what the anatomy will look like at the time of surgical exposure. Hasty preparation will lead to longer operative time and a much more frustrating learning curve with this technique.

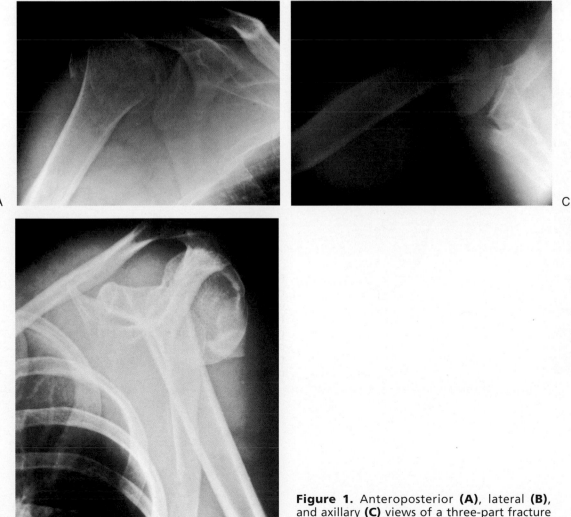

A

C

B

Figure 1. Anteroposterior **(A)**, lateral **(B)**, and axillary **(C)** views of a three-part fracture of the right proximal humerus.

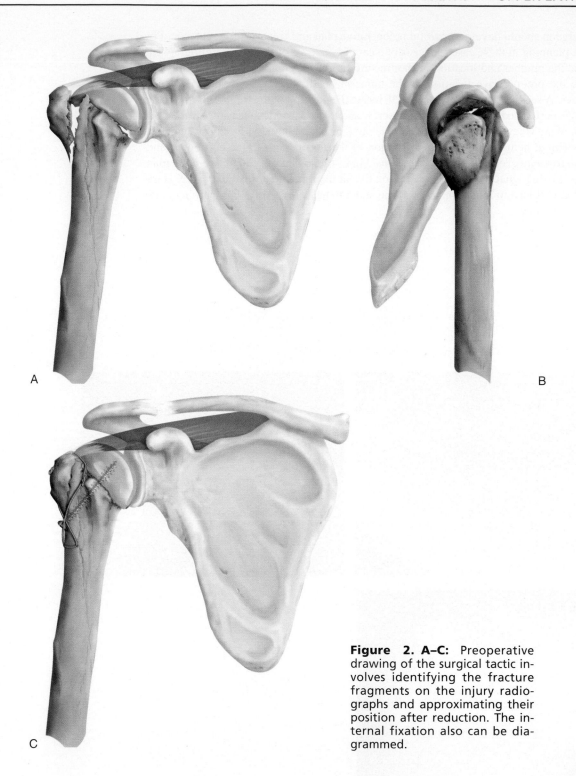

A

B

C

Figure 2. A–C: Preoperative drawing of the surgical tactic involves identifying the fracture fragments on the injury radiographs and approximating their position after reduction. The internal fixation also can be diagrammed.

SURGERY

Regional anesthesia is frequently used for this procedure. Interscalene block provides adequate anesthesia during the case and can provide postoperative pain relief if long-acting local anesthetics are used. The surgeon can supplement the block with local anesthetics and epinephrine to ensure adequate cutaneous anesthesia and to retard bleeding from the skin and subcutaneous tissues during the surgical exposure. General anesthesia is reserved for uncooperative patients and for those with severe chronic pulmonary disease. An interscalene block paralyzes the ipsilateral diaphragm, which can lead to respiratory distress in patients with severe preoperative pulmonary compromise.

For use of the image intensifier during the procedure, the patient must be carefully positioned. A radiolucent table and a "bean bag" are helpful. The patient is positioned in the beach-chair position with the head elevated 60 to 75 degrees. The patient is positioned so that the shoulder protrudes off the side of the table, allowing access for the image intensifier. The bean bag is necessary to secure this positioning. The affected arm is draped free with access for an extended deltopectoral incision (Fig. 3). An interscapular pad and careful molding of the bean bag are needed to allow manipulation of the arm and shoulder during the case (Fig. 3).

A deltopectoral incision is made, beginning at the edge of the acromion and extending distally to the level of the deltoid insertion. The cephalic vein is identified and can be sacrificed or, preferably, mobilized and medially retracted. We frequently release part or all of the deltoid insertion to facilitate exposure of the humeral head and retraction of the anterior deltoid. Failure to do this makes placement of the tension wire bands extremely difficult. The deltoid tendon is released subperiosteally in line with the long axis of the humerus, after which the shoulder is gently abducted. The clavipectoral fascia is incised, allowing entry into the subacromial space. Aufranc or Howman retractors are placed superiorly and laterally, exposing the humeral head, shaft, and rotator cuff (Fig. 4).

A pointed tenaculum clamp is used to grasp the humeral head, providing provisional control of the proximal fragment. The fracture site is debrided of hematoma and soft tissue. The head and shaft are then impacted, reducing the fracture and creating a stable configuration (Fig. 5A and B).

Fracture fixation is achieved by placing a 6.5- or 4.5-mm lag screw from the proximal lateral humeral shaft into the humeral head (Fig. 6). The screw size is based on the size of the bone and bone quality. Recently we found that 4.5-mm cortical screws inserted in a lag fashion achieve excellent purchase with little risk of additional comminution of the fragile

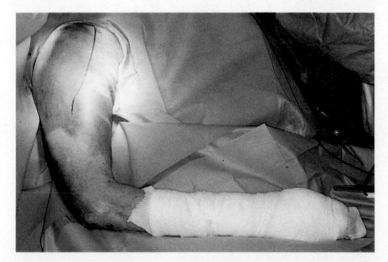

Figure 3. The patient is placed in the beach-chair position with the entire extremity draped free. An extended deltopectoral incision is made.

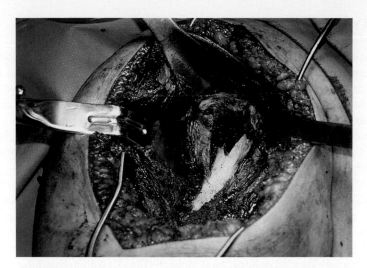

Figure 4. After development of the deltopectoral interval, the distal deltoid insertion is released subperiosteally in line with the humerus. After the clavipectoral fascia is opened, retractors can be placed in the subacromial space, exposing the fracture and humeral head.

humeral cortex. The lateral cortex is overdrilled with a 4.5-mm drill, and a countersink is used. If the tuberosities are displaced, they can now be reduced to the head and shaft and fixed with an additional lag screw or heavy suture into the humeral head (Fig. 7).

Two 18-gauge wires are then placed through a drill hole in the humeral shaft. The drill hole is placed 3 to 4 cm below the fracture site in intact cortex. A 3.2-mm drill bit is used. The hole is drilled from anterior to posterior. Two wires are then passed from anterior to posterior through this hole. One wire is passed beneath the supraspinatus tendon as a fig-

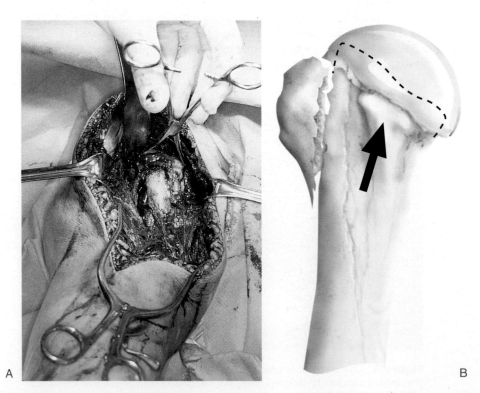

Figure 5. A: The humeral head is grasped with a pointed clamp and reduced to the shaft. **B:** The shaft is impacted into the humeral head.

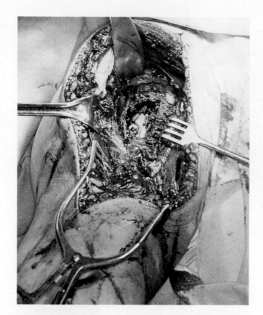

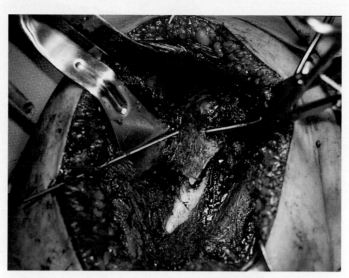

Figure 6. Initial stability is achieved by placing a 4.5- or 6.5-mm lag screw from the lateral humeral cortex into the humeral head.

Figure 7. In a three-part fracture, the greater tuberosity is reduced to the humeral head and shaft and held with a pointed clamp. A guide wire has been placed in preparation for insertion of a cannulated lag screw.

ure-eight tension band. The other wire is passed through the tuberosities, also in figure-eight fashion. A 14-gauge angiocatheter culposcopy needle can be used as a cannula to facilitate passage of the wires (Fig. 8). Two twists for tightening are used in each wire on each side of the shaft. Ideally the twists are placed at the level of the junction of the head and shaft to achieve maximal tightening of the wires (Fig. 9).

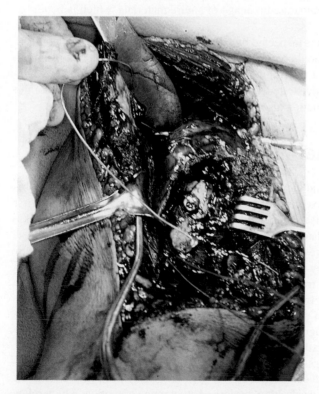

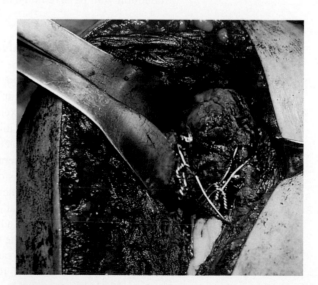

Figure 8. A 14-gauge angiocatheter is used as a wire-passing cannula. It is passed beneath the supraspinatus tendon just medial to its insertion on the greater tuberosity.

Figure 9. The figure-of-eight wires are passed and tightened by using two twists in each wire. The twists are placed close to the fracture site to achieve maximal tightening.

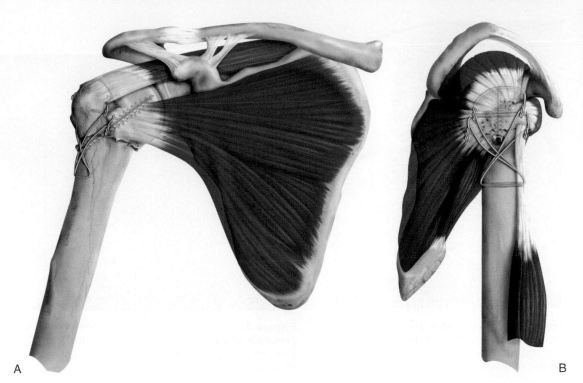

Figure 10. A, B: Anteroposterior and lateral drawings illustrating fracture reduction and placement of internal fixation.

Many surgeons may wish to substitute heavy Dacron suture or tape for the stainless steel wires. I prefer using wire because I believe that its greater stiffness allows it to be more securely tightened. In addition, sharp bone fragments and edges occur at the fracture site, which may lead to fretting and premature breakage of suture materials, which is better resisted by the steel wire.

When completed, the construct is inspected by using the image intensifier. The length of the screws in the humeral head should be verified and shortened if there is a risk of intrarticular protrusion. The position of the fragments and accuracy of the reduction are determined. An idealized construct is illustrated schematically in Figure 10. The stability of the reduction with passive range of motion also should be confirmed.

POSTOPERATIVE MANAGEMENT

A sterile dressing is applied, and the arm is immobilized in a sling or shoulder immobilizer. Gentle, passive pendulum exercises and active elbow exercises are started on the first postoperative day. Passive exercises are performed for the first four postoperative weeks. Active assisted exercises are initiated at week 3 or 4 and are continued until the sixth postoperative week. Thereafter, active range of motion and strengthening exercises are instituted. Supervised physical therapy is continued until maximal recovery is achieved, which on average requires 6 months of treatment. In the early postoperative period, patients are seen in the outpatient department frequently. Patients are asked to return every 2 weeks for the first 6 weeks for examination of the surgical wound and to determine the compliance with the exercise program. Radiographs are obtained to ensure no loss of fracture stability has occurred. Generally by the sixth postoperative week, adequate fracture healing has occurred to allow a progressive range-of-motion and muscle-strengthening program. The frequency of outpatient visits is reduced to monthly or greater. Nearly full passive range of motion should be recovered by 6 weeks after surgery. Active range of motion, which relies on adequate strength and coordination of the deltoid and rotator cuff, requires prolonged therapy. The goal for these patients should be overhead function of the arm with 120 degrees or more of forward flexion and adequate internal and external rotation. Return of the ability to perform activities of daily living is achieved in nearly all patients. Return to sports that require throwing or vigorous overhead use of the arm, as in tennis or swimming, is more difficult to achieve.

Hawkins et al. (5) reported treatment of a series of three-part fractures of the proximal humerus with the tension-band technique. Patients averaged 126 degrees of forward elevation, with eight of 15 patients subjectively scoring their results as functionally good to excellent. All but two patients had excellent pain relief. The two poor results occurred in a patient with a broken tension-band wire and in one patient with osteonecrosis of the humeral head. Both required secondary surgery.

In our own (3) experience with the technique in two- and three-part fractures, excellent results were achieved in 10 of 13 patients. Early aggressive range-of-motion exercises led to an average forward flexion of 160 degrees. This technique is ideal for the elderly patient with osteopenic bone. Properly done, the technique offers excellent fracture fixation, allowing early mobilization of the shoulder. In addition, the implants are small, avoiding subacromial impingement or devascularization of the humeral head that has been associated with T-shaped or cloverleaf plates. The incidence of avascular necrosis of the head is reported to be lower by using tension banding as compared with plates for three- and four-part fractures (7).

COMPLICATIONS

Injury to the axillary nerve has been reported after this procedure, and care must be taken to avoid injury to the nerve as it courses through the deltoid muscle. Most axillary nerve palsies are neuropraxias and carry a good prognosis for recovery. Electromyography is useful to monitor the course for recovery, especially in situations in which little return of function is noted by 3 months. Avascular necrosis occurs in approximately 15% to 20% of three-part fractures and between 50% and 75% of four-part fractures (2). Avascular necrosis usually leads to pain and a poor result. Prosthetic replacement of the humeral head or total shoulder replacement may be needed as salvage. Breakage of the tension-band wires is reported sporadically, and when it occurs, removal should be performed. If excessive comminution of the shaft occurs, excessive shortening above the deltoid insertion occurs, which can lead to pseudosubluxation and prolonged weakness of the rotator cuff. When significant comminution is present in the humeral metaphysis, a buttress plate is needed to maintain humeral height and length.

Residual shoulder stiffness and loss of shoulder rotation is a frequent complication after any shoulder injury. Perhaps the best defense against this complication is immediate postoperative rehabilitation, which is allowed by the screw–tension-band technique. When stiffness that limits function occurs, persistent but gentle range of motion is needed. Occasionally, a gentle manipulation under anesthesia may be performed in a patient who tolerates therapy poorly, provided the fracture appears well healed. Pain consistent with rotator-cuff impingement is frequently encountered, and subacromial corticosteroid injection will often ease the pain and improve the results of therapy. In our experience, arthroscopic decompression or lysis of adhesions has not been necessary. In most cases, patience and persistence generally provide the best results.

ILLUSTRATIVE CASE FOR TECHNIQUE

A 63-year-old woman tripped and fell onto her outstretched right hand and sustained a displaced two-part fracture of the right proximal humerus (Fig. 11). Open reduction and internal fixation was performed the following day by using a screw and two tension-band wires (Fig. 12). An immediate postoperative rehabilitation protocol was initiated, and the patient was discharged on postoperative day 2 after having demonstrated understanding of the exercise regimen. Passive shoulder range of motion and active elbow exercises were

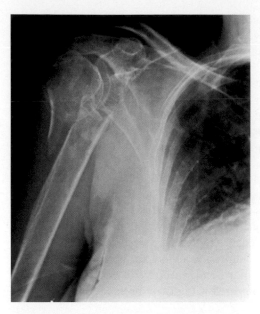

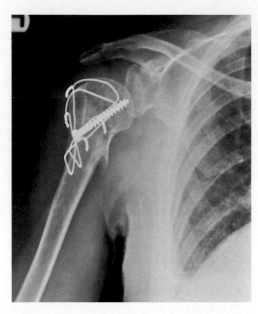

Figure 11. A radiograph of two-part prox-imal humerus fracture in a 63-year-old right-hand-dominant woman.

Figure 12. Postoperative radiographs af-ter open reduction and internal fixation.

conducted for 4 weeks. Active assisted exercises under the supervision of a therapist were started and progressed to active range-of-motion exercises and strengthening by 6 weeks. Therapy was continued for 6 months with a maintenance program of home exercises given thereafter. At 1 year, an excellent functional and pain-free shoulder resulted (Fig. 13). The patient achieved 160 degrees of forward flexion and had full overhead use of the arm. According to the functional-outcome scale described by Hawkins et al. (5), this patient achieved an excellent result.

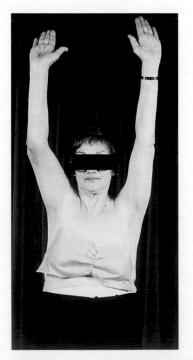

Figure 13. A clinical photo-graph demonstrating the shoulder motion in forward flexion at 1 year after surgery.

RECOMMENDED READING

1. Bigliani, L.U.: Treatment of two and three part fractures of the proximal humerus. *Instr. Course Lect.,* 38:231–244, 1989.
2. Brooks, C.H., Revell, W.J., and Heatley, F.W.: Vascularity of the humeral head after proximal humeral fracture. *J. Bone Joint Surg. [Br],* 75:132–136, 1993.
3. Cornell, C.N., Levine, D., and Pagnani, M.J.: Internal fixation of proximal humerus fractures using the screw-tension band technique. *J. Orthop. Trauma,* 8:23–27, 1994.
4. Hawkins, R.J, Bell, R.H., and Gun, K.: Three part fractures of the proximal part of the humerus. *J. Bone Joint Surg. [Am],* 68:1410–1414, 1986.
5. Hawkins, R.J., and Kiefer, G.N.: Internal fixation techniques for proximal humerus fracture. *Clin. Orthop.,* 223:77–85, 1987.
6. Szyskowitz, R., Seggl, W., Schleifer, P., and Condy, P.J.: Proximal humeral fractures: management and expected results. *Clin. Orthop.,* 292:13–25, 1993.
7. Young, T.B., and Wallace, W.A.: Conservative treatment of fractures and fracture dislocations of the upper limb of the humerus. *J. Bone Joint Surg. [Br],* 67:373–377, 1985.

Master Techniques in Orthopaedic Surgery,
FRACTURES, edited by D. A. Wiss,
Lippincott–Raven Publishers, Philadelphia © 1998.

4

Proximal Humeral Fractures: Arthroplasty

Louis U. Bigliani

INDICATIONS/CONTRAINDICATIONS

Proximal humeral replacement can be a useful surgical technique for acute displaced fractures of the proximal humerus (Fig. 1). The indications for the use of the prosthesis are (a) four-part fractures and fracture dislocations, (b) head-splitting fractures, (c) impression fractures involving more than 40% of the articular surface, and (d) selected three-part fractures in older patients with osteoporotic bone. The majority of severely displaced proximal humeral fractures occur in the older population, with a predominance in women. Other methods of treatment including closed reduction, open reduction–internal fixation, head excision, and fusion have been reported to have a high percentage of unsatisfactory results.

The contraindications for this procedure are active soft-tissue infection, chronic osteomyelitis, and paralysis of the rotator-cuff muscles. Deltoid paralysis is not a contraindication: adequate yet compromised function can be achieved in such a shoulder.

PREOPERATIVE PLANNING

A detailed history and physical are essential, although an adequate clinical evaluation of the injured limb may be difficult because of pain and swelling. It is important to establish whether the patient has lost consciousness or has had a seizure. The neurovascular status should be assessed with a high index of suspicion for injuries to the axillary nerve and artery. Injuries to the axillary artery are limb threatening and should be evaluated with emergency arteriography and a vascular surgery consultation. Injuries to the brachial plexus or peripheral nerves are initially treated conservatively. Electromyographic analysis should be planned 3 to 4 weeks after injury to help clarify the extent of the injury. A

L. U. Bigliani, M.D.: The Shoulder Service, The New York Orthopaedic Hospital, Columbia-Presbyterian Medical Center, New York, New York 10032.

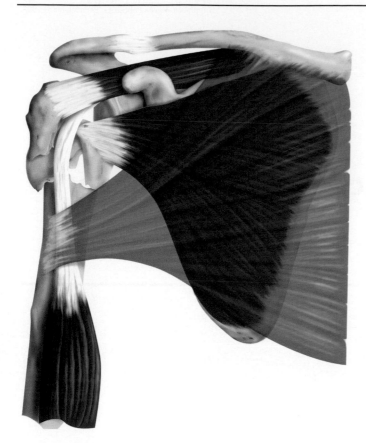

Figure 1. A four-part fracture of the proximal humerus. The humeral head is free-floating and displaced from both tuberosities and the shaft. The lesser tuberosity fragment is pulled medially by the subscapularis, the greater tuberosity fragment is pulled posteriorly and superiorly by the supraspinatus and infraspinatus, and the shaft fragment is pulled medially by the pectoralis major.

neurologic deficiency should not delay definitive management of the fracture. Most injuries are neuropraxias and will resolve over time sufficiently to allow adequate function. If there is not improvement in the neurologic status and a procedure to the axillary nerve is needed, this can be done within 3 months of injury without compromise.

To determine whether a humeral head replacement is the best treatment option for a displaced proximal humeral fracture, the fracture pattern must be clearly delineated. In the majority of cases, this can be achieved with a trauma series (Fig. 2A and B). This includes a true anteroposterior (AP) view of the scapula (taken 30 to 40 degrees oblique to the coro-

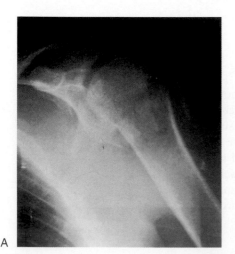
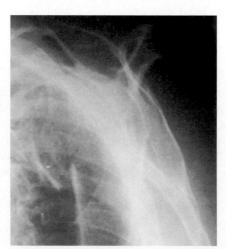
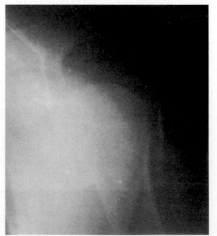

A   B, C

Figure 2. **A:** An anteroposterior radiograph of a four-part fracture. **B:** A lateral view in the scapular plane. **C:** A Velpeau axillary view.

nal plane of the body), a transscapular lateral or Y view, and an axillary view. The axillary view is taken by abducting the arm 20 to 30 degrees and placing the tube in the axilla with the radiographic plate above the shoulder; there is no need to abduct the arm fully. Often the surgeon must position the arm because of pain. Alternately, a Velpeau axillary view (Fig. 2C) can be obtained, with the patient remaining in the sling and leaning back over the plate, and the tube directed downward. If displacement cannot be determined, or if the status of the articular surface of the humeral head or the glenoid is not adequately delineated, then a computed tomography (CT) scan also may be used to clarify the situation.

Use of a preoperative scanogram of both the involved and the uninvolved arm often helps establish the proper length of the prosthesis relative to the remaining humeral shaft.

SURGERY

Patient Positioning

Proper patient positioning is the first step to a successful procedure, and its importance cannot be overemphasized. The goal is to have access to the superior, inferior, medial, and lateral aspects of the shoulder. This is achieved by having the involved shoulder elevated from the table and properly supported. We prefer interscalene regional-block anesthesia, as it provides excellent muscle relaxation, which facilitates exposure. Two small towels are placed under the medial border of the scapula so that the shoulder is elevated off the edge of the table. The patient should be brought to the edge of the table so that the lateral border of the scapula and thorax is at the edge of the table (Fig. 3). The head is supported by a headrest, and the top portion of the operating table is removed so that superior access is available. The operating table should then be placed in a modified beach-chair position. The table is first flexed fully so that there is knee flexion. The back of the operating table is then elevated so that the patient sits up at an angle of approximately 45 to 50 degrees. A small armboard is used at the level of the humeral shaft so that the elbow and forearm can be supported during the surgery. The armboard may need to be shifted superiorly to allow enough extension for the preparation of the shaft. Surgical drapes should be used to isolate the operative field superiorly to the midclavicle and inferiorly below the axilla so that the arm can be draped free and is able to be moved throughout the surgery.

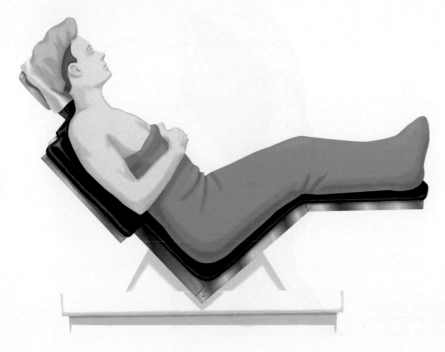

Figure 3. The patient is placed in a modified beach-chair position with the back flexed approximately 40 to 50 degrees, and the lateral border of the scapula and thorax is at the edge of the table.

Technique

Approach. A long deltopectoral approach is performed, starting just below the clavicle and extending over the lateral aspect of the coracoid to the deltoid insertion on the humeral shaft (Fig. 4). Large Gelpi retractors can be placed in the skin to provide exposure. The cephalic vein is identified in the deltopectoral interval and is usually retracted laterally. There are fewer tributary veins on the medial side than on the lateral side, so retracting the vein laterally decreases bleeding. Often, however, there is a large crossover vein superiorly, which should be cauterized so that superior exposure is not compromised. It is important to preserve the deltoid origin on the clavicle and acromion. Rarely is the deltoid origin removed. If more exposure is needed, the deltoid insertion may be partially elevated; however, the distal pectoralis insertion is usually detached for about half of its length (Fig. 5). This should be tagged with a suture and reattached during closure. At this stage, the coracoid and coracoid muscles should be identified. The coracoid is a lighthouse to the shoulder, and dissection should not be medial to this structure unless the head is displaced (Fig. 6). A broad retractor is placed beneath the lateral borders of the coracoid muscles. The coracoid muscles should not be cut or the coracoid process osteotomized, because they provide a barrier to protect the neurovascular bundle. The leading edge of the anterior portion of the coracoacromial ligament can be resected to facilitate exposure. It extends from the lateral aspect of the acromion to the lateral aspect of the coracoid. The surgeon should not remove a significant amount of the coracoacromial ligament, as this may compromise superior stability. Another retractor is placed underneath the deltoid, and the muscle is retracted laterally. The long head of the biceps should be identified distally and followed proximally, as this is an important structure that will lead us to the center of the shoulder at its glenoid insertion (Fig. 7).

Exposure of the Fracture. Once the retractors have been placed in the appropriate position, hemorrhagic bursa and fracture hematoma can be identified and gently removed. It is important not to remove large pieces of bone that may be used later to support the prosthesis on the shortened proximal shaft. The key to recognizing the various components of

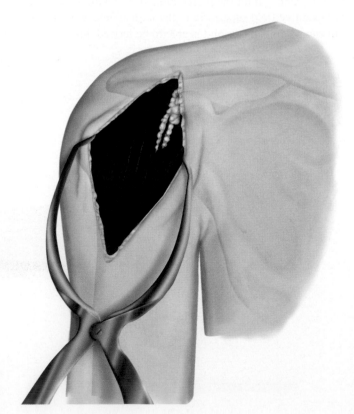

Figure 4. A long deltopectoral approach starts just below the clavicle and extends over the lateral aspect of the coracoid to the deltoid insertion on the humeral shaft.

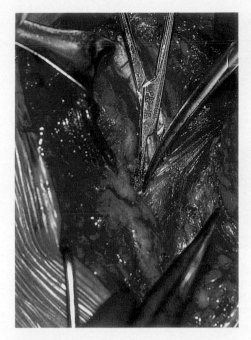

Figure 5. The superior insertion of the pectoralis major is usually detached to allow improved exposure.

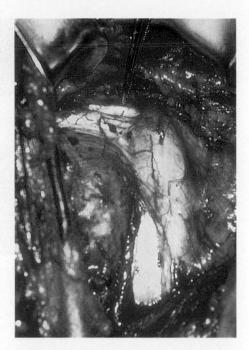

Figure 6. The coracoid should be readily identified, and dissection should not proceed medial to it. The leading edge of the coracoacromial ligament may be resected to improve exposure over rotator-cuff muscles.

the fracture is the long head of the biceps. As the biceps is followed proximally, the lesser tuberosity is on the medial side, and the greater tuberosity is usually on the lateral side (see Fig. 1). As a rule, the rotator interval can be split in the area of the bicipital groove, as this is often fractured. The head is usually between the tuberosities and can be removed (Fig. 8). If the head has been dislocated laterally, the greater and lesser tuberosities act almost as a hood and can be elevated intact. In this situation, the head can be removed, and the prosthesis can be placed in without disturbing the rotator interval, greater tuberosity, and lesser

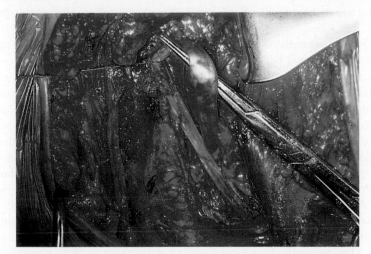

Figure 7. The distal portion of the long head of the biceps should be identified and approximated, as this will help to differentiate between the lesser and greater tuberosities and the area of the rotator interval. If possible, the long head of the biceps should be preserved to act as a head depressor.

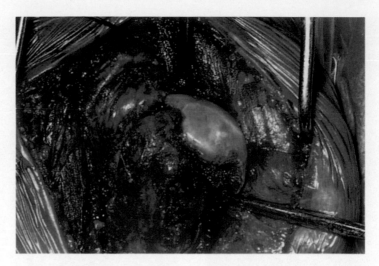

Figure 8. The humeral head is usually a free-floating fragment that can be easily removed by using a metal finger. It is important to evaluate the head for any soft-tissue insertion. The head may be used as bone graft if needed or to support the prosthesis.

tuberosity fragments. Generally, however, the interval must be opened in the area of the bicipital groove. Once again, it is important at this stage to preserve any loose fragments and pieces of bone to be used later in the procedure. The biceps tendon should be tagged with a nylon suture. Then both tuberosities are mobilized and tagged with no. 2 heavy nylon suture. I prefer to use swedged-on needles and place them into the tendon proximal to the tuberosity insertion. This preserves the integrity of the remaining bone attached to the tendon, avoiding fragmentation of the tuberosity. Adequate tuberosity mobilization should be done superiorly and medially. Often, superior exposure may be limited by the leading edge of the anterior fascicle of the coracoacromial ligament. As mentioned previously, the leading edge should be resected.

This is a good time to evaluate the patient for subacromial impingement. If there is a large subacromial spur in the ligament, or if the patient has an impingement configuration of the acromion, then it may be worthwhile to perform an anterior acromioplasty. This is not a routine part of the procedure. Also at this stage, it may be reasonable to evaluate the patient for a tear in the rotator cuff. Generally, the rotator cuff is intact in this group of patients.

If there is an anterior dislocation of the head below the coracoid and under the coracoid muscles, then this should be slowly and carefully dissected, especially if there has been more than a week's delay in performing the procedure, as significant adhesions and scarring may be present. In this instance, very gentle blunt dissection should be done from lateral to medial. Avoid placing any sharp instruments medial to the head without direct visualization. We prefer to use blunt retractors in this situation to avoid injuring the neurovascular bundle. If the head segment has been displaced posteriorly, the shaft and greater tuberosity are gently retracted laterally so that the head can be removed. If the head is scarred in posteriorly, it may need to be osteotomized into segments to facilitate removal.

Shaft Preparation and Prosthesis Placement. The proximal shaft of the humerus should be dealt with in a very gentle manner. Often there is osteoporotic bone, and sometimes there may be an undisplaced fracture of the shaft, which should not be disturbed. If there is a shaft component to the fracture, then fixation is important to do before prosthesis placement. This can usually be achieved with a cerclage wire and heavy nylon sutures. The addition of the prosthesis and cement usually provides a stable reconstruction with adequate support. Before exposure of the shaft, the armboard is moved up the table to allow the limb to be extended and externally rotated. This maneuver brings the shaft into the wound. The medullary canal is prepared with rasps and reamers (Fig. 9). Generally there is

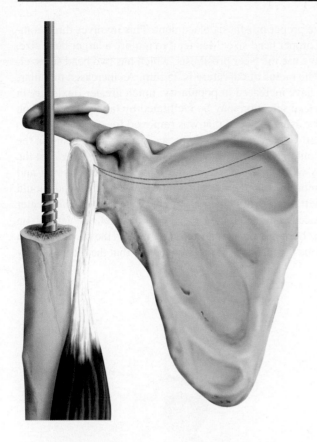

Figure 9. The medullary canal is prepared with rasps and reamers if cement is to be used.

not sufficient bone stock to allow a press-fit, and cement will be needed. In addition, when both of the tuberosities are fractured, rotational stability of the implant is often lost. The proximal part of the humerus should be prepared with drill holes to allow tuberosity fixation with nonabsorbable nylon sutures. Three or four holes should be placed in the area of the greater tuberosity (Fig. 10). I like to place no. 2 or no. 5 heavy nonabsorbable nylon sutures with a swedged-on needle through the shaft. These sutures are then tagged with a clamp.

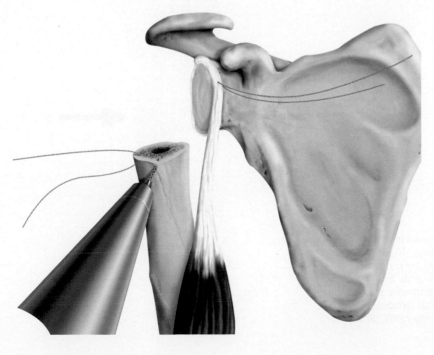

Figure 10. Drill holes should be placed in the proximal shaft for attachment of the tuberosities before cementing in the prosthesis. Three to four drill holes are placed in the greater tuberosity, and one to two holes in the lesser tuberosity.

Next it is important to determine proper prosthesis placement. This involves three components: retroversion, height, and proper head size. Men tend to require a larger head size, and women, a smaller head size. We use the Neer prosthesis, which has two head sizes, either a 22- or a 15-mm neck size. The radius of curvature is 25 mm. As increased modularity of humeral prosthetic systems have increased in popularity, much greater flexibility in humeral-head sizing exists now. Head selection may be facilitated by taking a radiograph of the contralateral shoulder and by using the head that was removed for comparison. It is important, however, not to overstuff or overtighten the joint, as stiffness may result in the postoperative period. The head should not be seated so deeply that it is placed against the remaining proximal shaft, as this will usually decrease the length of the humerus and shorten the myofascial sleeve, compromising deltoid function. Generally, the head should be elevated above the proximal shaft to a position that will allow space for both the greater and the lesser tuberosities to be placed underneath the head. This is crucial. The tension on the biceps tendon, if the tendon has been preserved, can act as a guide to the proper tension of the whole myofascial sleeve. If the prosthesis is inserted so deeply that the biceps is very

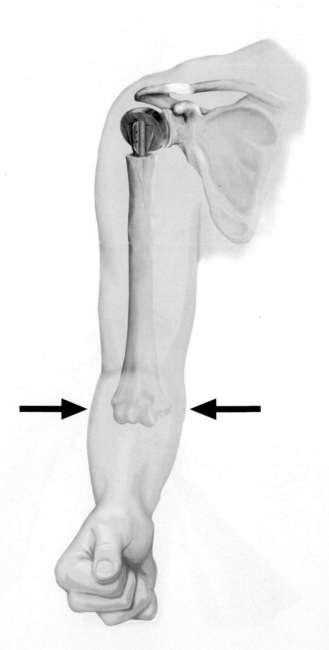

Figure 11. The prosthesis should be placed in a stable position, which is usually between 25 and 40 degrees of retroversion. Retroversion can be tested by palpating the distal humeral epicondyles with the thumb and forefinger. Also, the posterior fin of the prosthesis should be near the posterior aspect of the bicipital groove. In fractures, the distal portion of the groove may still be visualized.

slack in its anatomic position, then often the prosthesis has been placed too deeply into the medullary canal. If the biceps tendon is excessively taut, this usually suggests that the prosthesis is too proud. If the tuberosities are not placed below the head of the prosthesis, impingement will occur. Also, these tuberosities must be attached to the proximal shaft. If extra bone has been saved, it should be used between the prosthesis and the shaft before cementing.

The third important component is the determination of the proper amount of retroversion. A rule of thumb is that the lateral fin of the prosthesis should be in the area of the bicipital groove. Often the majority of the bicipital groove is not present in fractures, but sometimes the distal part of the groove may be identified. A useful maneuver is to stuff a sponge down the shaft, which allows me to support the stem of the prosthesis so that I may judge the retroversion. I generally like to use my forefinger and thumb distally at the elbow to feel the epicondyles of the distal humerus (Fig. 11). The head of the prosthesis should then be reduced on the glenoid to allow internal and external rotation to be assessed. If the prosthesis appears to be stable, with 40 to 50 degrees of external rotation and internal rotation with the arm at the side, then the retroversion is adequate. Generally the goal is to achieve approximately 20 to 30 degrees of retroversion. If there has been a posterior fracture dislocation, then the retroversion may be decreased by 5 to 10 degrees. If there is an anterior fracture dislocation, then the retroversion may be increased by 5 to 10 degrees. Therefore, as a rule, the retroversion should never be less than 20 or more than 40 degrees. At this stage, the prosthesis can be cemented into place with the shaft properly supported (Fig. 12). It is important to make sure that the nonabsorbable nylon sutures are through the holes in the proximal shaft.

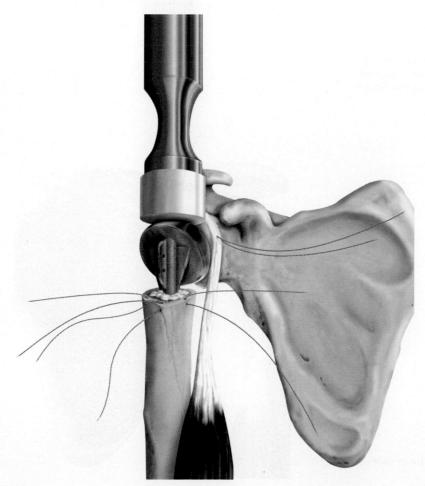

Figure 12. Cement might be needed to support the prosthesis if there is proximal bone loss.

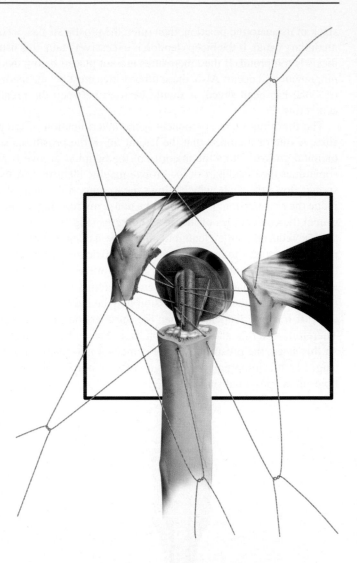

Figure 13. Tuberosity repair is an essential part of the procedure. Both tuberosities should be attached to the shaft and also to each other through the fin of the prosthesis.

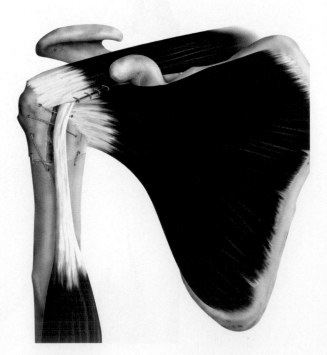

Figure 14. The biceps tendon should be preserved and placed in the rotator interval area.

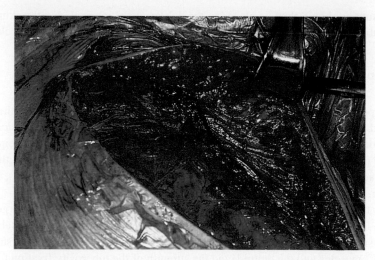

Figure 15. A meticulous deltoid closure with repair of the pectoralis major insertion should be performed.

Tuberosity Repair. Tuberosity repair is the next important step. Failure of tuberosity repair is one of the most common causes of failure of the procedure. It is important to attach the tuberosities both to the fin of the prosthesis and to the shaft of the proximal bone (Fig. 13). The nylon sutures that have been placed proximal to the tuberosities in the tendon can be used to mobilize the tendons and bring them forward. I generally reattach the greater tuberosity first, by using three to four heavy nylon sutures. Next, the lesser tuberosity is fixed with two heavy nylon sutures. The two sutures are placed through the fin of the prosthesis to both tuberosities and tightened. The arm should be supported in a slightly flexed and abducted position. The biceps tendon that has been preserved is now placed in its groove. The rotated interval that has been opened is now closed above the biceps tendon, so that the biceps tendon comes out at the distal aspect, which is now the bicipital groove (Fig. 14). The arm should now be gently internally and externally rotated and flexed to test the stability of the tuberosity repair.

Closure. Hemovacs should be used if there is excessive bleeding. These are generally kept in place for 12 to 14 h and should exit laterally in the proximal deltoid, avoiding injury to the axillary nerve. The insertion of the pectoralis major should be closed (Fig. 15).

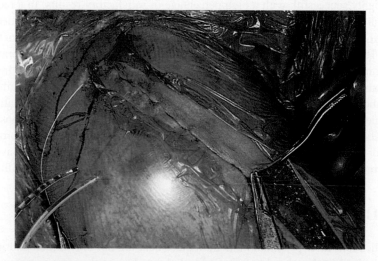

Figure 16. A subcuticular skin closure with either absorbable or nonabsorbable sutures can be performed.

Multiple sutures should then be placed in the deltopectoral interval, and the skin is closed in a subcuticular fashion (Fig. 16). Steri-strips are used to promote a cosmetic closure.

POSTOPERATIVE MANAGEMENT

Proper postoperative rehabilitation is essential because adequate motion of the shoulder is required for optimal function. The patient's ability to participate in the physical therapy and to understand the restrictions on activity are crucial. In general, the principles are to gain early passive motion until the fracture has healed and then to begin strengthening exercises. Radiographs should be taken in the recovery room at 1 week, 6 weeks, 3 months, and 1 year.

Passive motion is begun early, usually on the first postoperative day. The surgeon determines the limits of early motion, based on the intraoperative assessment of stability after the tuberosity reconstruction. Consideration is given to the quality of bone, the status of the rotator-cuff muscles and the deltoid, and the strength of the tuberosity fixation to the shaft and the prosthesis. On the first day, the surgeon usually raises the scapular plane to approximately 80 to 90 degrees. On the second, gravity-assisted pendulum exercises are done first to allow warm-up and obtain the patient's confidence. After this, assisted forward elevation and supine external rotation with a stick are performed. The patient, after gaining some early motion with the help of a therapist, may lie supine and raise the arm by using the uninvolved contralateral arm. These three exercises are generally done for the first 6 weeks until adequate tuberosity healing has occurred. The goal before discharge from the hospital should be 140 degrees of forward elevation in the scapular plane and 30 degrees of external rotation. Radiographs should be taken before discharge to see that tuberosity displacement has not occurred. Furthermore, radiographs should be repeated at 6 weeks to see whether the tuberosities have healed.

When there is evidence of tuberosity healing at approximately 6 to 8 weeks, active assistive elevation with a pulley and isometric strengthening exercises for the rotator cuff and deltoid are initiated. After this, in 2 to 3 weeks, progressive resistive and strengthening exercises are added. Activities of daily living such as personal hygiene and eating are allowed, and these help to build early muscle strength and endurance. Gentle strengthening should be the early part of every exercise routine and is an important part of the prolonged physical-therapy program. The patient is encouraged to perform the exercises on a daily basis for at least 6 months, preferably 1 year, to achieve optimal results.

The overall success of prosthetic replacement for humeral fractures depends on proper evaluation, surgical technique, and rehabilitation. If proper steps are followed, this procedure is highly successful, with a high percentage of satisfactory results. In a recent series of humeral head replacements performed at our hospital, 95% of patients had adequate pain relief, with 73% being essentially pain free. Overall, 82% of patients had a satisfactory result, and 18% had an unsatisfactory result. The impact on favorable or unfavorable results is predominantly from the range of motion achieved by the patient rather than from the degree of pain. The majority of failures in our series reflected weakness and inability to raise the arm above horizontal. In addition, the single most important variable in a patient's ability to achieve a satisfactory result was found to be patient compliance in the postoperative rehabilitation program. Thus it can be expected that at the end of 1 year after prosthetic insertion for a four-part fracture, most patients will be free of pain but will have variable range of motion and strength, often dependent on the adequacy of their rehabilitation.

COMPLICATIONS

Complications after proximal humeral replacement are not uncommon and in most instances can be directly related to failure of technique. Among the most common complications reported are the following.

Tuberosity Displacement

This usually involves the greater tuberosity rather than the lesser tuberosity, and it often involves the older patient with osteopenic bone. The problems with greater tuberosity displacement are much greater, as the attached supraspinatus, infraspinatus, and teres minor are critical for satisfactory motion and strength in the shoulder, and if the grater tuberosity is displaced, these tendons are rendered ineffective. In addition, with superior displacement of the greater tuberosity, there may be a mechanical block to motion, as the tuberosity occupies a portion of the subacromial space. Although displacement of the lesser tuberosity is not so problematic, because the weakness in the subscapularis may be made up for by other muscles, displacement may result in a mechanical block as the arm is internally rotated. In addition, wide displacement of the lesser tuberosity and associated subscapularis may result in postoperative anterior instability. The critical factor in eliminating the potential for tuberosity displacement is the healing of the tuberosity to the shaft of the humerus. Secure fixation of the greater tuberosity to both the prosthesis and the shaft of the humerus, combined with bone graft between the tuberosity and shaft, will maximize the potential for tuberosity shaft healing if the patient is adequately protected from active motion postoperatively. If there is displacement of the greater tuberosity postoperatively, consideration should be given for early reattachment and regrafting, if the patient is in need of satisfactory function of the shoulder. Whereas nonunion is often a far greater problem in terms of motion and strength, malunion of the greater tuberosity, either superiorly or posteriorly, frequently results in pain, either from impingement in the subacromial space or from the mechanical block caused by the displaced tuberosity. If the patient is symptomatic and malunion exists, strong consideration should be given to osteotomy and repositioning of the tuberosity.

Prosthetic Loosening

The bony support in the proximal humerus is often not ideal because of osteopenia. With loss of the rotatory stability of the implant because of loosening, there may be a change of version of the prosthesis and secondary pain, instability, or destruction of the previously normal glenoid. Whereas loosening caused by poor bone stock in an uncemented implant could have been avoided if cement had been used at implantation, loosening also may occur with a cemented implant. With humeral loosening in a cemented implant, the standard workup should include examination for infection and mechanical loosening, and revision of the prosthesis should be considered.

Malposition of the Prosthesis

Malposition may involve abnormal version, an abnormally proud prosthesis, or an abnormal depth of prosthesis. Mistakes in cementation of the implant in abnormal version are not uncommon, as the landmark for correct version, the bicipital groove, is usually involved in the fracture. There are three basic guides that can be used to place the prosthesis in the proper amount of retroversion (20 to 40 degrees):

1. The prosthetic fin should be placed just lateral to the position of the bicipital groove.
2. The prosthetic fin should be 20 to 40 degrees retroverted relative to the transverse axis of the elbow, as judged by palpation of the medial and lateral epicondyles.
3. With the elbow bent 90 degrees and the arm at the side in 0 degrees of internal or external rotation, the implanted humeral head should face directly toward the glenoid fossa.

If the malpositioned prosthesis is too proud, there may be impingement against the residual glenoid fossa. If the humeral head is inserted too deeply into the intramedullary canal, instability of the humeral head may result because of inadequate tension in the myofascial sleeve. In addition, insertion of the prosthesis to too great a depth makes the greater tuberosity relatively proud and may result in greater tuberosity impingement on the acromion.

Postoperative Stiffness

This is an important complication because it is almost entirely preventable. Attention to the details of surgery, early passive motion postoperatively, and patient cooperation with rehabilitation all play critical roles in avoiding postoperative stiffness. It must be emphasized to the patients that lack of compliance or understanding of the postoperative rehabilitation program is the single most common factor associated with rehabilitation failure and postoperative stiffness.

Infection

This is a less-common complication,, but it poses all of the problems with treatment and decision making that infection in an implant will pose.

ILLUSTRATIVE CASE FOR TECHNIQUE

A 56-year-old skier fell while negotiating a turn and complained of severe and incapacitating pain in the shoulder. Initial examination showed exquisite pain with any movement of the arm, palpable crepitus, and marked ecchymosis and swelling. The axillary nerve was normal to testing. Radiographs revealed a four-part anterior fracture dislocation of the humerus (Fig. 17A–C).

Three days after the injury, he was taken to the operating room, where a proximal humeral prosthesis was inserted with reconstruction of the greater tuberosity to the fin of the prosthesis and the shaft of the humerus. Early passive range-of-motion exercises were begun. When radiographic signs of union of the greater tuberosity were present, a program of progressively resistive strengthening exercises was instituted. A postoperative radio-

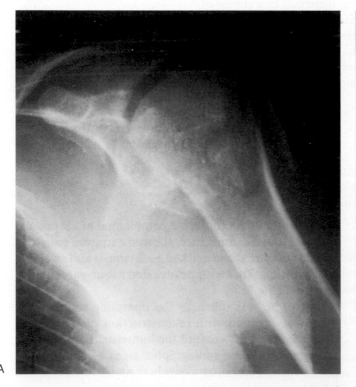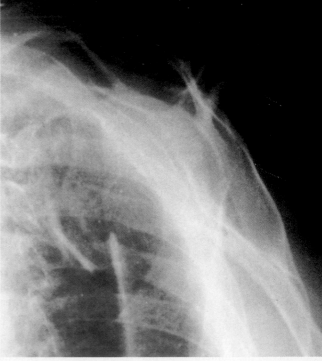

A   B

Figure 17. A: Anteroposterior (AP) radiograph showing impaction and lateral displacement of the head with the greater tuberosity displaced. **B:** A transscapular view showing displacement of the lesser and greater tuberosities.

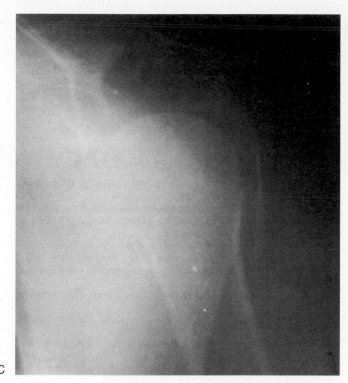
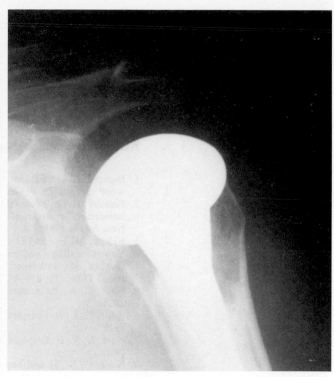

C   D

Figure 17. (*continued*) **C:** A Velpeau axillary view taken in the shrug, which depicts the position of the head and glenoid as well as the tuberosity displacement. **D:** An AP view showing adequate fixation of the tuberosities to both the shaft and humeral head. It is important to note that the greater tuberosity is below the head of the prosthesis.

graph shows satisfactory healing of the greater and lesser tuberosities to the shaft of the humerus, good position of the humeral implant relative to the glenoid, and a slight amount of asymptomatic hetertopic bone (Fig. 17D). At 1 year after surgery, the patient had no pain, passive forward flexion to 160 degrees, and active forward elevation to 150 degrees. The patient was pleased with the result and has returned to recreational skiing.

Acknowledgment

This chapter is reprinted from Craig, E.V. (ed.): *Master Techniques in Orthopaedic Surgery: The Shoulder.* Lippincott–Raven Publishers, Philadelphia, 1997, pp. 259–272.

RECOMMENDED READING

1. Bigliani, L.U.: Fractures of the shoulder. In Rockwood, C.A., Jr., and Green, D.P. (eds.): *Fractures in Adults,* 3rd ed. J.B. Lippincott, Philadelphia, 1990.
2. Bigliani, L.U., Nicholson, G.P., and Flatow, E.L.: The management of fractures of the proximal humerus. In Friedman, R.J. (ed.): *Arthroplasty of the Shoulder.* Thieme Medical Publishers, New York, 1993.
3. Bloom, M.H., and Obata, W.G.: Diagnosis of posterior dislocation of the shoulder with use of Velpeau axillary and angle-up roentgenographic views. *J. Bone Joint Surg. [Am],* 49:943–949, 1967.
4. Hughes, M., and Neer, C.S.: Glenohumeral joint replacement and post-operative rehabilitation. *Phys. Ther.,* 55:850–858, 1975.
5. Neer, C.S., II: Articular replacement of the humeral head. *J. Bone Joint Surg. [Am],* 37:215–228, 1955.
6. Neer, C.S., II: Displaced proximal humerus fractures, Part I. *J. Bone Joint Surg. [Am],* 52:1077–1089, 1970.
7. Neer, C.S., II: Displaced proximal humerus fractures, Part II. *J. Bone Joint Surg. [Am],* 52:1090–1103, 1970.
8. Neer, C.S., II, and McIlveen, S.J.: Remplacement de la tete humerale avec reconstruction des tuberosities et de la coiffe dan les fractures desplacees a 4 fragments. Resultats actuels et techniques. *Rev. Chir. Orthop.* 74(SII):31–40, 1988.
9. Tanner, M.W., and Cofield, R.H.: Prosthetic arthroplasty for fractures and fracture—dislocations of the proximal humerus. *Clin. Orthop.* 179:116–128, 1983.

Master Techniques in Orthopaedic Surgery,
FRACTURES, edited by D. A. Wiss,
Lippincott–Raven Publishers, Philadelphia © 1998.

5

Humeral Shaft Fractures: Open Reduction Internal Fixation

Peter J. O'Brien, Pierre Guy, and Piotr A. Blachut

Historically, humeral shaft fractures have been classified by fracture location, fracture pattern, associated soft-tissue injuries, and the quality of the bone. The Orthopaedic Trauma Association adopted Müller's alphanumeric system for classification of long-bone fractures. This system is easily remembered and gives the treating surgeon a precise anatomic description of the fracture. The humerus is designated by the number 1, and the segment (diaphysis) is 2. The fracture types are A, simple; B, wedge; or C, complex. Subgroups are further defined based on fracture geometry. Figure 1 is a schematic drawing of this widely used classification scheme.

INDICATIONS/CONTRAINDICATIONS

Open reduction and internal fixation (ORIF) is an excellent technique for treating selected humeral shaft fractures. As numerous authors and studies have shown, the majority of humeral shaft fractures can be treated nonoperatively. High rates of union and excellent functional results usually occur after nonoperative treatment of these fractures. However, there are specific clinical settings where open reduction and plate fixation is favored over closed functional methods. Although there are no absolute indications for plate fixation, we favor its use in some patients based on the fracture structure or the presence of concomitant injuries (8; Table 1).

P. J. O'Brien, M.D., F.R.C.S.C.: Department of Orthopaedics, University of British Columbia, Vancouver Hospital and Health Sciences Center, Vancouver, British Columbia, V5Z 4E3, Canada.

P. Guy, M.D., F.R.C.S.C.: Department of Orthopaedic Surgery, McGill University Health Center, Montreal, Quebec, H3G 1A4, Canada.

P. A. Blachut, M.D., F.R.C.S.C.: Department of Orthopaedics, Division of Orthopaedic Trauma, University of British Columbia, Vancouver Hospital and Health Sciences Center, Vancouver, British Columbia, V5Z 4E3, Canada.

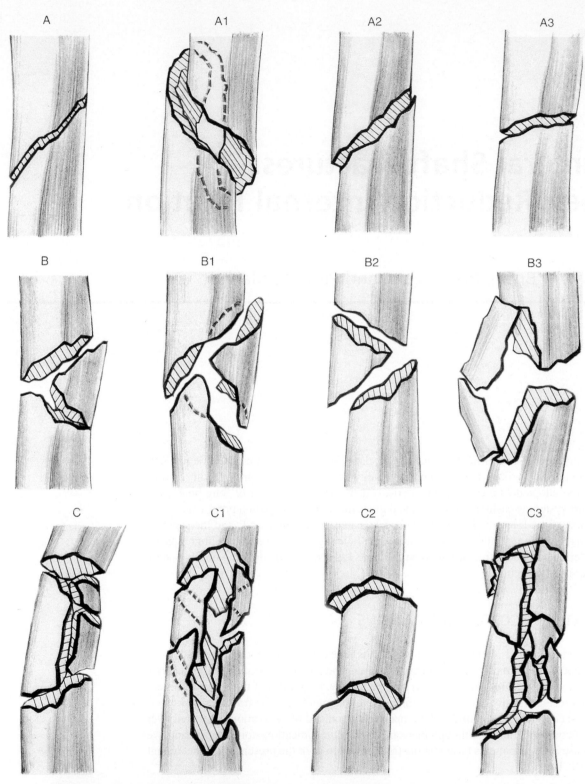

Figure 1. The alphanumeric classification for humeral diaphyseal fractures as used by AO and Orthopaedic Trauma Association.

TABLE 1. *Indications for ORIF*

Early	Late
Failure of closed Rx	Nonunion
Multiple injuries, patient	Malunion
Multiple injuries, limb	
Open fracture	
Pathologic fracture	
Associated arthrodesis	
Periprosthetic fracture	

ORIF, open reduction internal fixation; Rx, treatments.

Morphologic Considerations

Internal fixation is indicated in patients with closed fractures in which a satisfactory reduction cannot be achieved or maintained. The most common cause of a poor reduction in an otherwise healthy individual is interposition of soft tissue. Failure to maintain an acceptable closed reduction sometimes occurs in obese patients or women with large breasts. In these situations, surgical intervention may be necessary. Other indications include segmental fractures and periarticular fractures. The latter can be difficult to control, and the prolonged immobilization of the adjacent joint can lead to loss of motion.

Open fractures require surgical debridement and bony stabilization to allow optimal soft-tissue management. After thorough debridement, ORIF of the humerus is a good method of fracture stabilization for most Grade I, II, and IIIA injuries with limited bony defects. It produces a stable limb, improving postoperative wound management. With extreme comminution or bone loss, acute shortening or up to 5 cm is usually well tolerated (10). However, if the cortex is continuous, conservation of length and a delayed bone grafting is preferred. Grade IIIB and IIIC injuries, as well as some gunshot wounds, are better treated with an external fixator by using ring or unilateral frames.

Experience has taught us that nonoperative treatment of pathologic humeral fractures frequently results in nonunion and persistent pain. There is widespread agreement that patients with a pathologic humeral fracture as a result of metastatic disease benefit from surgical stabilization. Usually these fractures are best managed with a locked intramedullary nail. Occasionally, a fracture is not amenable to intramedullary nailing and is better managed with a long-spanning plate.

Fractures above or below an elbow or shoulder arthroplasty frequently require internal fixation. Fractures that occur around the stem of an implant occasionally require revision of the prosthesis.

Delayed union and nonunion are additional indications for ORIF of a humeral fracture. Delayed union is generally accepted as failure of the fracture to unite within 2 to 3 months, whereas nonunion is present when the process is delayed or arrested beyond 4 to 6 months. Nonunions can occur because of fracture instability, poor bone vascularity, or marked displacement. In nonunion after an open fracture or a fracture that has been operated on, infection must be ruled out (12).

Malunion is rarely an indication for surgical intervention because angular deformity is often well tolerated after closed treatment. The amount of malalignment that can be accepted varies between patients and is influenced by level of activity and cosmesis. Most patients tolerate up to 20 to 30 degrees of varus, 20 degrees of anterior angulation, and 5 cm of shortening (10).

Concomitant Injuries

Internal fixation of humeral shaft fractures also is indicated in a variety of circumstances due to concomitant injuries.

The polytrauma patient with multiple injuries is the most common candidate for operative treatment of humeral shaft fractures (3,4,8). When patients sustain injuries to multiple body systems [central nervous system (CNS), pulmonary, abdominal, etc.] early surgical stabilization of long-bone fractures may be lifesaving. Fixation should be undertaken early to reduce analgesic needs, allow early mobilization, and facilitate nursing care.

Patients with ipsilateral injuries to the shoulder, elbow, or forearm often require operative treatment of the humeral fracture. In bilateral humeral fractures or any contralateral upper-extremity injury, fixation is necessary to allow activities of daily living and self-care. Humeral shaft fractures associated with a fracture of both forearm bones require fixation of both the forearm and the humerus to allow early range of motion. Finally, rehabilitation of injuries to the lower extremities can be accelerated by fixation of the humerus, which allows use of crutches through the stabilized humerus.

An axillary or brachial artery injury associated with a closed fracture should be stabilized at the time of vascular repair. Internal fixation of the humerus through the vascular approach is recommended to protect the vascular repair, to facilitate ongoing assessment, and allow rehabilitation of the limb. Brachial plexus or peripheral nerve injuries in the ipsilateral limb are often an indication for internal fixation of a humeral fracture. One study reported that concomitant brachial plexus injuries may be associated with high rates of delayed union, nonunion, and malunion of the humeral shaft when treated closed (6). To prevent these complications and to facilitate rehabilitation, operative treatment can be considered with this combination of injuries.

The management of humeral fractures with associated radial nerve injury remains controversial (1,5,7,13,14). The incidence of radial nerve injury in humeral fractures is approximately 10%, with a range reported between 2% and 26%. Humeral shaft fractures seen with a radial nerve injury (primary radial nerve injury) do not usually require nerve exploration. If the fracture reduction can be maintained, closed treatment will result in fracture healing and a good outcome with a greater than 80% chance of spontaneous nerve recovery. The majority of cases are neuropraxias, which should show signs of recovery by 3 to 4 months, with improvements in muscle grade up to 2 years after injury (4).

Some studies have shown that with modern microsurgical techniques and late exploration of radial nerve palsies, better than 90% recover (1,13). Therefore, we recommend initial observation and late exploration for nerve injuries that do not resolve. The injury should be documented clinically and electrophysiologically with electromyogram/nerve-conduction study (EMG/NCS) in the early stages. The hand should be splinted, and an intensive physiotherapy program should be initiated to maintain mobility at the elbow, wrist, and fingers. Patients are evaluated monthly and have a follow-up EMG/NCS at 6 and 12 weeks. If after 4 to 6 months there is no sign of radial nerve recovery, we explore the nerve.

More controversial is the management of secondary radial nerve palsy. Most commonly this occurs after closed reduction of a humeral fracture. Traditionally, a nerve palsy occurring in such a circumstance was considered an indication for nerve exploration and internal fixation. Although some have shown that the nerve can be trapped between the fracture fragments and intuitively it would seem reasonable to explore the nerve and free it from any ongoing compression, there is no scientific evidence that the outcome is improved by early surgery. Secondary radial nerve palsy, however, continues to be an accepted indication for early exploration.

Relative contraindications to plate fixation of humeral shaft fractures include Grade IIIB open fractures with massive soft-tissue injury or extensive bone loss, soft-tissue or bone infection, or severe osteoporosis that would preclude fixation.

PREOPERATIVE PLANNING

As with all injured patients, a careful history and physical examination are mandatory. Associated injuries should be identified and carefully assessed. Physical examination should include a careful examination of the chest, neck, shoulder, arm, elbow, forearm, wrist, and hand. The physical signs of fracture are usually obvious after humeral shaft fractures. The neurologic examination of the limb must be meticulous. Radial nerve injury is the most commonly associated neurologic injury, but any peripheral nerve, including the brachial plexus, can be injured in association with a humeral diaphyseal fracture. The vascular assessment includes palpation of the axillary, brachial, and radial pulses and an assessment of tissue perfusion at the level of the hand. The soft-tissue compartments of the arm and forearm should be evaluated for compartment syndrome.

Good-quality radiographs of the humerus are essential. Anteroposterior (AP) and lateral views of the humerus should be obtained that include the shoulder and elbow joints (Fig. 2A). The anatomic location of the fracture, the fracture pattern, and the expected bone quality are critical when developing a preoperative plan.

Once a decision is made to operate on a humeral fracture, a surgical tactic should be developed, which includes the patient position, the surgical approach, the steps necessary for fracture reduction, temporary fixation, and the implant to be used for final fixation. A preoperative tracing and cutout of the humeral fracture pattern is often useful for planning the steps of reduction and fixation (Fig. 2B and C). Postoperative radiographs are obtained to ensure accomplishment of the preoperative plan (Fig. 2D).

There are four basic approaches to the shaft of the humerus. Three of these (the anterolateral, the posterior, and the straight lateral) are most often used for ORIF. The anteromedial approach to the humerus is rarely used in humeral shaft fracture treatment. The decision about which surgical approach to use is based on the fracture location, the extent of the fracture, and the patient's general condition. The most commonly used technique of exposure is the anterolateral approach (15). Fractures located anywhere in the proximal two thirds of the humerus can be successfully managed through this approach. The anterolateral approach, however, does not allow adequate exposure of the distal one third of the humerus and therefore cannot be used if the fixation must be extended into the distal diaphysis/metaphysis. The posterior approach can be used for fractures that involve the distal half of the humeral shaft. In fractures involving the distal two thirds of the humerus, with an associated radial nerve injury that requires surgery, we prefer the straight lateral approach to the humerus. This approach can be extended into the anterolateral approach and, therefore, is the only approach that gives access to the entire humerus.

The steps necessary for fracture reduction and temporary fixation before final fixation must be carefully considered. In most cases direct reduction techniques are appropriate. The fracture hematoma is evacuated, and the fracture surfaces are anatomically reduced. For spiral or oblique fracture patterns, temporary fixation can usually be accomplished with the Weber pointed reduction forceps. Transverse fractures can usually be stabilized temporarily with K-wires. Some comminuted fractures that still have cortical contact between the main proximal and distal pieces cannot be temporarily stabilized satisfactorily. In those cases, the appropriate plate is secured to one fragment, the fracture is then reduced under the plate, and fixation is completed. Severely comminuted fractures may be amenable to indirect reduction techniques. The femoral distractor is used to secure the reduction, which is confirmed under image intensification. The appropriate plate is then secured to the main proximal and main distal fragments. The soft-tissue attachments to the comminuted intercalary fragments are left intact. Bone grafting is not added when the indirect reduction technique is used.

When planning plate fixation, interfragmentary compression is desirable. In oblique or spiral fractures, this can be done by using interfragmentary lag screws inserted outside (Fig. 3) or through the plate (Fig. 4). Interfragmentary screws alone are insufficient fixation for humeral shaft fractures and must be supplemented with a neutralization plate.

Unfortunately, interfragmentary screws cannot always be used, particularly in transverse fracture patterns. In such cases, interfragmentary compression is accomplished by using a dynamic compression plate (DCP). The plate must be prestressed (prebending) to avoid a gap in the far cortex (Fig. 5). In general, the plate of choice is a broad 4.5-mm DC plate (Fig. 4). This is a strong plate with a wide surface contact, combined with offset screw holes to prevent longitudinal splitting of the shaft from colinear screws. In acute fractures, at least six cortices of fixation above and six below the fracture (more in cases of osteoporotic bone or when treating nonunions) are required. Bone grafting should be planned with commin-

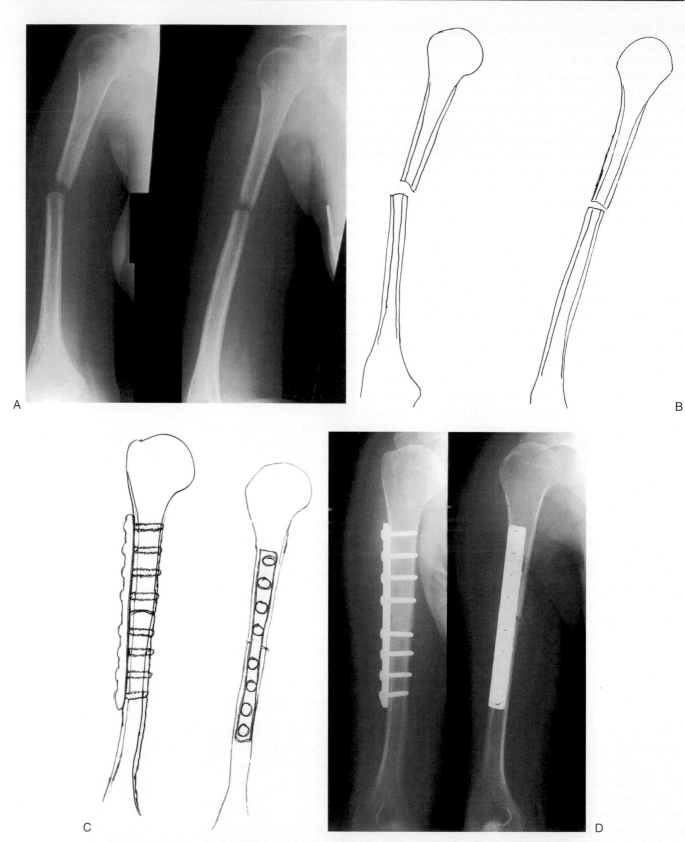

Figure 2. Preoperative planning to establish a surgical strategy. **A:** Anteroposterior (AP) and lateral radiograph of a 20-year-old woman with a delayed union of a transverse humeral shaft fracture. **B, C:** Tracing of the fracture, its reduction, and location of a prebent 4.5-mm eight-hole DCP. **D:** Postoperative radiographs showing accomplishment of the preoperative plan.

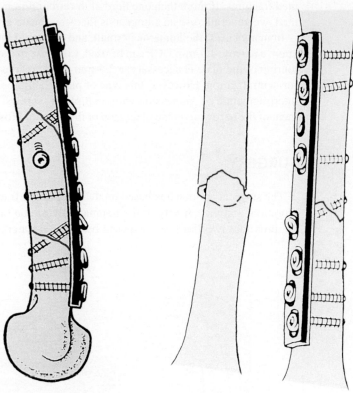

Figure 3. Initial fixation is accomplished with an interfragmentary screw. This is supplemented by a neutralization plate.

Figure 4. Interfragmentary fixation through the plate.

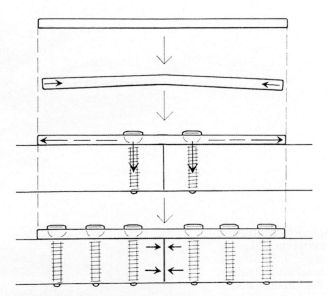

Figure 5. Transverse fracture pattern in which interfragmentary compression is achieved by using a prebent plate.

uted fractures. If more than one third of the circumference of the humeral shaft is comminuted, we generally use an autogenous iliac-crest bone graft.

In many cases, the humerus is small, and the broad DCP cannot be used. In such a situation, a narrow 4.5-mm DCP can be used. Likewise in the distal shaft, where extensive contouring of the plate is necessary, a 3.5-mm pelvic reconstruction plate is occasionally used for neutralization. However, this type of plate should be used only when there is excellent interfragmentary compression with multiple lag screws. It is important to avoid encroachment of the hardware in the olecranon or the coronoid fossa when fixing the distal humerus.

SURGERY

The surgical approach is based on the level of the fracture, the need for radial nerve exploration, and the severity of the trauma (polytrauma or isolated). In general, fractures in the proximal two thirds are exposed by an anterolateral approach (Fig. 6A). We use the

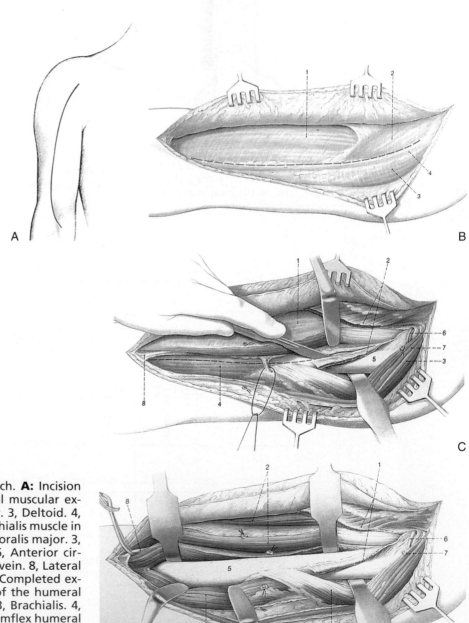

Figure 6. The anterolateral approach. **A:** Incision for anterolateral approach. **B:** Initial muscular exposure. 1, Biceps. 2, Pectoralis major. 3, Deltoid. 4, Cephalic vein. **C:** Splitting of the brachialis muscle in the line of its fibers. 1, Biceps. 2, Pectoralis major. 3, Deltoid. 4, Brachialis. 5, Humerus. 6, Anterior circumflex humeral vessels. 7, Cephalic vein. 8, Lateral cutaneous nerve of the forearm. **D:** Completed exposure of the proximal two thirds of the humeral shaft. 1, Pectoralis major. 2, Biceps. 3, Brachialis. 4, Deltoid. 5, Humerus. 6, Anterior circumflex humeral vessels. 7, Cephalic vein. 8, Lateral cutaneous nerve of the forearm.

straight lateral approach when radial nerve exploration is indicated; and we prefer to have the patient supine (anterolateral, lateral approaches) if the patient has polytrauma. A sterile tourniquet is used if the fracture is in the middle or distal one third.

The anterolateral approach is done with the patient in the supine position with a pad beneath the scapula (Fig. 7). The arm is free draped, allowing access to the neck (subclavian vasculature), the shoulder, the elbow, and the forearm. The shoulder is abducted 45 to 60 degrees. Surface landmarks from proximal to distal are the coracoid process, the deltopectoral groove, the lateral bicipital sulcus, and the lateral epicondyle. These are marked with a sterile pen (Fig. 7).

Depending on the proximal extension of the fracture, the proximal extent of the incision is based 1 to 3 cm distal to the coracoid (Fig. 6). It courses distally along the deltopectoral groove. The belly of the biceps is identified, and its lateral border mobilized. The incision is extended longitudinally 1 cm lateral to the biceps, exposing the brachialis muscle (Fig. 6B). Distally the incision can extend down to about 6 cm from the lateral epicondyle. Care is taken to avoid injury to the cephalic vein proximally and the lateral cutaneous nerve of the forearm medially and distally. The biceps is retracted medially, and the deep dissection is done longitudinally through the brachialis muscle, lateral to its midline and down to bone, aiming for the middle of the humeral shaft (Fig. 6C). In doing so, the radial nerve (lateral to brachialis) is protected, and the innervation of the lateral portion of the brachialis (radial) is preserved (Fig. 6D). Flexion of the elbow, along with partial (anterior) detachment of the deltoid insertion and of the medial brachialis origin is done to allow reduction and plating of the anterolateral surface of the humerus (Fig. 8).

The posterior approach is used in cases of isolated fractures in the distal half of the humerus (2). The patient is placed prone and brought to the edge of the operating table. The arm is free-draped to allow access to the whole arm and the elbow. The shoulder is abducted 90 degrees in neutral flexion and supported distally at the elbow by a modified Mayo stand (Fig. 9A). This stand was altered by cutting a hole at the edge of the tray and padding the exposed rim of the stand. During the procedure, the forearm and hand are dropped into the hole, which is lined by a sterile C-arm pack protecting the forearm from contamination by its low-lying position. An additional advantage is the ability to place instruments on the Mayo stand.

The exposure itself is longitudinal and in-line between the posterolateral corner of the acromion and the olecranon (Fig. 9B). It extends from the distal border of the posterior deltoid, along the lateral edge of the long head of the triceps, to the tip of the olecranon. These surface landmarks are drawn on the skin before incision. The long head can be identified as a mobile mass on the posteromedial aspect of the arm. Skin, subcutaneous tissue, and

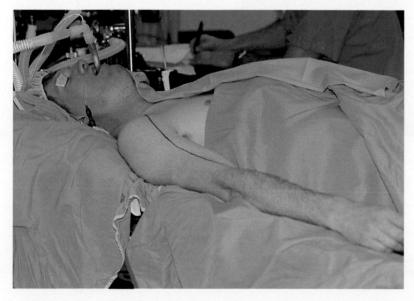

Figure 7. Positioning and landmarks for the anterolateral approach.

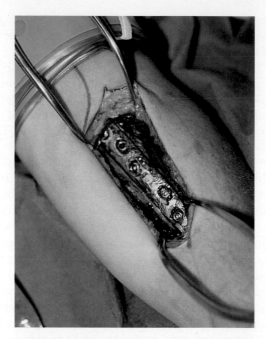

Figure 8. Prebent, broad, 4.5-mm dynamic-compression plate applied to a transverse fracture through an anterolateral approach.

fascia are incised, and the distal, thick, white triceps tendon is identified. Proximally, the interval between the long and the lateral heads of the triceps is identified and dissected bluntly. Distally, these two superficial heads are sharply dissected by division of the triceps tendon (Fig. 10A and B). Careful blunt dissection is carried out to identify the radial nerve and the deep head of the triceps (Fig. 11A and B). A rubber sling is placed around the ra-

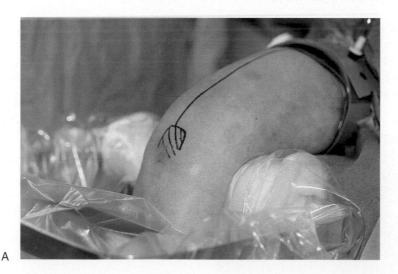

A

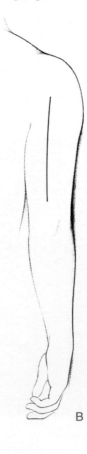

B

Figure 9. A: Positioning and landmarks for the posterolateral approach with modified Mayo stand. **B:** Skin incision for posterior approach.

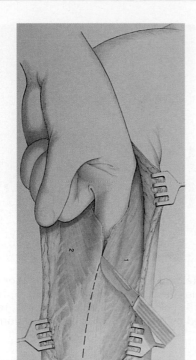
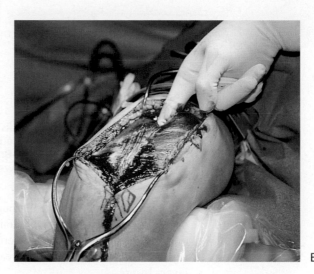

A

B

Figure 10. The posterior approach. **A, B:** Identification of the long and lateral heads of the triceps. 1, Long head of triceps; 2, Lateral head of triceps.

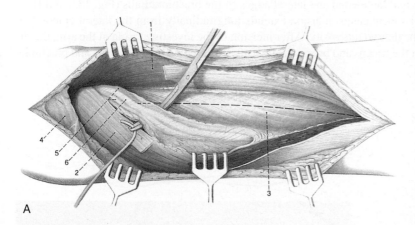

A

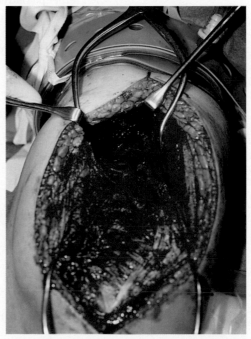

B

Figure 11. A, B: Exposure of the deep head of the triceps and radial nerve. **A:** 1, Long head of tricep. 2, Lateral head of triceps. 3, Deep (medial) head of triceps. 4, Deltoid. 5, Deep brachial artery. 6, Radial nerve.

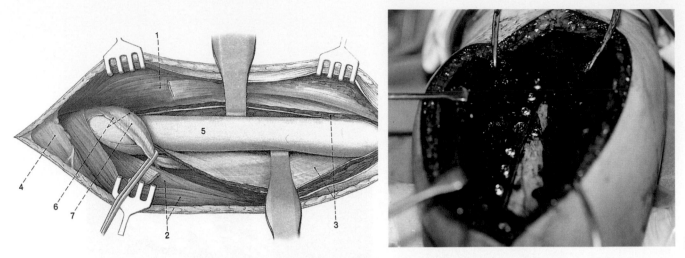

A   B

Figure 12. A: Exposure of the distal half of the humeral shaft. 1, Long head of triceps. 2, Lateral head of triceps. 3, Medial head of triceps. 4, Deltoid. 5, Humerus. 6, Deep brachial artery. 7, Radial nerve. **B:** By using the posterior approach, reduction and lag-screw fixation is achieved, followed by placement of a neutralization plate.

dial nerve, which is protected throughout the case. The lateral intermuscular septum can be divided. The deep triceps is split longitudinally in its midline, and its medial and lateral portions elevated, exposing the humerus (Fig. 12A). Reduction and fixation can now proceed (Fig. 12B). The closure includes reapproximation of the triceps aponeurosis and superficial layer closure.

The straight lateral approach requires careful dissection and excellent visualization of the radial nerve and adjacent structures (2). It is ideal for exploration of the radial nerve and fixation of the distal humerus in a multiply injured patient. With the patient supine, the shoulder and arm are draped as for an anterolateral approach. The arm is kept adducted along the patient's side. The following surface landmarks are identified and drawn: the lateral epicondyle and the medial and lateral edges of the brachioradialis (Fig. 13A and B).

The skin and subcutaneous incision extends longitudinally from the lateral epicondyle proximally to the deltoid tuberosity. After incision of the investing fascia of the arm, the intervals between the triceps and brachialis proximally and the brachioradialis and brachialis

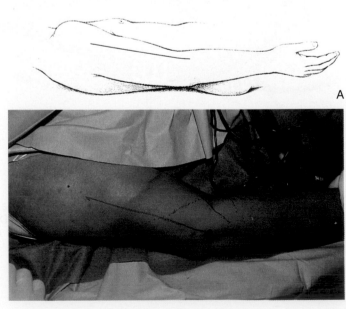

A

B

Figure 13. A, B: Positioning and skin incision for the straight lateral approach to the distal humerus.

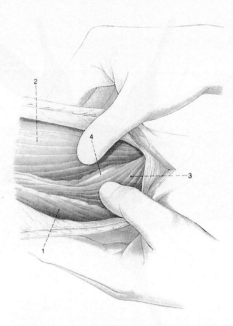

Figure 14. The radial nerve is identified in the interval between the brachialis and the brachioradialis. 1, Triceps. 2, Brachialis. 3, Brachioradialis. 4, Radial nerve.

distally are identified (Fig. 14). The distal interval is first developed bluntly as described by Henry (9): ". . . place well-gloved thumbs, lengthwise and parallel, on each belly (brachialis and brachioradialis), and open the plane like a book on your knee. The nerve marks the place." The radial nerve is isolated, looped with a rubber sling and protected. The nerve is retracted laterally while the proximal dissection is completed. The periosteum anterior to the intermuscular septum is split longitudinally, and subperiosteal elevation progresses medially and proximally with direct visualization and protection of the nerve at all times. This can be gently elevated if further access is required. As the nerve courses posteriorly and proximally, one might need to incise the intermuscular septum to mobilize the nerve and visualize its relation to the fracture. The nerve is retracted anteriorly, and the dis-

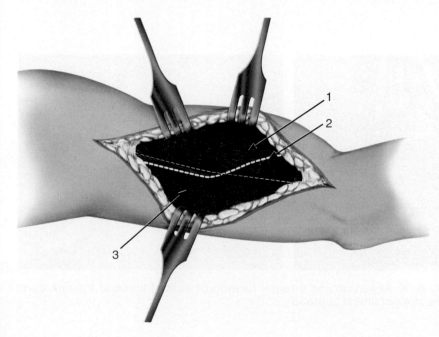

Figure 15. The interval between brachialis and triceps proximally and between brachioradialis and triceps distally is developed. 1, Biceps brachii muscle. 2, Radial nerve. 3, Triceps brachii muscle.

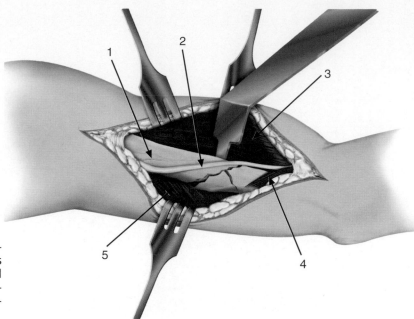

Figure 16. The brachialis and brachioradialis are retracted anteriorly and the triceps posteriorly, exposing the distal humeral shaft. 1, Humerus. 2, Radial nerve. 3, Brachialis muscle. 4, Brachioradialis muscle. 5, Triceps brachii muscle.

tal dissection is completed. Distally, the plane between the brachioradialis and the triceps is identified (Fig. 15). This plane is incised sharply, and the brachioradialis is reflected anteriorly, protecting the distal portion of the nerve. The entire distal humerus is exposed laterally and anterolaterally (Fig. 16). Reduction and internal fixation of the fracture progress by following the principles previously described. A narrow 4.5-mm plate placed laterally is often the best implant with this exposure. Screws are directed from lateral to medial, and the plate is often quite distal; therefore one must avoid screw placement in the coronoid/olecranon fossa (Fig. 17A and B).

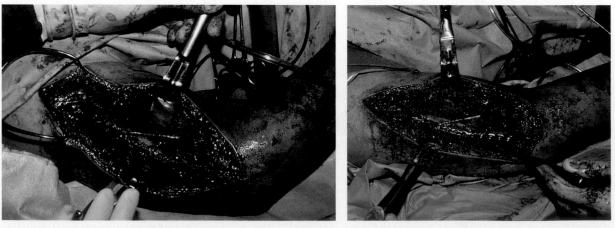

Figure 17. A, B: Reduction and internal fixation of a distal humeral fracture done through the straight lateral approach.

POSTOPERATIVE MANAGEMENT

Prophylactic antibiotics are used. In addition to a single preoperative dose, prophylaxis is generally continued for 24 h postoperatively. Cephazolin, 1 g i.v., 1 h before surgery and every 8 h for three doses postoperatively is our usual protocol. Patients with a penicillin allergy receive vancomycin, 1 g i.v., 1 h before surgery and 500 mg i.v., every 12 h postoperatively for 24 h. Open fractures require 72 h of prophylactic antibiotic administration.

Postoperatively, patients are placed in a sling, which is removed to permit active range-of-motion exercises of the shoulder and elbow within a day or two of surgery. Full elbow and shoulder motion should be obtained within 1 month of surgery. Patients are seen in the clinic 2 weeks after their surgery. They are then seen on a monthly basis until the fracture is united and they have returned to normal activity. Radiographs are obtained at each visit. The patients are carefully assessed for shoulder, elbow, wrist, and hand function. The radiographs are studied for signs of fracture healing and any evidence of implant failure. In rigid fixation, fracture union is often difficult to assess. If follow-up radiographs show maintenance of the reduction, light weights are usually allowed at 6 weeks and regular weights at 12 weeks. At 12 weeks, patients can begin returning to normal activities. Heavy work can be started by 16 weeks. Sporting activities, such as tennis and golf, can also be started about 4 months after surgery.

COMPLICATIONS

Most complications can be avoided by adhering to basic principles.

Failure of fixation occurs in up to 4% of patients and can be avoided by careful preoperative planning, implant selection, and limited soft-tissue dissection. When using a plate, interfragmentary compression either with lag screws and a neutralization plate, or with a compression plate alone, is essential. At least six cortices of fixation on each side of the fracture must be obtained. If the fixation fails, revision ORIF is necessary, usually with a longer plate and bone graft. Immobilization with a fracture sleeve before revision of fixation is rarely successful in securing union and is rarely used.

Nonunion after plate osteosynthesis occurs in 3% to 5% of cases. Factors thought to contribute to nonunion include open fractures, middle-third transverse fractures, pathologic fractures, alcohol abuse, or a technical error in the index procedure. Factors that can be controlled by the surgeon include accurate fracture reduction, stability of fixation, minimizing soft-tissue stripping, and bone grafting. Nonunion is treated by revision ORIF and autogenous cancellous bone grafting. A longer plate must be used at the revision procedure. Intramedullary nailing is not a good option for treatment of nonunion after plate fixation (11). The biology of the blood supply to bone does not allow an extraosseous procedure (plate removal) and an intraosseous procedure (intramedullary nailing) to be done at the same time and still result in bone healing.

With few studies assessing function in detail, loss of motion of the shoulder or elbow is probably underreported. Several studies reported that 15% to 20% of patients have decreased shoulder and elbow motion after ORIF. Etiologic factors include fracture with extensive soft-tissue injuries or with ipsilateral bone or joint injury. Stable fixation and early motion are recommended. If significant stiffness is identified, a more vigorous physiotherapy program is initiated. We have not had to use any surgical modalities (arthroscopy, manipulation, etc.) to deal with joint stiffness after ORIF of humeral shaft fractures in our practice.

Infection occurs in up to 6% of cases after ORIF. From a preventive point of view, the routine use of perioperative antibiotics, limited soft-tissue dissection, careful hemostasis, and thorough debridement of open fractures may reduce the rate of infection after ORIF. If infection develops, careful workup and identification of the organism is mandatory. This is followed by assessing and correcting problems with stability, fragment approximation, vascularity, and soft-tissue coverage. The infected site should be incised, drained, and thoroughly debrided. The area is packed with antibiotic-loaded acrylic cement beads. Systemic parenteral antibiotics also are used. The choice of local and systemic antibiotic depends on the Gram-stain findings and the final culture and sensitivities. Parenteral antibiotics are generally continued for 6 weeks. The local antibiotic depot is usually removed at 7 to 10 days at the time of repeated debridement and irrigation. If the fixation is rigid, it is left in place. If, on the other hand, the fixation is loose, it is revised, and rigid fixation is obtained.

Radial nerve palsy most frequently occurs at the time of injury. Iatrogenic radial nerve palsy occurs in about 5% of surgical cases. An intraoperative laceration should never occur, but if it does, it should be repaired immediately by a trained microsurgeon. A postoperative nerve palsy after identification and protection of the nerve should be observed, and full functional recovery anticipated.

ILLUSTRATIVE CASE FOR TECHNIQUE

A 30-year-old woman had an isolated humerus fracture after a fall from a horse. She had a spiral humeral shaft fracture and was neurologically intact. After closed reduction and application of a hanging cast, she developed a complete radial nerve palsy. Furthermore, radiographs in the cast demonstrated an unacceptable reduction (Fig. 18A). Because of malreduction and secondary nerve palsy, she underwent nerve exploration and internal fixation. Because of the fracture location (distal one third), it was thought that an anterolateral approach would not provide enough distal exposure. The posterior approach was ruled out because of the fracture geometry and the expected anterolateral location of the nerve injury. ORIF was done through a straight lateral approach. At the time of exposure, the radial nerve and the brachialis muscle were both found to be entrapped between the fracture fragments. Anatomic reduction was obtained and held with two large fragment-reduction clamps. Stable internal fixation was achieved with three interfragmentary compression screws. In the presence of excellent interfragmentary fixation, a 3.5-mm reconstruction plate was contoured and applied as a neutralization plate. Postoperative mobilization was started immediately. Fracture healing occurred radiographically by 12 weeks (Fig. 18B). The radial nerve recovered completely, and the patient returned to full activities.

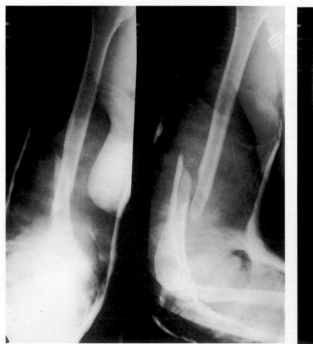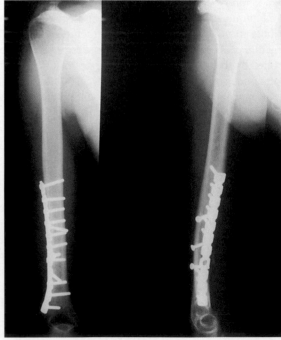

A   B

Figure 18. A: Radiograph showing failure of closed management of a humeral shaft fracture at the junction of the middle and distal third. **B:** The straight lateral approach is used in this illustrative case. This allows isolation of the nerve and reduction and fixation of fractures in the distal two thirds of the humerus. Fixation was achieved through lag screw and a neutralization reconstruction plate. Radiographic signs of healing were apparent at 12 weeks.

RECOMMENDED READING

1. Amillo, S., Barrios, R.H., Martinez-Peric, R., et al.: Surgical treatment of the radial nerve lesions associated with fractures of the humerus. *J. Orthop. Trauma* 7:211–215, 1993.
2. Bauer, R., Kerschbaumer, F., and Poisel, S.: *Operative Approaches in Orthopedic Surgery and Traumatology.* 1st ed. Thieme Verlag, New York, 1987.
3. Bell, M.J., Beauchamp, C.G., Kellam, J.K., et al.: The results of plating humeral shaft fractures in patients with multiple injuries: the Sunnybrook experience. *J. Bone Joint Surg. [Br],* 67:293–296, 1985.
4. Bleeker, W.A., Nisten, M.W., and ten Duis, H-J.: Treatment of humeral shaft fractures related to associated injuries: a retrospective study of 237 patients. *Acta. Orthop. Scand.* 62:148–153, 1991.
5. Böstman, O., Bakalim, G., Vainionpää, S., et al.: Radial palsy in shaft fracture of the humerus. *Acta. Orthop. Scand.* 57:316–319, 1986.
6. Brien, W.W., Gellman, H., Becker, V., et al.: Management of fractures of the humerus in patients who have an injury of the ipsilateral brachial plexus. *J. Bone Joint Surg. [Am],* 72:1208–1210, 1990.
7. Dabezies, E.J., Banta, C.J., II, Murphy, C.P., et al.: Plate fixation of the humeral shaft for acute fractures, with and without radial nerve injuries. *J. Orthop. Trauma* 6:10–13, 1992.
8. Heim, D., Herkert, F., Hess, P., et al.: Surgical treatment of humeral shaft fractures: the Basel experience. *J. Trauma* 35:226–232, 1993.
9. Henry, A.K.: *Extensile Exposure.* 1st ed. E.S. Livingstone, Edinburgh, 1945.
10. Klenerman, L.: Fractures of the shaft of the humerus. *J. Bone Joint Surg. [Br],* 48:105–111, 1966.
11. McKee, M.D., Miranda, M.A., Reimer, B.L., et al.: Management of humeral nonunion after the failure of locking intramedullary nails. *J. Orthop. Trauma* 10:492–499, 1997.
12. Rosen, H.: The treatment of nonunions and pseudoarthroses of the humeral shaft. *Orthop. Clin. North Am.* 21:725–742, 1990.
13. Samardzic, M., Grujicic, D., Milinkovic, Z.B.: Radial nerve lesions associated with fractures of the humeral shaft. *Injury* 21:220–222, 1990.
14. Sarmiento, A., Horowitch, A., Aboulafia, A., et al.: Functional bracing for comminuted extra-articular fractures of the distal-third of the humerus. *J. Bone Joint Surg. [Br],* 72:283–287, 1990.
15. Vander Griend R., Tomasin, J., and Ward, E.F.: Open reduction and internal fixation of humeral shaft fractures: results using AO plating techniques. *J. Bone Joint Surg. [Am],* 68:430–433, 1986.

Master Techniques in Orthopaedic Surgery,
FRACTURES, edited by D. A. Wiss,
Lippincott–Raven Publishers, Philadelphia © 1998.

6

Humeral Shaft Fractures: Intramedullary Nailing

Barry L. Riemer

INDICATIONS/CONTRAINDICATIONS

Most low-energy isolated fractures of the humeral shaft can be treated nonoperatively. However, functional bracing of humeral fractures is much less effective in patients with high-energy closed fractures, open fractures, and multiple injuries. In these patients, the advantages of surgical stabilization probably outweigh its risks. The indications for operative treatment of humeral shaft fractures include pathologic and impending pathologic fractures, displaced segmental fractures, ipsilateral forearm fractures (floating elbow), fractures with arterial injuries, open fractures, and any fracture with significant soft-tissue injuries that requires wound care. Some patients with low- or intermediate-level injuries cannot tolerate brace treatment because of pain, fracture instability, or body habitus. Women with large breasts are often difficult to brace because of angular deformity. Patients with excessive shortening of more than 2.5 cm or angulation of more than 25 degrees may be surgical candidates.

Multiply injured patients with humeral fractures require special consideration. Internal fixation is particularly important when orthopaedic injuries require weight bearing on the injured arm with crutches or a walker. In patients with significant head or chest trauma, humeral stabilization is indicated to facilitate pulmonary care, especially when a chest tube is required.

Plate fixation is the most common technique used when internal fixation of a humeral fracture is necessary. However, locked intramedullary nailing has several advantages compared with plate osteosynthesis. With closed nailing, the fracture site is not exposed, and the fracture hematoma is minimally disturbed, thereby enhancing fracture healing. Comminuted fractures can be stabilized through small incisions, minimizing blood loss and cosmetic deformity, fixation in osteopenic bone can be achieved, and weight bearing can be done on the injured extremity postoperatively.

B. L. Riemer, M.D.: Department of Orthopaedic Surgery, Orthopaedic Trauma Division, Allegheny University of the Health Sciences, Pittsburgh, Pennsylvania 15212-4734.

Contraindications to humeral nailing include fractures of 5 to 7 cm of the shoulder or elbow joints, adolescents and children with open epiphyses, patients with narrow medullary canals or preexisting deformity that precludes closed nailing, and certain highly contaminated Grade IIIB open fractures acutely.

PREOPERATIVE PLANNING

An accurate history and careful physical examination is necessary in patients with humeral shaft fractures because associated injuries are common. In patients with multiple trauma, a multidisciplinary approach to evaluation and treatment is essential. Aggressive resuscitation and treatment of life- or limb-threatening conditions are the first priority. Virtually all conscious patients with a displaced humeral fracture are first seen with pain, swelling, and inability to use the arm. The extremity should be inspected for open wounds, abrasions, or hematomas. Because of the vulnerability of the radial nerve after fracture, a detailed neurovascular examination is mandatory. The axillary, brachial, and radial pulses should be palpated. The axillary, radial, median, and ulnar nerve function should be assessed. In some patients with high-energy injuries, a detailed examination of the brachial plexus is necessary. An isolated radial nerve palsy that is present at the time of initial examination is not an indication alone for nerve exploration and internal fixation. These are usually neuropraxias and resolve spontaneously in 3 to 4 months. On the other hand, a patient with an intact radial nerve who develops a progressive deficit after casting or splint should undergo nerve exploration with plate osteosynthesis. In patients with multiple trauma, head injury or drug or alcohol intoxication with a humeral fracture are problematic. In patients with altered consciousness, a complete neurologic examination is frequently impossible, and it is important to document that an adequate neurovascular examination could not be performed. The humerus is also a common site for metastatic and myeloplastic disease. In the absence of a history of significant trauma, a pathologic fracture should be considered.

In a patient with a suspected fracture, an anteroposterior (AP) and lateral radiograph of the entire humerus should be obtained. If the fracture extends into the shoulder or elbow joints, separate plain films or computed tomography (CT) scans of these areas may be helpful. High quality radiographs are imperative so that medullary-canal diameter can be estimated. Because the humerus does not tolerate reaming well, a clear delineation of canal diameter is imperative. The Seidel nail (Howmedica, Inc.), for example, is available in only one size, 9 mm. The distal canal, allowing 10% magnification error, must measure at least 10 mm on both AP and lateral radiographs to accommodate the nail.

If surgery is delayed, the arm is placed into a coaptation or long-arm splint. A coaptation splint with an elastic wrap from the hand to the upper humerus, supported by a sling, is an effective way of reducing pain and swelling from the humerus while awaiting surgery. In patients who are bedridden because of other injuries, the weight of the arm resting against the edge of the splint can erode skin. In this patient population, we prefer long-arm splints.

Unlike the femur or tibia, specific humeral nails have different indications and advantages. Nails with a curved upper segment are inserted through the greater tuberosity and require at least 5 or 6 cm of intact proximal bone to guide the nail into the diaphysis. Therefore they should not be used in very proximal fractures. Nails that are straight in the anteroposterior plane, inserted in line with the medullary canal, can stabilize more proximal fractures but violate the rotator cuff and lateral articular cartilage. Nails that do not use locking screws for distal stability avoid the potential hazards of an injury to the neurovascular structures and the difficulty of locking in dense cortical bone, but do so at the expense of rotational stability. All nails require proximal locking to avoid migration proximally beneath the acromion. The humerus does not tolerate reaming well, so small-diameter nails designed to be inserted without reaming must be available. Ideally, a surgeon should be familiar with several different nails and understand the indications for different implants. It is important to fit the nail to a specific fracture and not the fracture to any nail.

SURGERY

Surgery is performed under general endotracheal anesthesia rather than regional techniques whenever possible. Because linear access to the medullary canal is needed, the head is rotated toward the contralateral shoulder. An interscalene block can be used in patients with serious anesthetic risks; however, positioning of the head can be uncomfortable. In closed fractures, a cephalosporin antibiotic is administered. With open fractures, an aminoglycoside is added.

Patient Positioning

The patient is positioned so that the surgeon and assistant have easy access to the proximal humerus and are able to reduce the fracture, and the fluoroscope should arc around the arm without impeding the surgeon's ability to work. Unlike nailing in the lower extremity, the surgeon must contend with the chest when performing humeral nailing. A fracture table is never used because iatrogenic brachial plexus injuries have been reported with excessive static longitudinal traction.

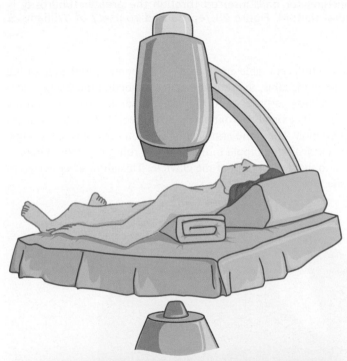

A

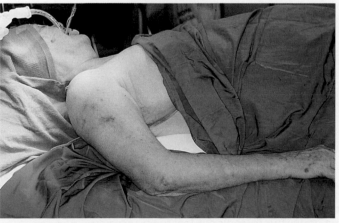

B

Figure 1. A,B: With the patient positioned to the contralateral side of the table, the radius of the fluoroscope can reach the operative humerus, allowing the surgeon and the assistants to remain stationary. A roll is placed behind the ipsilateral shoulder to bring the humeral head out from underneath the acromion for an articular starting point and to allow circumferential access to the humeral shaft. Figure 1A reproduced courtesy of Howmedica, Rutherford, NJ.

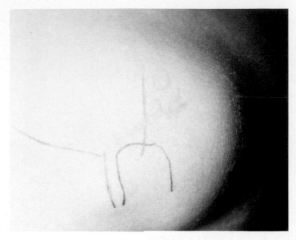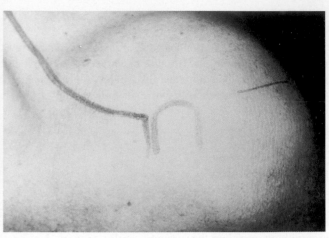

A   B

Figure 2. A: The incision for straight nails is made over the anterior edge of the acromion in line with the medullary canal of the humerus. This starting point is directly above the coracoacromial ligament, which must be released to avoid impingement. The oblique line labeled RC is the point and orientation of the rotator-cuff incision. This incision also brings the osseous entry portal in line with the lateral edge of the articular cartilage. **B:** The incision for nails inserted through the greater tuberosity is through the superior lateral deltoid. Figure 2B reproduced courtesy of Williams & Wilkins, Baltimore, MD.

The patient is placed on a radiolucent table and moved to the contralateral edge of the table. If the arm is left resting on the table, the shoulder cannot extend or the fracture adequately be manipulated for reduction purposes. A roll is placed under the operative scapula (Fig. 1). The shoulder should easily extend approximately 30 degrees to bring the humeral head out from beneath the acromion. The entire arm is prepped from fingertips to the angle of the mandible proximally and from the nipple to the shoulder roll posteriorly. Draping should expose the entire arm to the medial third of the clavicle. This allows free access to the arm and nail-insertion site.

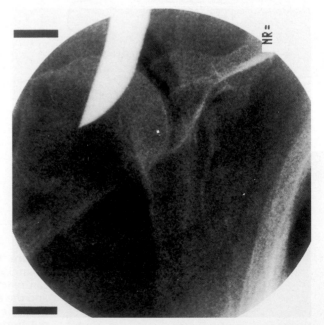

Figure 3. An awl is inserted into the humeral head. A sufficiently large hole to accommodate the Seidel nail (9 mm) is created in line with the humeral diaphysis. This is done under fluoroscopic control to ensure accuracy.

Entry Portal

When a straight humeral nail is used, an incision is made anterior to the midportion of the acromion (Fig. 2A). This point is in line with the humeral medullary canal. It is important to incise the coracoacromial ligament, which is easily palpated on the undersurface of the acromion. This minimizes the problems of impingement and shoulder stiffness. The rotator cuff should be incised in line with its fibers, avoiding its avascular portion near the greater tuberosity. On the other hand, curved nails are inserted through the greater tuberosity. A lateral incision is made, the deltoid is split, and the tuberosity is entered with an awl (Fig. 2B). The nail should not be inserted through the rotator-cuff insertion, just medial to the greater tuberosity. Nails inserted through this portal have been associated with unacceptable rates of shoulder complications with the rotator cuff retracted. The humeral head is entered with an awl and enlarged to accommodate the nail (Fig. 3).

The humerus is manually manipulated to reduce the fracture. A guide wire is inserted through the humeral head, crossing the fracture site under fluoroscopic control (Figs. 4 and 5). It is imperative to avoid excessive longitudinal traction during nailing, which can cause neurologic injury. Nails are inserted with a closed technique unless a radial nerve injury is present. Patients with radial nerve palsies should have open nailing or plating. If crepitus cannot be felt with fracture manipulation, soft-tissue interposition with risk to the radial nerve must be suspected, and an open reduction of the fracture should be performed.

The nail is assembled on the proximal driving and targeting device (Fig. 6). In the case of the Seidel nail, distal control is accomplished by an internal distal-locking mechanism. The distal nail is cut into three phalanges. A ball-tipped screw is retracted into the substance of the nail, spreading the phalanges, gaining an interference fit with the endosteal bone. This provides adequate axial control. Rotational control has been less consistent but usually adequate to achieve union. The distal spreading screw is inserted into the end of the nail and finger-tightened so that it contacts the phalanges of the distal end of the Seidel nail. The round end of the spreading screw acts as a blunt tip, facilitating passage of the nail across the fracture site. The nail is inserted over a guide wire (Fig. 7). A mallet can be used to impact the nail but only by gently tapping the proximal aiming device locking bolt (Fig. 8A and B).

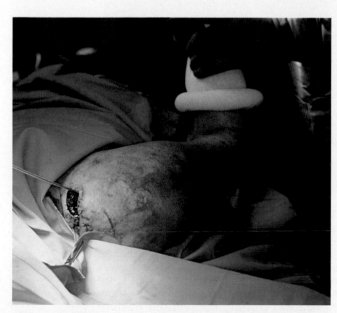

Figure 4. The fracture is reduced, and a guide pin for nail insertion is inserted.

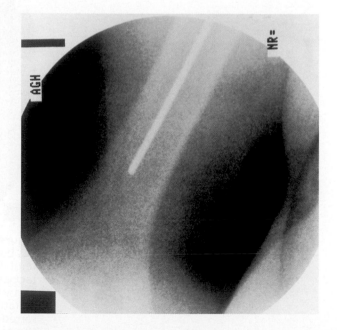

Figure 5. The guide pin is inserted, and its distal position is checked fluoroscopically.

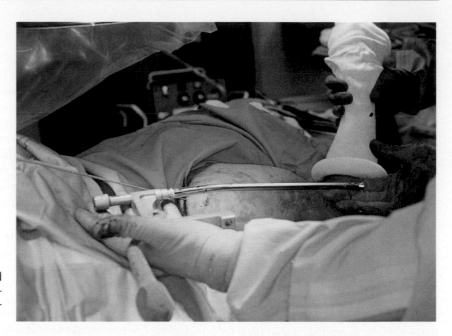

Figure 6. The Seidel nail is assembled with its proximal aiming device. The 7-degree bend is positioned with the apex anterior.

Because the entry portal for many humeral nails is intraarticular, it is imperative to bury the nail within the substance of the humeral head. Because the nail is inserted eccentrically into a sphere, multiple fluoroscopic images must be obtained to ascertain that the proximal end of the nail is below the horizon of the cortical bone (Fig. 9).

With the Seidel nail, distal interlocking precedes proximal locking. A long screwdriver is inserted through the upper nail, engaging the spreading screw (Fig. 10). The screw is

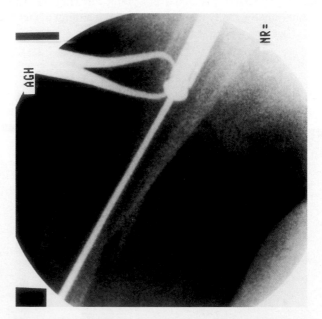

Figure 7. The distal locking screw of the Seidel nail has been inserted into the end of the nail and turned until the ball of the spreading device has come in contact with the phalanges of the nail without spreading. This creates a rounded nail end, reducing the chances of iatrogenic fracture comminution. The nail is inserted over the guide pin. Fluoroscopic images show the rounded nail end crossing the reduced fracture over the guide pin.

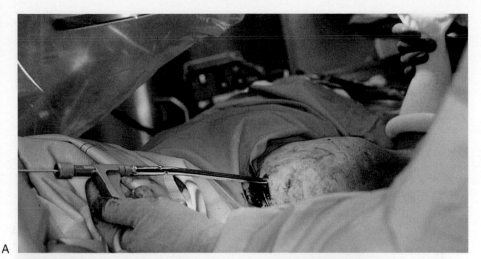

A

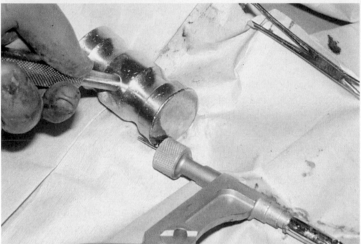

B

Figure 8. A: The nail is inserted as far as possible by hand. **B:** A mallet may be used to apply gentle taps to the insertion device.

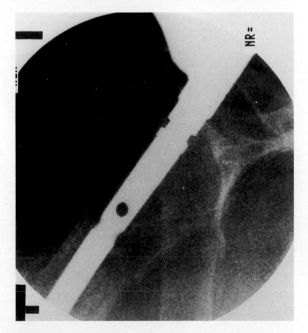

Figure 9. The nail is inserted until, under fluoroscopic control, the proximal end of the nail is clearly within the substance of the humeral head. This often requires multiple oblique and tangential views.

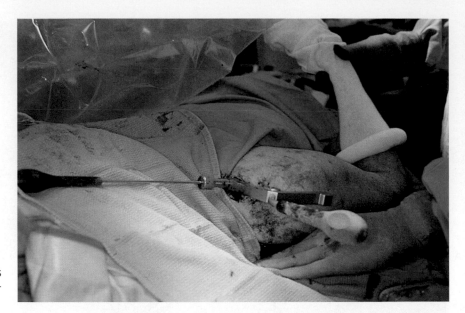

Figure 10. The spreading screwdriver is inserted through the proximal nail, engaging the distal spreading device.

turned counterclockwise until it is tight, retracting the ball into the phalanges of the nail, spreading them apart. A popping sound is often heard and signals the end of tightening. Spreading can often be seen fluoroscopically (Fig. 11A and B). At other times, bone interdigitates into the phalanges of the nail, creating a stable construct that prevents spreading. In either case, once adequate purchase is obtained, the same sense of tightening of the distal spreading screw and popping are appreciated.

Most humeral nails achieve rotational control with distal locking screws. Screws are inserted from anterior to posterior. An incision is made lateral to the biceps tendon (Fig. 12). The only neurovascular structures in this area are the terminal branches of the musculocutaneous nerve, the lateral antebrachial cutaneous nerves. The brachialis muscle is spread, exposing the distal humerus. Standard fluoroscopic techniques are used to locate the hole

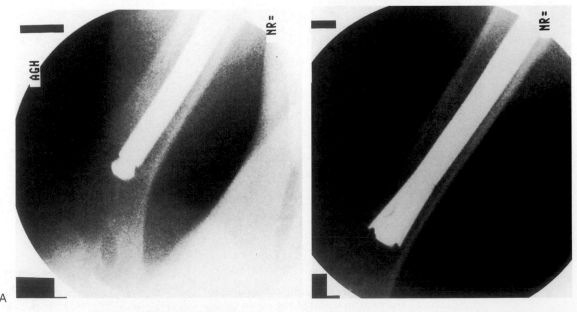

A   B

Figure 11. A: The distal spreading screw is engaged but not retracted. **B:** The distal spreading device is retracted proximally by turning the screwdriver counterclockwise, spreading the phalanges against the endosteal bone, completing distal locking.

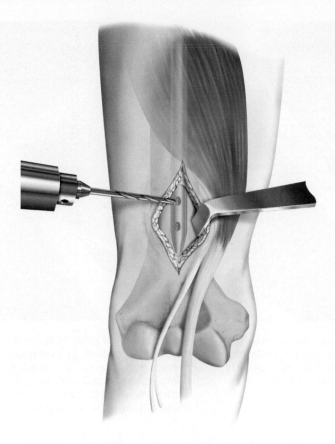

Figure 12. The incision for insertion of distal locking screws in the humerus requires an incision lateral to the biceps tendon. An incision is needed sufficient to retract the tendon and branches of the lateral antebrachial cutaneous nerves. The freehand technique is used. Note that the nail must be rotated such that access to the locking holes is lateral to the biceps tendon. Figure 12 reproduced courtesy of Howmedica, Rutherford, NJ.

in the nail. Unlike distal locking in the femur or tibia, which is performed in soft metaphyseal bone, distal humeral locking is performed in dense cortical bone, and the surface is sloped. The drill must be centered exactly over the hole to be successful. When inserting a nail that uses distal locking, care must be taken to rotate the nail so that the distal locking screw will remain lateral to the biceps tendon.

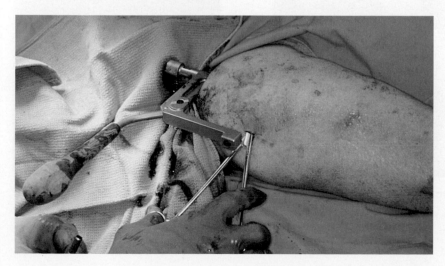

Figure 13. The proximal locking device has marked the incision for the lateral-to-medial screw. A hemostat has been passed through the incision, spreading longitudinally to the bone, sweeping branches of the axillary nerve out of the surgical field.

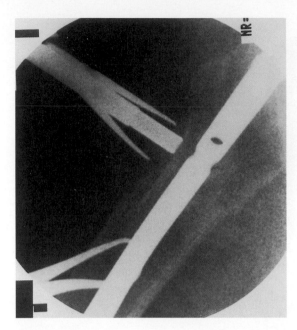

Figure 14. A drill guide has been inserted through the open hemostat, engaging the lateral cortex. This prevents branches of the axillary nerve from reentering the surgical field.

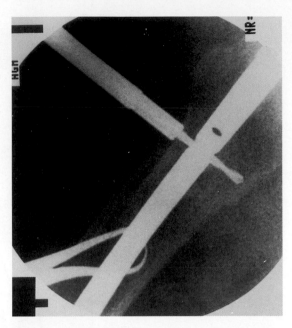

Figure 15. The pilot hole for the proximal locking screw is drilled. In osteopenic bone or when there is potential for an unrecognized fracture, it is imperative to drill under fluoroscopic control to avoid overpenetration with drillpoints, which could damage the axillary artery and vein.

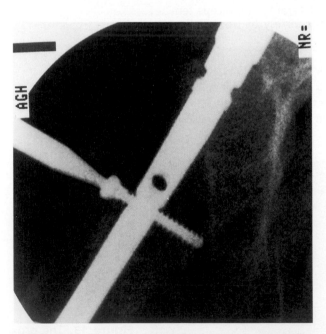

Figure 16. The proximal locking screw is inserted.

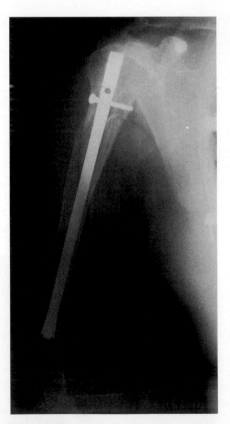

Figure 17. Postoperative radiographs showing excellent alignment of this comminuted fracture.

Little experience has been reported with nails that use lateral-to-medial distal locking screws. Iatrogenic injury to the radial nerve from anterior retraction and to the ulnar nerve from overpenetration of drill points or screws are theoretic concerns.

Proximal locking requires a sound knowledge of the neurovascular structures. The axillary nerve courses along the posterior neck of the humerus where it lies in close contact to the bone. An injury to the axillary nerve can paralyze a portion of the deltoid muscle. Anterior-to-posterior screws in the proximal humerus, therefore, should be avoided.

Distal to the surgical neck, the axillary nerve branches into two to four segments. Injury to one of these segments is unlikely to cause significant shoulder dysfunction. An attempt, however, should be made to protect as much of the nerve as possible. This is accomplished by inserting a hemostat through the soft tissue and sliding the drill guide between the teeth of the hemostat (Figs. 13 and 14). The drill guide is held in place, preventing the branches of the axillary nerve from entering the surgical field. The proximal locking screw is inserted (Figs. 15–17), and the insertion equipment is disassembled. When the rotator cuff has been incised longitudinally, a simple side-to-side repair is often all that is necessary. Some surgeons recommend inserting a nonabsorbable suture to mark the entry point to facilitate nail removal. The deltoid requires no repair. The skin and subcutaneous tissue are closed at the surgeon's discretion.

POSTOPERATIVE MANAGEMENT

Incisions are minimal and require very little care. The arm is maintained in a sling until the patient is comfortable. In multiply injured patients, sufficient stability is obtained in the immediate postoperative period to abduct the arm from the chest for pulmonary care.

Postoperative rehabilitation is extremely variable. Some patients are able to abduct and elevate the arm on the day of surgery, whereas others require extensive rehabilitation to regain shoulder motion. Active rehabilitation of the shoulder and elbow are begun as soon as the patient is comfortable, generally within 1 week. Exercises involving rotational movements should be avoided for 3 weeks when inserting a nail that locks distally without cross-screws.

Crutch or bed-to-chair ambulation can be initiated in the immediate postoperative period, often within the first several days. Even patients who have a very slow return of shoulder function can bear weight on their arm with crutches.

Physical therapy is maintained until a plateau is reached. Reports of final shoulder function have been inconsistent, varying from no problems to a 50% rate of permanent shoulder impairment. It is clear that many patients will have a permanent measurable loss of shoulder motion, particularly with an articular starting point. It has been our experience, however, that significant functional impairment of the shoulder is very uncommon with proper surgical technique.

Follow-up is mandated by associated injuries and the progress of that particular patient. Shoulder stiffness is a particular concern. Patients who regain shoulder motion early can be followed up at a 2-week interval for wound care and then be seen at 4- to 6-week intervals until union. Those patients who have difficulty with shoulder motion, however, must be followed up more frequently, as often as every 2 weeks.

COMPLICATIONS

Complications of humeral nailing differ from those of other locked intramedullary nails used in the femur or tibia. There have been no reported cases of secondary shoulder infections. All humeral nails start in or in very close proximity to the shoulder joint. All have the potential to violate the shoulder either directly or by damaging the rotator-cuff insertion onto the greater tuberosity. An infection after humeral nailing can, theoretically, track along the nail, causing a septic arthritis of the shoulder.

The major complication after humeral nailing is compromised shoulder function. Whether nails are inserted through the greater tuberosity as an extraarticular starting point or through the rotator cuff, shoulder difficulties have been reported. The greater tuberosity starting point can elevate a ridge of bone around the rotator-cuff insertion that impinges on the acromion with abduction. Oblique proximal locking screws that enter the upper greater tuberosity, inserted in an attempt to avoid injury to branches of the axillary nerve, also can lead to impingement.

The potential for shoulder complications increases with an articular starting point. Damage to the rotator cuff has the potential to permanently injure the shoulder. The medullary canal is in line with the lateral edge of the articular surface of the humeral head. An axial, articular starting point, therefore, will violate the rotator cuff and damage at least a small portion of the articular surface. These problems can be minimized by decompressing the shoulder on nail insertion by transecting the coracoacromial ligament. The lateral articular damage may account for the loss of the last few degrees of full abduction that is often seen.

If a patient with an intact radial nerve awakens with a postnailing palsy, urgent surgical exploration is indicated. A lacerated nerve should be repaired, whereas a nerve entrapped or impaled on a sharp bone spike may improve after extrication.

Nonunions after humeral nails pose special problems. The bone of the distal humerus is thin and hard, and the canal tapers. A true isthmus of the humerus does not exist. There is no rich layer of endosteal bone to be morselized by reamers and dispersed into the fracture site to act as an internal bone graft. When nails loosen, significant distal bone is eroded, making subsequent fixation difficult. When a fracture fails to heal with a primary nailing, exchange nailing alone is not adequate to achieve union but must be supplemented by a bone graft. Fixation with very long plates, spanning not only the nonunion site but the site of distal erosion, with extensive bone grafting, sometimes of both areas, has been reported.

ILLUSTRATIVE CASE FOR TECHNIQUE

An obese 67-year-old woman with a heavy arm sustained multiple injuries including a closed comminuted humeral fracture in a motor vehicle accident. Her neurovascular status was normal. A flail chest necessitated the use of a ventilator, and an ipsilateral chest tube required abduction of her arm for pulmonary toilet. A comminuted intertrochanteric/subtrochanteric fracture was stabilized with an intramedullary nail, necessitating weight bearing on her humerus. Comminution in osteopenic bone made her an ideal candidate for intramedullary humeral nailing.

A comminuted proximal shaft fracture extended close to the surgical neck of the humerus, making proximal fixation precarious (Fig. 18A and B). The fracture was too proximal for a nail inserted through the greater tuberosity, eccentric to the medullary canal. Her distal medullary canal measured 12 mm in diameter. The Seidel nail, being straight in the anteroposterior plane, was selected for this proximal humerus. It is indicated only in patients who can accommodate a 9-mm nail without reaming, such as this geriatric, osteopenic woman.

The nail was inserted without difficulty. Adequate axial control for elevation of her arm and weight bearing was achieved in the immediate postoperative period. Sufficient rotational control for healing was achieved, and the fracture united without incident at 8 weeks (Fig. 19). Within 4 months, she regained all but the last 10 degrees of shoulder elevation, without functional deficit.

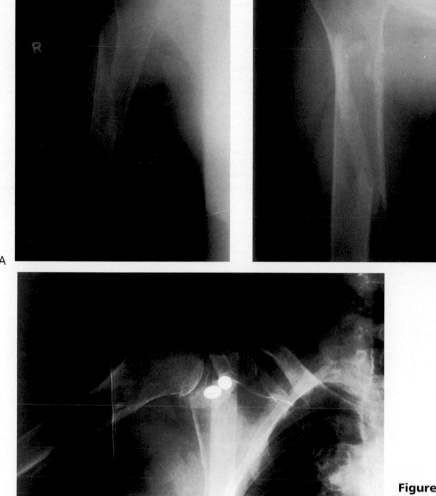

Figure 18. A: Internal- and external-rotation radiographs demonstrate a highly comminuted proximal humeral shaft fracture with proximal extension into the head. Note an undisplaced fracture line into the greater tuberosity. **B:** A radiograph centered on the shoulder fails to show any displacement of the humeral head fracture.

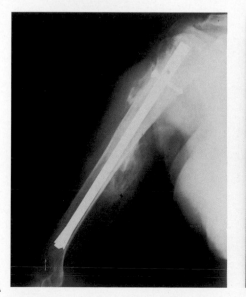
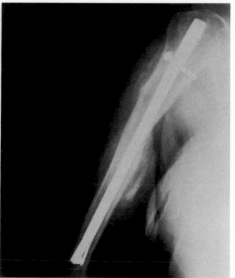

Figure 19. A,B: The fracture has united. Note that the fracture of the greater tuberosity and head remain undisplaced.

RECOMMENDED READING

1. Henley, M.B., Monroe, M., and Tencer, A.F.: Biomechanical comparison of methods of fixation of a midshaft osteotomy of the humerus. *J. Orthop. Trauma,* 5:14–20, 1991.
2. McKee, M.D., Miranda, M.A., Riemer, B.L., et al.: Management of humeral nonunion after the failure of locking intramedullary nails. *J. Orthop. Trauma,* 10:492–429, 1996.
3. Riemer, B.L., Butterfield, S.L., D'Ambrosia, R., and Kellam, J.: Seidel intramedullary nailing of humeral diaphyseal fractures: a preliminary report. *Orthopaedics,* 14:239–246, 1991.
4. Riemer, B.L., D'Ambrosia, R., Kellam, J., Butterfield, S.L., and Burke, C.J., III: The anterior acromial approach for antegrade intramedullary nailing of the humeral diaphysis. *Orthopaedics,* 16(11):1219–1223, 1993.
5. Riemer, B.L., Foglesong, M.E., Burke, C.J., III, and Butterfield, S.L.: Complications of Seidel intramedullary nailing of narrow diameter humeral diaphyseal fractures. *Orthopaedics,* 17:19–29, 1994.
6. Robinson, C.M., Bell, K.M., Curt Brown, C.M., and McQueen, M.M.: Locked nailing of humeral shaft fractures. *J. Bone Joint Surg. [Br],* 74:558–561, 1992.

Master Techniques in Orthopaedic Surgery,
FRACTURES, edited by D. A. Wiss,
Lippincott–Raven Publishers, Philadelphia © 1998.

7

Distal Humerus Intraarticular Fractures: Open Reduction Internal Fixation

Jesse B. Jupiter

INDICATIONS/CONTRAINDICATIONS

As the techniques and implants designed for stable fixation of the articular and metaphyseal skeleton have improved, it has become evident that the majority of intraarticular fractures of the distal humerus are best treated by open reduction and internal fixation. The favorable results of operative treatment compared with those associated with skeletal traction or cast immobilization have been well documented (1–6,8). Operative reduction affords the opportunity to accurately reduce the disrupted trochlea and restore its congruous relation to the olecranon, thereby ensuring the intrinsic stability of the humeroulnar relation. Even the more complex distal humeral fractures such as those associated with comminution, open fractures, or ipsilateral fractures of the limb are now equally effectively treated by surgical means.

Yet the surgical anatomy of the distal humerus can prove treacherous, as the fragile articulations are supported by a meager amount of subchondral bone and no soft tissue. With such a fracture in the elderly, the ability of the bone to support stable fixation with screws and plates proves to be problematic. In such cases, the surgeon must feel secure in his or her ability to provide stable fixation. Alternatives to operative fixation in these situations include nonoperative immobilization, skeletal traction, and in some cases, total elbow arthroplasty.

J. B. Jupiter, M.D.: Department of Orthopaedic Surgery, Massachusetts General Hospital, Boston, Massachusetts 02114.

PREOPERATIVE PLANNING

Awareness of the common pitfalls of surgical intervention should be considered preoperatively. Given the complex architecture of the distal humerus, routine radiographs often fail to provide the true extent of the intraarticular fracture. An anteroposterior (AP) radiograph obtained with traction on the forearm, once anesthesia has been induced, will reveal a more accurate representation of the fracture anatomy. There is little place for other imaging techniques such as computed tomography (CT) or magnetic resonance imaging (MRI) scan in the preoperative evaluation of the intraarticular fracture of the distal humerus. Severe comminution of the supracondylar columns should alert the surgeon to the availability of a bone graft.

SURGERY

Because the operative procedures can be lengthy, in most cases, general endotracheal anesthesia is preferred. The patient is placed in the lateral position with the involved limb supported over bolsters, keeping it off the chest wall (Fig. 1). This position permits ready access to the iliac crest for autogenous bone graft. A sterile pneumatic arm tourniquet offers the possibility of a wider sterile field and the ability to reapply the tourniquet as needed.

Technique

Although a number of surgical procedures have been described (see Exposures) and offer adequate exposures to most T and Y fractures, my preference has been to use the transolecranon approach, particularly for comminuted fractures. Through a straight, longitudinal skin incision (Fig. 2), the osteotomy is made a shallow V or chevron fashion in the center of the olecranon sulcus (Fig. 3). This area, with the smallest zone of articular cartilage in the olecranon location, will be best identified by elevation of the anconeus muscle off the olecranon to directly visualize the articular surface. A sponge is placed from lateral

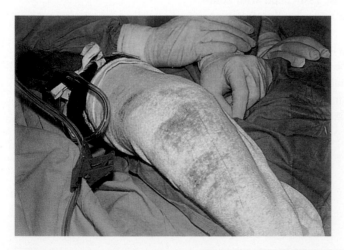

Figure 1. The patient is placed in the lateral position. A sterile pneumatic tourniquet is preferred.

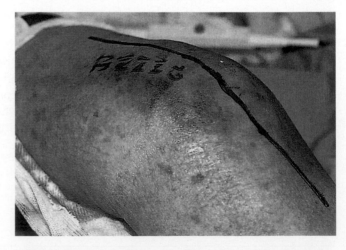

Figure 2. A straight longitudinal skin incision is used.

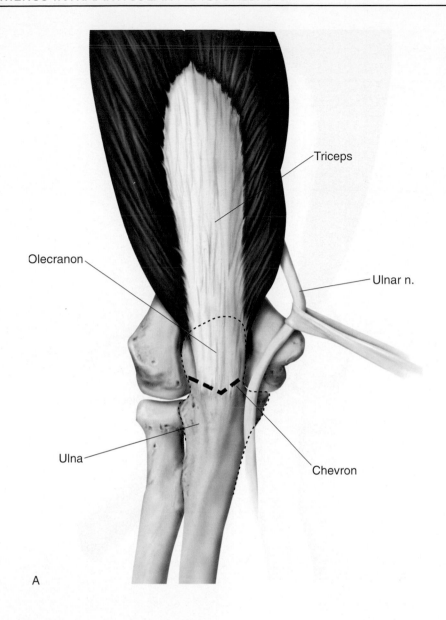

Triceps

Olecranon

Ulnar n.

Ulna

Chevron

A

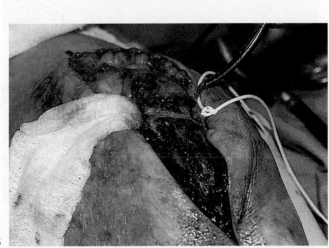

B

Figure 3. A: The olecranon osteotomy is marked out in the shape of a shallow V or chevron. CET, common extensor tendon. **B:** The anconeus muscle is elevated off the lateral aspect to permit a sponge to be placed as countertraction.

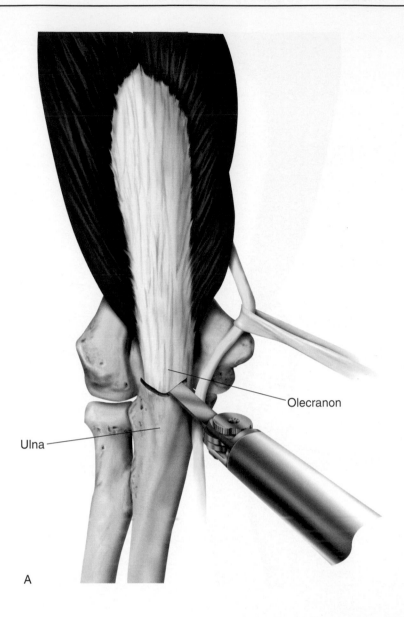

Olecranon

Ulna

A

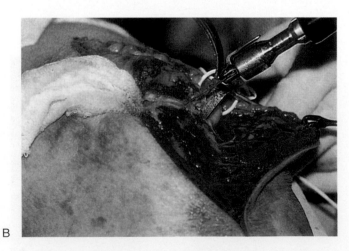

B

Figure 4. A, B: A thin-bladed oscillating saw is used to start the osteotomy.

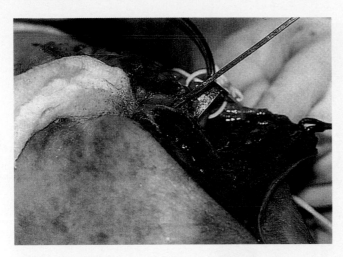

Figure 5. The olecranon osteotomy is completed with a thin-bladed osteotome, creating an uneven joint surface that will facilitate realignment.

to medial and used as a countertraction as the osteotomy is created with a thin-bladed oscillating saw (Fig. 4) and completed with a thin-bladed osteotome (Fig. 5).

Before the olecranon osteotomy is created, the ulnar nerve should be exposed. The fascia over the flexor carpi ulnaris is longitudinally split over 6 cm to enhance the nerve's mobility. In doing this, there is less chance for the nerve to become surrounded by fibrosis in the cubital tunnel.

The osteotomized olecranon fragment is elevated proximally, leaving a margin of triceps tendon on either side to suture on completion of the surgery (Fig. 6). The exact nature of the intraarticular fracture pattern may reveal itself only at this juncture. The fracture hematoma should be cautiously removed by using a small dental pick or pulsed lavage, as the articular fragments may lack soft-tissue or bony attachments (Fig. 7).

Once the fracture anatomy is confirmed, the goal is to reduce the articular fragments onto the bony columns of the distal humerus, initially holding the reduction with provisional Kirschner-wire (K-wire) fixation (Fig. 8).

In some instances, the intraarticular fracture of the trochlea may be found to be present in both the sagittal and coronal planes (Fig. 9). In these cases, Herbert screws have been of particular use, as the threads can be buried under the articular surface (Fig. 10). An alternative to the Herbert screw is the fine-threaded K-wires. If a defect exists in the subchondral bone, one should plan to support the articular fragment with autogenous cancellous bone graft.

Definitive skeletal fixation in the majority of these fractures begins with interfragmentary screw fixation of the sagittal fracture of the trochlea. One or two 3.5-mm cortical or 4.0-mm cancellous screws will be sufficient to provide a firm hold of the fragments. In those cases in which comminution is present in the sagittal plane, these screws should not be placed as interfragmentary screws but rather placed without "overdrilling" the near cortex to prevent overcompressing the fragments, which will tend to narrow the trochlea, thus threatening the intrinsic stability of the trochlea–olecranon relation (Fig. 11). With certain fracture patterns, the surgeon may find that the articular reconstruction may be facilitated by securing one of the articular components directly to one of the bony columns of the distal humerus. This would be followed by restoration of the remaining articular element to this stable skeletal and articular unit.

Caution must be exercised with regard to the presence of either the tip or head of the screws in the cubital tunnel. In such cases, the ulnar nerve is best further mobilized by releasing the distal part of the medial intermuscular septum to allow the nerve to sit more freely in the subcutaneous tissues.

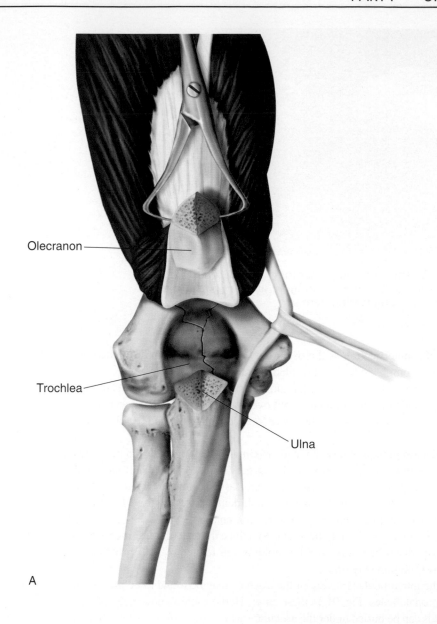

Olecranon

Trochlea

Ulna

A

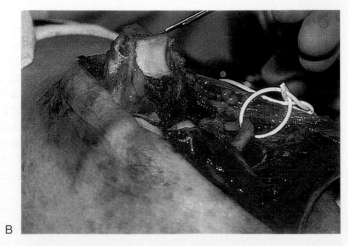

B

Figure 6. A, B: The osteotomized proximal olecranon fragment is elevated proximally. Note the ulnar nerve has been isolated and mobilized and protected with the rubber loop.

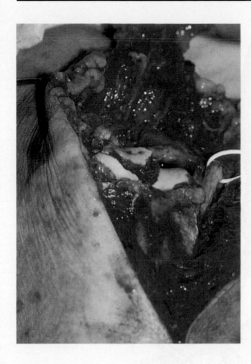

Figure 7. The fracture hematoma is carefully removed by using a small dental pick or pulsatile lavage.

Stable fixation of the articular fragments to the humeral bony columns is preferentially accomplished with strategically placed plates. Mechanical strength will be enhanced by placing the plates and respective screws as close to 90 degrees to each other as possible. For the majority of T or Y fractures that split the bony columns of the distal humerus well proximal to the olecranon fossa, the plates can be applied to the medial ridge of the medial column and along the posterior aspect of the lateral column. The topographic anatomy of the distal humerus is most amenable to this, as the articular cartilage of the capitellum does not extend onto the posterior part of the distal humerus (Fig. 12).

There are occasions in which the fracture lies primarily in the very distal part of the bony columns below the level of the medial epicondyle. A plate applied along the ridge of the medial bony column would be ineffective in supporting the articular fragments. In these cases, several options exist for the surgeon. By using 3.5-mm reconstruction plates, the plate can be contoured to bend around and "cradle" the medial epicondyle (Fig. 13). The very distal screws can be directed into the medial epicondyle and angulated from each other to afford an "interlocking" relation between the screws. An alternative to this is to direct the distal screw proximally to secure fixation into the lateral column (Fig. 14).

Yet another option is to place a plate directly onto the lateral aspect of the lateral skeletal column (Fig. 15). This would require elevation of the origin of the brachioradialis and wrist extensor muscles, which can be sutured back into place. This placement provides an opportunity to gain a further hold on the trochlea fragments through a screw placed transversely from the most distal screw hole into the trochlea (Fig. 16). Defects beneath the plate should be reconstructed with autogenous iliac crest graft.

At this juncture, the elbow should be put through a range of motion visually to control the stability of the internal fixation. If motion of the fracture fragments is observed to exist, it would be best to revise or alter the fixation at this point by using the alternative plate application described previously.

The olecranon osteotomy is reduced under direct vision. My preference for internal fixation continues to be tension-band wires with two obliquely placed K-wires providing rotational control (Fig. 17). Care is taken to bend the proximal ends of the K-wires and seat them onto the proximal olecranon both to prevent proximal migration and to avoid the

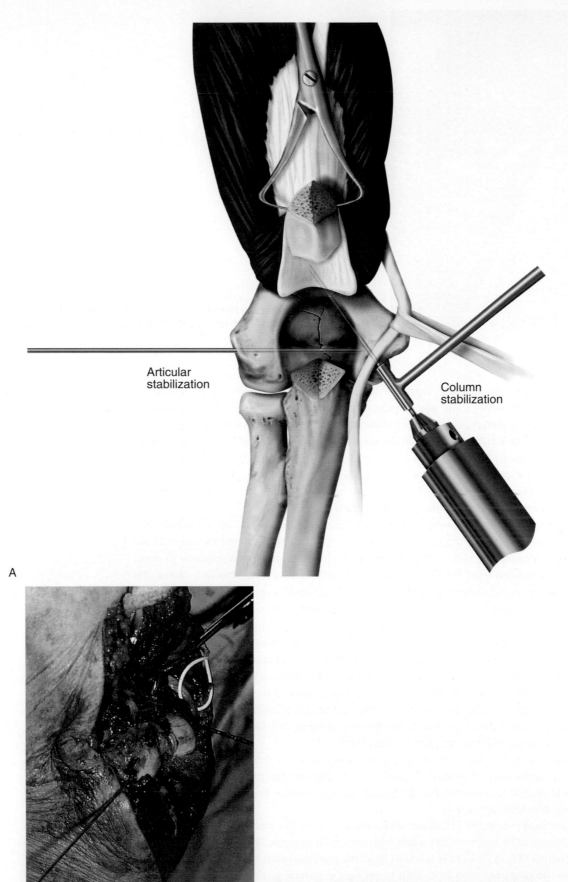

Articular
stabilization

Column
stabilization

A

B

Figure 8. A, B: The fracture is reduced and provisionally secured with K-wires.

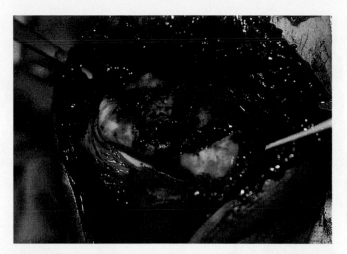

Figure 9. Intraarticular fractures of the trochlea in the coronal plane are especially difficult to secure.

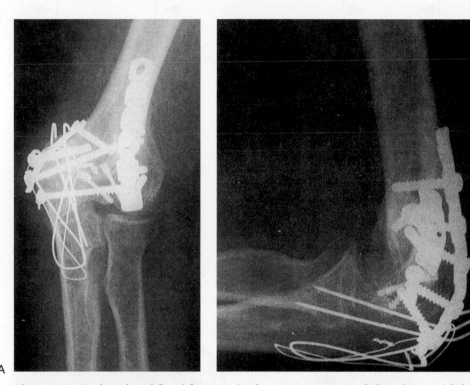

A   B

Figure 10. Reduced and fixed fracture in the anteroposterior **(A)** and lateral **(B)** projection. The Herbert screw may be used for articular fragments.

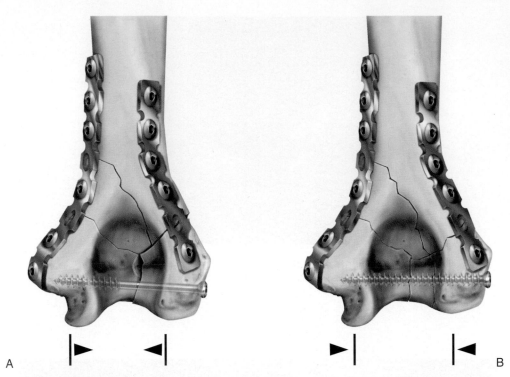

A   B

Figure 11. A,B: When intraarticular comminution exists, a full-threaded, but not a lag screw, is best placed without compressing the fragments.

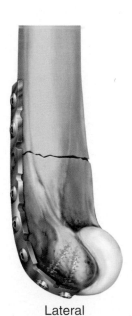

Lateral

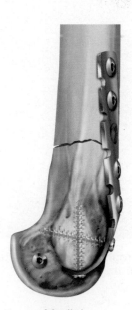

Medial

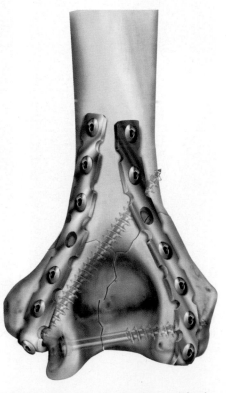

Figure 12. The plate on the lateral bony column can extend distally, as the articular cartilage of the capitellum does not extend posteriorly.

Figure 13. With complex "low" fractures, a plate can be constructed to bend around the medial epicondyle with screws directed into the medial epicondyle from different directions providing and "interlock" between the screws.

Figure 14. An alternative, with the contoured plate bent around the medial epicondyle, is to pass a screw through the plate and into the lateral column.

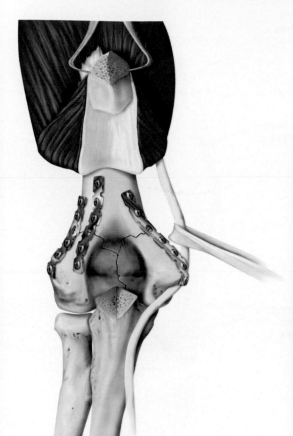

A

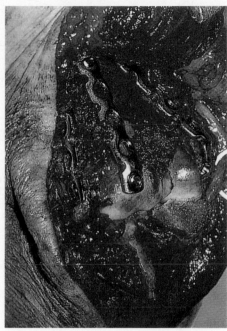

B

Figure 15. A, B: Another option is to place three plates with one along the lateral column, one posterior on the lateral column, and one bent around the medial epicondyle.

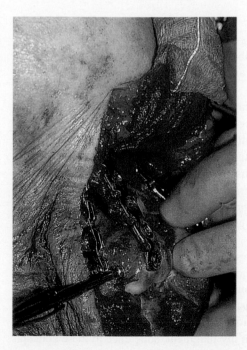

Figure 16. A transverse screw is placed through the lateral plate and across the trochlear fracture fragments.

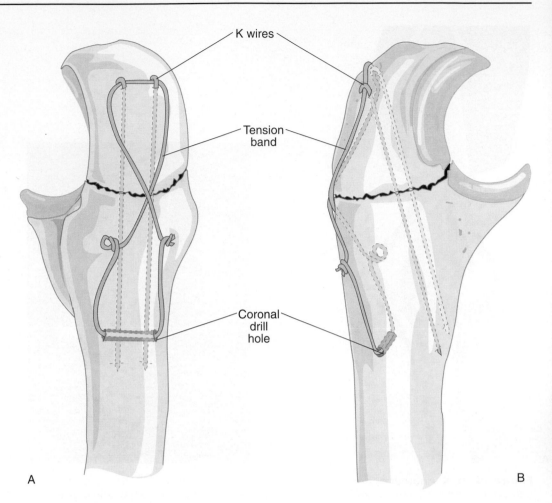

Figure 17. A, B: The olecranon osteotomy is secured with oblique K-wires and a tension-band wire.

prominence of the wire interfering with full elbow motion (Fig. 18). At the completion of the fixation, the elbow is again put through a range of motion to test the security of the internal fixation.

The tourniquet is let down and hemostasis carefully secured. Over a large suction drain, the wound is closed in layers. A bulky dressing with Dacron batting is applied, and a resting splint of plaster applied to the elbow in full extension. Given that one will often see a residual flexion contracture after the elbow trauma, I have found providing a resting splint for nighttime use only, with the elbow in extension, helps to lessen these problems.

The most common pitfalls of this type of surgery relate to the operative approach to the distal humerus: inadequate exposure, ulnar nerve mobilization, unrecognized articular comminution, fractures of the bony columns just above the articular surfaces, and stable plate fixation.

To address these pitfalls, I would emphasize several specific aspects of the exposure and procedure: extensile exposure through olecranon osteotomy, wide mobilization of the ulnar nerve, careful identification and provisional fixation of articular fragments, custom placement of plates distal on the posterior aspect of the lateral bony column and bent around the medial epicondyle, direct screws into the cortical bone of the bony columns, and careful fixation of the olecranon osteotomy. In my judgment, adherence to these concepts makes the difference between a successful and an unsuccessful procedure.

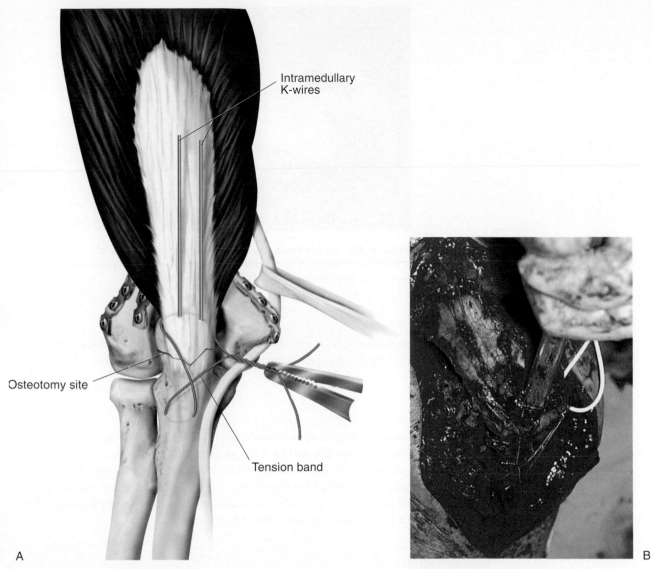

Intramedullary
K-wires

Osteotomy site

Tension band

A   B

Figure 18. A, B: Attention should be paid to tapping the bent ends of the K-wires into the proximal olecranon to diminish local discomfort.

POSTOPERATIVE MANAGEMENT

Active motion is initiated on the first postoperative day. The patient is instructed to lie supine and forward flex the involved shoulder to bring the elbow overhead. With the uninjured arm supporting the involved forearm, gravity is used to assist elbow flexion. A similar approach is used for elbow-extension exercises, but in this case, the patient sits upright and gently assists the forearm into extension (Fig. 19).

Active and patient-assisted flexion–extension exercises are continued throughout the first 3 to 4 weeks. A splint is applied only for the first few weeks and only during sleep with the elbow extended. Radiographs should be obtained frequently to assess the stability of the internal fixation. It is imperative that the surgeon monitor the patient and coordinate the rehabilitation process. A trained physical therapist can be helpful similarly to serve as a monitor, but passive activities and resisted exercises are to be avoided.

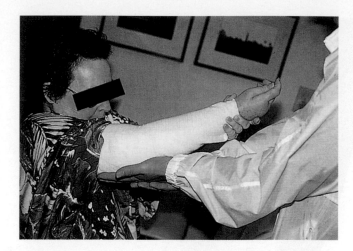

Figure 19. Postoperatively, active motion is begun by the patient under the guidance of a physical therapist. Gravity is used to assist elbow flexion and extension.

At 6 weeks postoperatively, if radiographic union is progressing satisfactorily, the patient may begin light resisted exercises to restore muscle tone and strength.

Results

In predicting outcome, both in elbow motion and function, it is often the nature of the injury rather than the treatment that will have the greatest influence. Most activities of daily living can be performed in a range of motion from 30 to 130 degrees, with lack of full extension more easily compensated for than a loss of flexion. With current techniques, approximately 80% can attain an adequate arc of flexion even after severe fractures. Typically, pronation and supination are unaffected by this fracture.

Rehabilitation

Rehabilitation after distal humerus fractures should be expected to require between 12 and 16 weeks *after* fracture union. Muscle strengthening and endurance form the basis of a supervised exercise program. Typically, not too infrequently, lack of full extension exists, and I often treat this with dynamic or static types of splints or both. Once fracture union has been assured, the use of passive therapy modalities can be initiated.

COMPLICATIONS

Failure of fixation most commonly results from a lack of secure fixation of the implants at the time of surgery. Clinically, fixation instability is heralded by pain, limited motion, and ultimately confirmed by radiographic documentation of implant loosening or breakage. If suspected within the initial 6 weeks, consideration for reoperation or referral to an individual or center with extensive experience is appropriate. Cast immobilization is appealing to many but all too often results in an extremely limited range of motion.

Nonunion is being more frequently seen as the operative approach to these fractures becomes more widely accepted. Management is difficult and includes rigid fixation with two or even three plates, decompression of the ulnar nerve, and release of the anterior capsule. When this occurs in the older patient, the disability may be profound. In this patient, Morrey (7) reported reliable salvage with joint-replacement arthroplasty.

Nonunion of an olecranon osteotomy occurs in about 5% and has been associated with a variety of techniques of internal fixation. This is in part the sequela of the osteotomy having "smooth" fracture planes and thus being intrinsically unstable. The use of a chevron-shaped osteotomy should minimize this problem.

Infection, although uncommon and more often associated with open fractures, can prove catastrophic. If suspected, extensive wound debridement, lavage, and parenteral antibiotics are to be instituted immediately. If the internal fixation is stable, it is advisable to retain the fixation, as fracture union can take place even in the face of active infection.

Ulnar nerve palsy is a common problem that can be prevented or minimized by mobilizing the nerve proximally and distally at the time of surgery. If seen postoperatively and not responsive to rest and corticosteroid injection, early exploration can offset the profound disability that may be associated with a progressive motor deficit associated with ongoing ulnar nerve ischemia.

ILLUSTRATIVE CASE FOR TECHNIQUE

An 85-year-old practicing attorney fell, landing on her left nondominant upper extremity. Radiographs revealed a complex, multifragmented intraarticular fracture of the distal humerus. Anteroposterior and lateral radiographs revealed a low, multifragmented, intraarticular fracture of the distal humerus (Fig. 20). Through an olecranon osteotomy, the articular surface was reduced and secured back onto the bony columns of the distal humerus with three strategically placed plates (Fig. 21). Autogenous iliac-crest bone graft was used (Fig. 22). The comminuted extraarticular fragments were secured under the plates, with attention taken to preserve soft-tissue attachments. Anteroposterior and lateral radiographs demonstrated bony union along with maintenance of the articular anatomy (Fig. 23). The patient was able to return to functional activities within 6 weeks after surgery (Fig. 24). She recovered 110 degrees of elbow flexion and lacked 40 degrees of elbow extension.

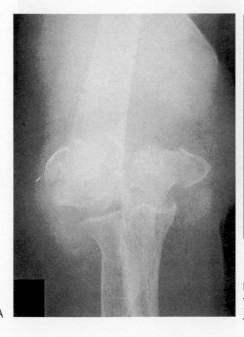
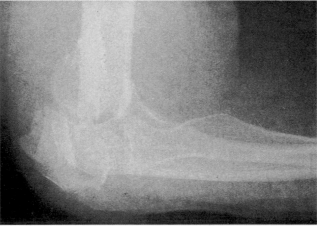

A

B

Figure 20. Comminuted Y condylar fracture in elderly woman seen on anteroposterior **(A)** and lateral **(B)** projections.

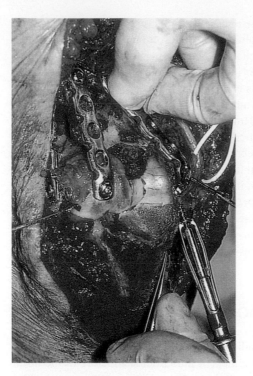

Figure 21. These plates were used to stabilize fracture distally.

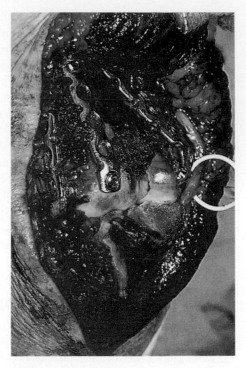

Figure 22. The comminution was treated with autogenous iliac bone graft.

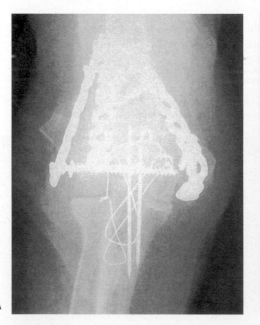

A

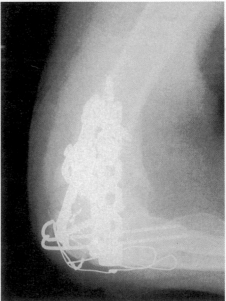

B

Figure 23. Near-anatomic restoration is seen on the anteroposterior **(A)** and lateral **(B)** projections.

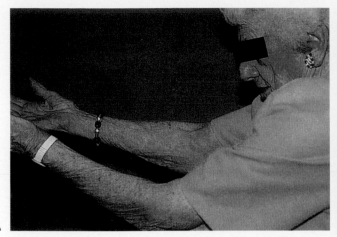

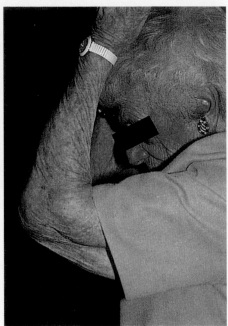

Figure 24. A useful arc of motion from 40 degrees **(A)** to 110 degrees **(B)** was obtained.

Acknowledgment

This chapter is reprinted from Morrey, B.F. (ed.): *Master Techniques in Orthopaedic Surgery: The Elbow*. Raven Press, New York, 1994, pp. 53–70.

RECOMMENDED READING

1. Aitken, G.K., and Rorabeck, C.H.: Distal humeral fractures in the adult. *Clin. Orthop.*, 207:191–197, 1986.
2. Gabel, G.T., Hanson, G., Bennett, J.B., Noble, P.C., and Tullos, H.S.: Intraarticular fractures of the distal humerus in the adult. *Clin. Orthop.*, 216:99–107, 1987.
3. Jupiter, J.B., and Mehne, D.K.: Fractures of the distal humerus. *Orthopaedics,* 15:825–833, 1992.
4. Jupiter, J.B., and Morrey B.L.: Fractures of the distal humerus. In Morrey, B.F. (ed.): *The Elbow and Its Disorders.* W.B. Saunders, Philadelphia, 1993, pp. 328–336.
5. Jupiter, J.B., Neff, U., Holzach, P., and Allgower M.: Intercondylar fractures of the distal humerus. *J. Bone Joint Surg. [Am],* 67:226–239, 1985.
6. Mehne, D.D., and Jupiter, J.B.: Fractures of the distal humerus. In Browner, B. (ed.): *Skeletal Trauma.* W.B. Saunders, Philadelphia, 1991, pp. 1146–1176.
7. Morrey, B.F.: Distal humeral non-unions treated by total elbow arthroplasty. AAOS annual meeting, San Francisco, February, 1993.
8. Perry, C.R.: Transcondylar fractures of the distal humerus. *J. Orthop. Trauma,* 3:98–106, 1989.

Master Techniques in Orthopaedic Surgery,
FRACTURES, edited by D. A. Wiss,
Lippincott–Raven Publishers, Philadelphia © 1998.

8

Olecranon Fractures: Open Reduction Internal Fixation

Gregory J. Schmeling

INDICATIONS/CONTRAINDICATIONS

Olecranon fractures are a result of direct or indirect forces, or a combination of both (9). Direct forces drive the olecranon into the distal humerus, whereas indirect forces are applied through contraction of the triceps muscle. Indirect forces generally produce transverse or short oblique fracture patterns. Direct forces produce comminuted fractures, often with a joint-depression component similar to a tibial plateau fracture.

Olecranon fractures can be nondisplaced (elbow-extensor mechanism intact) or displaced (elbow-extensor mechanism disrupted). Nondisplaced fractures have less than 2 mm of joint gap or step-off, active elbow extension is intact, and there is no significant fragment motion with deep elbow flexion. Fractures are displaced if they do not meet these criteria (9).

The treatment objectives for olecranon fractures are reconstruction of the articular surface, restoration or preservation of the elbow-extensor mechanism, preservation of elbow motion and function, and prevention or avoidance of complications (12). The indications for operative treatment include displaced fractures, injuries with elbow-extensor mechanism disruption, and open fractures. Contraindications for operative treatment include nondisplaced fractures, injuries with the elbow-extensor mechanism intact, and poor overall medical condition of the patient.

Operative treatment options include open reduction and internal fixation (tension-band principle or lag screw/neutralization principle) or excision with elbow-extensor mechanism reconstruction (12,18). In displaced fractures, the goals of treatment are met most often with open reduction and internal fixation.

Olecranon fractures are usually isolated injuries but can be one of the many skeletal injuries in the polytrauma patient. In isolated fractures, elbow pain is the presenting com-

G. J. Schmeling, M.D.: Division of Orthopaedic Trauma, Department of Orthopaedic Surgery, MCW Clinics at FMCH East, Milwaukee, Wisconsin 53226.

plaint. Physical examination reveals an elbow effusion, and in displaced fractures, a palpable defect is often identified. Crepitus with elbow motion is also present. The inability to extend the elbow against gravity suggests loss of elbow-extensor mechanism integrity. Neurovascular evaluation includes particular attention to the ulnar nerve. The proximity of the ulnar nerve places it at risk for injury, especially when the direct forces are involved.

Essential radiographs for evaluation of the injury include an anteroposterior view and a true lateral view. When the olecranon fracture is part of an elbow fracture–dislocation, traction radiographs are used to evaluate the injury as well. The lateral radiograph reveals the extent of the fracture and the presence of comminution or joint depression. The integrity of the radial head–capitellar articulation is examined, and subluxation or dislocation of the semilunar notch from the trochlea is noted. The anteroposterior radiograph is examined for sagittal fracture lines that are not well displayed on the lateral view. The integrity of the radial head–capitellar and semilunar notch–trochlea articulation also are determined on this view. Comparison radiographs are helpful in complex fracture patterns.

PREOPERATIVE PLANNING

A preoperative plan is drawn, and a surgical tactic developed. The preoperative plan begins with a tracing of the fracture fragments. The fragments are then reduced on paper. The need for bone graft to support depressed intraarticular fragments is determined. The proposed fixation is added. The method of fixation chosen is dependent on the fracture personality and the experience of the surgeon. The surgical tactic is a sequential outline of the planned procedure and is added to the drawing (Fig. 1).

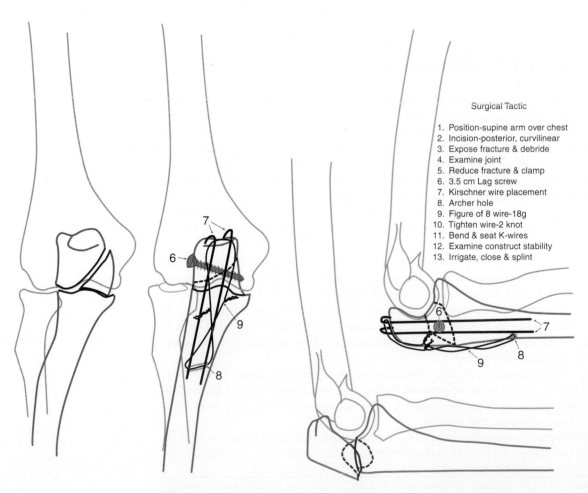

Surgical Tactic

1. Position-supine arm over chest
2. Incision-posterior, curvilinear
3. Expose fracture & debride
4. Examine joint
5. Reduce fracture & clamp
6. 3.5 cm Lag screw
7. Kirschner wire placement
8. Archer hole
9. Figure of 8 wire-18g
10. Tighten wire-2 knot
11. Bend & seat K-wires
12. Examine construct stability
13. Irrigate, close & splint

Figure 1 Preoperative plan of illustrative case. This is a tracing from the radiographs. Blue, ulna; red, fixation; black, humerus/radius.

I prefer to classify olecranon fractures after the method of Schatzker (18; Fig. 2). Displaced fractures are extraarticular or intraarticular. Intraarticular fractures are further divided into transverse, oblique, comminuted, or fracture–dislocation. Transverse fractures are simple or complex (associated joint depression). Oblique fractures are proximal (tip to the midpoint of the semilunar notch) or distal (midpoint of the semilunar notch to the coronoid process). Comminuted fractures have multiple fracture lines and may be associated with a radial head fracture or elbow dislocation.

Methods of fixation follow two principles of fracture fixation: tension band or lag screw/neutralization (1,2,4,8,10,11,14,16,17,20). A tension-band construct may consist of two Kirschner wires (K-wires) with a figure-of-eight wire, or an intramedullary screw with a figure-of-eight wire, or a lag screw and dorsal plate (3.5-mm semitubular or reconstruction; Fig. 3A–C). A figure-of-eight wire alone does not provide sufficient stability to resist physiologic loading (16). The advantages of the lag screw/dorsal plate technique include less operative time, more anatomic reductions, fewer hardware symptoms, less postoperative loss of reduction, and lower incidence of infection (10). The lag screw/neutralization construct consists of a lag screw across the fracture and a radial or ulnar neutralization plate (semitubular, reconstruction, or compression). Two K-wires with a figure-of-eight wire will also neutralize the lag screw (Fig. 3D).

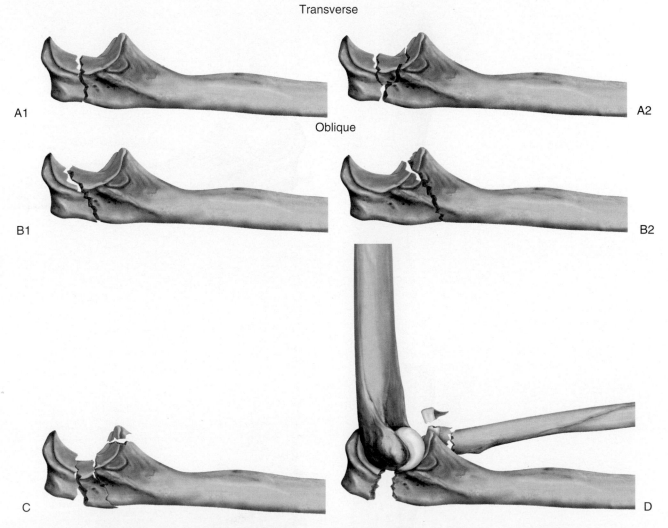

Transverse

A1   A2

Oblique

B1   B2

C   D

Figure 2. Modification of the Schatzker classification of olecranon fractures: **A:** transverse; **A1**, simple; **A2**, complex; **B:** oblique; **B1**, proximal; **B2**, distal; **C:** comminuted; **D:** fracture–dislocation (From McKee, M.D. and Jupiter, J.B.: Trauma to the adult elbow and fractures of the distal humerus. In Browner, B.D., Jupiter, J.B., Levine, A.M., and Trafton, P.G. (eds.): *Skeletal Trauma.* W.B. Saunders, Philadelphia, 1992, pp. 1455–1522; Fig. 41-16.).

Ultimately the choice between two K-wires with a figure-of-eight wire, or a medullary screw with a figure-of-eight wire, or a lag screw with either a tension-band plate or a neutralization plate for fixation of the transverse or oblique fracture patterns comes to surgeon experience. All three of these fixation techniques will provide enough stability for early motion. Outcomes for each technique are similar if complications are avoided (4,16).

The tension-band techniques are used for simple and complex transverse fracture patterns. Complex transverse fractures also require joint elevation and bone graft. Larger joint depressions may require fixation besides the tension-band construct. Miniscrews, K-wires, and absorbable pins all are used. A lag screw neutralized with either a 3.5-mm plate (semitubular or reconstruction) or two K-wires with a figure-of-eight wire are used for proximal

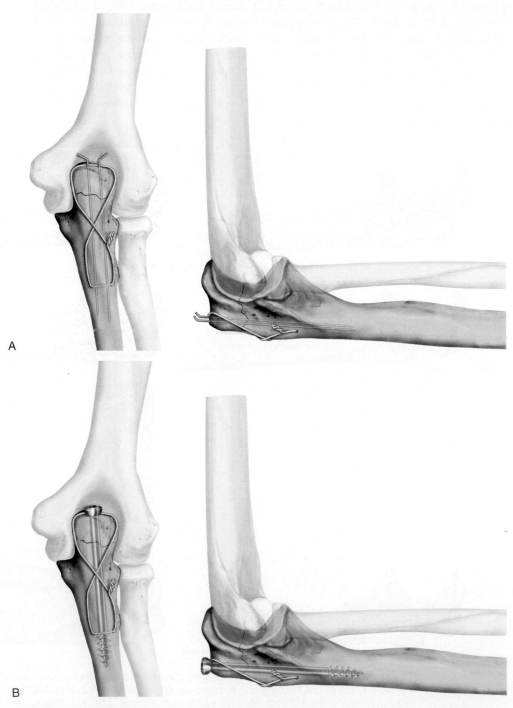

Figure 3. Tension-band constructs. **A:** Two K-wires with a figure-of-eight wire. **B:** Medullary screw with a figure-of-eight wire.

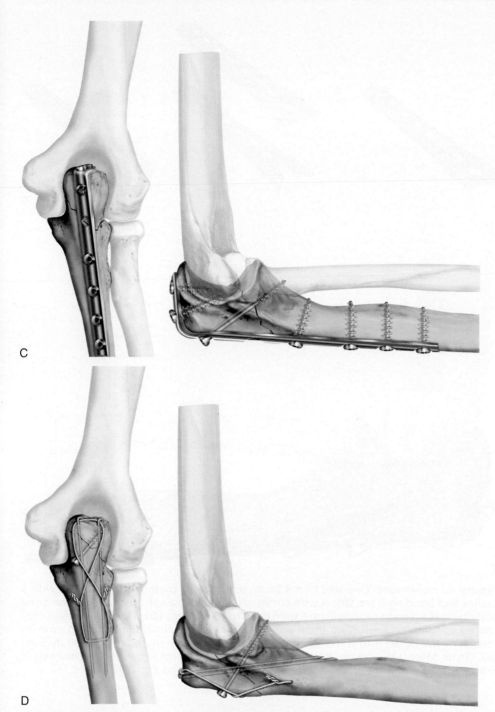

Figure 3. *(continued)* **C:** Dorsal plate with lag screw. **D:** Two K-wires that engage the anterior cortex plus lag screw. [Parts A and B from ref. 20; parts C and D from Helm, U.: Forearm and hand/mini-implants. In Müller, M.E., Allgöwer, M., Schneider, R., and Willeneger, H. (eds): *Manual of Internal Fixation*. Springer-Verlag, Berlin, 1991, pp. 453–484; Fig. 8.6.]

oblique fractures. A lag screw neutralized with a 3.5-mm plate (reconstruction or compression) is used for distal oblique fractures. Bone graft, lag screws, and a dorsal-neutralization 3.5-mm plate [semitubular hook plate (Fig. 4D), reconstruction plate, or compression plate] all are required for comminuted fractures. Repair or reconstruction of the associated injuries in comminuted olecranon fractures is also required.

Excision and triceps advancement is done if the preoperative plan shows significant bone loss. Additionally, it is considered if the fracture cannot be reduced or the bone is of such poor quality that planned fixation is inadequate (3,5,15,19).

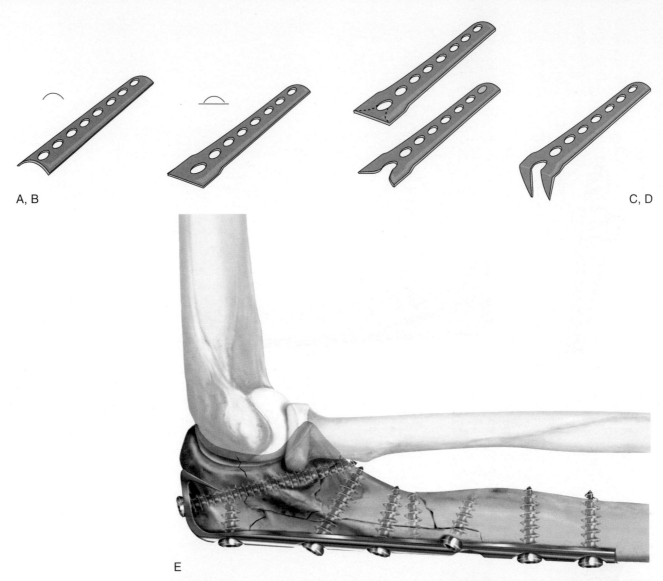

A, B

C, D

E

Figure 4. Hook plate. One end of a 3.5-mm semitubular plate **(A)** is flattened with a mallet and bending irons **(B)**. A wire cutter is used to cut away a portion of the distal plate hole **(C)**. The two cut ends are then bent to 90 degrees **(D)**. The plate is then contoured to the olecranon. Two holes are placed in the proximal olecranon to ease insertion of the hooks into the fragment. Cut portions of the plate are bent 90 degrees **(E)**. (From Mast, J.W., Jakob, R., and Ganz, R.: *Planning and Reduction Techniques in Fracture Surgery*. Springer-Verlag, Berlin, 1989; Fig. 3.17 and Fig. 4.37.)

SURGERY

Simple Fractures

The patient is placed supine on the operating table and anesthesia is administered. In my experience, either regional (Bier or axillary block) or general anesthesia is acceptable. A tourniquet is applied, and the arm is placed in an arm holder across the patient's chest (Fig. 5). The patient receives preoperative antibiotics. Cefazolin is used for closed injuries. Gram-negative or anaerobic coverage (aminoglycoside or penicillin or both) are added to cefazolin in open injuries.

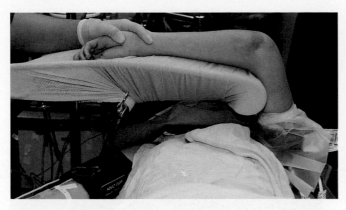

Figure 5. The patient's arm is placed across the chest on an arm holder. A tourniquet is applied.

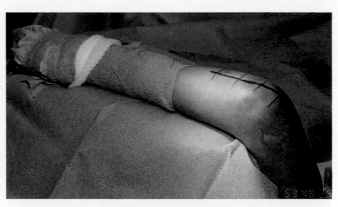

Figure 6. The patient's arm is prepped and draped for surgery and placed on the arm holder.

The arm is then prepped and draped (Fig. 6). A sterile Kerlex dressing is wrapped around the wrist, and a weighted speculum attached to the end of the Kerlex is passed off the table (Fig. 7). The weighted speculum provides enough traction to maintain the arm on the arm holder with the dorsal surface exposed. This eliminates the need for an assistant to hold the arm. An iliac crest is also prepped and draped if the preoperative plan determined the need for a bone graft.

The limb is exsanguinated, and the tourniquet inflated. The incision begins distally on the subcutaneous border of the ulna (Fig. 8). It is continued proximally in line with the subcutaneous border of the ulna to the olecranon area, where it is curved radially around the tip of the olecranon and then extended proximally in the midline 3 to 5 cm.

The incision is developed down to the fascia. A subcutaneous flap is elevated over the tip of the olecranon from radial to ulnar. The dorsal component of the fracture line is now usually visible (Fig. 9). Two millimeters of periosteum is reflected from either side of the fracture lines to simplify visualization and fracture reduction. Distally, muscle origins are reflected extraperiosteally as needed. The fracture lines are cleaned of clot and debris. The joint is visualized by retracting the proximal fragment. The joint is cleaned of clot and debris.

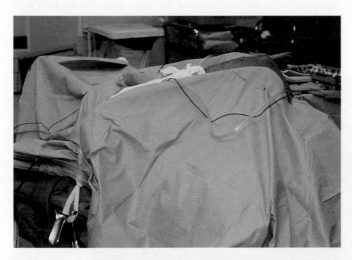

Figure 7. A sterile Kerlex (Kendall Healthcare Products, Mansfield, MA) is wrapped around the patient's forearm. A weighted vaginal speculum is attached to the Kerlex. The traction holds the arm on the arm holder.

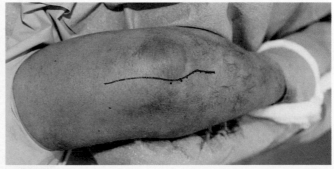

Figure 8. The skin incision begins distally along the ulnar subcutaneous border and is curved radially around the tip of the olecranon and extended proximally in the midline.

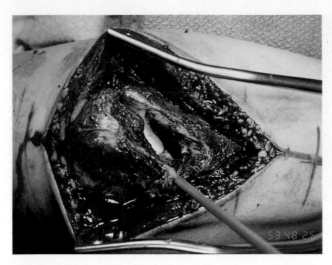

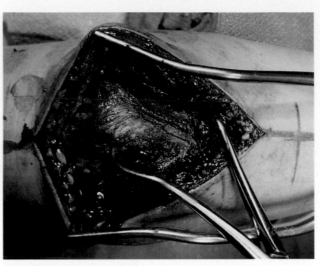

Figure 9. The incision is carried down to the fascia and periosteum. A subcutaneous flap is developed radially with the skin over the tip of the olecranon. The dorsal component of the fracture line is now visible.

Figure 10. The fracture is reduced and held in place with a pointed reduction clamp. In this case, one lag screw is placed across the fracture.

Fracture reduction begins with elevation of any depressed articular component, if present. Bone graft is used if necessary to support the depressed fragments. Small screw fixation can be added if necessary. The fracture is then reduced and temporarily held in place with K-wires or reduction clamps. Additional lag screws are used if needed (Fig. 10). The fixation determined by the preoperative plan is then added.

If a tension-band construct with K-wires was chosen, two 1.6-mm K-wires are placed by using a parallel drill guide (Fig. 11). The K-wires are overinserted 1 to 1.5 cm and then are backed out to ease seating to the final depth. The K-wires are placed down the intramedullary canal of the ulna. Alternately, the K-wires engage the anterior cortex of the ulna (Fig. 3D). Engaging the anterior cortex may diminish pin migration. I have found both techniques of K-wire placement (intramedullary or engaging the anterior ulnar cortex) to have identical outcomes and therefore recommend either one. Intraoperative radiographs are obtained to verify the reduction and fixation position.

A 2-mm hole is drilled perpendicular to the long axis of the ulna approximately 3 to 4 cm distal to the fracture (distal anchor hole). This drill hole is approximately halfway be-

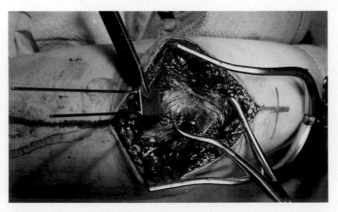

Figure 11. The preoperative plan in this case included a tension-band construct with K-wires and a figure-of-eight wire. Two 1.6-mm K-wires are placed across the fracture site with a parallel drill guide.

tween the volar and dorsal surfaces of the ulna. Anterior placement of this drill hole has been advocated based on a mathematical analysis (17). The anchor hole may be drilled before or after fracture reduction and K-wire placement. I have not had any problems drilling the anchor hole after K-wire placement. Drilling the distal anchor hole before K-wire placement avoids the potential complication of the drill hitting the K-wires but does not eliminate the possibility that the K-wires may prevent the tension-band wire placement in the distal anchor hole.

An 18- or 20-gauge wire (figure-of-eight wire) is passed through this drill hole. This wire is then crossed over the dorsal surface of the olecranon. A small loop is added to the wire proximal to the point where the wire crosses the dorsal olecranon surface on the radial side (Fig. 12). A 14-gauge angiocatheter is then passed from ulnar to radial side between the triceps tendon and the tip of the olecranon to help avoid injury to the ulnar nerve. The needle is removed. The radial limb of the figure-of-eight wire is inserted into the angiocatheter (Fig. 12). While I push gently on the figure-of-eight wire, the angiocatheter is pulled back out (Fig. 13). The figure-of-eight wire is now located anterior to the triceps insertion, which has been shown to be the optimal position (1). This portion of the wire is twisted to the other end of itself. Two knots are now present in the wire, one knot on each side of the ulna.

The wire knots are then tightened simultaneously. This provides more uniform tension to the bone-implant construct. The knots are cut to a length of 3 to 4 mm, bent down, and buried in the soft tissues if possible (Fig. 14). The K-wires are bent dorsally just past 90 degrees with a metal suction tip (Fig. 15) and cut, leaving 3 to 4 mm of wire remaining past the bend. By using a wire pliers, the K-wires are bent over to 180 degrees (Fig. 16) and rotated until the short portion of the bent wire is anterior. The K-wires are then seated with a mallet and nail set (Fig. 17).

I have recently begun using a 1.6-mm stainless steel Dall Miles cable (Howmedica, Inc., Rutherford, NJ) instead of a wire as the figure-of-eight wire. The cable sleeve is placed along the ulna so that the soft tissues can easily cover it, making it less prominent. The theoretic advantage of the cable is the ability to achieve greater tension in a more symmetric fashion. Stable constructs have been achieved intraoperatively. Long-term follow-up is not available to date, but initial review determined that overtensioning of the cable can occur,

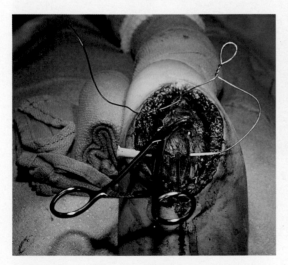

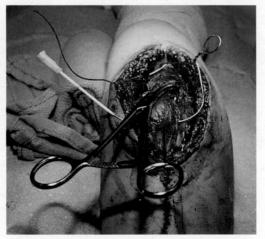

Figure 12. The figure-of-eight anchor hole is placed in the distal fragment. A wire is passed through the hole and crossed over the dorsal cortex of the ulna. A twist with a loop is placed into the limb of the wire that is now radial. A 14-gauge angiocatheter is passed from ulnar to radial side anterior to the triceps tendon along the tip of the olecranon. The needle is removed. The radial limb of the wire is put into the angiocatheter.

Figure 13. With gentle pushing on the wire, the angiocatheter is removed. The figure-of-eight wire now lies anterior to the triceps tendon on the tip of the olecranon. This end of the wire is twisted to itself.

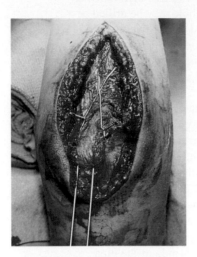

Figure 14. By using two needle holders, the figure-of-eight wire is tightened by twisting the loop on the radial side and the knot on the ulnar side. The twists are cut to a length of 3 to 4 ml.

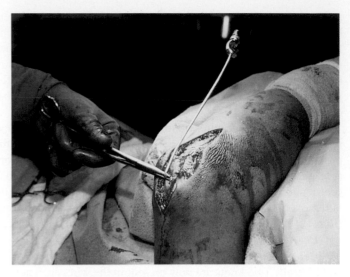

Figure 15. The two K-wires are bent dorsally to 90 degrees with a metal suction tip and a heavy needle holder.

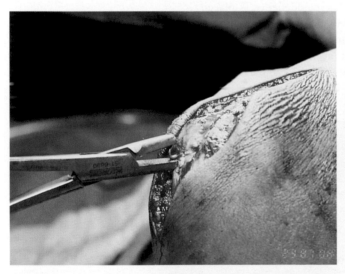

Figure 16. The K-wires are then cut, leaving 3 to 4 ml past the bend. A heavy needle holder is used to bend the K-wires to 180 degrees.

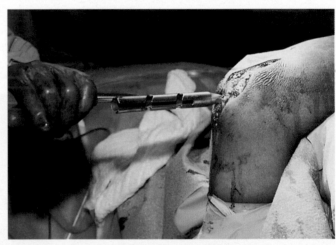

Figure 17. The bent K-wires are rotated 180 degrees so that the short end of the bend is now anterior. The Kirschner wires are seated with a nail set.

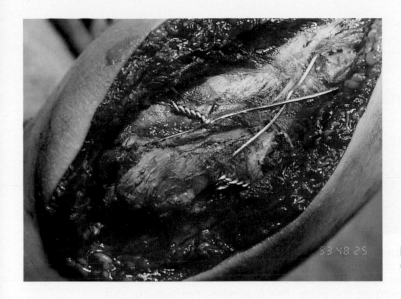

Figure 18. The reduction and quality of fixation is evaluated as the arm is placed through a range of motion.

resulting in crushing of the fragments and loss of reduction. The cable should not be overtensioned if chosen for fixation.

The tourniquet is released. Final radiographs are obtained. The fracture is examined through a full range of elbow motion to verify stability (Fig. 18). The wound is irrigated and closed in layers. A drain is not used if adequate hemostasis is obtained after tourniquet release. The arm is placed into a posterior plaster splint. Antibiotics are continued for 24 h.

Alternative Constructs

Medullary Screw with a Figure-of-Eight Wire. A medullary screw can substitute for the K-wires in the previously described technique (Fig. 3B). Advocates of this technique point out that static and dynamic compression are applied, that the screw is less likely to back out, and that this fixation is the strongest biomechanical construct (4,11,16). Disadvantages include prominent hardware and loss of reduction as the screw engages the distal ulnar canal, causing fragment translation.

The medullary screw is placed after fracture reduction. A 6.5-mm cancellous (32-mm thread length) or 4.5-mm malleolar screw is used. A washer is used to help anchor the figure-of-eight wire proximally. The triceps tendon is split in line with its fibers. The pilot hole is drilled, starting at the tip of the olecranon, down the canal. The pilot hole is tapped. An alternative method is to leave the fracture displaced and to drill the pilot hole retrograde into the proximal fragment. The fracture is then reduced and held in place with clamps. The pilot hole is identified in the proximal fragment and the drill bit inserted through it into the distal fragment.

As the screw engages the distal ulna, translation of the proximal fragment can occur. Before final seating of the screw, the figure-of-eight wire is inserted as described. The wire is passed around the screw below the triceps tendon. After the wire is tightened, the screw is seated. The washer is located on the bone deep to the triceps tendon. This avoids injury to the triceps tendon at final seating of the screw. The procedure continues as described.

Lag Screw and Tension-Band Plate. This technique involves placing a lag screw, usually through the plate, across the fracture, and placing a plate on the dorsal surface of the olecranon (Fig. 3C). It is especially useful with oblique fractures in the sagittal plane. The lag screw is usually inclined from just distal to the tip of the olecranon to the coronoid process. The plate is bent around the tip of the olecranon, and two screws are placed proximally. The plate is tensioned by first placing a screw distal to the end of the plate. One limb

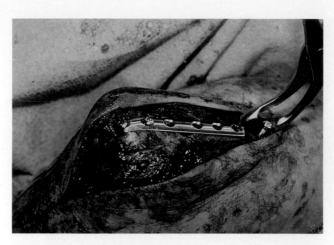

Figure 19. The fracture is reduced and a plate applied. A screw is placed into the ulna. A Verbrugge clamp is applied to the screw and the plate. Closing the clamp puts tension on the plate. This is unmeasured tension, and care must be taken so the fracture is not displaced.

of a Verbrugge clamp is then placed around the screw head, and the other hooks the last hole in the plate (Fig. 19). Closing the clamp applies tension to the plate. Alternatively, an articulated tensioning device can be used to tension the plate. Three to four screws are then added distally. The procedure continues as described previously.

Comminuted Fractures

The surgical exposure described previously is used for comminuted fractures. Care is taken to avoid devascularization of bone fragments. Reduction proceeds in a step-wise fashion. Temporary fixation is achieved with K-wires. The quality of the reduction, proposed final fixation, and bone is now assessed. If the fracture cannot be reduced, the planned fixation will not be stable, or if the bone is severely osteopenic, the temporary fixation is removed, the fragments excised, and the triceps tendon advanced.

If adequate fixation can be achieved with an anatomic reduction, final fixation is applied. K-wires are replaced with lag screws. Bone graft is used to support osteochondral fragments. A dorsal plate is then applied to neutralize the lag screws. A pelvic reconstruction plate is shaped to fit dorsally to the tip of the olecranon. Alternatively, a 3.5-mm semitubular plate is fashioned into a hook plate (Fig. 4A–C) and shaped to fit dorsally to the tip of the olecranon (Fig. 4D). The hooks engage the olecranon at the most proximal point. This supplies additional points of fixation. The quality of fixation is assessed by moving the elbow neutral to 120 degrees. Closure continues as previously described.

Open Fractures

Open fractures are taken to the operating room immediately, where irrigation and debridement are completed. The open wounds are extended as needed. Fixation proceeds as previously described. Part of the wound is left open, but the joint may be closed over a suction drain. The wound and joint are returned to the operating room on postinjury days 2 and 4 for irrigation and debridement. Wound closure is completed on postinjury day 4. Wound closure is accomplished by delayed primary closure, skin graft, local rotational flap, or free tissue transfer as needed. Antibiotics are used for 24 h after each wound manipulation.

POSTOPERATIVE MANAGEMENT

The postoperative rehabilitation is divided into three phases: initial, motion, and strengthening. Initially, the limb is splinted at 90 degrees for 3 to 5 days to promote soft-tissue healing. The second phase (motion) depends on the fixation used. Fractures fixed with the tension-band principle begin early active motion on day 5. A cast brace is used as needed, based on fixation quality and patient reliability. Fractures fixed with the lag screw/neutralization principle are placed in a long-arm cast for a total of 2 to 3 weeks. A cast brace is used for an additional 3 to 4 weeks. Active and active assisted motion exercises continue until the patient enters phase three. Isometric and isotonic exercise are started early, based on patient tolerance.

Phase three consists of strengthening. The prerequisites for entering this phase are radiographic evidence of progression to union, clinical evidence of union (no pain with physiologic stress), and an active range of motion of at least 75% of the contralateral elbow (75% of normal with bilateral injuries). The patient begins a progressive-resistance program designed to strengthen the entire upper extremity. Functional-capacity evaluations are used for return to work for manual laborers.

The rehabilitation protocol is tempered by the quality of fixation and the intraoperative stability achieved. If stable fixation is achieved, even in comminuted fractures, the protocol continues as described. If the quality of fixation will not withstand early motion, then the arm is splinted for 3 weeks. The rehabilitation protocol then continues as described and is adjusted if needed.

RESULTS

A union rate of 76% to 98% can be expected with functional results generally good to excellent (5,7,8,10,15,20). The patient is told to expect some loss of motion and strength (extension loss of 10 degrees, flexion loss of 5 degrees, and pronation and supination loss of 5 degrees each). Strength is decreased compared with the contralateral limb but may be functionally insignificant (5). Factors that negatively influence outcomes include age, malreduction, delayed operative treatment when indicated, and comminution.

COMPLICATIONS

The most frequent complications of internal fixation of olecranon fractures are related to the hardware. Hardware symptoms are present in 22% to 80% of cases (6–8,10,13,15,20). K-wire migration occurs in up to 15% of the cases. Hardware removal is required in 34% to 66% of fractures. Hardware failure occurs in 1% to 5% of cases.

When a K-/figure-of-eight wire construct is used, several steps may help avoid symptoms related to the implants. K-wires are overinserted 1 cm and then backed up to ease deep final seating. The K-wires are bent 180 degrees before final seating so that the bent portion of the wire penetrates the tip of the olecranon, making the wires less prominent. K-wires that engage the anterior cortex may prevent the wires from backing out. The figure-of-eight wire knots should be buried in the surrounding muscle to avoid their prominence. Hardware prominence, symptoms, and removal may be unavoidable in this very superficial area. The preoperative discussion should include a description of the hardware-related symptoms and the frequent necessity for hardware removal.

Infection occurs in 0 to 6% of cases. The risk of infection is reduced with the use of perioperative antibiotics and in open fractures with attention to the soft tissues and wound closure. Acute infection is managed with irrigation and debridement as needed, antibiotics, and wound closure or soft-tissue reconstruction (tissue transfer).

Ulnar neuritis is present postoperatively in 2% to 12% of the cases. The ulnar nerve is not routinely exposed during open reduction and internal fixation, but constant awareness of its location minimizes the possibility of injury. Observation is usually all that is required as symptoms either quickly resolve or improve with time. Late neurolysis may reduce symptoms in some patients.

Heterotopic ossification occurs in 2% to 13% of fractures. Indomethacin is recommended to help prevent heterotopic ossification in fractures at risk (associated severe soft-tissue injury, elbow dislocation). Significant heterotopic ossification is treated with delayed resection and prophylactic irradiation.

ILLUSTRATIVE CASE FOR TECHNIQUE

The patient was a 17-year-old female involved in a motor vehicle accident. She was complaining of left hip and elbow pain. Initial evaluation revealed a nondisplaced transverse acetabular fracture and a distal oblique olecranon fracture (Fig. 20A and B). A preoperative plan was drawn and surgical tactic developed (Fig. 1). On postinjury day 2, the patient

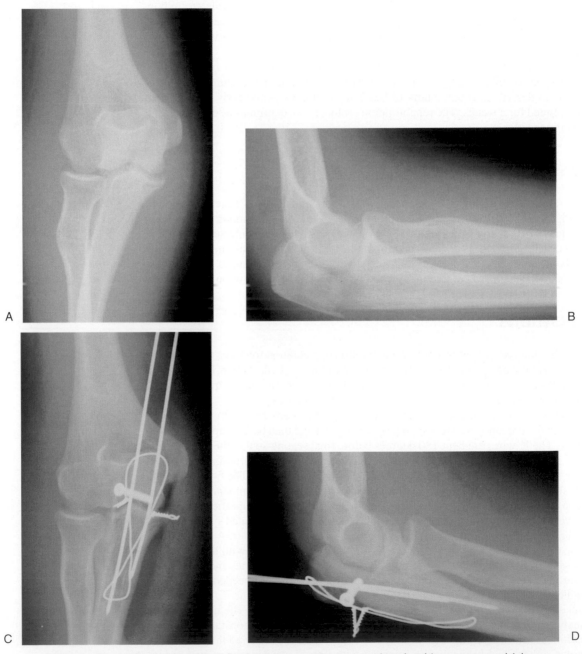

Figure 20. Oblique olecranon fracture in a young woman involved in a motor vehicle accident. Preoperative anteroposterior **(A)** and lateral **(B)** radiographs. Intraoperative anteroposterior **(C)** and lateral **(D)** radiographs.

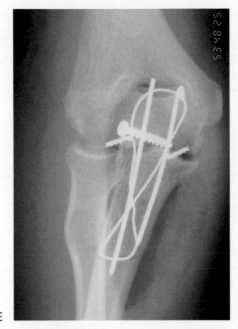

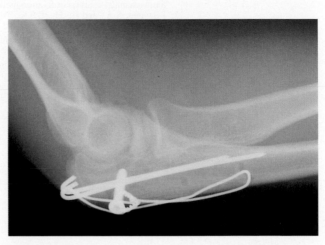

E   F

Figure 20. (*continued*) Final follow-up anteroposterior **(E)** and lateral **(F)** radiographs.

was taken to the operating room where open reduction and internal fixation was done (Fig.
20C and D). The fracture was reduced and held with a pointed reduction clamp. A lag screw
was placed across the fracture. K-wires and a figure-of-eight wire were then added (Fig.
2D). The fracture was stable through a full range of elbow motion. The wound was closed,
and the elbow splinted.

Physical therapy began on postoperative day 5 with active and active-assisted range-of-
motion exercises. The patient had nearly a full, painless range of motion by the end of postoperative week 3. At final follow-up, the patient's elbow had a range of motion equal to the
contralateral side (Fig. 20E and F). The patient had only minor symptoms related to the
hardware. Hardware removal is planned for 18 months after injury.

RECOMMENDED READING

1. Coleman, N.P., and Warren, P.J.: Tension-band fixation of olecranon fractures: a cadaver study of elbow extension. *Acta. Orthop. Scand.*, 62:58–59, 1990.
2. Colton, C.L.: Fractures of the olecranon in adults: classification and management. *Injury,* 5:121–129, 1973.
3. Fern, E.D., and Brown, J.N.: Olecranon advancement osteotomy in the management of severely comminuted
   olecranon fractures. *Injury,* 24:267–269, 1993.
4. Fyfe, I.S., Mossad, M.M., and Holdsworth, B.J.: Methods of fixation of olecranon fractures: an experimental
   mechanical study. *J. Bone Joint Surg. [Br],* 67:367–372, 1985.
5. Gartsman, G.M., Sculco, T.P., and Otis, J.C.: Operative treatment of olecranon fractures: excision or open reduction with internal fixation. *J. Bone Joint Surg. [Am],* 63:718–721, 1981.
6. Helm, R.H., and Miller, S.W.M.: The complications of surgical treatment of displaced fractures of the olecranon. *Injury,* 18:48–50, 1987.
7. Holdsworth, B.J., and Mossad, M.M.: Elbow function following tension band fixation of displaced fractures
   of the olecranon. *Injury,* 16:182–187, 1984.
8. Horne, J.G., and Tanzer, T.L.: Olecranon fractures: a review of 100 cases. *J. Trauma,* 21:469–472, 1981.
9. Hotchkiss, R.N., and Green, D.P.: Fractures and dislocations of the elbow. In Rockwood, C.A., Jr., Green,
   D.P., and Bucholz, R.W. (eds.): *Rockwood and Green's Fractures in Adults,* 3rd ed. Lippincott, Philadelphia,
   1991, pp. 795–805.
10. Hume, M.C., and Wiss, D.A.: Olecranon fractures: a clinical and radiographic comparison of tension band
    wiring and plate fixation. *Clin. Orthop.,* 285:229–235, 1992.
11. Johnson, R.P., Roetker, A., and Schwab, J.P.: Olecranon fractures treated with AO screw and tension bands.
    Orthopedics, 9:66–68, 1986.
12. Jupiter, J.B., and Mehne, D.K.: Trauma to the adult elbow and fractures of the distal humerus. In Browner,
    B.D., Jupiter J.B., Levine, A.B., and Trafton, P.G. (eds.): *Skeletal Trauma,* 1st ed. Philadelphia, W.B. Saun-
    ders, 1992, pp. 1125–1176.

13. Macko, D., and Szabo, R.M.: Complications of tension-band wiring of olecranon fractures. *J. Bone Joint Surg. [Am],* 67:1396–1401, 1985.
14. Montgomery, R.J.: A secure method of olecranon fixation: a modification of tension band wiring technique. *J. R. Coll. Surg. Edinb.,* 31:179–182, 1986.
15. Murphy, D.F., Greene, W.B., and Dameron, T.B.: Displaced olecranon fractures in adults: clinical evaluation. *Clin. Orthop.,* 224:215–223, 1987.
16. Murphy, D.F., Greene, W.B., Gilbert, J.A., and Dameron, T.B.: Displaced olecranon fractures in adults: biomechanical analysis of fixation methods. *Clin. Orthop.,* 224:210–214, 1987.
17. Rowland, S.A., and Burkhart, S.S.: Tension band wiring of olecranon fractures: a modification of the AO technique. *Clin. Orthop.,* 277:238–242, 1992.
18. Schatzker, J.: Fractures of the olecranon. In Schatzker J., and Tile, M. (eds.): *The Rationale of Operative Fracture Care,* 1st ed. Springer-Verlag, New York, 1987, pp. 89–95.
19. Teasdall, R., Savoie, F.H., and Hughes, J.L.: Comminuted fractures of the proximal radius and ulna. *Clin. Orthop.,* 292:37–47, 1993.
20. Wolfgang, G., Burke, F., Bush, D., et al: Surgical treatment of displaced olecranon fractures by the tension band wiring technique. *Clin. Orthop.,* 224:192–204, 1987.

Master Techniques in Orthopaedic Surgery,
FRACTURES, edited by D. A. Wiss,
Lippincott–Raven Publishers, Philadelphia © 1998.

9

Radial Head Fractures: Open Reduction Internal Fixation

Bernard F. Morrey

INDICATIONS/CONTRAINDICATIONS

Three factors are considered important to define a candidate for radial head fixation after fracture.

Fracture type. The best indication for open reduction and internal fixation (ORIF) is a Mason Type II radial head fracture (3,5,7,11). This includes a fracture of less than 30% of the radial head, or the classic "slice fracture" that is displaced more than 3 mm.

Associated Injury Causing Instability (4,7). These complications include associated elbow dislocation, isolated medial collateral ligament disruption, and Essex–Lopresti injury.

Age. All Type II radial head fractures may be considered amenable for ORIF in those younger than 50 to 55 years. Type II fractures with associated instability should be fixed at virtually any age.

Type I radial head fracture is best treated without surgical intervention (5,7). Internal fixation also should not be used in Type III (comminuted) radial head fractures (5,8) in an older individual (older than 50 years), in an isolated injury, or in a fracture that is too comminuted to be fixed.

PREOPERATIVE PLANNING

Equipment. The AO miniset is adequate for most fractures (Fig. 1). The Herbert screw is available and might be used. It has the advantage of stabilizing the fracture before insertion of the screw, but it is expensive. It is not necessary to have both systems available (2).

B. F. Morrey, M.D.: Department of Orthopaedics, Mayo Medical School; and Department of Orthopaedics, Mayo Clinic and Mayo Foundation, Rochester, Minnesota 55905.

If the fracture is comminuted or primarily involves the radial neck, then an AO miniplate system should be available (6).

Associated Injury. It is of paramount importance to determine whether ligament injury has occurred. The effect of radial head fixation is usually adequate in most instances, so direct ligamentous repair is not necessary. If the elbow remains unstable after radial head–fracture fixation, one might be prepared for the concurrent application of a distraction device.

In an Essex–Lopresti injury, the status of the wrist must be assessed. After the radial head fracture has been treated, the injury at the wrist is managed either by reduction and splinting in full supination, by cross-pinning of the ulna, or by direct suture of the triangular fibrocartilage.

SURGERY

The patient is placed under a general anesthesia, and the extremity is prepared and draped with a nonsterile tourniquet. An arm table may be used. I prefer the position described for other reconstructive procedures with the patient in the supine position and the arm being brought across the chest.

Technique

A classic Kocher's or "distal J-incision" is made (Fig. 2), and the interval between the anconeus and extensor carpi ulnaris identified and entered (Figs. 3 and 4). A portion of the extensor carpi ulnaris is elevated sufficiently to allow exposure of the lateral collateral ligament complex (Fig. 5). If it has not been torn by the injury, an incision is made in the capsule anterior to the lateral complex that attaches to the ulna (Fig. 6). If the elbow is stable, sufficient reflection of the common extensor tendon is necessary to allow adequate exposure of the radial head. A band is used to reflect the common extensor tendon, and a small rake retracts the inferior posterior aspect of the capsule.

The wound is cleared of hematoma. If there are loose fragments without soft tissue, they may be removed from the wound and the surface cleansed with a water pik (Fig. 6). If the soft tissue remains on any of the loose fragments, great care is taken to maintain this as a source of blood supply to the fragment. If there is a single-slice fracture, it is readily fixed

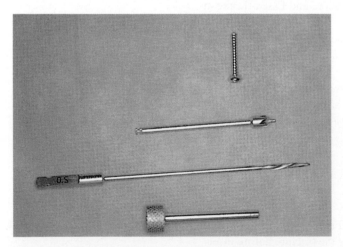

Figure 1. Most fractures are managed with the 2.7-mm miniscrew system, which includes a countersink to lessen the likelihood of screw-head prominence.

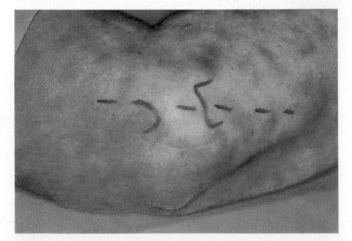

Figure 2. With the patient in a supine position with the arm brought across the chest, the distal portion of the Kocher's incision is made over the radial head and over the lateral epicondyle.

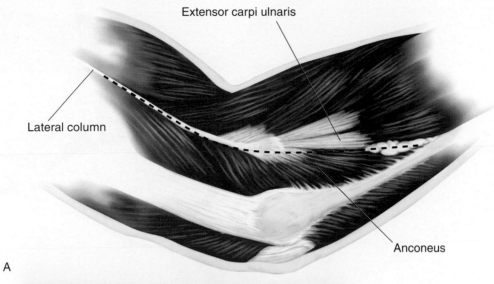

Extensor carpi ulnaris

Lateral column

Anconeus

A

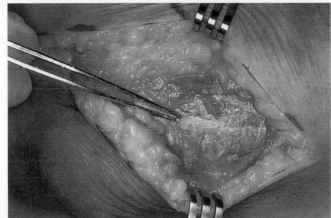

B

Figure 3. A, B: The interval between the anconeus and extensor carpi ulnaris is well visualized here.

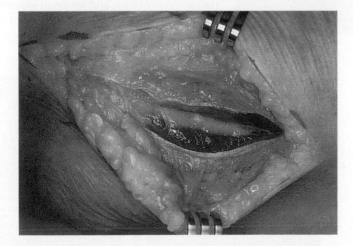

Figure 4. The interval is entered, and the muscles are retracted.

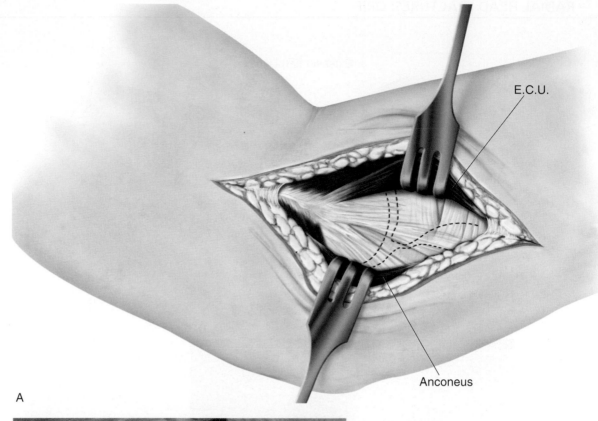

A

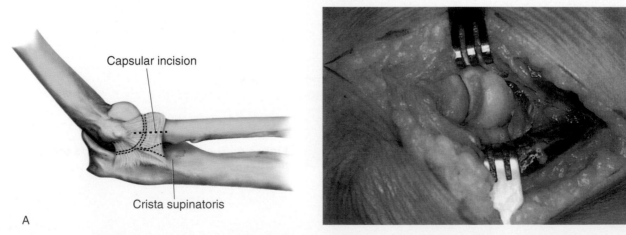

E.C.U.

Anconeus

B

Figure 5. A, B: Sharp dissection of the extensor carpi ulnaris and minimal elevation of the anconeus by a periosteal elevator reveal the lateral capsule.

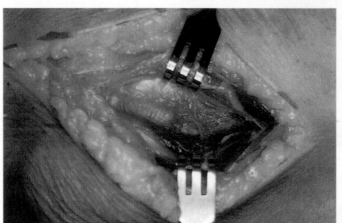

Capsular incision

Crista supinatoris

A

B

Figure 6. The lateral capsule is opened just anterior to the lateral complex, which originates at the humerus and attaches to the ulna **(A)**. The fracture has been identified, and the hematoma cleaned with a water pik **(B)**.

to the remaining portion of the radial head. The articular surface is reduced anatomically and held with a tenaculum (Fig. 7). The cortical elements are likewise reduced anatomically. It should be noted that, as with tibial plafond fractures, there may be a plastic deformation of the articular surface such that the articular surface and the cortical margins may not simultaneously appear to be anatomically reduced. In this instance, preference is, of

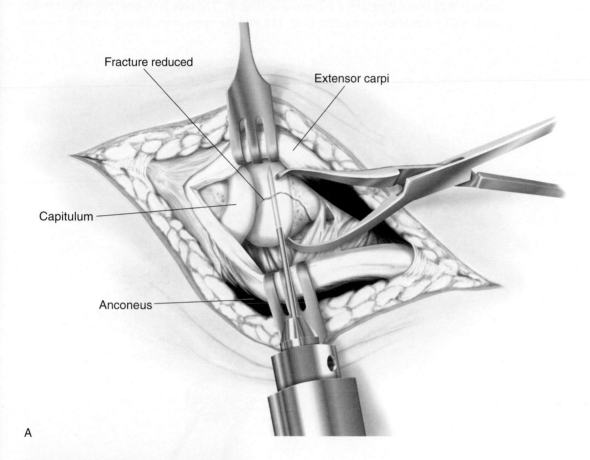

Fracture reduced

Extensor carpi

Capitulum

Anconeus

A

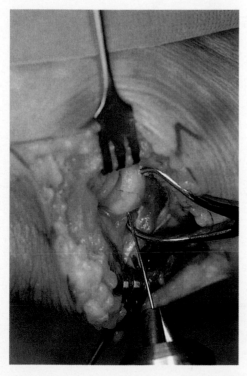

B

Figure 7. A, B: The fracture has been reduced. A Kirschner wire (K-wire) is used to secure the fracture, and it is placed in the anterior half of the fracture fragment.

course, given to the anatomic reduction of the articular surface. The reduced fracture fragment is stabilized with a single 0.425 Kirschner wire (K-wire). This is placed through the anterior half of the fragment (Fig. 7). The forearm is then rotated to expose the remainder of the fractured segment. A 2.0-mm hole is first drilled with a tissue protector (Fig. 8). The precise depth of the screw hole is determined with the depth gauge, and the fracture fragment is then overdrilled with a 2.7-mm drill (Fig. 9). The hole is tapped (Fig. 10), countersunk with a hand-held instrument (Fig. 11), and the appropriate-length screw is inserted

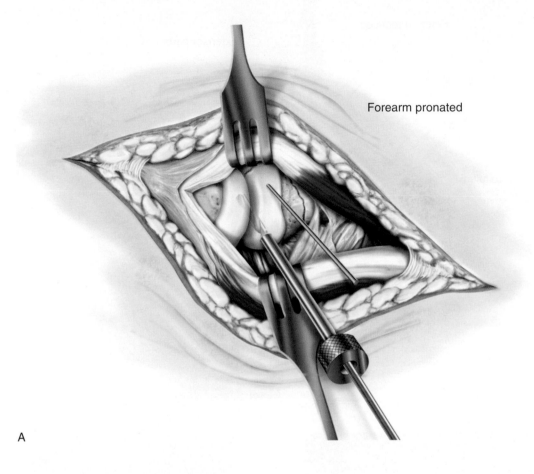

Forearm pronated

A

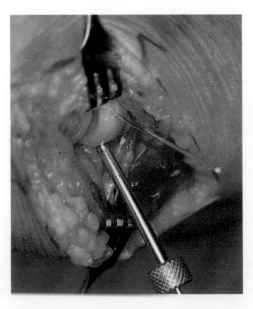

B

Figure 8. A, B: The forearm is slightly pronated, exposing the posterior half of the fracture fragment. A drill sleeve and a 2.0-mm drill bit are used.

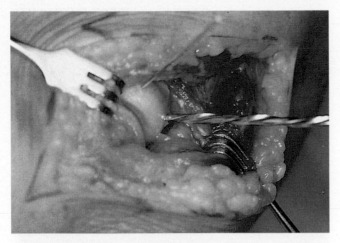

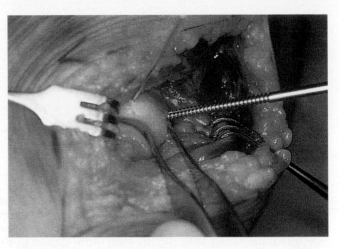

Figure 9. A 2.7-mm drill bit is then used to overdrill the fracture fragment to receive the 2.7-mm screw. Care should be taken not to split small slice-fracture fragments with the overdrilling process.

Figure 10. The screw hole is tapped to receive the 2.7-mm screw.

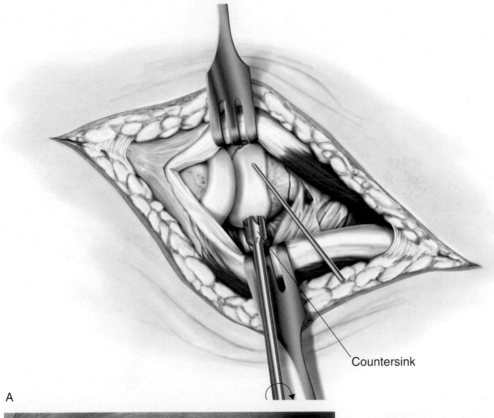

Countersink

A

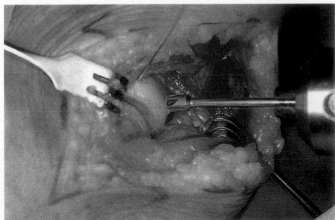

B

Figure 11. A, B: So the screw head will fit flush with the surface of the fracture fragment, a hand-held countersink instrument is used.

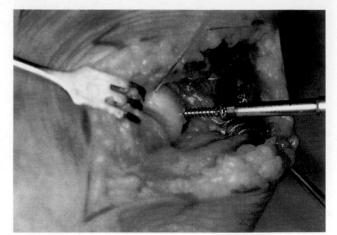

Figure 12. A 2.7-mm screw is then inserted across the fracture fragment, preferably perpendicular to the fracture surface. The errors in screw length should be with the screw slightly short rather than slightly long. Anticipation of the slightly increased depth of insertion after the countersink should also be taken into consideration.

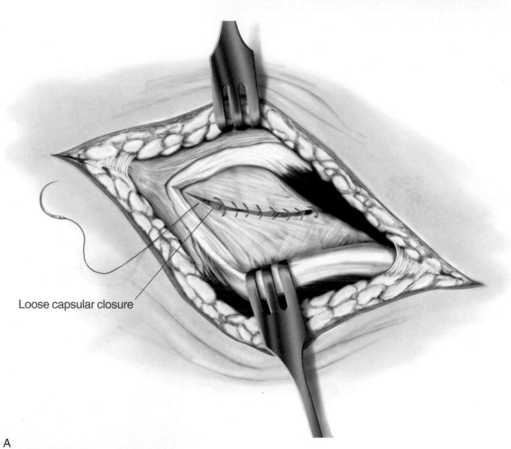

Loose capsular closure

A

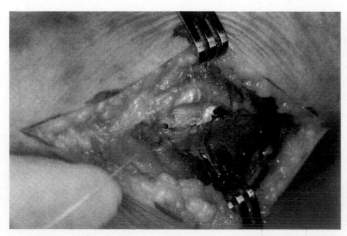

B

Figure 13. A, B: The annular ligament is only loosely closed. Great care should be taken not to overlap the structure, as it may be a source of irritation, with subsequent pronation and supination.

(Fig. 12). The forearm is slightly supinated, the K-wire is removed, and an identical technique is used to insert a second screw parallel to the first in the region of the K-wire.

If the fracture is comminuted, the small center fragments are first reduced and stabilized by reduction to the larger fragment. This may then be stabilized with a small K-wire or a bone-holding clamp. A sharp towel clip also may be used. The mini-AO screws are used to compress the fracture fragments to the stable column. Particular care is taken to avoid the screw extending past the cortex on the opposite side.

Special care is taken to close the rent over the incision in the lateral capsule. This should not be so close or tight as to cause restriction of pronation and supination. This should be tested after closure of the capsule to ensure there is not excessive friction or compression with the radial head (Fig. 13). An intraarticular drain is placed, and absorbable sutures are used to close the Kocher's interval. Subcutaneous tissue and skin are closed in a routine fashion.

It is worth noting that the slice fracture typically occurs with the forearm partially pronated. The slice thus occurs through the part of the radial head that does not articulate with the lesser sigmoid notch (Fig. 14). This slight prominence of the screws is of little con-

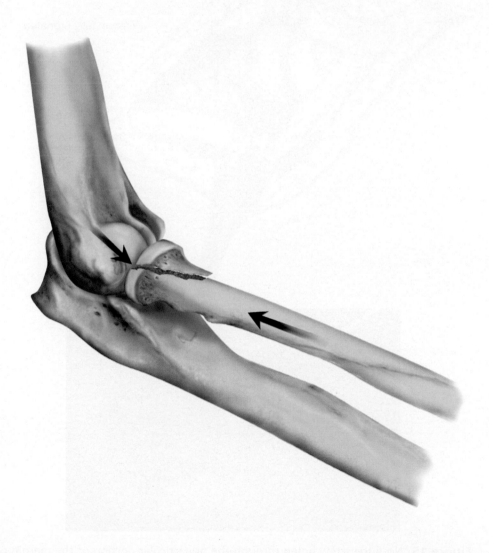

Figure 14. The slice fracture occurs with the forearm slightly pronated, and thus the fracture fragment is through the nonarticular portion of the margin of the radial head.

sequence, as the screw heads are off the articular surface (Fig. 15) and do not articulate with
the ulna (Fig. 16).

POSTOPERATIVE MANAGEMENT

If absolute rigidity has been obtained with the fixation device, a posterior splint is applied for 3 days, and a portable continuous passive motion (CPM) machine is used for ap-

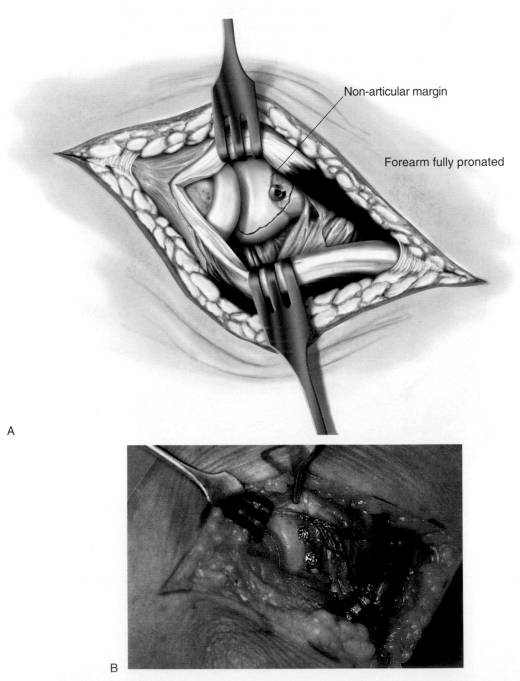

Figure 15. Note the screw going through the nonarticular portion of the margin of
the radial head with the broader portion that articulates with the lesser sigmoid notch
appearing below **(A)**. Both screws have been inserted and are flush with the surface,
and they are not a source of irritation **(B)**.

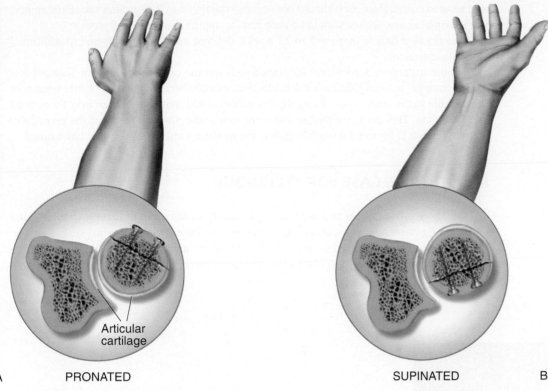

A   PRONATED   SUPINATED   B

Figure 16. The fixation can be applied through a margin of the radial head that does not articulate with the ulna either in full pronation **(A)** or in full supination **(B)**.

proximately 2 to 3 weeks. Patients are cautioned to avoid active motion because this causes increased pressure on the radiohumeral joint. Radiographs are taken at 3 weeks. If the fracture is stable, then gentle active motion is allowed, and passive pronation and supination is encouraged, avoiding flexion in pronation as this causes increased stress on the fracture (9). Radiographs are taken again at 6 weeks. It is anticipated that early healing should have begun by this time. A period of 3 months is typically required for complete fracture healing to have taken place.

Results

There are several reports, but no large series, of long-term follow-up after this procedure (5). For the Type II fracture, approximately 90% appear to have a united fracture with a satisfactory result (10,11). The results of Type III radial head fractures are less commonly reported (9). Success ranges from that comparable to the slice fracture to as low as 30% to 33%. A recent study in our laboratory demonstrated improved functional results with strength approaching normal in the uncomplicated fracture (1). The strength of the ORIF group was superior to that of both those having resection and those treated without surgery.

COMPLICATIONS

The most common complication of radial head fixation is failure of fixation. This is seen particularly in those fractures with comminution or with collateral ligament insufficiency causing increased stresses on the repaired fracture fragment. The treatment is delayed radial head excision. Resection should not occur in the first 5 to 7 days after the initial injury, but if displacement occurs, should be deferred for approximately 3 to 4 weeks.

If the fracture fails to unite in 8 to 12 weeks, delayed excision is preferred to additional attempts at fixation.

In some instances, particularly if fixation was not the only procedure, or fixation followed attempts at manipulation or debridement, ectopic bone may occur. Little treatment is available in the acute stage. Typically the process must mature and then may be excised at a later date. This does complicate and compromise the ultimate result of the procedure, and prevention is far more desirable than is the treatment after ectopic bone has formed.

ILLUSTRATIVE CASE FOR TECHNIQUE

This 38-year-old patient sustained a valgus injury to the elbow, disrupting the medial collateral ligament, causing a compression fracture of the neck of the radius (Fig. 17). The technique described was used to insert a miniplate at the margin of the radial head after the fracture was reduced (Fig. 18). At 1 year the fracture has healed (Fig. 19), and the patient

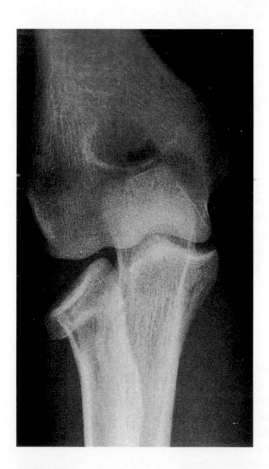

Figure 17. Valgus stress resulted in a radial neck fracture in this 38-year-old woman. Depression to this extent can occur only with disruption of the medial collateral ligament.

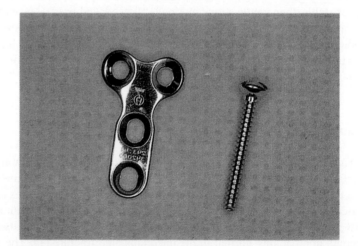

Figure 18. At reduction, the radial head was intact, and a miniplate was used with a 2.0-AO cortical screw.

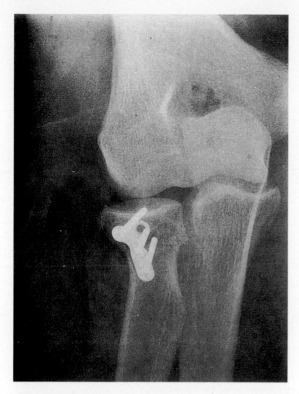

Figure 19. One year after treatment, the patient's fracture was healed with minimal depression, and the patient has a near-normal arc of motion.

has range of motion of 10 to 145 degrees, flexion of 70 degrees, and supination of 80 degrees. There is no pain.

Acknowledgment

This chapter is reprinted from Morrey, B.F. (ed.): *Master Techniques in Orthopaedic Surgery: The Elbow*. Raven Press, New York, 1994, pp. 97–111.

RECOMMENDED READING

1. Boulas, J., and Morrey, B.F.: Functional results of different treatment modalities for radial head fractures (in preparation).
2. Bunker, T.D., and Newman, J.H.: The Herbert differential pitch bone screw in displaced radial head fractures. *Injury*, 16:621, 1985.
3. Heim, U., and Trub, H.J.: Erfahrungen mit der Primaren Osteosynthese von Radius-Kopfchenfrakturen. *Helv. Chir. Acta.*, 45:63, 1978.
4. King, G.J.W., Evans, D.C., and Kellam, F.J.: Open reduction and internal fixation of radial head fractures. *J. Orthop. Trauma*, 5:21, 1991.
5. Konlic, E., and Perry, C.R.: Indications and technique of open reduction and internal fixation of radial head fractures. *Orthopedics*, 15:837–842, 1992.
6. Leung, K.S., and Tse, P.Y.T.: A new method of fixing radial neck fractures: brief report. *J. Bone Joint Surg. [Br]*, 71:326, 1989.
7. Morrey, B.F.: Radial head fracture. In Morrey, B.F. (ed.): *The Elbow and Its Disorders*, 2nd ed. W.B. Saunders, Philadelphia, 1993.
8. Odenheimer, K., and Harvey, J.P., Jr.: Internal fixation of fractures of the head of the radius. *J. Bone Joint Surg. [Am]*, 61:785, 1979.
9. Sanders, R.A., and French, H.G.: Open reduction and internal fixation of comminuted radial head fractures. *Am. J. Sports Med.*, 14:130, 1986.
10. Shmueli, G., and Herold, H.Z.: Compression screwing of displaced fractures of the head of the radius. *J. Bone Joint Surg. [Br]*, 63:535, 1981.
11. Soler, R.R., Tarela, J.P., and Minores, J.M.: Internal fixation of fractures of the proximal end of the radius in adults. *Injury*, 10:268, 1979.

Figure 19. One year after treatment, the patient has regained full flexion (A), full extension (B), and pronation (C) and supination (D).

RECOMMENDED READING

Master Techniques in Orthopaedic Surgery,
FRACTURES, edited by D. A. Wiss,
Lippincott–Raven Publishers, Philadelphia © 1998.

10

Forearm Fractures: Open Reduction Internal Fixation

Brendan M. Patterson

INDICATIONS/CONTRAINDICATIONS

Virtually all displaced diaphyseal forearm fractures in adults benefit from operative management. Several series noted the problems associated with closed management of these skeletal injuries (1,3,4). Plate fixation of diaphyseal forearm fractures has led to a dramatic improvement in functional outcomes and is considered the "gold standard" with which other methods are compared (1,3,5,9,10).

The indications for nonoperative management of forearm fractures include isolated fractures of the ulnar shaft resulting from a direct blow (i.e., the "nightstick" fracture), nondisplaced fractures of the forearm in which the anatomic bow of the radius can be maintained with interosseous molding, and most pediatric fractures. Isolated fractures of the ulna with significant comminution or displacement greater than 50% may benefit from internal fixation because of the higher incidence of nonunion compared with the classic minimally displaced nightstick variant. Fractures in the distal third of the ulna require close observation if nonoperative treatment is selected to assure that the distal radioulnar joint remains well reduced.

The severity of the soft-tissue injury plays a critical role in determining operative management. Open fractures in which the initial debridement produces a relatively clean wound can usually be managed with immediate plate fixation. Wounds in which there is considerable devitalization and contamination may not be amenable to immediate internal fixation with plates. Provisional stabilization with external fixation and delayed plate osteosynthesis, with or without early flap closure, may be necessary for severe open injuries of the forearm.

Fractures of the forearm with associated dislocations of the elbow or wrist will usually require fixation of the forearm to facilitate reduction of the adjacent dislocation. In Mon-

---

B. M. Patterson, M.D.: Department of Orthopaedic Surgery, MetroHealth Medical Center, Case Western Reserve University School of Medicine, Cleveland, Ohio 44109.

teggia's fractures, in which there is a fracture of the proximal ulna and a dislocation of the radial head, the radial head cannot be maintained in a reduced position without stabilization of the ulna. Conversely, fracture of the distal third of the radius with dislocation of the distal radioulnar joint, Galeazzi's fracture, is often termed the "fracture of necessity," as surgical stabilization of the radius is required to effect reduction of the distal radioulnar joint.

PREOPERATIVE PLANNING

Successful surgical management is based on sound preparation of the patient and a plan of treatment. In the awake, cooperative patient, a concise history of the mechanism of injury and thorough examination of the upper extremity are essential. Concurrent, ipsilateral injuries to the upper arm, wrist, and hand should be determined clinically, and radiographs are obtained on the basis of the examination. Severe pain, weakness, or paresthesias may be indicative of ischemia. Careful assessment of the soft-tissue envelope, forearm compartments, neurologic function, and vascular supply to the hand must be performed and documented before surgery. The neurologic examination should include motor assessment of the radial, posterior interosseous, medial, and ulnar nerves and sensory evaluation of the radial, median, and ulnar nerves. The axillary, brachial, radial, and ulnar pulses should be palpated.

An impending or established compartment syndrome mandates immediate fasciotomy with skeletal stabilization. The diagnosis of compartment syndrome in the awake patient is based on classic symptoms and physical findings. Pain out of proportion to the injury, tenderness with passive extension of the fingers, and firm, tender compartments with palpation are common findings. Measurement of compartment pressures in an awake, cooperative patient does not contribute significantly to decision making, as patients with classic signs and symptoms of compartment syndrome require immediate fasciotomy. In the obtunded patient, the diagnosis of compartment syndrome requires a high degree of clinical suspicion and careful serial assessment. In the unconscious patient, compartment-pressure measurement may be the only reliable indicator, and repeated measurements may be required. In these patients, the threshold for decompression may be lower. The critical pressure measurement that dictates a forearm fasciotomy remains controversial. Early studies recommended fasciotomy based on an absolute tissue pressure. However, as tissue perfusion is more important, recommendations based on the differential between mean diastolic pressures and compartment pressures are considered to be more reliable than absolute compartment pressures. Heckman et al. (6) suggested a tissue pressure within 20 to 30 mm Hg of the mean diastolic blood pressure as an indicator of a compartment at increased risk of irreversible ischemia.

High-quality orthogonal radiographs that include anteroposterior (AP) and lateral views of the forearm are essential. The plain radiographs should include the elbow and wrist joints to evaluate the injured forearm appropriately. If optimal care is to be provided, associated wrist or elbow pathologic conditions must be diagnosed. Separate views of the elbow, the wrist, and the hand may be required to complement the forearm views. The location of the fracture, its obliquity, the degree of comminution, and the presence of an associated proximal or distal soft-tissue injury are important for surgical planning. The decision to perform intraoperative stress fluoroscopy is based on the initial examination and plain radiographs of the wrist. This dynamic evaluation may be useful to diagnose an associated carpal instability that may benefit from early treatment.

Small-fragment compression plates with 3.5-mm screws are recommended for most diaphyseal fractures of the forearm. Templates for the compression plates are available for preoperative planning. Inadequate plate length and unbalanced fixation, with too many holes on one side of the fracture and not enough on the other, are two of the most common errors that can lead to compromised results. These mistakes can often be avoided by careful preoperative planning.

Early operative treatment of these injuries improves outcomes. Delay in surgical treatment beyond the first several days after injury increases the difficulty of reduction and frequently increases the amount of soft-tissue dissection. In patients whose surgery is delayed more than 2 weeks after injury, exposure of both fracture sites before fixation of either the radius or the ulna may be necessary.

SURGERY

After satisfactory general or regional anesthesia, the patient is placed supine on the operating room table with the extremity placed on a hand table. A tourniquet is applied to the upper arm, and the arm is prepped and draped in a standard fashion. A first-generation cephalosporin is administered before inflation of the tourniquet. The iliac crest should be prepared in those cases in which autogenous graft may be required. In those cases in which there is a single surgeon, the ipsilateral iliac crest is generally more convenient. Harvest of the ipsilateral crest localizes the patient's pain to a single side, allows the patient to lie on the contralateral side in the postoperative period, and eliminates the need for the surgeon to change positions during the procedure. In those instances in which there is a second surgeon, the contralateral iliac crest may be used to expedite the case. Grafting should be performed in fractures with extensive comminution or segmental patterns. One should consider bone grafting for diaphyseal fractures in which more than one third of the circumference is comminuted. It is very important to maintain soft-tissue attachments to comminuted fragments by using an indirect method of reduction to decrease the need for iliac-crest bone graft.

The surgical incisions are planned and drawn on the volar and dorsal aspects of the forearm with a skin marker (Fig. 1). The extensile volar approach of Henry is recommended for most fractures of the radius (7). The Henry approach is especially useful for fractures in the distal half of the radius because a plate is easily applied to the flat, volar surface of the radius in this area. The volar approach can be extended proximally to the radial head and the anterior aspect of the elbow joint. The subcutaneous anatomy of the ulna allows ready exposure through a posterior approach with the arm in a flexed position (Fig. 2).

The arm is elevated and exsanguinated by gravity or an Esmarch bandage. In most cases, the volar approach to the radius is made initially. Depending on the level of the fracture, the skin incision traverses the elbow crease at an angle and then extends distally from the lateral aspect of the biceps tendon toward the wrist joint along the course of the flexor carpi

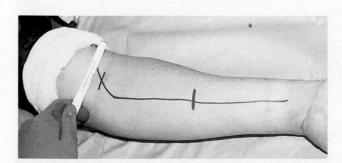

Figure 1. The skin incision for the Henry approach is marked on the volar aspect of the forearm. The patient is supine on the operating table, the elbow is extended, and the forearm is held in supination.

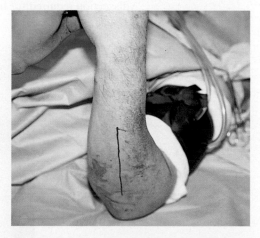

Figure 2. The subcutaneous approach to the ulna is marked with the elbow flexed and the forearm in neutral rotation. The fracture site should be palpated to determine the midpoint of the incision.

Radial Sensory Branch

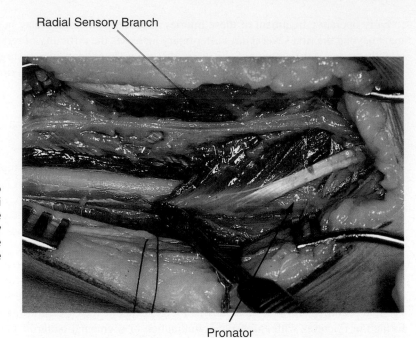

Pronator

Figure 3. The volar fascia is opened sharply to expose the brachioradialis and the flexor carpi radialis muscles. The interval between these muscles is developed bluntly. The sensory branch of the radial nerve courses beneath the brachioradialis and pierces the volar fascia in the distal third.

radialis (Fig. 3). For fractures in the proximal or middle third of the radius, the fascia is incised along the lateral aspect of the biceps, and the volar compartment is opened along the ulnar side of the brachioradialis muscle. Care must be taken to avoid injury to the posterior interosseous branch of the radial nerve as it passes through the supinator proximally and to the superficial sensory branch as it emerges from beneath the brachioradialis distally. The pronator teres may be elevated for middle-third fractures of the radius (Fig. 4). The recurrent radial artery and vein are ligated, which allows better exposure to the supinator. Periosteal dissection in the zone of injury is minimized by carefully selecting the surface of the bone to which the plate will be applied. The approach may be extended proximally to the elbow joint (Fig. 5). Comminuted fracture fragments are teased into position with a dental pick and provide "cortical reads" to determine rotational, angular, and longitudinal alignment. The fracture ends are exposed with small reduction clamps and right-angle retractors (Fig. 6). The use of the pointed or serrated small-fragment reduction clamps provides excellent control of the proximal and distal fracture segments without the soft-tissue dissection required for insertion of broad surface clamps or levering retractors.

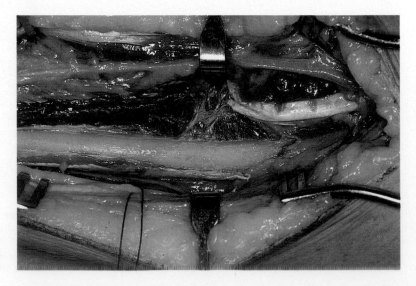

Figure 4. The pronator teres has been elevated sharply to expose the middle third of the radius.

Biceps Tendon   Leash of Henry

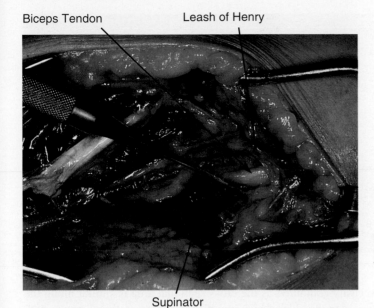

Supinator

Figure 5. The Henry approach can be extended to the proximal third of the radius if needed. The probe shows the insertion of the bicipital tendon.

The radius is usually reduced under direct visualization. The principles of compression-plate fixation are then used. For fractures in the distal third of the radius, a plate applied distally and volarly requires little contouring (Fig. 7). Prebending the plate may be necessary in the middle and proximal thirds and is mandatory for plates applied to the dorsal, bowed surface of the radius. The first cortical screw is placed in a neutral position, and then a second screw is placed eccentrically on the opposite side of the fracture to allow compression when tightened. In oblique fracture patterns, an interfragmentary lag screw may be placed through the plate to enhance stability. Most short oblique fractures are amenable to lag-screw fixation. Screws are then placed at the end of the plate, and the remaining screw holes are used as needed. In young patients with good-quality bone, the length of the plate is more important than the number of screws or cortices engaged. In elderly patients with poor bone stock, one needs to maximize stability by ensuring at least four screws/eight cortices proximal and distal to the fracture site. Newer plate designs, such as the low-contact dynamic-compression plates, have a modified undersurface to reduce the contact of the plate against the bone, which may reduce bone ischemia. These plates, available in titanium and stainless steel, have beveled screw holes that provide greater angles of insertion for screw place-

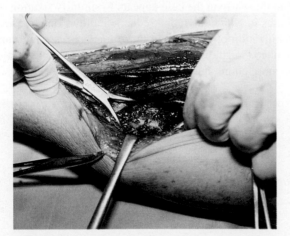

Figure 6. Exposure is facilitated through the use of right-angle retractors and small Weber clamps. Extensive dissection of soft tissue with wide exposure of the fracture site is avoided.

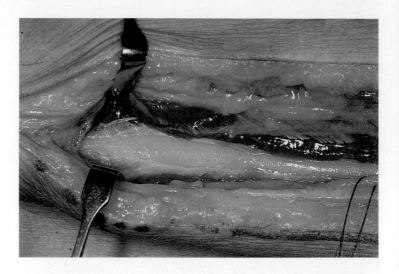

Figure 7. The distal third of the radial shaft is exposed with retraction of the brachioradialis radially and flexor carpi radialis ulnarly. The radius is relatively flat in this zone, and the plate generally needs minimal contouring.

ment. The plates are also easily contoured as the cross-sectional area is similar along the length of the plate, as opposed to the older design in which the cross-sectional area varied. Sharp drill bits and irrigation of the bone during drilling are recommended to reduce the potential for thermal necrosis around the hole.

The dorsal, Thompson approach to the radius is often useful for fractures in the proximal third of the radius. The skin incision for the dorsal approach begins just anterior to the lateral epicondyle of the distal humerus and extends distally toward the ulnar side of Lister's tubercle (Figs. 8 and 9) The internervous plane between the extensor carpi radialis brevis (ECRB) and the extensor digitorum communis (EDC) is developed (Fig. 10). Proximally the supinator should be exposed and elevated with the forearm in supination to protect the posterior interosseous nerve (Fig. 11). Supination of the forearm moves the posterior interosseous nerve away from the area of dissection (Fig. 12). The dorsal approach is not recommended for fractures in which the distal end of the plate extends beyond the abductor pollicis longus, as the implant can lead to inflammation in this area.

When surgery is performed within the first week after injury, the radius can be stabilized before exposure and reduction of the ulna. If surgery is delayed beyond 7 to 10 days, it may be necessary to expose and mobilize the radius and ulna before fixation of either bone. The decision of which bone to fix first is usually based on surgeon preference. In cases in which both fractures are simple short oblique or transverse patterns, my preference is initially to stabilize the radius. Exposure of the radius is generally more complicated than that of the ulna, and performing this early in the case appears to simplify fixation of the ulna. This is especially true in cases in which the radial reduction allows one to use an indirect reduction method for stabilization of the ulna. In those fractures in which one bone is significantly more comminuted than the other, internal fixation of the lesser fragmented bone may aid reduction of the more comminuted fracture.

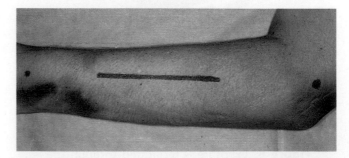

Figure 8. The dorsal approach to the radius is marked along a line from the lateral humeral epicondyle to the ulnar side of Lister's tubercle.

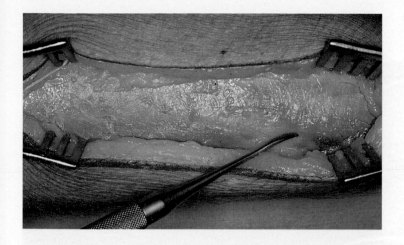

Figure 9. The dorsal investing fascia is examined to define the interval between the extensor carpi radialis brevis (ECRB) and the extensor digitorum communis (EDC).

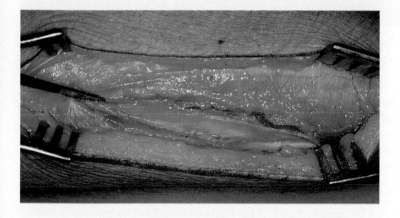

Figure 10. The dorsal fascia is incised along this interval. The abductor pollicis longus (APL) crosses the dorsal surface of the radius obliquely in the distal portion of the exposure.

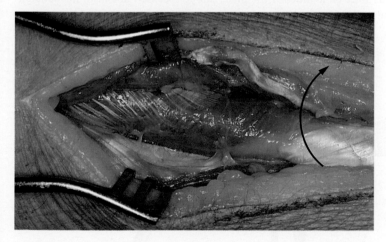

Figure 11. In the proximal aspect of the dorsal approach, the supinator overlies the radius.

PIN (nerve)

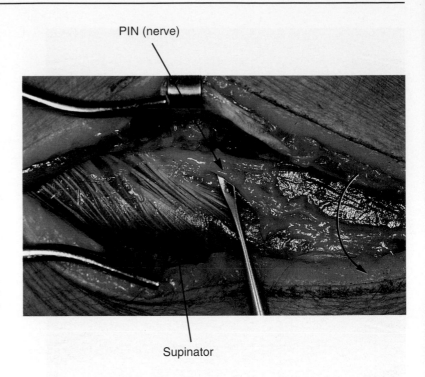

Supinator

Figure 12. The forearm is pronated, which brings the posterior interosseous nerve (PIN) closer to the operative field and may increase the risk for injury.

Once the radius has been stabilized, the elbow is flexed, and the ulna is exposed. A straight dorsal approach along the subcutaneous border is performed. The osseous anatomy and subcutaneous location of the ulna make it ideal for fixation with indirect reduction methods. It is preferable to place the ulnar plate on the dorsal surface beneath the extensor carpi ulnaris. The plate can be fixed to one side of the fracture with a screw and then "pushed" by using a bone spreader placed between the plate and a screw placed outside the plate as a post (Fig. 13). Comminuted fracture fragments are reduced with the use of a dental pick and compressed by partial release of the laminar spreader. The fracture is further compressed by use of the eccentric drill guide and compression plate. Late symptoms related to the ulnar plate may be avoided if the plate can be recessed dorsal to the subcutaneous border of the ulna (Fig. 14).

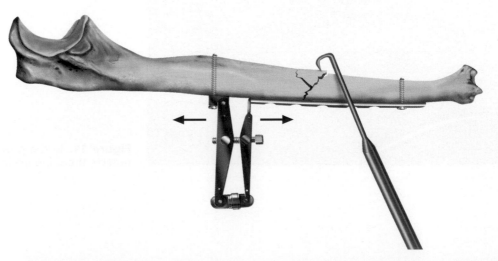

Figure 13. Indirect reduction of the ulna is depicted. A laminar spreader and screw are used for distraction of the fracture. The dental pick is used to tease the wedge fragment into position. The laminar spreader is then gradually released, and the fracture is compressed with an eccentric screw.

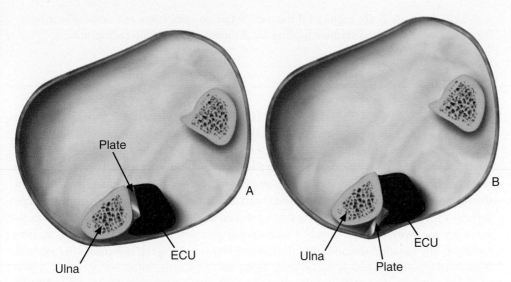

Figure 14. A, B: The plate along the subcutaneous border of the ulna should be placed so that it lies beneath the extensor carpi radialis brevis (ECRB) and is recessed dorsal to the subcutaneous border of the ulna. This reduces symptoms related to the plate's being painfully prominent, especially when the forearm is placed on a rigid surface.

After internal fixation of the radius and ulna, forearm alignment and rotation are clinically assessed. Failure to restore the radial bow and angulation reduces pronation and supination of the forearm (11). Full-length intraoperative films of the forearm are obtained to assess the adequacy of reduction and fixation. The location of the plate relative to the fracture site, screw length, and screw position are critically analyzed.

The wounds are closed by reapproximation of the skin with simple nylon sutures for the volar wound. The tourniquet may be released for a short period just before closure to identify sources of excessive bleeding. Closure of the fascia on the volar side is not necessary nor is it advised. The fascia may be closed on the ulnar side if the soft-tissue swelling is not excessive. This is done because patients may complain of muscle herniation along the ulnar border. The tourniquet is released, and a compressive, above-elbow, postoperative plaster splint is applied.

POSTOPERATIVE MANAGEMENT

Plate osteosynthesis of the forearm allows early postoperative rehabilitation of the injured extremity. Finger motion is instituted on the day after surgery. The plaster splint is removed 3 to 5 days after surgery. Shoulder, elbow, forearm, and wrist motion is encouraged after removal of the splint. The patient is instructed in active and active-assisted range-of-motion exercises. Active-assisted supination and pronation exercises are emphasized. A soft compressive dressing is used until the wound seals. Sutures are removed at approximately 10 days.

The need for occupational or physical therapy is based on the progress in the early postoperative period. Motivated patients with isolated low-energy injuries can often be treated with a self-administered home exercise program after initial instruction by the surgeon or the therapist. Patients with multiple injuries or with associated ipsilateral arm or hand injuries who show no improvement or lose range of motion in the first 2 to 3 weeks after treatment should participate in a therapy program. Most patients who require open reduction on a delayed basis will need postoperative occupational therapy.

The patient is advised to perform most activities of daily living with the affected extremity. Restrictions include heavy lifting, antigravity pushing, and sports. Radiographs are recommended as clinically indicated. Routine radiographic evaluation of the forearm at 6-

to 8-week intervals is not required if the patient has no symptoms and activity is increasing. The most useful to determine healing are 3-month and 6-month radiographs.

COMPLICATIONS

Early complications include nerve palsy, compartment syndrome, and wound infection. Nerve palsies after surgery are most commonly the result of traction or severe swelling. Injury to the superficial sensory branch of the radial nerve may cause a painful neuroma. Patients should be closely observed postoperatively to avoid missing an evolving compartment syndrome. Patients with severe pain unrelieved by usual doses of narcotic medication should have a careful necrologic assessment and direct palpation of the compartments. Tenderness with passive extension of the fingers should be sought. The patient should be evaluated for pain with passive stretch. Compartment-pressure measurements should be performed if any question remains after the clinical assessment. Deep infection after internal fixation of closed fractures is uncommon. However, if an acute infection occurs, it is best managed with irrigation, debridement, retention of the initial plates, and culture-specific intravenous antibiotics.

Late complications involve nonunion, refracture after plate removal, and synostosis (2,8,12). Most patients do not require removal of the hardware after open reduction and internal fixation of the forearm. A prominent, painful plate on the ulna may be an indication for its removal. Dissection to remove plates on the radius is demanding, and the risks of surgery probably outweigh the benefits for most patients (2,8). Forearm nonunion develops in fewer than 5% of cases managed with compression-plate fixation (1,3,4,9,10). Treatment consisting of replating with autogenous bone grafting is usually successful. Synostosis after internal fixation is a difficult problem. The results of late reconstruction for posttraumatic synostosis are often disappointing. Factors affecting the outcome include the severity of the initial injury, the time elapsed between injury and reconstruction, and the location of the synostosis in the forearm. Resection for synostosis in the middle forearm appear to have better outcomes than do distal or proximal resections (12).

ILLUSTRATIVE CASE FOR TECHNIQUE

A 45-year-old man had a both-bone forearm fracture with an ipsilateral humeral shaft fracture in a motor vehicle accident. The humerus was plated through an anterolateral approach before the forearm procedure. Radiographs of the forearm fracture are shown in Figure 15.

The radius was approached through a volar incision. Deep dissection was performed medial to the brachioradialis. The radius was exposed proximally, and the fracture fragments were mobilized with small-fragment Weber clamps. The radius fracture was reduced and stabilized with a seven-hole stainless steel LC-DC plate. The elbow was flexed, and the ulna was exposed through a straight dorsal approach, and the ulna was secured with an identical plate. The postoperative radiographs are shown in Figure 16A and B.

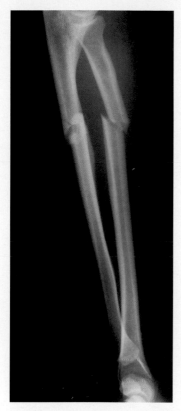

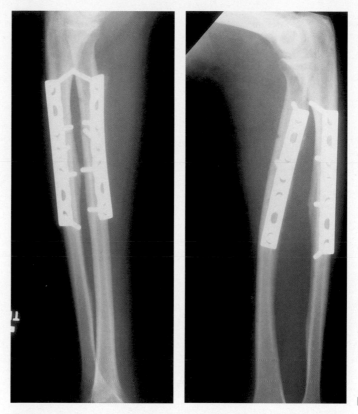

A

B

Figure 15. Injury film of forearm fracture of the proximal radius and ulna.

Figure 16. Postoperative anteroposterior **(A)** and lateral **(B)** views of the forearm after rigid internal fixation with two LC-DC plates.

RECOMMENDED READING

1. Anderson, L.D., Sisk, T.D., Tooms, R.E., and Park, W.I., III: Compression-plate fixation in acute diaphyseal fractures of the radius and ulna. *J. Bone Joint Surg. [Am]*, 57:287–297, 1975.
2. Beaupre, G.S., and Csongradi, J.J.: Refracture risk after plate removal in the forearm. *J. Orthop. Trauma*, 10:87–92, 1996.
3. Burwell, H.N., and Charnley, A.D.: Treatment of forearmfractures in adults with particular reference to plate fixation. *J. Bone Joint Surg. [Br]*, 46:404–425, 1964.
4. Chapman, M.W., Gordon, J.E., and Zissimos, A.G.: Compression-plate fixation in acute diaphyseal fractures of the radius and ulna. *J. Bone Joint Surg. [Am]*, 71:159–169, 1989.
5. Duncan, R., Geissler, W., Freeland, A.E., and Savoie, F.H.: Immediate internal fixation of open fractures of the diaphysis of the forearm. *J. Orthop. Trauma*, 6:25–31, 1992.
6. Heckman, M.M., et al.: Compartment pressure in association with closed tibia fractures. *J. Bone Joint Surg. [Am]*, 76:1285–1292, 1994.
7. Henry, W.A.: *Extensile Exposures*, 2nd ed. Churchill Livingstone, New York, 1973, p. 100.
8. Langkamer, V.G., and Ackroyd, C.E.: Removal of forearm plates: a review of complications. *J. Bone Joint Surg. [Br]*, 72:601–604, 1990.
9. Mih, A.D., Cooney, W.P., Idler, R.S., and Lewallen, D.G.: Long-term follow-up of forearm bone diaphyseal plating. *Clin. Orthop.*, 299:256–258, 1994.
10. Moed, B.R., Kellam, J.F., Foster, J.R., et al.: Immediate internal fixation of open fractures of the diaphysis of the forearm. *J. Bone Joint Surg. [Am]*, 68:1008–1017, 1986.
11. Schemitsch, E.H., and Richards, R.R.: The effect of malunion on functional outcome after plate fixation of both bones of the forearm in adults. *J. Bone Joint Surg. [Am]*, 74:1068–1078, 1992.
12. Vince, K.G., and Miller, J.E.: Cross-union complicating fracture of the forearm. *J. Bone Joint Surg. [Am]*, 69:640–653, 1987.

Master Techniques in Orthopaedic Surgery,
Fractures, edited by D. A. Wiss,
Lippincott–Raven Publishers, Philadelphia © 1998.

11

Forearm Fractures: Intramedullary Nailing

Daniel M. Zinar

INDICATIONS/CONTRAINDICATIONS

Diaphyseal fractures of the forearm in adults are relatively common injuries that usually occur after intermediate or high-energy trauma. With widespread dissemination of the methods of fixation advocated by the AO/ASIF, plate fixation of these injuries has become the gold standard. Numerous authors have shown high rates of union and excellent functional outcomes after plate osteosynthesis of these fractures. The chief drawbacks with this method of fixation are the long incisions and wide exposure necessary to reduce and fix the fractures. Radial nerve palsies are not uncommon after open reduction and internal fixation, particularly in the proximal one third. Furthermore, the resultant scar can be a significant cosmetic deformity, particularly in female patients.

Intramedullary nailing of forearm fractures is not meant to replace conventional plate fixation. Rather, it is indicated in a subgroup of patients in whom nailing may be advantageous to plate osteosynthesis. The indications for intramedullary nailing of the radius and ulna include segmental fractures, gunshot fractures with severe comminution, refracture of the forearm after plate removal, fracture occurring above or below an existing plate, and fractures occurring in athletes who participate in contact sports.

Nailing is contraindicated in children or adolescents to avoid injury to the growth plate during nail insertion. Forearm nailing is also contraindicated in adults whose intramedullary canal measures less than 3 mm at the narrowest point. Fractures less than 3 cm from the proximal or distal end of the bone should not be nailed because of inadequate fixation of the short segment of bone (Fig. 1). Nailing should be avoided in patients with preexisting deformity of the forearm that would preclude nailing without an osteotomy. Finally, nailing is not the fixation method of first choice to stabilize corrective osteotomies or treat nonunions.

D. N. Zinar, M.D.: Department of Orthopaedic Surgery, Los Angeles County-Harbor—University of California at Los Angeles Medical Center, Torrance, California 90509.

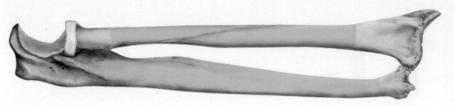

Figure 1. Portion of radius and ulna that can be treated with interlocking forearm nail. At least 3 cm of intact bone on either end must be present.

PREOPERATIVE PLANNING

Forearm fractures may occur as an isolated injury or after multiple trauma. In the severely injured patient, basic and advanced advanced trauma life support (ATLS) and a full trauma evaluation and resuscitation are mandatory. Once life- and limb-threatening injuries have been addressed, the injured arm is carefully evaluated. The entire upper extremity is inspected for open wounds, ecchymosis, abrasion, deformity, and so on. The limb is palpated from shoulder to fingers, looking for areas of tenderness or fracture crepitus. Ipsilateral injuries to the shoulder, upper arm, elbow, wrist, and hand commonly occur after high-energy trauma. The arm is critically examined to ensure that a compartment syndrome does not exist. If there is any doubt, the compartment pressure should be measured. The forearm is the second most common site for a compartment syndrome, after the lower leg. The axillary, brachial, radial, and ulnar pulses should be palpated and compared with those of the opposite side. The sensory and motor components of the radial, medial, and ulnar nerves must be documented. In patients with proximal injuries, the function of the brachial plexus requires evaluation. If the fracture is open, the wounds should be sterilely dressed, the limb splinted, and intravenous antibiotics administered. The patient should be brought to the operating room as soon as possible for irrigation and debridement.

Anteroposterior (AP) and lateral radiographs of the entire injured and uninjured forearm are obtained to determine proper nail length, diameter, and radial bow. There are three methods of determining correct nail length: First, the patient's uninjured arm is measured with a tape measure from the tip of the olecranon to the ulnar styloid, and 1 cm subtracted; second, a nail of known length is placed against the affected bone intraoperatively while applying traction to keep the bone out to the appropriate length, and it is checked fluoroscopically; or third, preoperatively, by using radiographic templates with known magnification parameters. Because the radial head is often difficult to palpate, the radial length can be determined by subtracting 2 cm from the ulnar length.

Special projections, such as oblique radiographs, computed tomography (CT) scanning, or other imaging modalities, are not helpful in preoperative planning.

SURGERY

General anesthesia is preferred over regional anesthesia because the relaxation obtained improves the chances of achieving a closed reduction. Closed nailing is more successful if surgery is done within 72 h of injury. The patient is placed supine on an operating table equipped with a radiolucent arm with the arm draped free (Fig. 2). A mobile C-arm image intensifier is brought in from the head of the table. The surgeon sits in the axilla while the assistant is positioned at the end of the hand table. For ulnar nailing, the shoulder is abducted and internally rotated, and the elbow is flexed to 90 degrees (Fig. 3).

Reduction of the fractures can be accomplished by a closed or open method. Closed nailing is preferable, as it preserves blood supply and enhances fracture healing. Closed reduction is achieved by longitudinal traction or direct pressure at the fracture site. Traction devices using finger traps have not been successful. The surgical assistant should wear sterile lead gloves to minimize radiation exposure to their hands. When the fracture fragments are locked in bayonet apposition, a miniopen technique through a 2- to 4-cm incision may be used to reduce the fragments (Fig. 4).

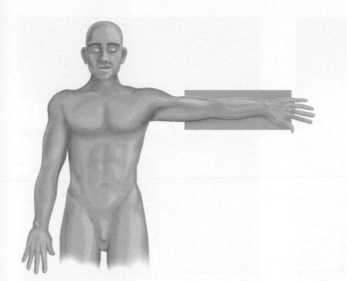

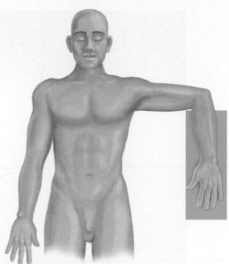

Figure 2. The patient positioned supine with a radiolucent arm board. The surgeon sits facing the axilla, while the image intensifier comes in from the head of the table.

Figure 3. With nailing of the ulna, the elbow is bent 90 degrees for access to olecranon for entry portal.

Entry Portal

A tourniquet is used whenever possible to minimize blood loss. If both bones are fractured, the radius is approached first. However, both bones are prepared for nailing before nailing either fracture. A 1.5-cm incision is made just lateral to Lister's tubercle at the distal radius (Fig. 5). The extensor pollicis longus tendon is identified and released from its sheath around Lister's tubercle (Fig. 6). The interval between the short and long wrist extensors is then identified (Fig. 7). It is important to identify the distal edge of the radius to avoid inadvertent insertion through the scaphoid. The medullary canal is entered obliquely through a 2.0-mm pilot drill hole at the dorsal margin of the radius (Fig. 8). Flexion of the wrist over a stack of towels is helpful to prevent inadvertent perforation of the volar cortex (Fig. 9). The entry portal is enlarged with a cannulated 6.0-mm reamer (Fig. 10).

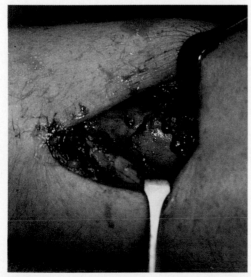

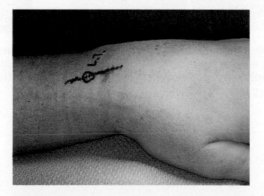

Figure 4. A 4-cm "miniopen" incision used to reduce a completely displaced fracture of the radius.

Figure 5. A 2-cm incision centered over Lister's tubercle for entry portal into radius.

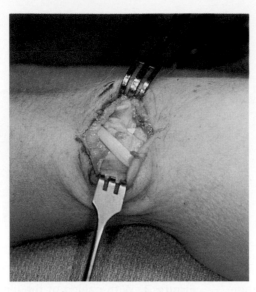

Figure 6. Extensor retinaculum is divided to expose the extensor pollicis longus (EPL) tendon. The EPL tendon is then released from its surrounding sheath.

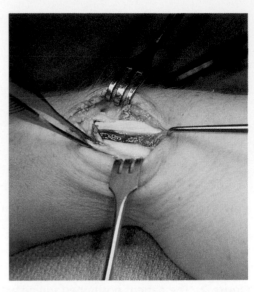

Figure 7. Interval between the extensor carpi radialis longus (EECRL) is developed. The extensor pollicis longus (EPL) is retracted radially with the ECRL.

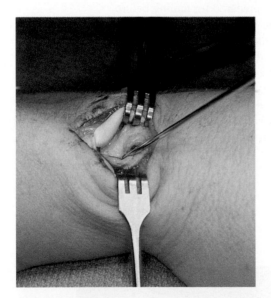

Figure 8. The 2.0-mm guide pin is introduced at a point 5 mm from the distal edge of the radius. The pin is started vertically to gain entry into the bone.

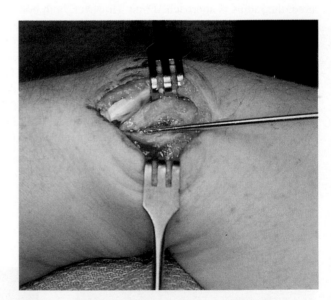

Figure 9. The wrist is then flexed, and the pin is brought into a more horizontal direction to avoid penetration of the volar cortex.

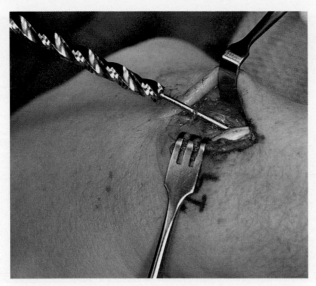

Figure 10. A 6-mm cannulated reamer is introduced over the 2.0-mm trochar wire to enlarge the entry portal.

Because the ulna bows toward the radius in the proximal third, the point of insertion for the ulna is toward the radial side of the olecranon, approximately 5 mm from the lateral cortex. A 1-cm incision is used with the same 2.0-mm drill, followed by a 6-mm cannulated reamer.

Canal Preparation

Proper size reamers are essential for successful nailing. Both hand and power reamers are available (Fig. 11). Small end-cutting and side-cutting reamers are manufactured by Biomet (Warsaw, IN, U.S.A.) and Smith and Nephew Richards (Memphis, TN, U.S.A.). The narrowest portion of the intramedullary canal may range from 3 to 7 mm. Preoperative canal sizing determines whether reaming is necessary before nail insertion. The medullary

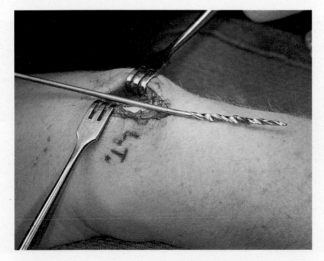

Figure 11. A hand reamer is demonstrated with a 15-degree bend to help "skate" off the volar cortex. Reamers are available in sizes from 3.0 to 5.5 mm in 5-mm increments.

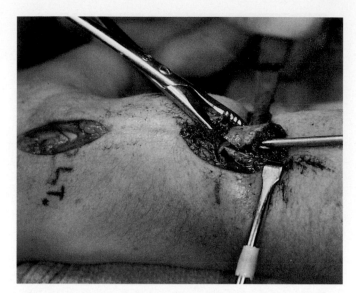

Figure 12. Power reamer is demonstrated during an open nailing to prepare the canal at the fracture site.

canal should be overreamed by 0.5 to 1 mm to prevent nail incarceration, fracture comminution, or distraction at the fracture site.

Whether open or closed nailing is performed, both fractures should be reduced and prepared before either bone can be nailed; otherwise, the stability of the nailed bone may make reduction of the other fracture difficult. When closed nailing is performed, the rotational control obtained by the interference fit of the nail is less important than it is with open nailing. If open nailing is performed, the canal may be reamed from the fracture site (Fig. 12). After the last reamer is used, it is replaced with a 2.4-mm straight guide rod. The radius is reduced and temporarily stabilized with a guide rod. The ulna is prepared in a fashion similar to that of nailing.

Forearm nails are manufactured in several different materials and shapes. Some are made of stainless steel, and others of titanium. Some are prebent to conform to the normal dorsoradial bow of the radius and lateral ulna bow. Other nails are straight and must be contoured before insertion with a rod bender. The radial nail should be contoured with respect to the normal dorsoradial bow. This can be determined by obtaining radiographs of the un-

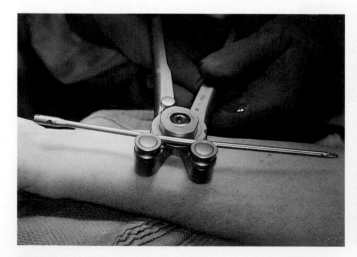

Figure 13. A nail vender is used to contour the radial nail.

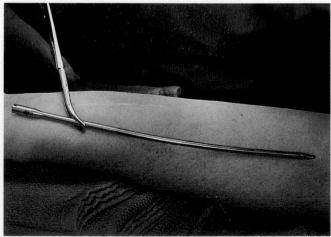

Figure 14. The nail is bent to recreate the dorsoradial bow. The amount of bow can be determined by measuring the radiographs of the uninjured radius preoperatively.

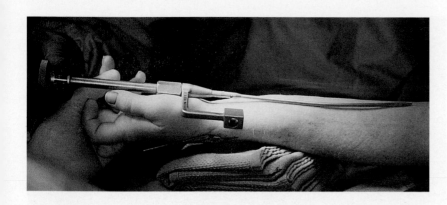

Figure 15. The nail driver and proximal targeting guide is assembled. Orientation of the nail in relation to normal dorsal radial bow is shown.

injured forearm to help assess the amount the nail should be bent. This process is similar to the process of bending reconstruction plates before implantation (Fig. 13). After proper nail contouring (Fig. 14), orientation of the implant with respect to anatomy is important. After assembly of the nail on the driver and drill guide (Fig. 15), the nail is inserted with hand pressure or light hammering. Proper rotational alignment is confirmed by the use of the image intensifier. Orientation of the bicipital tuberosity and the radial styloid are helpful in confirming correct rotation of the radius. In addition, at the completion of the procedure, an intraoperative check of the arc of forearm rotation is essential to prevent malreduction. The nail is seated so that the driving end is countersunk just below the cortex (Fig. 16).

Interlocking Screw Insertion

The nail can be locked statically (screws at both ends) or dynamically (screws at one end only). Fracture stability, expected patient compliance, and postoperative immobilization all must be considered. For unstable fracture patterns, possible noncompliant patients, and patients who desire to be free of any postoperative immobilization, static locking should be performed for optimal rotational control and maintenance of length. If the surgeon has any doubt about the length or rotational stability of the fracture, static interlocking should be done.

A 2.0-mm drill is used to prepare both the distal and proximal interlocking screws (Fig. 17). One 2.7-mm fully threaded locking screw is placed through a targeting guide on the

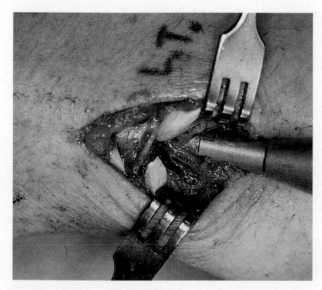

Figure 16. The nail is seated so that the female end is countersunk just below the cortex to avoid irritation of the extensor tendons.

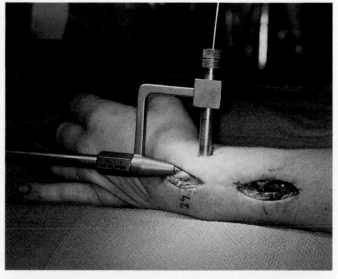

Figure 17. A 1.5-cm incision is made to insert the driving-end interlocking screw. Drill and screw guides must be placed onto bone to avoid injury to the superficial branch of the radial nerve.

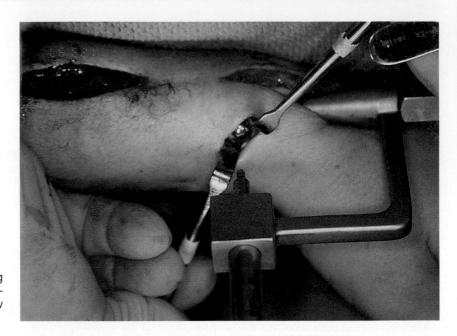

Figure 18. Driving-end interlocking screw is shown seated on bone. Image intensification is used to verify that screw has engaged the hole in the nail.

driving end of the nail. In the radius, this screw is placed from radial to ulnar through a 1-cm incision (Fig. 18). The soft tissues are spread to make sure the drill guide is firmly on bone to avoid injury to the superficial branch of the radial nerve. In the ulna, the driving end screw is placed from ulnar to radial through a 1-cm incision to avoid injury to the ulnar nerve. Interlocking the far end of the nail is difficult. It is done with the aid of an image intensifier. A perfect circle view of the hole is obtained. An incision is necessary to expose the bone in the proximal radius to avoid injury to the posterior interosseous nerve. The arm should be kept in neutral position with the hole no more than 3 cm from the end of the radius to decrease the possibility of injury to the posterior interosseous nerve. The length of the screw is measured from a calibrated drill, and a unicortical 2.7-mm screw is inserted.

After placement of the screws, the range of motion of the arm is checked, and the arc of

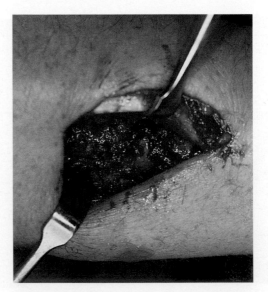

Figure 19. Bone graft obtained from reamer at entry portal is used to pack around the fracture site through the "mini-open" incision.

rotation is recorded. Both screw holes are checked to ensure proper position of the nail and screws by using the image intensification.

Bone Grafting

With closed nailing, bone grafting is not usually necessary. If nailing is done as an open procedure, a primary bone graft should be done, especially if there is comminution, a bone defect, or any distraction or gap at the fracture site. Frequently, sufficient bone from the reamers at the entry portal may be used if the amount of bone needed is small (Fig. 19). Cancellous bone from the distal radius or proximal ulna can also be used. If larger amounts of bone are needed, an iliac-crest bone graft should be obtained. We have no experience with the use of bone-bank grafts or synthetic bone used in conjunction with forearm nailing.

POSTOPERATIVE MANAGEMENT

If secure fixation is achieved in a compliant patient, then a long-arm posterior splint or sugar-tong splint is applied for 2 weeks (Fig. 20). In noncompliant patients or in patients whose nailing was done as an open procedure or dynamically locked, nails are immobilized for 4 to 6 weeks. Heavy lifting and twisting should be avoided for 3 months. Patients are followed up at monthly intervals to determine clinical outcomes and radiographic healing. Recreational activities such as golf or tennis are permitted at approximately 6 months. Hardware removal is not recommended unless the patient is severely symptomatic.

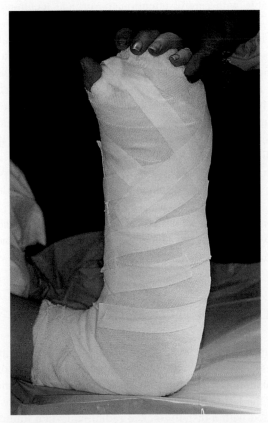

Figure 20. A postoperative bulky hand dressing is incorporated with a sugar-tong splint to provide even compression to reduce swelling and control pain. The dressing is removed at 2 weeks for suture removal.

At Los Angeles County-Harbor—University of California at Los Angeles Medical Center, both retrospective and prospective reviews have been done to evaluate forearm nailing. Union rates of 97% have been reported with good and excellent results in 25 patients. This compares favorably with results of other series of forearm fractures treated with plating. All studies emphasized the need for proper patient selection and careful surgical technique with attention to detail (6–8). Ulna nailing was described successfully by De Pedro (1).

Marek (3) reported no nonunions or infections in his series of patients treated with intramedullary nailing. Street (5) reported a 93% union rate in his series of patients treated with a square forearm nail. Studies have correlated accuracy of reduction and restoration of radial bow in forearm fracture with return of function (4).

COMPLICATIONS

The most common complications of forearm nailing include nail incarceration, iatrogenic comminution of the fracture, fracture distraction, nonunion, and cortical perforation during reaming or nail insertion. Successful nailing eliminates the problem of refracture after implant removal, which has been reported with plating of forearm fractures. The major complication of nonunion can be minimized if (a) closed nailing is done whenever possible, (b) distraction at the fracture site is avoided, and (c) bone grafting is done when open nailing is necessary in comminuted fractures. Radiographic consolidation at the fracture can be slow and should not limit restoration of function. Technical problems such as nail incarceration, fracture distraction, iatrogenic comminution, and cortical perforation are preventable with careful attention to surgical technique and preoperative planning.

Nail incarceration is the most common complication. It can be avoided by making sure that the nail advances with each blow of the hammer. A change in pitch also should alert the surgeon that the nail may be too tight. Removal of the nail with a vise grip or splitting of the cortex may be necessary to remove an incarcerated nail. This is followed by overreaming of the canal by 1 mm and reinsertion of the nail with static locking.

Fracture distraction and iatrogenic comminution also can be prevented by proper canal preparation. Overreaming by 0.5 to 1 mm will minimize this problem. If either of these occurs during open nailing, then bone grafting is recommended.

Nonunion is best managed by compression-plate osteosynthesis. Hypertrophic nonunion does not require bone grafting. Atrophic nonunion should be plated with supplemental cancellous bone grafts.

Cortical perforation usually occurs during the entry portal into the radius. Flexion of the wrist to 90 degrees over a stack of towels will prevent the drill or reamer or both from exiting through the volar cortex.

ILLUSTRATIVE CASE FOR TECHNIQUE

A 43-year-old woman had a Galeazzi fracture of the left forearm treated by plate osteosynthesis. At 2 years after injury, the plate was removed because of local discomfort. Three months after plate removal, the patient was lifting a package and noted immediate pain and swelling of the left forearm. Radiographs show a refracture (Fig. 21A and B). The patient was treated with a distally locked radial nail via a limited open incision at the fracture site. The fracture healed at 10 weeks with full restoration of function (Fig. 22).

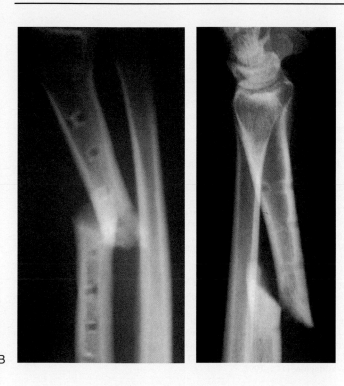

, B

Figure 21. Anteroposterior **(A)** and lateral **(B)** radiograph of radius, which show a refracture after plate removal.

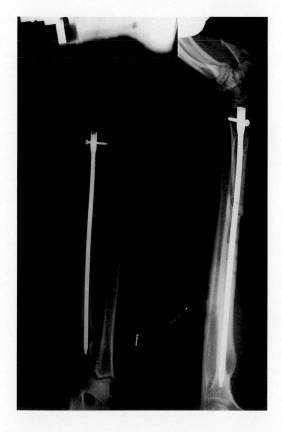

Figure 22. Postoperative radiograph showing completed forearm nailing with dynamic interlock (only driving end was locked).

RECOMMENDED READING

1. Amit, Y., Salai, M., Checkik, A., et al.: Closing intramedullary nailing for the treatment of diaphyseal forearm fractures in adolescence: a preliminary report. *J. Pediatr. Orthop.*, 5:143–146, 1985.
2. Anderson, L.D., Sisk, T.D., Tooms, R.E., Park, W.I. III: Compression-plate fixation in acute diaphyseal fractures of the radius and ulna. *J. Bone Joint Surg. [Am]*, 57:287, 1975.
3. Chapman, M.W., Gordon, J.E., Zissimos, A.G.: Compression-plate fixation of acute fractures of the diaphyses of the radius and ulna. *J. Bone Joint Surg. [Am]*, 71:159, 1989.
4. DePedro, J.A., Garcia-Navarette, F., DeLucas, F.G., Otero, R., Oteo, A., Stern, L.L.: Internal fixation of ulnar fractures by locking nail. *Clin. Orthop.*, 283:81, 1992.
5. Hidaka, S., and Gustilo, R.B.: Refracture of bones of the forearm after plate removal. *J. Bone Joint Surg. [Am]*, 66:1241, 1984.
6. Langkamer, V.G., and Ackroyd, C.E.: Safe forearm plate removal: fact or fallacy? *J. Bone Joint Surg. [Br].*, 71:875, 1989.
7. Marek, F.M.: Axial fixation of forearm fractures. *J. Bone Joint Surg. [Am]*, 41:1099, 1961.
8. Rush, L.V., and Rush, H.L.: Technique for longitudinal pin fixation of certain fractures of the ulna and of the femur. *J. Bone Joint Surg.*, 21:619, 1939.
9. Schemitsch, E., and Richards, R.: The effect of malunion on functional outcome of fractures of both bones of the forearm in adults. *J. Bone Joint Surg. [Am]*, 74:1068, 1992.
10. Smith, H., and Sage, F.P.: Medullary fixation of forearm fractures. *J. Bone Joint Surg. [Am]*, 39:91, 1957.
11. Street, D.: Intramedullary forearm nailing. *Clin. Orthop.*, 212:219, 1986.
12. Street, D., Plut, J., Wood, W.: Intramedullary forearm nailing. American Academy of Orthopaedic Surgeons Exhibit, 1979.
13. Street, D.M.: Medullary nailing of forearm fractures. *J. Bone Joint Surg. [Am]*, 39:715, 1957.
14. Wolgin, M., and Zinar, D.M.: Intramedullary fixation of forearm fractures using the Street square forearm nail. American Academy of Orthopaedic Surgeons meeting, New Orleans, 1990.
15. Zinar, D.M., Wolgin, M., et al.: Prospective evaluation of forearm i.m. nailing. American Academy of Orthopaedic Surgeons Meeting, Washington, D.C., 1992.

Master Techniques in Orthopaedic Surgery,
FRACTURES, edited by D. A. Wiss,
Lippincott–Raven Publishers, Philadelphia © 1998.

12

Distal Radial Fractures: External Fixation

Thomas F. Varecka

INDICATIONS/CONTRAINDICATIONS

Fractures of the distal radius are among the most common skeletal injuries cared for by orthopaedic surgeons. However, there is no consensus as to the best method of treatment. Considerable controversy exists over which treatment method (i.e., cast, external fixation, percutaneous pinning, or internal fixation) is ideal (1,4–6,8,9,11,13,14,17,20,21,28).

The use of external fixation has many advantages. It is relatively easy to use, adaptable, relieves pain, and is well accepted by most patients. Furthermore, it is versatile, provides access to the wrist, and can be converted to other forms of treatment, if necessary. For these reasons, external fixation has gained widespread acceptance in the management of difficult distal radius fractures (3–6,8,9,11–13,15,17,18,20,21).

Recent recognition that even small degrees of malalignment can adversely affect functional outcomes has stimulated a search for better methods of treating distal radial fractures. Casting is frequently inadequate in preventing loss of reduction and late collapse in comminuted and unstable fracture patterns (2,5,8,11–14,16,19–21). To avoid these problems, the practice of incorporating percutaneously inserted pins into plaster casts was introduced. This method of treatment had the advantage of preventing some of the collapse seen in comminuted distal radial fractures but hindered soft-tissue access. External fixation, as the direct descendent of the pins-in-plaster technique, is most useful in the treatment of unstable fractures of the distal radius. If the principles of external fixation are to be applied rationally, the surgeon should understand the factors associated with instability after distal radius fractures and learn how to identify them clinically and manage them surgically, to achieve a satisfactory outcome.

Initially, a thorough and accurate history and physical examination is performed. In the case of distal radius fractures, the history can shed light on the mechanism of injury, the energy involved, the patient's reaction to the injury, and his or her lifestyle and activity level. Furthermore, factors such as occupation, hand dominance, and presence of confounding

---

T. F. Varecka, M.D.: Department of Orthopaedic Surgery, University of Minnesota, Hennepin County Medical Center, Minneapolis, Minnesota 55415.

factors or comorbidities (e.g., preexisting arthritis, neuromuscular disease) may influence treatment and results. These factors can have a significant impact on whether external fixation is indicated, or some other method of treatment is used (4,6,7,10,13,15,17,21).

Similarly, a good physical examination is indispensable. The magnitude of deformity may provide clues as to whether the fracture is minimally displaced and stable or markedly displaced and unstable. The degree of swelling correlates with the extent of soft-tissue damage, suggesting wide initial displacement and resultant instability (Fig. 1A and B). It is important to document the status of the radial, median, and ulnar nerves, the flexor and extensor tendons, and the radial and ulnar arteries at the time of initial evaluation. The presence or absence of neurovascular deficits often has medicolegal ramifications and must be documented. The clinical evaluation of the injured wrist and hand is sometimes painful for patients or tedious for physicians, especially with high-energy injuries or when the patient's mental status is altered. Nonetheless, this information should never be omitted. A complete physical evaluation is mandatory to rule out other injuries, be they regional or systemic.

Last, a full set of good-quality radiographs should be obtained. Routine views include anteroposterior (AP), lateral, and oblique projections of the injured wrist and AP and lateral views of the forearm, including the elbow. These views usually provide an adequate assessment of angulation, shortening, displacement, comminution, and articular involvement. Care should be taken to obtain a true lateral of the wrist and forearm and not a semisupinated lateral. Comparison views of the opposite wrist and forearm are frequently helpful in determining normal skeletal parameters. Rarely are specialized studies, such as computed tomography (CT) scans or magnetic resonance imaging (MRI), necessary in the acute setting. A critical analysis of the plain radiographs is the most important factor in determining fracture stability.

Radiographic findings that have proven most predictive of instability after distal radius fractures are

1. radial shortening of more than 10 mm or loss of radial inclination of more than 20 degrees (Fig. 2A);
2. loss of, or reversal of, volar articular inclination of more than 20 degrees (Fig. 2B);
3. radial displacement of more than 4 to 6 mm;
4. comminution of more than 50% of the diameter of the radius, as seen on the lateral radiograph; or
5. intraarticular fracture extension or displacement or both of more than 2 mm.

Each of these factors is associated with loss of structural integrity and often leads to loss of reduction after closed manipulation and casting. When the sum of historic factors (e.g., high-energy injury), physical findings (e.g., early severe swelling), and radiographic changes (e.g., radial shortening) portends instability, a plaster cast will almost always fail and is contraindicated (2,4,8,11,14,20). Unfortunately, these conditions of instability are

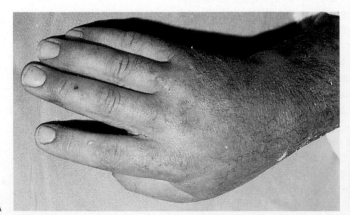
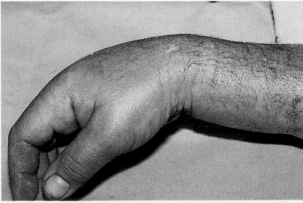

A   B

Figure 1. A: The right hand and wrist of a 37-year-old construction worker who fell from a height of about 15 ft., landing on his outstretched hand. **B:** Notice swelling and extension deformity of the wrist.

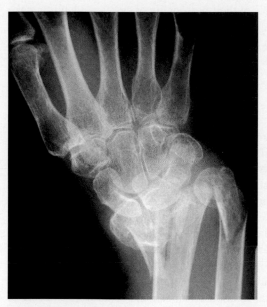
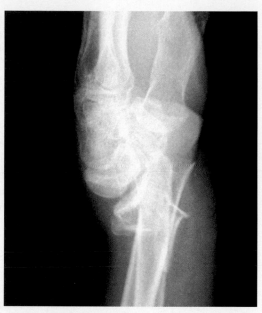

A   B

Figure 2. A: Anteroposterior (AP) radiograph showing marked shortening and displacement consistent with high-energy injury and fracture instability. **B:** Lateral radiograph showing dorsal displacement and reversal of normal volar inclination of distal articular surface.

frequently ignored or unrecognized; thus after a good initial reduction, the fracture collapses and redisplaces, often by the time of the first follow-up visit. The resultant deformity ultimately results in pain, decreased motion, decreased grip strength, and, eventually, lessened hand function (2,8,11,16,19,21).

Unbalanced and deforming mechanical forces after fracture must be neutralized to prevent redisplacement. Neutralization of these forces can be achieved with a rigid *exoskeletal* system, such as an external fixator. External fixation relies on the biomechanical principle of "ligamentotaxis," a technique of restoring length and alignment by the use of sustained traction. This method of treatment uses the ability of the soft tissues to bring about reduction of bone fragments when placed under tension (3,10). The soft tissues are tightened and consequently pull displaced fragments into anatomic alignment. Moreover, by maintaining such soft-tissue tension, the external fixator resists the tendency for redisplacement by neutralizing deforming forces generated by muscle contraction, functional use, or even gravity.

The principal indication for using an external fixator is a patient with a displaced, mechanically unstable distal radius fracture in whom achieving and maintaining an anatomic reduction is necessary (1,2,4,6–9,11–13,15,17,18,20,21). Young patients with high-demand, strenuous jobs or vigorous hobbies are excellent candidates for external fixation, as are older individuals whose fractures will predictably collapse after casting and who cannot tolerate functional loss resulting from malalignment. The presence of bilateral upper-extremity injuries, in which bilateral long-arm casts would severely hamper self-care or independence, is another indication for external fixation. Last, open fractures of the distal radius, in which access to the wound is vital, is a strong indication for external fixation.

A relative indication for external fixation includes the desire to maintain an anatomic appearance of the hand and wrist, when a cast alone is likely to lead to redisplacement of the fracture fragments and clinical deformity.

When making decisions about distal radius fractures, emphasis should be placed on the patient's functional status, physical needs, and desires for optimal recovery as opposed to relative factors such as age or bone density.

Because of its versatility, few contraindications exist to external fixation. The external fixator is not an obstacle to other necessary treatment of the hand or wrist. In certain instances, local skin conditions may be so badly compromised that external fixation may not be suitable. In some patients, idiosyncrasies of their personality or emotional lability make it difficult or impossible to manage their fractures in an external fixator, which should be avoided. The presence of a simple, stable, low-energy distal radius fracture rarely requires external fixation because a cast is suitable (6,17,20).

PREOPERATIVE PLANNING

Preoperative planning begins with the initial assessment of the injury. The patient should be readied for the operating room (OR) after ensuring that there are no other traumatic or systemic contraindications to surgery. It is important to explain to the patient the implications of external fixation and its advantages and disadvantages. It is also useful to explain postoperative protocols, stressing the importance of regaining motion of the fingers, forearm, elbow, and shoulder.

The OR should be informed of the planned surgery so that appropriate equipment is available. Equipment should include a standard set of operating instruments; the preferred external-fixation system; a power driver, if desired, for inserting the fixator pins; an operating table that allows application of intraoperative traction; and a C-arm image intensifier with monitor. To be complete, the external-fixation system should come with a variety of pins, connectors, clamps, bars, wrenches, and so on, to allow assembly in a variety of configurations. It is important to personally review the equipment to ensure that an entire set of fixator components is available before the surgery actually begins. Additionally, the surgeon should direct how the patient will be positioned, the location of the image intensifier, and where OR personnel will stand or sit to be of optimal assistance. The injury radiographs should be in full view while surgery is performed. Intraoperative reference to these radiographs is helpful in determining where pins will be placed, how the external fixator will be positioned to neutralize deforming forces, reduction maneuvers, and whether supplemental Kirschner wires (K-wires) are needed. Careful preoperative planning makes the procedure run more smoothly, allows the assistants to understand what tasks they will be expected to perform, and frees the surgeon's mind to concentrate completely on the surgical tasks required to reduce and stabilize the fracture. Although not done in every case, drawing and measuring the angles of radial inclination and volar tilt, as well as constructing the amount of radial length, on radiographs of the contralateral wrist is a helpful exercise, particularly for the less experienced surgeon.

Although the fracture reduction and fixator application can be accomplished with a variety of anesthetic techniques, general anesthesia is favored. Anxiety and fear on the part of patients may significantly interfere with regional anesthesia. The muscle relaxation achieved with general anesthesia usually improves the ability to reduce the fracture.

SURGERY

The patient is positioned on the operating table in a supine position with a radiolucent arm table attached ipsilateral to the fractured extremity (Fig. 3A and B). The preferred arm table is one that does not need a lateral supporting leg, as such supports tend to interfere with C-arm access. Also, the arm table should have built in, or readily accept, an intraoperative traction device (Fig. 4A–C).

Once the patient is anesthetized, a tourniquet is placed on the upper arm. Although not routinely used, it can prove very useful if unexpected bleeding should arise during external fixator application or if an open procedure is required.

At this time, a trial reduction is done to verify that the fracture can be reduced and that the planned maneuvers are effective in accomplishing this task. Often, a complete reduction cannot be accomplished at this stage, and the importance of intraoperative traction becomes self-evident. The patient's arm is now sterilely prepped and draped. The intraoperative traction apparatus is applied to the patient's hand/arm, and its effectiveness in aiding reduction of the fracture can be assessed with the C-arm (Fig. 5A and B).

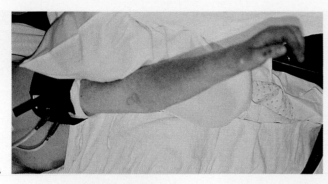
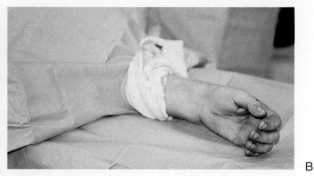

Figure 3. A: Patient in supine position with extremity positioned on arm table. **B:** Patient's arm draped and ready for operative procedure.

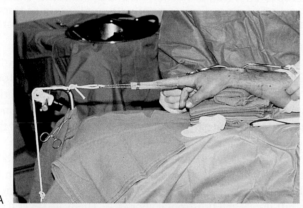

Figure 4. A: Patient in sidearm traction; traction applied through use of finger traps and sterile rope hung over a pulley and attached to 3 to 5 kg of weight. **B:** Intraoperative traction setup. **C:** C-arm is easily positioned after traction has been applied.

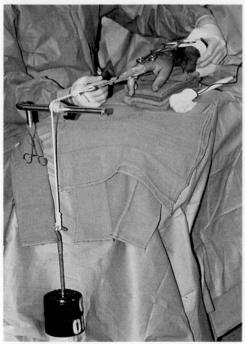

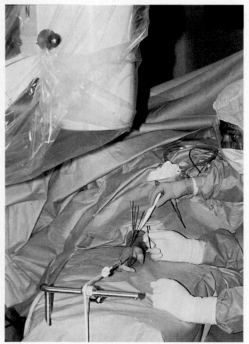

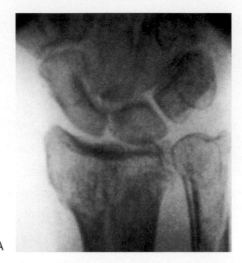
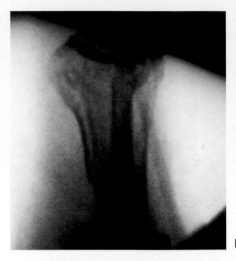

A   B

Figure 5. A: Anteroposterior (AP) projection on image intensifier showing restoration of length and correction of gross displacement with application of traction. **B:** Lateral projection on image intensifier showing acceptable correction of deformity with traction.

The surgeon is now ready to begin insertion of the fixator pins in the forearm, wrist, or hand. Depending on the configuration of the fracture, it may be appropriate to span the wrist with the fixator, thus requiring insertion of the pins into the second metacarpal; alternatively, and in the absence of metaphyseal comminution, only spanning the fracture may be necessary; therefore no metacarpal pins would be required.

In the forearm, the so-called *bare area* of the radius can be palpated about 10 to 12 cm proximal to the radial styloid and at about a 45-degree dorsal inclination to the midaxial frontal plane. With the proximal pins in this region, they will be in a plane approximately midway between a full-dorsal and full-frontal approach. There are several advantages with this location and position:

1. The likelihood of impaling muscle or tendon is minimized;
2. Injury to the dorsal branch of the radial nerve is minimized;
3. The area is sufficiently far from the zone of injury that chances of pin-tract complications are reduced; and
4. Pins placed in this position provide good mechanical stability for the fracture.

Concern over the integrity of the superficial radial nerve, and avoidance of iatrogenic damage to it, usually requires a formal, open approach for forearm pin placement. Such exposure is particularly necessary with fixator systems using a single, rigid tube design, or those with a segmental design, but rigidly connected by ball-and-socket adjustment modules. Both configurations are meant for application in the radial midaxial position, thereby placing the radial nerve at risk (Fig. 6A and B). In this instance, a 3- to 5-cm skin incision is made, with a formal exposure of the cortex of the radius and direct visualization and retraction of the radial nerve. Understanding that the radial nerve is first deep to, and then volar to, the brachioradialis tendon (this tendon also being volar to the so-called *bare area* of the radius) allows more-limited dissection. Insertion of pins through a 1-cm "stab" wound can be safely undertaken if the radial bare area is used, as the insertion sites remain dorsal to the brachioradialis tendon and away from the nerve (Fig. 7A and B). Almost all external fixator systems now use drill and pin sleeves to further minimize the risk of soft-tissue damage.

The actual mechanics of pin insertion will depend on the nature of the pins used. Some fixator systems have self-drilling, self-tapping pins, and these are usually inserted with a power drill. Other systems use a predrilling technique, which allows drilling the hard cortical bone with a sharp drill bit and inserting the pins manually.

The pins are advanced until they have completely engaged the opposite cortex of the radius. Excessive advancement can lead to irritation of the interosseous membrane, neu-

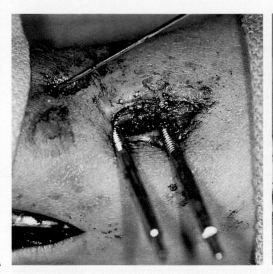
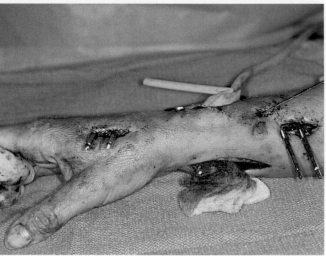

A   B

Figure 6. A: Incision required for exposure of radial cortex, when placing proximal fixator pins. **B:** View of entire forearm, showing both proximal and distal pin sites. Note that proximal and distal pins are not coplanar, which can lead to a supination deformity at the fracture site.

rovascular structures, or other tissues. Overadvancement requires partial removal, which can lead to premature pin loosening, especially with tapered pins used in certain fixator systems. The two proximal pins should have starting points approximately 3 to 5 cm apart on the radial cortex of the radius; in rigid or segmental fixators, these are placed in parallel fashion. In modular or component fixators, pins are placed to theoretically converge approximately 1 to 1.5 cm ulnarward to the ulnar surface of the radius. Proper positioning is confirmed with the image intensifier.

For most distal radius fractures, a spanning fixator construction is indicated. In these instances, the entry sites for the distal pins are on the radial surface of the second metacarpal. The major problem encountered in placing these pins is the possible penetration of the first dorsal interosseous muscle. To avoid this, gentle palmarward displacement of the muscle is accomplished with the thumb of the surgeon's nondominant hand, while the dominant hand is used to place the pin. The more proximal pin is placed through the proximal metaphyseal portion of the metacarpal and advanced until engaging not only the ulnar cortex of

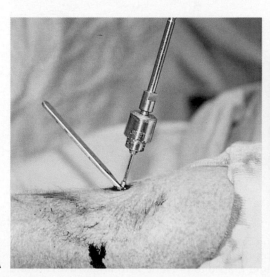
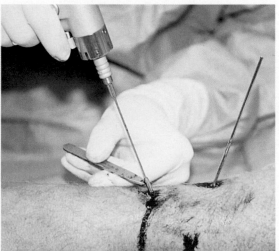

A   B

Figure 7. A: Insertion of proximal pins through stab incision in the bare area of radius. **B:** Insertion of second of the two proximal pins.

the second metacarpal but also the radial cortex of the third. The relative thinness of the cortical bone at this level is associated with mechanical weakness, thus necessitating engaging three cortices to prevent premature loosening or accidental pullout of the pin. Because of the need to seat the pin into the third metacarpal, the line of orientation of the pin relative to the radial cortex of the second metacarpal will be coplanar with the midfrontal plane of the bone itself. The more distal pin is placed with a somewhat more dorsal orientation and with a 35- to 40-degree distally directed inclination. The starting point should be just distal to the junction of the middle and distal thirds of the metacarpal. Such placement and orientation of this pin puts it in cortical bone without the pin holes being diametrically opposed to each other, but rather offset. This minimizes force concentration and helps to avoid pin complications. Final pin placement is checked with the C-arm.

The fixator is now ready for assembly. My preferred system is that of a component-style fixator that allows complete versatility in application. A single small bar is connected to each of the pin sets at this time (Fig. 8A and B). Because of the component nature of the preferred fixator system, care must be taken to place the appropriate number and type of clamps on the fixator bars as they are applied to the fixator pins. It is easy to overlook this step, which then requires disassembly of the fixator or retrofitting of clamps, which may be awkward. A modular assembly is favored, with initial application of shorter bars to the separate proximal and distal pairs of pins. This allows a sequential assembly to be carried out while continuous traction, manipulation, and ligamentotaxis are implemented, redirected, or otherwise altered. The fracture remains incompletely reduced while the fixator is being assembled.

Having assembled short bars to the pins, two longer bars (usually 80 to 120 mm) are coupled with a bar-to-bar clamp and then assembled to the proximal and distal bar-to-bar clamps of the modular portions of the frame (Fig. 9A and B). The previously determined reduction maneuvers are now carried out, and all clamps securely tightened. Alignment of the fracture can be evaluated with the C-arm.

Quite commonly, radial length and dorsal displacement are adequately and anatomically corrected with the traction and simple manipulation. The most difficult deformities to deal with are residual dorsal angulation and depression of articular fragments. Achieving complete restoration of volar tilt is ideal, but difficult. A common mistake is to assume that the failure to correct the dorsal angulation is somehow related to insufficient traction and ligamentotaxis. In fact, the contrary is frequently the case. Anatomic studies have shown that the stout volar ligaments will preferentially tighten versus the dorsal ligaments. Further ap-

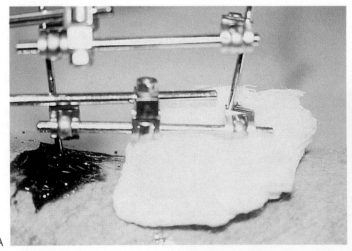
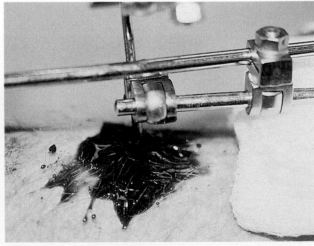

A   B

Figure 8. A: Modular assembly, showing two percutaneously placed pins and a short bar, connected by two bar-to-pin clamps, having a longer bar connected by a bar-to-bar clamp. Note the stack of gauze sponges placed to prevent pistoning of skin around the pins. **B:** Close-up view of the bar-to-pin and bar-to-bar clamps.

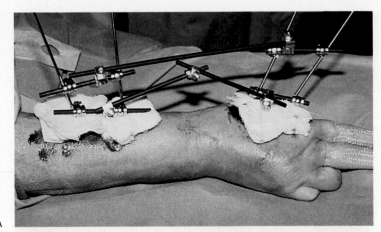

A

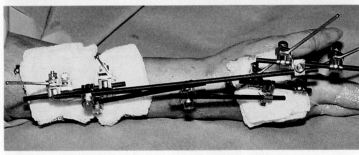

B

Figure 9. A: Dorsal view of fully assembled frame, with gauze dressings. Extreme positioning of wrist is not necessary. **B:** Lateral view of fully assembled frame. Note that proximal pins are placed dorsoradially to avoid the radial nerve.

plication of traction can paradoxically worsen the dorsal angulation, rather than correct it (3,10). In this circumstance, indirect reduction cannot be achieved, and a more direct maneuver is needed. The residual dorsal angulation is best addressed by percutaneously inserting 1.8- to 2.0-mm K-wires into the distal fragment(s) and using them as joysticks to manipulate the fragment(s) into a neutral position, or 0 degrees of dorsal angulation (18; Fig. 10A–H). Similarly, depressed articular fragments cannot be reduced by traction alone, because they have no soft-tissue attachments to draw them into alignment. These fragments are frequently impacted into the metaphysis from the compressive forces generated at the moment of injury. These fragments also must be reduced by direct means through a small dorsal incision. With a small osteotome or periosteal elevator in the fracture site, the depressed fragment can usually be teased back into place with gentle pressure under fluoroscopic control. Recently wrist arthroscopy has been used to assist with this maneuver. However, the acute hematoma, combined with the small joint volume and modest visual field, can make such arthroscopic efforts difficult. If the articular fragment is large enough, it may be secured with a K-wire. If the involved joint surface is small or consists of multiple pieces, bone graft should be inserted under the fragment(s) for support (12–14,18). Both autogenous and banked bone graft have proven effective in this situation. The use of bone-graft substitute, such as coralline hydroxyapatite or synthetic bone matrix (Norian SRS), for supporting depressed articular fragments shows promise. As more experience with these materials is gained, they may become the materials of choice for supporting such depressed fragments. With care and experience, a near-perfect restoration of articular congruence and distal radial anatomy can be achieved.

At this time, attention is directed to the distal radioulnar joint (DRUJ). After the fracture is reduced, full pronation and supination through the DRUJ should be passively achievable on the operative table (Fig. 11A and B). A mechanical block suggests an unreduced fragment or residual DRUJ subluxation. If a loose fragment is present, it can sometimes be brought back into place with a K-wire joystick, which is the preferred option. Alternatively, if small, it may be excised. When DRUJ subluxation is present, supination of the forearm will usually reduce the incongruity; however, cross-pinning of the distal radius and ulna for 3 weeks is recommended. Again, final alignment is verified by C-arm.

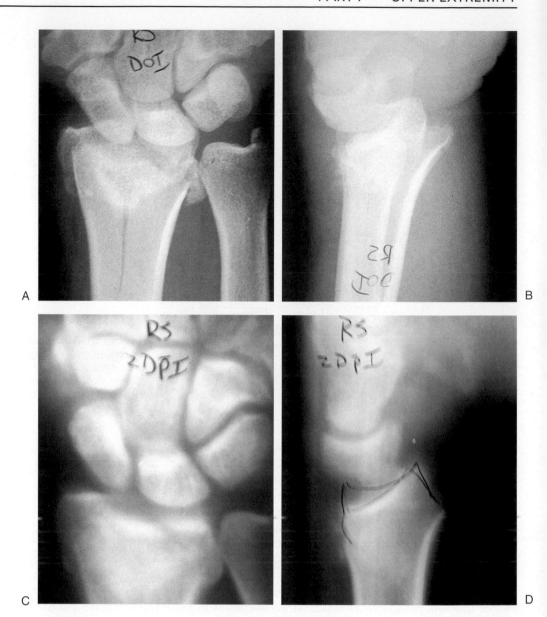

Figure 10. A: Anteroposterior (AP) radiograph view of a patient with a high-energy distal radius fracture. **B:** Lateral radiograph view of same patient. **C:** AP tomograms, after fixator application, demonstrating failure of traction and ligamentotaxis to reduce depressed articular fragments. **D:** Lateral tomograms, after fixator application, demonstrating failure of traction and ligamentotaxis to reduce dorsal angulation.

With a satisfactory reduction, the rigidity of the fixation is enhanced by the addition of one final bar. This usually measures 180 to 220 mm and connects to the proximal and distal modular constructs by means of a second set of short rods, which have been stacked onto the proximal and distal sets of pins.

The pin sites are dressed with an iodine-based or antibiotic ointment and a small stack of gauze sponges. The sponges are placed about the pins in sufficient quantity such that they are gently wedged between the skin and the lowermost bar as it is connected to the pins. Such wedging provides a gentle compressive effect on the skin adjacent to the pins. This prevents a "pistoning" phenomenon of the pin within the skin as swelling subsides. With prevention of the ebb and flow of edema about the pin sites, the incidence of pin-tract infections has been reduced. Having been sterilely placed at the time of surgery, the pin dress-

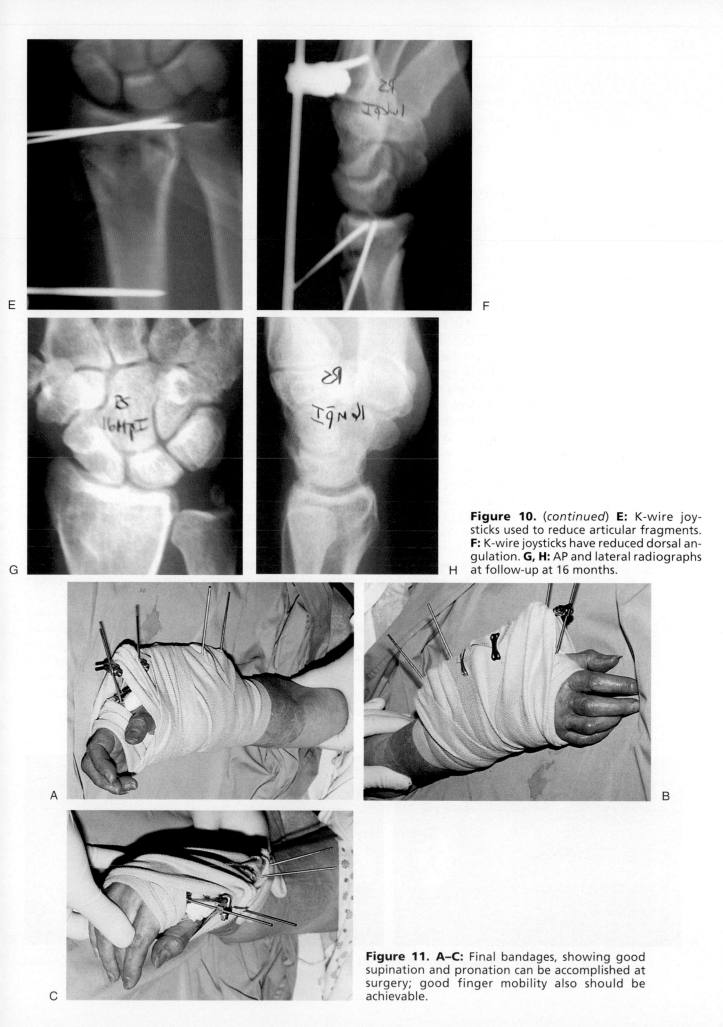

Figure 10. (*continued*) **E:** K-wire joysticks used to reduce articular fragments. **F:** K-wire joysticks have reduced dorsal angulation. **G, H:** AP and lateral radiographs at follow-up at 16 months.

Figure 11. A–C: Final bandages, showing good supination and pronation can be accomplished at surgery; good finger mobility also should be achievable.

ings can be left undisturbed until pin removal. It has also been found that periodic dressing changes are not necessary if the pin sites are otherwise kept clean and dry. A bulky dressing of gauze fluffs, gauze rolls, and an elastic wrap is then applied to complete the bandage. One final check is made to ensure that full finger motion is achievable, the thumb is not restricted in any way, and that full supination and pronation can be accomplished.

POSTOPERATIVE MANAGEMENT

Having discussed with the patient preoperatively the postoperative plan, we can initiate rehabilitation almost immediately. The patient's initial therapy is a self-directed program of finger exercises. The patient is seen at approximately 1 week for the first postoperative visit. At this time, the patient should have full active finger extension and nearly 50% to 60% of finger flexion (Fig. 12A). Pronation should be near complete, and supination of at least 20 to 25 degrees should be attainable. If these goals have been met, encouragement is offered to keep working aggressively on motion activities. If motion is lagging, edema is excessive, or pain seems to be an impediment, the patient is referred to a formal program of hand therapy. In either case, the patient is seen at 2 weeks after injury to reassess mobility and progress. Any lag in motion at this point is dealt with through an aggressive therapy program.

Patients are reevaluated, and radiographs obtained at weeks 1, 4, and 8. Any loss of reduction is usually noted by the first visit and should be dealt with immediately by adjustment of the fixator or revision surgery. However, when reduction has been anatomically achieved and secured at first treatment, loss of reduction is unusual. Any problems with the pins will be easily recognized by the time radiographs are obtained at 4 weeks. By 8 weeks, the fracture should be sufficiently healed that the fixator can be removed. Ordinarily, this is easily and comfortably carried out in the clinic and without the need for anesthesia.

While in the fixator, the patient is strongly encouraged to use the affected hand for routine activities of daily living, taking care only to avoid getting the hand and dressing wet (Fig. 12B). Refraining from using the hand for any lifting more than 5 lbs and avoiding all types of impact activities (e.g., hammering, pounding) is recommended. For patients with lower-extremity injuries, the hand and arm can be used to assist with ambulation by using a platform crutch.

Controversy exists regarding the optimal duration of treatment with an external fixator (4,6,7,9,10,13,15,17,20). When the energy of the trauma is severe enough to mandate the use of a fixator, then the fracture usually requires 8 weeks of immobilization and support (Fig. 13A and B). No detrimental effects have been noted as long as the carpus has not been overdistracted because of excessive traction. Such distraction will usually lead to a radiographic picture of diffuse osteopenia and subsequent clinical arthrofibrosis. Adequate ligamentotaxis and fracture reduction can be achieved without overdistraction.

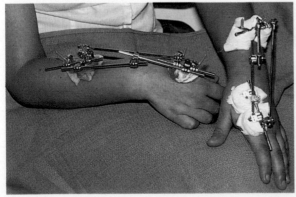
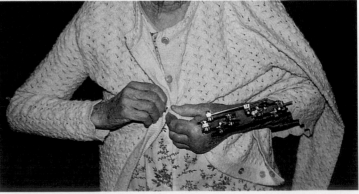

A   B

Figure 12. A, B: Patients should be able to use the extremity for functional activities.

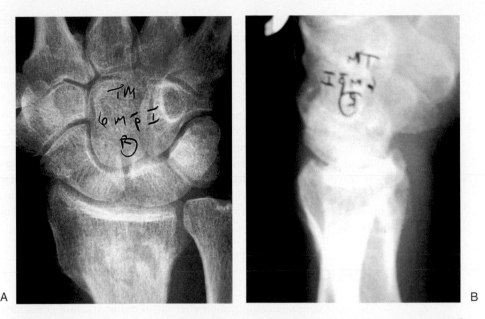

Figure 13. A, B: Patient at 6-month follow-up showing good maintenance of reduction, in spite of severe initial displacement.

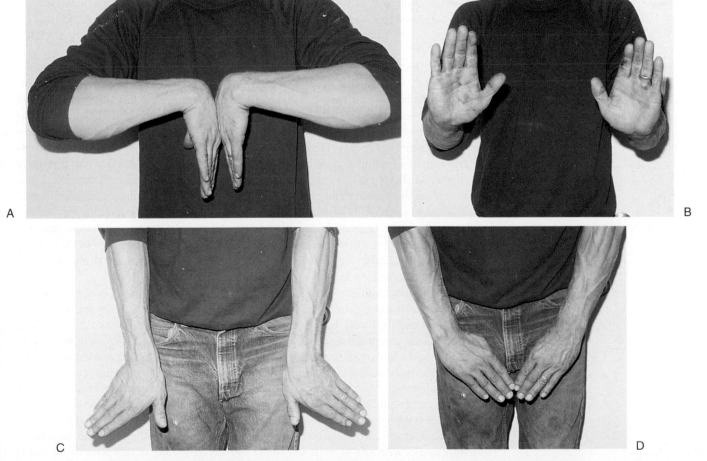

Figure 14. A, B: Patient demonstrating flexion and extension. **C, D:** Patient demonstrating ulnar and radial deviation. At this time, he had returned to light duty at his construction job and eventually resumed full activity.

After removal of the fixator, rehabilitation begins in earnest. Formal therapy sessions are almost always warranted to help patients recover wrist motion and hand strength. During this period, patients are frequently reluctant to use the hand or wrist vigorously for fear of reinjury. Most patients require repeated reassurance and much encouragement to maintain the motivation for achieving optimal recovery. Maximal recovery frequently is not seen until 6 to 8 months after injury (Fig. 14A–D). In the interim, patients must be encouraged to continue to use their hand and wrist as much, and as well, as possible. With perseverance and hard work, recovery of 50 to 70 degrees of extension, 40 to 45 degrees of flexion, full pronation, and 60 to 80 degrees of supination should be recovered. Grip strength of 70% to 100% of normal can be regained, if excessive posttraumatic shortening of the radius has been prevented. Although these values are not completely normal, they are sufficient to allow patients to perform virtually all their activities of daily living and allow return to almost all occupational duties, with the possible exception of those used in the heavy building trades.

COMPLICATIONS

The most common complication after distal radius fracture is secondary loss of reduction (1,2,8,11,17,21). If the fracture heals with deformity, the patient may develop a weakened grip, pain, decreased function, as well as a cosmetic deformity (16,19). The best treatment for this is prevention through stable fixation of the fracture. When such fixation is achieved, loss of reduction is much less likely. However, if loss of reduction occurs, early corrective osteotomy is recommended to reduce morbidity and improve function. Osteotomy of the radius is a technically demanding procedure and requires a careful analysis of the deformity, as well as meticulous preoperative planning. Iliac-crest bone grafting and internal fixation are almost always required. Frequently an arthroplasty of the DRUJ is indicated.

One of the most devastating complications after distal radial fracture is reflex sympathetic dystrophy (RSD). RSD is a broad spectrum of abnormal vasomotor responses, presumably mediated through excessive sympathetic nervous system discharge, resulting in swelling, pain, stiffness, and loss of function. Any patient can develop RSD, and a high degree of suspicion must be maintained if signs and symptoms develop, regardless of how simple the fracture may seem. The onset of RSD can occur as early as 5 to 7 days after injury and consist of nothing more than a subjective sense of paresthesia. Pain, excessive swelling, and difficulty in achieving good finger motion may be other early warning signs, long preceding the classic changes in skin color and texture or sudomotor activity. A presumptive diagnosis of RSD demands aggressive treatment, with physical therapy; antidepressant, antianxiety, or analgesic agents or a combination of these; and stellate ganglion blocks. Corticosteroids and transcutaneous electrical nerve stimulation (TENS) units have had mixed results. Early recognition and prompt treatment are necessary if compromised hand function is to be avoided.

Another common problem is median nerve compression. Compromise of the carpal tunnel as a result of fracture displacement often leads to increased pressures within the carpal tunnel. This, combined with increased tissue pressure from hemorrhage and swelling, can produce an acute compressive neuropathy of the median nerve. Left untreated, this condition causes pain and may in fact precipitate RSD. Treatment is decompression of the median nerve. In many instances, this simply consists of reducing the fracture, even if this is done preliminarily in the emergency department. If neurologic symptoms or signs persist or progress, acute surgical release of the carpal tunnel is warranted (Fig. 15A–F). Acute carpal tunnel syndrome can often develop within hours after internal or external fixation of distal radial fractures and is another reason to avoid regional anesthesia for the surgery.

Arthrofibrosis with loss of wrist and finger motion frequently occurs after distal radius fractures. Tight bandages, impingement on the finger joints by the fixator or bandages, and failure to encourage early finger movement can lead to significant digital stiffness. Overdistraction of the carpus with a fixator can cause profound stiffness in the wrist. Early, aggressive therapy in the convalescent phase is mandatory if this complication develops.

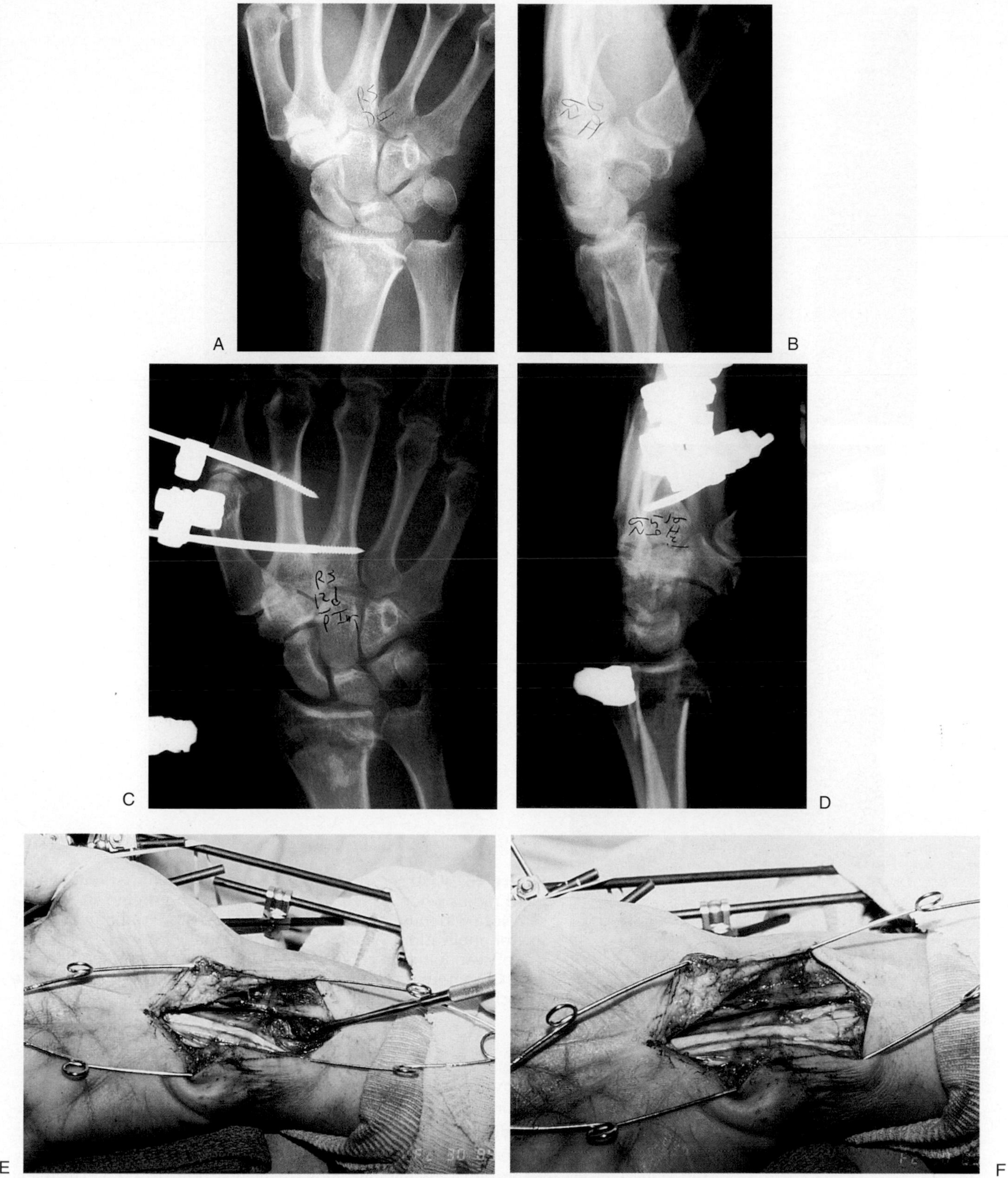

Figure 15. A, B: Anteroposterior (AP) and lateral radiographs of patient with high-energy distal radius fracture. **C, D:** AP and lateral radiographs of patient after fixator application. Note failure of volar fragment to reduce. At approximately 72 h after surgery, the patient began to complain of intense medial nerve paresthesias. **E:** Median nerve decompression. Large volar bone fragment, seen at end of periosteal elevator, was tenting the median nerve. **F:** Volar fragment reduced, decompressing the median nerve.

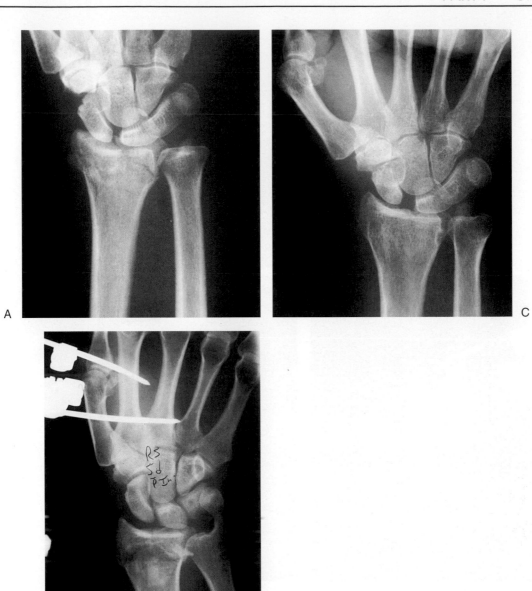

Figure 16. **A:** Anteroposterior (AP) radiograph of patient who injured radius when he fell from his bicycle, after being struck by a car. Note widening of scapholunate space. **B:** AP radiograph after fixator application. Widening of radiocarpal joint space, as well as loss of scapholunate congruence, suggest significant ligament injury. **C:** Same patient at 6 months, showing severe scapholunate dissociation on clenched-fist view.

Carpal instability can develop as a consequence of distal radius fractures and is often aggravated by external fixators (16,19). Acute instability, most often seen when the distal radial fracture has a longitudinal or vertical component extending into the articular surface, is exacerbated by distraction after external fixation. Recognition of this problem and a careful analysis of the intraoperative radiographs allows detection (Fig. 16A–C). Treatment consists of lessening the traction/distraction, followed by reduction of the instability pattern, either by open or closed methods, with appropriate pinning or repair. Late instability patterns involve principally the midcarpal joints and are almost always the consequence of failure to correct or to maintain normal volar tilt.

Finally, pin-tract problems, specifically drainage or infection, are always potential complications after external fixation (17). With good dressing techniques, pin-tract pathology can be minimized. If simple drainage and irritation develop, cleansing of the pin sites, opening of the skin surrounding the pins, and administration of antibiotics will usually suffice. In true infection, with purulent drainage, a more formal irrigation and debridement with change of pin location are necessary. Long-term antibiotics may be indicated if there is evidence of osteomyelitis.

Unstable, high-energy, comminuted fractures of the distal radius can be very effectively managed with the use of external fixation. Where excessive residual dorsal angulation or depression of intraarticular fragments represents an unacceptable postreduction alignment, percutaneously inserted K-wires can be used to achieve a satisfactory correction. Alternatively, limited open procedures, sometimes supplemented by the use of bone graft, will usually allow restoration of normal or near-normal skeletal architecture. Sterile dressings, applied at the time of surgery, and properly maintained, can be left in place until fixator removal. A high level of vigilance should be maintained for any postoperative complications, and these should be dealt with promptly. When all phases of treatment have been rendered with practiced care, satisfactory clinical results and patient outcomes can be routinely expected.

RECOMMENDED READING

1. American Academy of Orthopaedic Surgeons: *Clinical Policies: Colles' Fracture.* July 1991:14.
2. Bacorn, R.W., and Kurtzke, J.F.: Colles' fracture: a study of two thousand cases from the New York State Workman's Compensation Board. *J. Bone Joint Surg. [Am],* 35:643, 1953.
3. Bartosh, R.A., and Saldana, M.J.: Intraarticular fractures of the distal radius: a cadaveric study to determine if ligamentotaxis restores radiopalmar tilt. *J. Hand Surg. [Am],* 15:18, 1990.
4. Cooney, W.P. III: External fixation of distal radius fractures. *Clin. Orthop.,* 180:44, 1983.
5. Dias, J.J., Wray, C.C., Jones, J.M.: The radiologic deformity of Colles' fracture. *Injury,* 18:304, 1987.
6. Frykman, G.K., Tooma, G.S., Boyko, K., et al.: Comparison of eleven external fixators for treatment of unstable wrist fractures. *J. Hand Surg. [Am],* 14:247, 1989.
7. Horesh Z., and Volpin G.: The surgical treatment of severe comminuted intraarticular fractures of the distal radius with the small AO external fixation device: a prospective three-and-one-half year follow-up study. *Clin. Orthop.,* 263:147, 1989.
8. Hove, L.M., et al.: Prediction of secondary displacement in Colles' fracture. *J. Hand Surg. [Br],* 19:731, 1994.
9. Jakim, I., Pieterse, H.S., Sweet, M.B.E.: External fixation for intraarticular fractures of the distal radius. *J. Bone Joint Surg. [Br],* 73:302, 1991.
10. Kaempffe, F.A., Medige, J., Colluci M.: Biomechanical effects of wrist distraction: a cadaveric study. Presented at the Annual Meeting of the American Academy of Orthopaedic Surgeons, San Francisco, 1993.
11. Kongsholm, J., and Olerud, C.: Plaster cast versus external fixation for unstable intraarticular Colles' fractures. *Clin. Orthop.,* 241:57, 1989.
12. Leung, K.S., Shen, W.Y., et al.: Ligamentotaxis and bone grafting for comminuted fractures of the distal radius. *J. Bone Joint Surg. [Br],* 71:838, 1989.
13. Leung K.S., Shen W.Y., Tsang H.K., et al.: An effective treatment of comminuted fractures of the distal radius. *J. Hand Surg. [Am],* 15:11, 1990.
14. McBirnie, J., Court-Brown, C.M., McQueen M.M.: Early open reduction and bone grafting for unstable fractures of the distal radius. *J. Bone Joint Surg. [Br],* 77:571, 1995.
15. McQueen, M.M., Michie, M., Court-Brown, C.M.: Hand and wrist function after external fixation of unstable distal radial fractures. *Clin. Orthop.,* 283:200, 1992.
16. O'Flanagan, S.J., Ip, F.K., Roberts, C.J., Chow, S.P.: Carpal malalignment following intraarticular fractures of the distal radius in a working population. *Injury,* 26:231, 1995.
17. Sanders, R.A., Keppel, F.L., Waldrop, J.I.: External fixation of distal radial fractures: results and complications. *J. Hand Surg. [Am],* 16:385, 1991; *J. Bone Joint Surg. [Br],* 69:635, 1991.
18. Seitz, W.H. Jr., Froimson A.I., Leb R., et al.: Augmented external fixation of unstable distal radius fractures. *J. Hand Surg. [Am],* 16:1010, 1991.
19. Taleinik, J., and Watson, H.K.: Midcarpal instability caused by malunited fractures of the distal radius. *J. Hand Surg.,* 9:350, 1984.
20. Van der Linden, W., and Ericson, R.: Colles' fracture: how should its displacement be measured and how should it be immobilized? *J. Bone Joint Surg. [Am],* 63:1285, 1981.
21. Villar, R.N., Marsh, D., Rushton, N., Greatorex, R.A.: Three years after Colles' fracture: a prospective study. *J. Bone Joint Surg. [Br],* 69:635, 1987.

Master Techniques in Orthopaedic Surgery,
FRACTURES, edited by D. A. Wiss,
Lippincott–Raven Publishers, Philadelphia © 1998.

13

Distal Radial Fractures: Open Reduction Internal Fixation

Alan E. Freeland and William B. Geissler

INDICATIONS/CONTRAINDICATIONS

We define primary instability of distal radius fractures to include one or more of the following radiographic parameters: (a) more than 5 mm of radial shortening, (b) greater than 20 degrees loss of lateral inclination, (c) more than 2 mm of articulator step-off, and (d) comminution extending beyond the midaxial line. Outcomes of distal radial fractures parallel anatomic restoration. The goal for both reduction and result should include restoration of radial length to no more than 2 mm of shortening, no greater than 10 degrees loss of lateral inclination, no more than 2 mm of articular incongruity, and no more than 2 mm of dorsal or volar translation.

Closed manipulation alone is usually insufficient to maintain a reduction in unstable distal radial fractures. Unstable distal radial fractures that are reduced and casted frequently collapse. Therefore, some type of skeletal stabilization should be considered for unstable fractures after reduction. We prefer percutaneous or limited open Kirschner-wire (K-wire) fixation for these fractures.

When unstable distal radial fractures cannot be reduced or require bone grafting to fill and stabilize defects caused by comminution and impaction, the fracture is opened, reduced, bone grafted when required, and a plate is used for primary fixation. Plate fixation allows functional wrist positioning and early wrist and digital motion and rehabilitation while minimizing the risk of loss of reduction that may occur when K-wires or external fixation is removed. One or more K-wires still may be helpful in achieving or securing the overall construct in some patients.

A. E. Freeland, M.D., and W. B. Geissler, M.D.: Department of Orthopaedic Surgery and Rehabilitation, University of Mississippi Medical Center, Jackson, Mississippi 39216.

185

K-wires, external fixation, or combinations may be more appropriate to secure reduction in osteopenic bone and in instances of severe soft-tissue loss. They may be necessary in addition to plating when stability is uncertain after plate application and in cases in which there is cortical comminution on the surface opposite the plate. External fixation is initially used for distal radial fractures with severe articular comminution or loss. If the articular surface cannot be satisfactorily restored, early reconstruction may be indicated.

PREOPERATIVE PLANNING

The more severe the initial fracture displacement, the greater the need to restore normal anatomy. A thorough neurovascular examination is essential to identify arterial injuries or neurologic compromise or both. Palpation of the radial and ulnar pulses, as well as an assessment of color, warmth, and capillary filling of the hand, is helpful. An Allen test can be useful but is frequently limited because of pain. A motor and sensory examination should be performed distal to the fracture site. The median nerve is especially vulnerable to contusion and traction after displaced distal radial fractures. If an acute carpal tunnel syndrome or forearm compartment syndrome is identified, median nerve decompression should be considered at the time of fracture reduction, stabilization, or fasciotomy.

The distal radioulnar joint also should be assessed. Ulnar styloid fractures are common in severe distal radial fractures. These are more likely to be present when there is more than 2 mm of radial shortening. If the ulnar styloid fragment is large and displaced, it should probably be reduced and stabilized at the time of distal radial fracture treatment. The distal radioulnar joint can be clinically and radiographically examined after stabilization of the distal radial fracture, and in some instances, arthroscopic evaluation may be helpful.

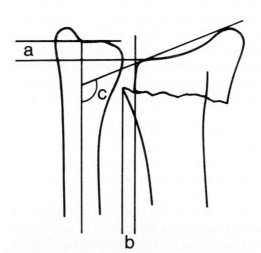 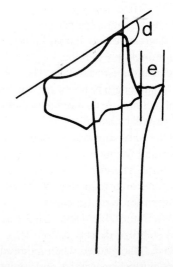

Figure 1. Anteroposterior radiographic parameters. Radial shortening **(a)**: the difference in level between the distal ulnar surface and the ulnar part of the distal radial surface. Radial displacement **(b)**: the displacement of the distal fragment in relation to the radial shaft. Radial angle **(c)**: the angle of the distal surface in relation to the long axis of the radius. (Reproduced with permission from ref. 1.)

Figure 2. Lateral radiographic parameters. Dorsal angle **(d)**: the angle of the distal radial surface in relation to the long axis of the radius. Dorsal displacement **(e)**: the distance of the distal radial fragment in relation to the radial shaft. (Reproduced with permission from ref. 1.)

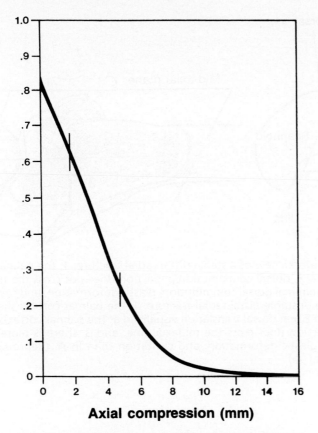

Figure 3. Estimated probability of an acceptable final anatomic position of a Colles' fracture as a function of radial axial shortening. (Reproduced with permission from ref. 1.)

Similarly, the carpus and intercarpal spaces can be evaluated on conventional wrist radiographs. Further evaluation such as stress radiographs or arthroscopy can be considered on an individual basis, remembering that the more severe the distal radius fracture, the more likely that an associated carpal or intercarpal injury may be present.

In all patients with significant wrist injuries, conventional posteroanterior and lateral radiographs should be obtained. If a distal radius and ulnar fracture is identified, the posteroanterior radiograph is evaluated for axial shortening, radial displacement, and radial angle/inclination (Fig. 1). The lateral radiograph is evaluated for dorsal angle/inclination and dorsal displacement (Fig. 2). Fractures with radial shortening of 2 mm or more are frequently unstable. Those with more than 5 mm displacement are almost always unstable (Fig. 3). Two mm or more of dorsal translation at the palmar cortex of the distal fragment has a high correlation with instability (positive shelf sign). Similarly, comminution or impaction extending past the midaxial line on lateral radiograph is highly correlated with instability (Fig. 4). Intraarticular displacement greater than 2 mm should be restored to minimize the chance of posttraumatic arthritis. The rule of two's is helpful in remembering these radiographic criteria (Table 1).

The principles of treatment of displaced extraarticular distal radial fractures are (a) anatomic or near anatomic fracture reduction; (b) bone grafting any significant defect (crossing the midaxial line) caused by comminution or impaction; and (c) stabilization of the fracture with a plate, K-wires, or a combination of the two. Continuous traction is instrumental in achieving and maintaining reduction.

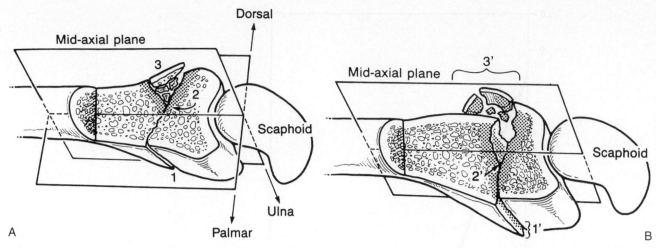

Figure 4. A: Lateral view of a stable distal radial fracture: 1, the palmar cortical shelf sign is negative; 2, dorsal comminution/impaction does not cross the midaxial plane; and 3, there is minimal dorsal comminution, plastic deformation, and cavitation. **B:** Lateral view of an unstable distal radial fracture: 1, the palmar cortical shelf sign is positive (more than 2-mm dorsal translation visualized at the palmar cortex); 2, dorsal comminution/impaction does cross the midaxial line; and 3, there is more severe dorsal comminution, plastic deformation, and cavitation than in **A**. (Reproduced with permission from ref. 4.)

Autogenous bone graft is most reliably obtained from the iliac crest. Small incisions minimize morbidity. The proximal ipsilateral olecranon is another source of autogenous bone. There is a small but very real risk of secondary fracture through the cortical defect at the ulnar donor site. Bone graft substitutes show great promise to decrease morbidity, hospitalization, and cost without compromising results, but currently neither number of cases nor the length of follow-up allows a firm unqualified endorsement in the distal radius. We have avoided allografting because of concerns of risk of infection and reliability and quality of bone healing.

In displaced *intraarticular* distal radial fractures, it is important to restore both the metaphysis and the articular surface. Once this is accomplished, the fracture is then evaluated and treated much as is an extraarticular fracture.

Palmarly displaced distal radial fractures with short oblique components are inherently unstable and require open reduction and internal fixation for optimal results. This is also true for the displaced distal medial ulnar die-punch fragments.

Although normal average parameters can be used for fracture restoration, posteroanterior and lateral radiographs of the uninvolved wrist often provide an excellent template for fracture repair.

TABLE 1. *Maximum allowable displacement leading to probable instability*

Intraarticular displacement	2 mm
Shortening	2 mm
Dorsal displacement (translation)	2 mm

Two millimeters or more in any one or more of these parameters probably signifies significant fracture instability. If it is not improved or restored, the probability of arthritis or functional deficit increases.

SURGERY

The patient is brought to the operating room and placed supine. An intravenous dose of a cephalosporin is administered to nonallergic patients. If the patient has an allergy, an alternative antibiotic is used. The patient is given a general or regional anesthetic for safety and comfort. The injured extremity is elevated and exsanguinated by using an Ace or Esmarch bandage before intravenous regional anesthesia or after general anesthesia. The extremity is prepped and draped in the usual routine sterile fashion.

Dorsally Displaced Distal Radial Fractures

A traction-assisted manipulative reduction of the distal radial fracture is performed. Traction is then applied manually through a pulley system applied through finger traps placed on the index and long fingers (Fig. 5A and B).

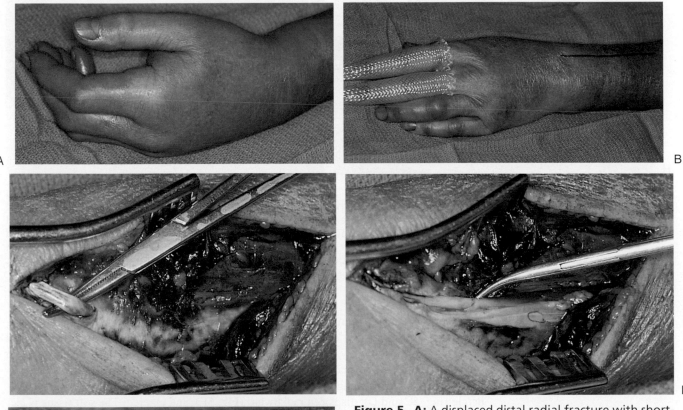

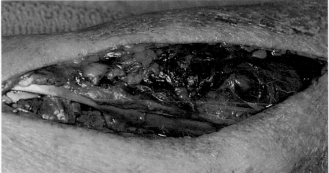

Figure 5. A: A displaced distal radial fracture with shortening, dorsal displacement, and swelling. **B:** Finger traps have been applied to the index and middle fingers and attached to a table-based traction apparatus. A closed manipulative reduction has been performed. The incision is outlined over the dorsum of the distal radius. **C:** The tendon sheath of the extensor pollicis longus has been opened just distal to the wrist retinaculum. The tendon has been identified and is isolated by a hemostat. **D:** The roof of the third dorsal compartment has been incised, exposing the extensor pollicis longus. A hemostat identifies the extensor pollicis longus just proximal to the wrist retinaculum. **E:** The extensor pollicis longus is allowed to displace radially outside the third dorsal compartment.

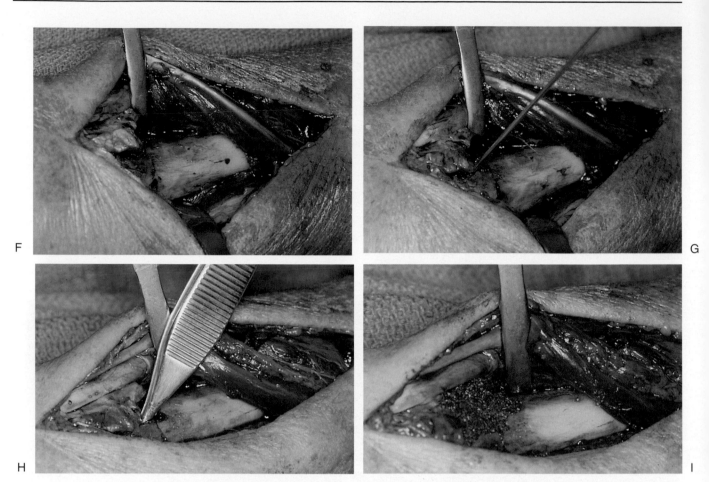

Figure 5. *(continued)* **F:** The floor of the third dorsal compartment is incised taking the surgeon directly to the fracture site. Subperiosteal dissection of the second and fourth dorsal compartments further exposes the fracture. The distal fragments still have some dorsal displacement and are not completely reduced. **G:** A K-wire is applied in the distal fragment for leverage and assistance with reduction. **H:** After reduction of the distal fragment, a bone cavity has been formed by comminution and impaction. **I:** The cavity is filled with compacted cancellous bone.

An approximately 10-cm incision is made on the dorsal radial side of the distal forearm, extending to the dorsal wrist crease. This is made over the midaspect of the distal radius with the aid of fluoroscopy, just lateral to Lister's tubercle. The incision is carried through the subcutaneous tissue, and bleeding is controlled with electrocoagulation. The third dorsal compartment containing the extensor pollicis longus is incised just ulnar to Lister's tubercle (Fig. 5C and D), displaced radialward (Fig. 5E), and entered. The soft tissue is elevated from the distal radius to both sides, reflecting the fourth dorsal compartment and its tendons, including the extensor digitorum communis and the extensor indicis proprius ulnarward and the second dorsal compartment containing the extensor carpi radialis brevis and longus radialward (Fig. 5F). The periosteal dissection is continued radialward and a small Hohmann retractor is placed to enhance exposure. The retractor is placed beneath the periosteum protecting the abductor pollicis longus and extensor pollicis brevis in the first dorsal compartment and the adjacent brachioradialis muscle. Similarly, a small Hohmann retractor may be placed subperiosteally on the ulnar side near the distal radius to protect the extrinsic finger extensors.

Bone-reduction clamps, small smooth K-wires, a bone distractor, or an external fixator may be used to help manipulate extraarticular distal radial fractures into alignment (Fig. 5G). Sometimes these maneuvers are sufficient to reduce intraarticular fragments as well.

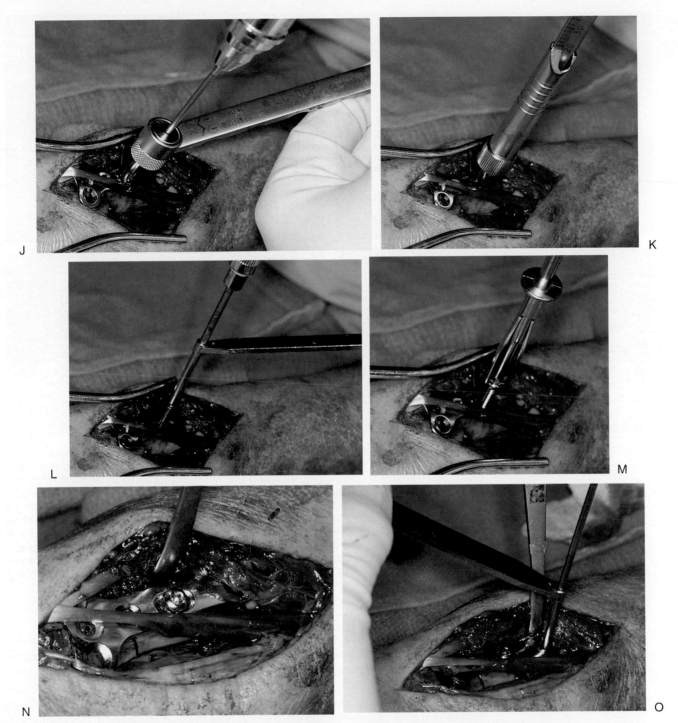

Figure 5. *(continued)* **J:** A neutral drill guide (color-coded green) is used from the small fragment set to center the drill in the elliptic hole in the stem of the T-plate. A 2.5-mm hole is drilled. **K:** A calibrated depth gauge is used to determine the depth of the screw hole. **L:** The screw hole is tapped with a 3.5-mm tap. **M:** A 3.5-mm screw is applied, securing the plate at its elliptical hole on the stem. C-arm fluoroscopy can be used and final adjustments made in the position of the T-plate. **N:** The T-plate coapted to the distal radius, buttressing and securing the distal fracture fragment. The extensor pollicis longus overlies the T-plate. *(figure continues)*

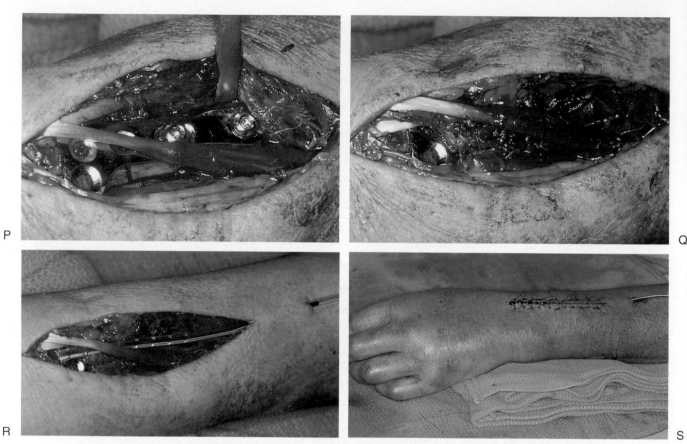

Figure 5. *(continued)* **O, P:** A round drill guide is used to drill a hole in the proximal stem. The process of the screw-hole preparation is completed and a second screw applied. The fracture is now secure, allowing the wrist and forearm to be taken through a full range of motion. Because the metaphysis was somewhat osteopenic, we elected not to place any screws in the bar of the plate through the distal fragment, allowing it to act as a buttress. **Q:** The dorsal retinaculum is sutured over the T-plate, providing some protection to the overlying tendons. **R:** A small hemovac drain is placed deep in the incisional wound and brought out through a separate proximal and dependent stab. **S:** Suturing is completed in layers, leaving the deep dorsal fascia open. Note the correction of the deformity but the persistence of residual hand and digital swelling and ecchymosis.

K-wires, Steinmann pins, a dental pick, or bone impactors are often helpful in restoring displaced intraarticular fragments. Reduction can be monitored by C-arm fluoroscopy or arthroscopy or both. Bone defects caused by comminution and impaction should be bone grafted (Fig. 5H).

Cancellous bone can be harvested from the ilium through limited incisions by using trephination drills or currettes and gouges. The bone cylinders obtained in this fashion can be used directly, or the cancellous bone can be compacted by using a 10-ml syringe and compressing the plunger (Fig. 6A–C). Compacted cancellous bone can then be removed from the cylinder of the syringe with a long spinal needle (Fig. 6D). When the bone grafting is completed (Fig. 5I), the fracture is usually stabilized by a minifragment dorsal T-plate (Fig. 5J–P). The plate can be contoured with bending irons for precise coaptation to the dorsal distal radius (Fig. 7A–C). K-wires, regular screws, or cannulated screws can be used to secure intraarticular fragments. As an alternative or adjunct to plate fixation, K-wires may be used to secure the metaphysis to the diaphysis, especially in osteopenic bone. Whenever possible, the dorsal retinaculum of the wrist is repaired (Fig. 5Q). This protects the extensor tendons from direct abrasion over the plate and screws during wrist and digital motion. The extensor pollicis longus is left radially displaced outside of its compartment. A small

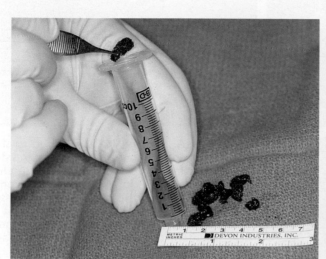

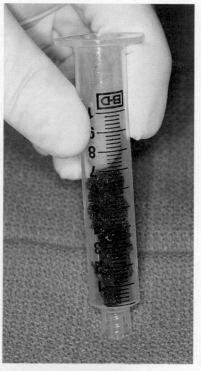

A

B

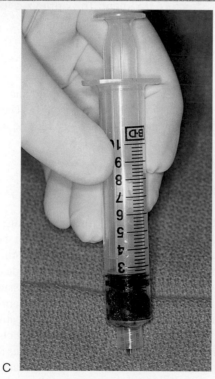

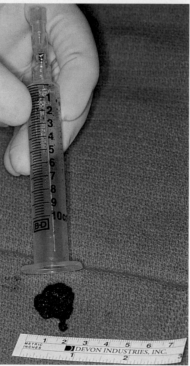

C

D

Figure 6. A: Pieces of cancellous bone taken by curettage from the ilium are placed in the barrel of a 10-ml syringe. **B:** The syringe is filled. **C:** The plunger compacts the cancellous bone. **D:** A no. 18 spinal needle is used to dislodge the compacted cancellous bone.

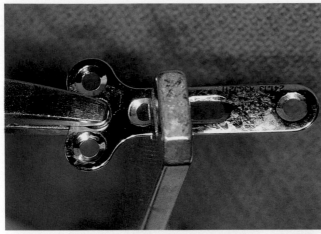

A

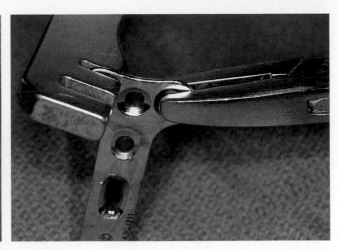

B

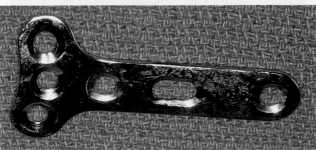

C

Figure 7. A: Bending irons are used to shape the T-plate and bend it between the bar and the stem. A bend should continually go in one direction. Bending forward and then backward in alternating directions decreases the fatigue life of the plate and weakens it. **B:** Two bending irons are used to shape the bar of the T-plate into a curve that will better approximate the distal fracture fragment. **C:** Contouring of the plate has been completed so that it has a very close fit over the reduced fracture fragment. This optimizes its stabilizing buttress function.

suction hemovac drain is placed deep in the operative wound and brought out proximally and dependently through a separate small incision (Fig. 5R). The deep fascia is not repaired. The subcutaneous tissue is reapproximated by using fine absorbable sutures. The skin is closed with fine nonabsorbable sutures (Fig. 5S).

Palmarly Displaced Distal Radial Fractures

Palmarly displaced short oblique distal radial fractures and displaced or rotated distal palmar ulnar die-punch fragments should be approached through a palmar incision. Either manual traction or traction applied through a pulley system by using finger traps is usually sufficient to achieve initial reduction. The palmar incision is made directly over the flexor carpi radialis (Fig. 8A). It is carried through the subcutaneous tissue, and bleeding is controlled with electrocoagulation. The palmar sheath of the flexor carpi radialis is incised longitudinally (Fig. 8B) and the tendon retracted. The posterior sheath of the flexor carpi radialis is incised longitudinally (Fig. 8C), exposing the flexor pollicis longus (Fig. 8D). The flexor pollicis longus and the radial artery and accompanying veins are retracted radialward (Fig. 8E). The median nerve and extrinsic flexor tendons are retracted ulnarward to expose the pronator quadratus. The insertion of the pronator quadratus is incised longitudinally along the palmar radial border of the distal radius at its insertion, leaving a small cuff of tissue that can be sutured during closure (Fig. 8F).

Again, K-wires, a dental elevator, an awl, or tenacular clamp may be helpful in completing the reduction (Fig. 8G). C-Arm fluoroscopy or arthroscopy or both, in cases of intraarticular fractures, also may be helpful. Once the reduction is achieved, K-wires are used for provisional fixation (Fig. 8H). A palmar small-fragment T-plate is then applied (Fig. 8I–L). The first screw is placed through the elliptical hole of the T-plate near the juncture of the stem and bar. This allows some freedom in adjusting the plate after application of the

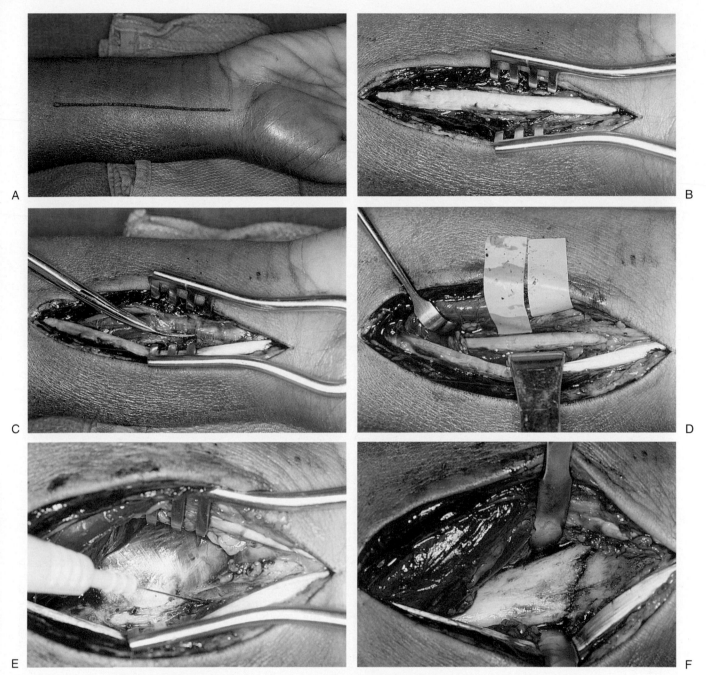

Figure 8. A: An incision is drawn over the distal portion of the flexor carpi radialis to approach a Thomas Type II or volar Barton's fracture. **B:** Subcutaneous tissue and anterior sheath over the flexor carpi radialis have been incised. **C:** The posterior sheath and deep antebrachial fascia are incised. **D:** The flexor pollicis longus and median nerve are identified. **E:** The flexor pollicis longus and median nerve are retracted and protected. The pronator quadratus is identified and incised along its radial insertion. **F:** The pronator quadratus is elevated from the periosteum of the distal radius, exposing the fracture.

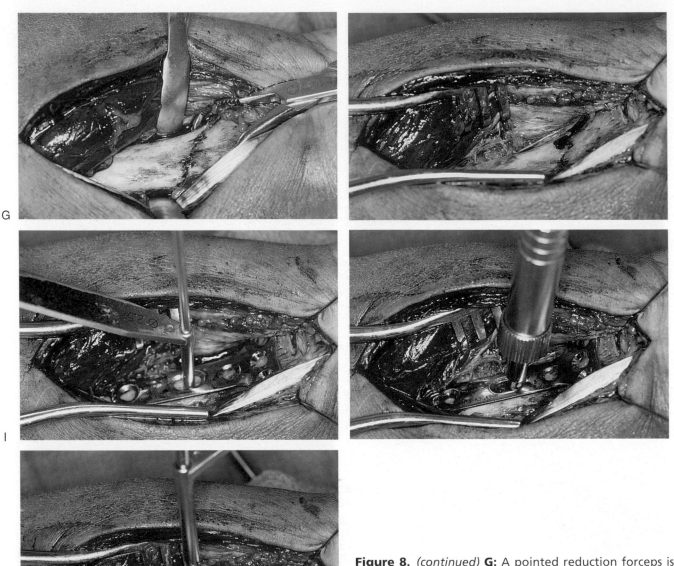

Figure 8. *(continued)* **G:** A pointed reduction forceps is used for fracture reduction. **H:** K-wires transfix the reduced fracture fragment. **I:** A contoured T-plate is placed over the fracture site. A hole is drilled in the elliptical hole of the stem by using the circular drill guide. **J:** The depth gauge identifies the screw length needed by measuring the depth of the drill hole. **K:** The screw hole is prepared with a 3.5-mm tap.

first screw. If necessary, contouring can be done with bending irons to ensure that there is good coaptation between the plate and the reduced fracture. The most proximal hole of the stem of the T-plate is aligned and secured with a screw. Screws may be placed through the bar of the plate to secure the fracture, although this is not always necessary (Fig. 8M). The screws nearest the fracture are usually angulated away from the fracture for more secure fixation. Screws are not placed directly into the fracture site. For displaced or rotated distal volar ulnar die-punch fragments, 2.7 minifragment T- or angle-plates are often useful.

Comminution and bone loss requiring bone grafting on the palmar side of the fractures are infrequent. Nevertheless, if there is bone loss or impaction of any consequence, cancellous bone grafting can be undertaken in a fashion similar to that of dorsally displaced distal radial fractures.

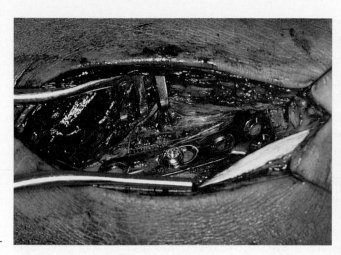

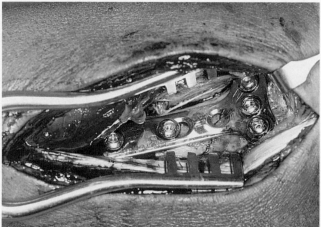

L

M

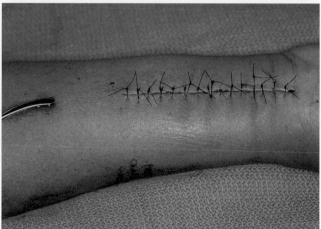

Figure 8. *(continued)* **L:** The plate is secured with a screw in the elliptical hole of the stem of the T-plate. Final adjustments can be made by using fluoroscopic C-arm control. **M:** The remainder of the screws are used to secure the plate with the fracture in a reduced position. The plate buttresses and stabilizes the fracture. **N:** A small hemovac drain is brought out proximally and dependently to the incision. The incision is closed in layers, leaving the deep fascia open.

N

Once reduction, fixation, and bone grafting are complete, the tourniquet is released, and hemostatis is obtained. Vascularization of the digits can be assessed during the period of reactive hyperemia. The wound is copiously irrigated with sterile saline containing antibiotics. The insertion of the pronator quadratus can be reapproximated by using interrupted absorbable sutures when this can be done without undue tension. We prefer to lay the pronator quadratus over the palmar surface of the distal radius without suturing it to avoid any vascular embarrassment of the muscle that might be caused by postoperative swelling. We have not seen any functional problems with this approach. A small hemovac suction drain is placed deep in the wound and brought out proximally and dependently through a separate small incision. Fine resorbable sutures can be used to reapproximate the subcutaneous tissue. The deep fascia is not repaired to avoid postoperative neurovascular embarrassment such as compartment syndrome. The skin is reapproximated. Interrupted or subcuticular nonabsorbable sutures are used (Fig. 8N). Steri-strips can be used to supplement subcuticular suturing. In some instances, staple sutures may be preferred.

POSTOPERATIVE MANAGEMENT

The patient is placed in a soft, sterile conforming hand dressing with extra padding over bony prominences and superficial neurovascular structures. This is carried above the elbow to prevent rotational forces at the fracture site. Padding is placed in the antecubital fossa, over the olecranon, and over the lateral and medial epicondyles to protect these structures and the underlying ulnar nerve. A long-arm posterior splint is applied with the elbow at 90 degrees of flexion, the forearm in neutral rotation, the wrist in 10 to 15 degrees of dorsiflexion (functional position), the thumb palmar abducted, and the thumb web space maintained. The fingers are free.

The patient is instructed to keep the arm at or above the level of the heart during the first 7 to 10 days. A sling is provided for ambulation, and some patients also use this when sitting down. Pillows on the side of a chair can be used as an alternative when the patient is sitting. When the patient is lying down, the wrist can be supported on the abdomen or chest with or without pillows or on pillows next to the patient. The drain is removed 24 to 48 h after surgery.

One of the most important advantages of open reduction, internal fixation, and bone grafting is that there is sufficient stability at the fracture site to place the wrist in a position of function. In this position, the digits can be rehabilitated more easily. We initially encourage 10 repetitions of progressive digital range-of-motion exercises within the patient's tolerance every hour while awake, if possible. We believe that restoration of good finger motion will positively influence wrist recovery. When full finger motion is achieved, the patient is able to use the hand and wrist after splint immobilization is discontinued. This will be an advantage in regaining wrist motion.

Rehabilitation of the wrist and digits is divided into arbitrary and overlapping stages. A knowledge and understanding of these stages is helpful to the patient, the family, the therapist, and the physician. These stages are (a) healing; (b) motion; (c) strength and power; (d) endurance; and (e) return to activities of daily living, work, and recreation.

Sutures are removed approximately 7 to 10 days after surgery. At this time, the long-arm plaster posterior splint is removed and replaced either with a volar wrist-support splint or a short-arm cast. The patient is asked not to rotate the forearm actively. Ordinarily, immobilization is continued for 3 weeks. Depending on the security of the fixation and the compliance of the patient, this period of protection can be adjusted to longer or shorter intervals. At 3 weeks, the patient is converted to a thermoplastic or prefabricated volar wrist-support splint. This allows the patient to maintain functional position of the wrist, preventing extensor tenodesis effect on the digits while allowing the patient to participate in finger rehabilitation. The patient is then started on warm-water soaks for 10 minutes 3 times a day. For the first 5 minutes, the patient is asked to concentrate on 10 repetitions of finger-motion exercises, wrist flexion and extension, wrist ulnar and radial deviation, and wrist circumduction. Pronation and supination also are carried out. Ten repetitions of each exercise are performed with the palm up, the palm down, and the thumb up. This moves and independently exercises wrist and digital flexors and extensors with and against gravity and with gravity eliminated. For the second 5 minutes, the patient is asked to start gentle progressive strengthening exercises by using a household sponge in the water.

Simultaneous edema and scar management is implemented. Elevation and digital range-of-motion exercises should help physically to pump edema fluid out of the extremity and to help circulation and prevent tendon adhesions. Retrograde massage, Coban wrapping, compression stockinette, Isotoner glove, or other compression garments and a Jobst pump or home Jobst pump can be used at the discretion of the physician and therapist.

Scar management is undertaken to soften, desensitize, and mobilize scar tissue. Massage is effective in this regard for up to 6 months from the time of injury or surgery. This is supplemented by vibration, soft polymeric silicone (Silastic) elastomer and Coban, and desensitization techniques as indicated.

As the patient's wrist motion improves, more aggressive resistance exercises can be advanced by using the hand helper and other grip strengtheners. At about 6 to 8 weeks, and depending on signs of fracture healing on radiograph, strengthening can be accomplished through the use of finger, wrist, and forearm curls and reverse curls. Endurance exercises begin with 10 repetitions and increase to 30 repetitions by using 50% of the patient's maximum lift. Once 30 repetitions have been reached, ½ to 1 pound can be added and the process repeated until the patient plateaus. Once the patient has plateaued, maintenance can be done 2 to 3 times a week.

Return to work requires striking a delicate balance between our primary responsibility to each patient and our responsibility to employers, third-party payors, and society. The patient responsibility is primal. Fulfill this conscientiously, and you will automatically and simultaneously fulfill the remaining responsibilities. The patient must be safe, within his or her pain tolerance, productive, and able to satisfy the employer before returning to work. Two factors affect this more than any others: whether the dominant or nondominant hand is injured, and the degree of physical demand of the job. Patients can expect to return to low-demand or self-paced professional or sales work at 2 to 4 weeks after injury. Injuries to the dominant hand may require 4 to 8 weeks longer, especially for craftsmen or surgeons. Laborers may require even longer (i.e., 3- to 4-month minimum) and may require work simulation, work hardening, and gradual phasing or ramping back to their job. Some laborers with severe fractures may have to retrain for lower demand occupations.

Athletes may return to throwing and catching at short distances at 1 to 2 months after injury. Velocity, distance, and frequency are integrated with a strength and conditioning program over the next 1 to 2 months and until full recovery is achieved. Impact activities such as short volleys (tennis), putting (golf), and bat contact (baseball) are started at 6 to 10 weeks after injury and increased as tolerated over the following 1 to 2 months. It takes 4 to 6 months on the average to achieve full motion and 1 year to achieve full strength with normal serves and ground strokes (tennis), driving and short iron games (golf), and full-swing contact (baseball).

Results

Outcomes, as measured by objective parameters such as range of motion, grip strength, and time to return to work and athletics, correlate highly first with fracture severity, second with anatomic restoration, and third with the physical demand of the patient's activities. Approximately one third of patients will have significant residual impairments. The majority of these are in patients with more severe fractures in which difficulty of restoration correlates with the fracture severity (6).

Outcome instruments such as a short-form general health survey (SF-36), the Arthritis Impact Measurement Scale (AIMS), and the Brigham and Women's Hospital carpal tunnel questionnaire are even more sensitive and comprehensive in assessing each patient's progress, problems, and result. These instruments should be a great help in treatment, rehabilitation, problem intervention, cost control, and rapport with patients, third-party payors, and employers.

COMPLICATIONS

Malunion

Early and late loss of reduction and consequent extraarticular malunion occurs in about 5% of patients (6). An unstable fracture that is reduced and casted will frequently lose reduction. An unstable fracture with a defect or impaction that is reduced and stabilized but not bone grafted may undergo a late loss of reduction. Consequently, it is important to identify those fractures that are inherently unstable. These fractures should be reduced, stabilized, and bone grafted. The bone grafting may in fact be the most critical of these three components.

Posttraumatic Arthritis

In addition to radial deformity, ulnar carpal impingement and carpal collapse resulting from radial shortening and loss of dorsal inclination can impair functional recovery and lead to posttraumatic arthritis. Intraarticular malunion can lead to posttraumatic arthritis in 90% of patients with 2 mm or more of articular incongruity as opposed to 10% with 1 mm or less of offset (12). Posttraumatic arthritis resulting from intraarticular malunion occurs with an incidence of about 6.5% of the total of distal radial fractures (6).

Median Neuropathy

Whereas the ulnar and radial sensory nerves should be carefully evaluated and monitored, the median nerve is most frequently injured in distal radial fractures. Up to 60% of distal radial fractures may have some symptoms of median nerve compromise (7). The initial injury can be from traction or compression; however, swelling and wrist positioning also play a role. Excessive wrist flexion and local anesthetic injections are problematic. Early fracture reduction and stabilization can minimize nerve damage and relieve symptoms of acute carpal tunnel or compartment syndromes. Carpal tunnel syndrome occurs in between 12% and 17% of distal radial fractures (15), whereas compartment syndrome has an incidence of 0.7% (6).

If the median neuropathy is initially complete or if it is progressive after reduction and stabilization, the nerve should be surgically decompressed and inspected. We prefer to decompress a compromised median nerve at the time of open reduction, internal fixation, and bone grafting. This prevents a catastrophic event with certainty, clarifies the exact condition of the nerve, and minimizes both the extent and duration of the nerve injury. Early carpal tunnel release does increase the total composite trauma to the wrist, hand, and extremity, and the risks of increased scarring, including tendon adhesions.

The median nerve carries 70% of the sympathetic fibers to the hand. Early decompression of persistent median neuropathies may alleviate or diminish sympathetic-mediated pain responses and their consequent dystrophic changes and complications, including persistent neuropathy (8% incidence), shoulder/hand syndrome (3.5% incidence), posttraumatic Depuytren's disease (11% incidence), and finger stiffness (1.5% incidence; 6,15).

Associated Carpal or Intercarpal Injuries

The carpal bones and intercarpal spaces should be examined on routine radiographs. Early concomitant repair of carpal fractures and wrist-ligament injuries at the time of distal radial fracture treatment usually provides the best opportunity for optimizing results. Arthroscopy after distal radial reduction and stabilization shows some promise in identifying and treating more occult lesions, especially those of the triangular fibrocartilage complex and the lunotriquetral ligaments.

Extensor Tendon Adhesions and Irritation

Extensor tendon ruptures, usually of the extensor pollicis longus, occur in about 1% of distal radial fractures (6). Extensor tendon adhesions are less well documented but do occur and are troublesome. These problems can result from dissection as well as plate application. New, lower profile plates that protect the tendons from both the plate and screw heads are currently under evaluation as a means to improve or minimize the problem. Extensor pollicis longus disruption can be prevented by anatomic reduction techniques and the avoidance of bone fragments or sharp edges near it. We have not seen any problems specifically from moving the extensor pollicis longus from its sheath and rerouting it radialward. Stable fracture fixation and early active wrist motion may be the best remedy for tendon adhesions and joint ankylosis.

Nonunion

Nonunion is rare in distal radial fractures but may occur in severe fractures. Soft-tissue loss, bone loss, comminution, and devascularization can play a role. Stable fixation and early bone grafting are usually necessary. Sometimes injury severity and osteopenia preclude successful treatment. Wrist fusion may be necessary for salvage.

Infection

Infection is rarely seen in closed distal radial fractures even after surgery. Injury severity or systemic compromise or both are usually implicated when infection does occur. Infection is identified by the classic signs of heat, redness, pain, and swelling. Fluctuance or drainage confirm the diagnosis when present. Treatment of cellulitis is by elevation and rest of the wrist and by intravenous or oral antibiotics. Purulence must be drained and any necrotic tissue debrided. Stable fixation should be continued until the fracture is healed.

ILLUSTRATIVE CASES FOR TECHNIQUE

Unstable Extraarticular Distal Radial Fracture with Dorsal Displacement

A 61-year-old woman fell while skating. She sustained a closed extraarticular distal radial fracture (Fig. 9A and B). There was 4 mm of radial shortening compared with the uninjured wrist. The lateral radiograph revealed 3 mm of dorsal translation, 30 degrees of loss of lateral inclination, and dorsal translation of the carpus on the distal radius. A bone defect could be seen on anteroposterior radiograph after fracture reduction (Fig. 9C) extending beyond the midaxial line on lateral radiograph (Fig. 9D), adding to fracture instability. After further restoration of lateral inclination by using K-wire manipulation, the defect was even larger (Fig. 9E).

A dorsal incision was made over the distal radius. Adjustments were made to achieve a final reduction that was near anatomic. Compacted cancellous bone graft was taken from the ilium, and the defect was filled. The fracture was stabilized with 3.5-mm small-fragment T-plate used in the buttress mode to complete the construct (Fig. 9F and G). Passive motion was recorded at the time of surgery to use as a guideline during rehabilitation.

Displaced Intraarticular Fracture with Bone Defect

A 42-year-old homemaker sustained a closed intraarticular fracture of the distal radius with a displaced and impacted midradial die-punch fragment (Fig. 10A and B). Articular displacement was 2 mm on AP radiograph and 3 mm on lateral radiograph. The distal radius was approached by a dorsal incision. A trephination drill was used to access the intramedullary canal of the distal radius proximal to the fracture (Fig. 10C and D). A bone impactor was introduced into the hole and advanced (Fig. 10E). With fluoroscopic control, the fragment was reduced by using the impactor (Fig. 10F–H). The visible bone defect (Fig. 10I) was filled by using pieces of compacted cancellous bone (Fig. 10J). These were ad-

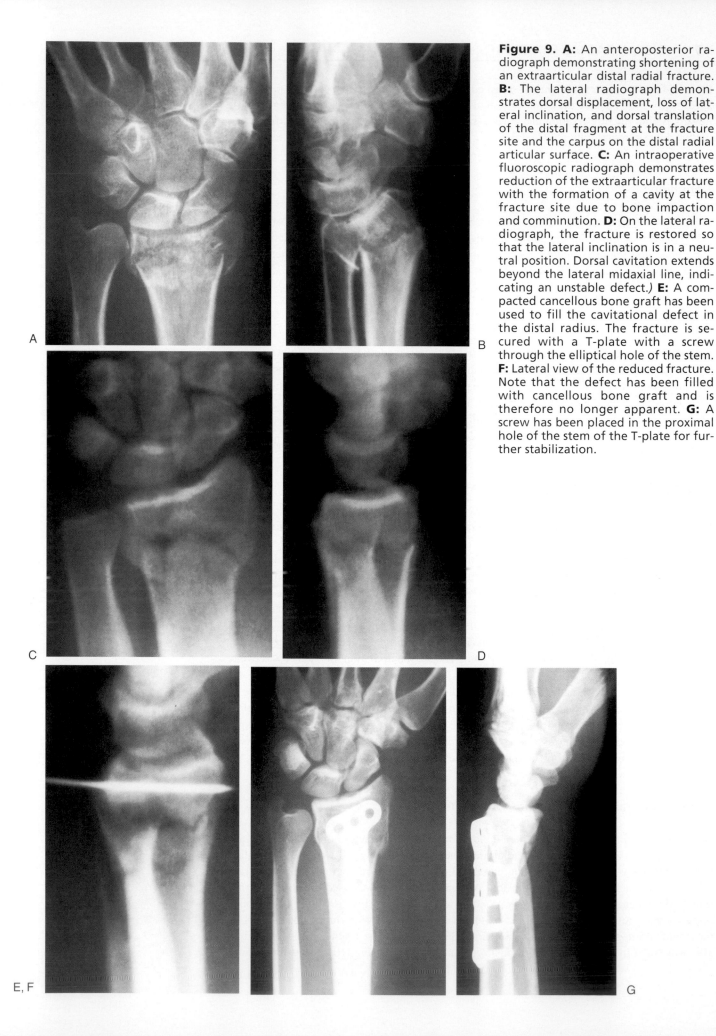

Figure 9. A: An anteroposterior radiograph demonstrating shortening of an extraarticular distal radial fracture. **B:** The lateral radiograph demonstrates dorsal displacement, loss of lateral inclination, and dorsal translation of the distal fragment at the fracture site and the carpus on the distal radial articular surface. **C:** An intraoperative fluoroscopic radiograph demonstrates reduction of the extraarticular fracture with the formation of a cavity at the fracture site due to bone impaction and comminution. **D:** On the lateral radiograph, the fracture is restored so that the lateral inclination is in a neutral position. Dorsal cavitation extends beyond the lateral midaxial line, indicating an unstable defect.) **E:** A compacted cancellous bone graft has been used to fill the cavitational defect in the distal radius. The fracture is secured with a T-plate with a screw through the elliptical hole of the stem. **F:** Lateral view of the reduced fracture. Note that the defect has been filled with cancellous bone graft and is therefore no longer apparent. **G:** A screw has been placed in the proximal hole of the stem of the T-plate for further stabilization.

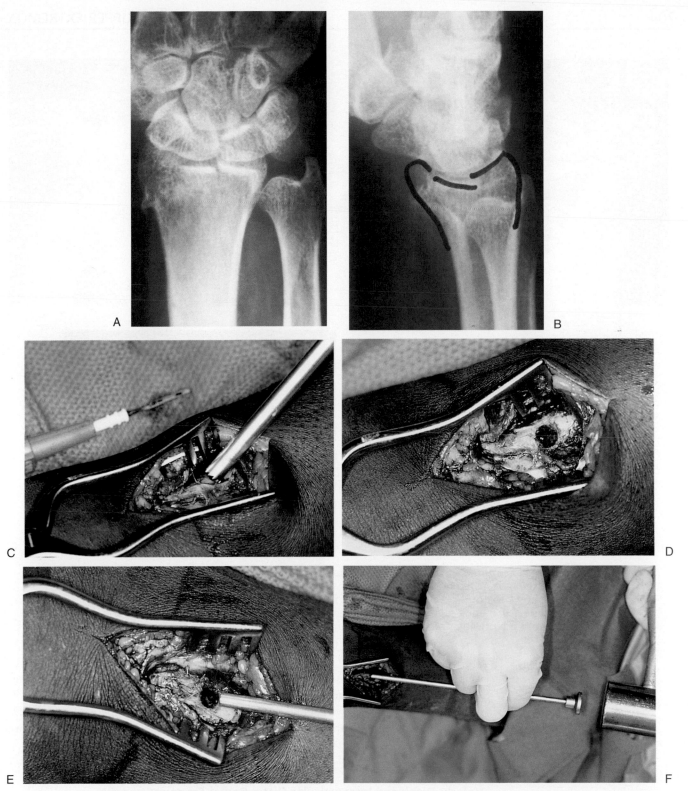

Figure 10. A: An anteroposterior (AP) radiograph of the wrist shows an intraarticular fracture of the distal radius with three major and nearly equal intraarticular fragments. The middle fragment, in particular, is impacted and displaced proximally. There is articular incongruity of 2 mm. **B:** On the lateral radiograph, there is an intraarticular distal radial fracture with impaction and loss of articular congruity of 3 mm. **C:** A trephination drill is used to access the intramedullary cavity of the distal radius proximal to the fracture site. **D:** The hole created by the trephine drill is visualized. **E:** A bone impactor is introduced into the trephinated hole. **F:** The impactor is advanced and held in position. The position of the impacted and displaced fracture fragment can be restored by manually transmitted pressure or with a mallet by using fluoroscopic radiographic control.

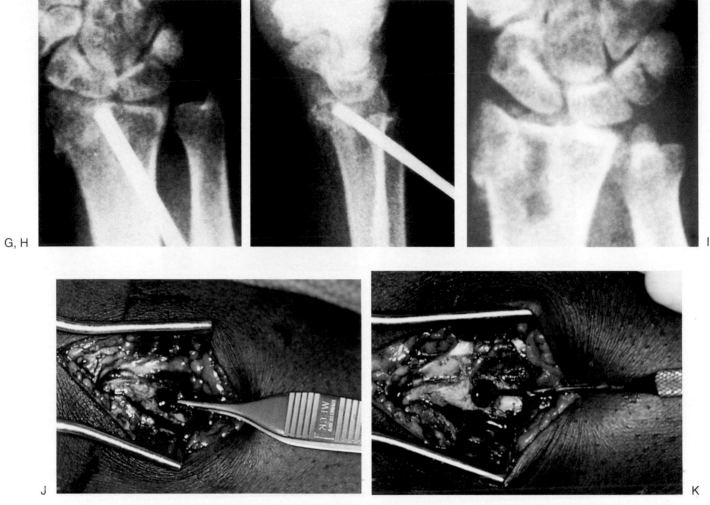

G, H

I

J

K

Figure 10. *(continued)* **G:** Fluoroscopic radiograph showing the depressed fracture fragment in a restored position after use of the impaction device. **H:** The lateral radiograph shows restoration of the displaced fracture fragment by using the bone-impaction device. **I:** Bone cavity underlying the restored intraarticular fragment. **J:** A bone graft is placed into the defect. **K:** A dental impactor is used to position the bone graft.

vanced and used to buttress and fill the defect by using a dental impactor (Figs. 10K and L). The fracture was further secured with a construct of two K-wires securing the styloid fragment to the shaft and two parallel K-wires placed parallel to the articular surface of the subchondral region of the three intraarticular fragments of the distal radius (Fig. 10M and N).

Volarly Displaced Intraarticular Distal Radial Fracture

A 29-year-old factory worker sustained a closed, volarly displaced, two-piece distal radius fracture in a motor vehicle accident (Fig. 11A and B). A palmar approach was used over the distal radius. Reduction was completed with a tenacular clamp (Fig. 11C and D). Provisional fixation was achieved with K-wires (Fig. 11E and F). A 3.5-mm small-fragment T-plate was contoured to the fracture and secured in the buttress mode (Fig. 11G and H). A screw hole overlying the fracture was left unfilled. Screws through the bar of the plate were applied in lag-screw fashion to achieve compression of the underlying fracture fragment (Fig. 11I and J).

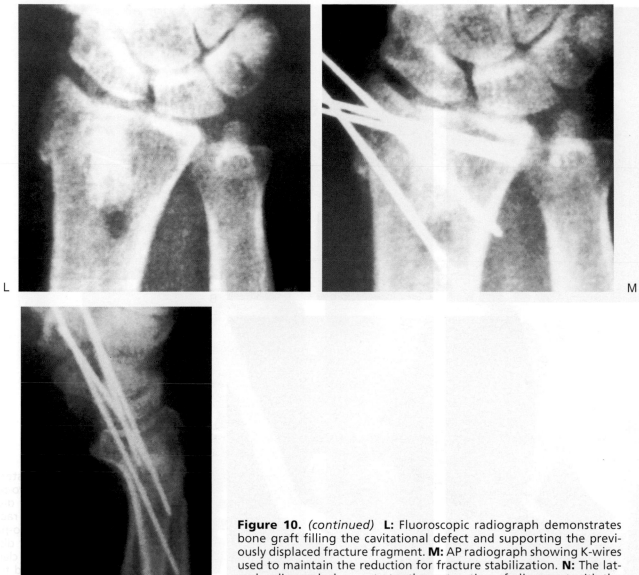

Figure 10. *(continued)* **L:** Fluoroscopic radiograph demonstrates bone graft filling the cavitational defect and supporting the previously displaced fracture fragment. **M:** AP radiograph showing K-wires used to maintain the reduction for fracture stabilization. **N:** The lateral radiograph demonstrates the restoration of alignment with the bone-grafted and K-wire–secured distal radial fracture.

RECOMMENDED READING

PART II

Lower Extremity

Master Techniques in Orthopaedic Surgery,
FRACTURES, edited by D. A. Wiss,
Lippincott–Raven Publishers, Philadelphia © 1998.

14

Femoral Neck Fractures: Open Reduction Internal Fixation

Marc F. Swiontkowski

INDICATIONS/CONTRAINDICATIONS

The indication for open reduction and internal fixation of a femoral neck fracture is a displaced femoral neck fracture in patients with adequate bone density, regardless of age. Nondisplaced or valgus impacted femoral neck fractures also may benefit from a limited anterior capsulotomy without complete visualization of the fracture. Open reduction of the femoral neck is done for two reasons. The first is to evacuate the intracapsular hematoma, which has been shown adversely to affect femoral head circulation. Because no significant blood supply is carried to the femoral head from the anterior hip capsule, an anterior approach to the femoral neck does no additional harm to the circulation of the femoral head (12). The second reason for open reduction is to optimize the reduction of the femoral neck before internal fixation. The accuracy of the reduction and density of the femoral head and neck have been shown to be the two most important factors in achieving stability after internal fixation of a femoral neck fracture. Even fractures that appear to be well reduced under fluoroscopic control can be markedly displaced on direct visualization, particularly in rotation. Because the femoral head is rendered relatively ischemic by the fracture and displacement, the internal fixation should be considered a relative orthopaedic emergency. Attempts to perform the surgery within 8 hours in the highest risk groups (patients younger than 50 years, including children) have improved outcome (10).

The contraindications for open reduction and internal fixation of a femoral neck fracture include rheumatoid arthritis or moderate osteoarthritis of the adjacent hip joint, poor bone density, limited life expectancy, and pathologic fractures related to metastatic disease. These patients are better treated by arthroplasty.

For purposes of patient selection, assessment of the primary and secondary compression and tension trabeculae on the admitting radiographs, as described by Singh (6), is helpful.

M. F. Swiontkowski, M.D.: Department of Orthopaedic Surgery, University of Minnesota Medical School, Minneapolis, Minnesota 55455.

However, the most critical element is a good history from the patient or family or both regarding the preinjury physical function. Multiple medical comorbidities or limited function or both direct the surgeon toward arthroplasty. Patients with major medical comorbidities benefit from evaluation and treatment of their associated medical condition for up to 48 hours before surgery. These elderly and often sick patients generally benefit from arthroplasty (3).

PREOPERATIVE PLANNING

After appropriate medical evaluation and treatment, the patient should semiurgently be brought to the operating room. Bucks traction has not been helpful in pain management before surgery, probably because it tightens the anterior hip capsule and limits capsular volume (1). An anteroposterior (AP) view and cross-table lateral radiographs are usually sufficient for diagnosis and planning treatment. However, an AP radiograph of the pelvis may be helpful in evaluating bone density, as well as helping to determine the neck–shaft angle if there is comminution at the femoral neck fracture site.

Multiple-injured patients must be fully evaluated in a rapid manner and cleared in terms of abdominal, chest, or head injury. In patients with multiple orthopaedic injuries, the femoral neck fracture should take priority over most other closed injuries. Approximately 3% to 5% of patients with diaphyseal fractures of the femoral shaft will have a concomitant ipsilateral femoral neck fracture (10). High-quality radiographs of the hip and knee must be included in the evaluation of all patients with femoral shaft fractures. Unfortunately, neither technetium 99 methyldiphosphate bone scans nor magnetic resonance imaging (MRI) can reliably differentiate patients who will develop posttraumatic osteonecrosis and are not useful, in the short term, in selecting patients for either open reduction and internal fixation or arthroplasty (7,9).

SURGERY

General, epidural, or spinal anesthesia may be used; however, spinal or epidural techniques are the best choices for older patients with medical problems. Patients may be positioned with the extremity draped freely in the supine position on a radiolucent table (Fig. 1A) or on a fracture table in the supine position. If the latter is chosen (which is the best method for obtaining high-quality lateral radiographs), only light traction should be applied to the limb, which allows some ability to manipulate the leg during surgery. If the former is chosen, the lateral image is obtained by externally rotating the limb after achieving temporary fixation.

The surgical approach is done through a straight lateral skin incision similar to that used for placement of a sliding hip screw in an intertrochanteric fracture. The incision must be curved anterior toward the gluteal pillar of the iliac crest in obese or muscular patients, which allows easier dissection of the distal interval between the tensor fascia and gluteus medius muscles (Fig. 1B).

The deep fascia is divided in line with the shin incision and the interval between the tensor fascia and gluteus medius muscles (Watson–Jones approach) developed (Fig. 1C and D). The hip capsule is identified by sweeping the pericapsular fat medially and inserting a Hohmann retractor along the anterior acetabular rim (Fig. 1E). The capsule is opened along the axis of the femoral neck (Fig. 1F). This can be done with minimal soft-tissue stripping, allowing the surgeon to assess the reduction of the femoral neck fracture directly and with biplane fluoroscopic control. A no. 15 blade on a no. 7 handle can be used under fluoroscopic control to limit the deep dissection.

An intracapsular hematoma under significant pressure is encountered in about 15% of patients, regardless of the amount of fracture displacement or age of the patient (2). The surgeon must be convinced that the femoral neck fracture is anatomic before using the lim-

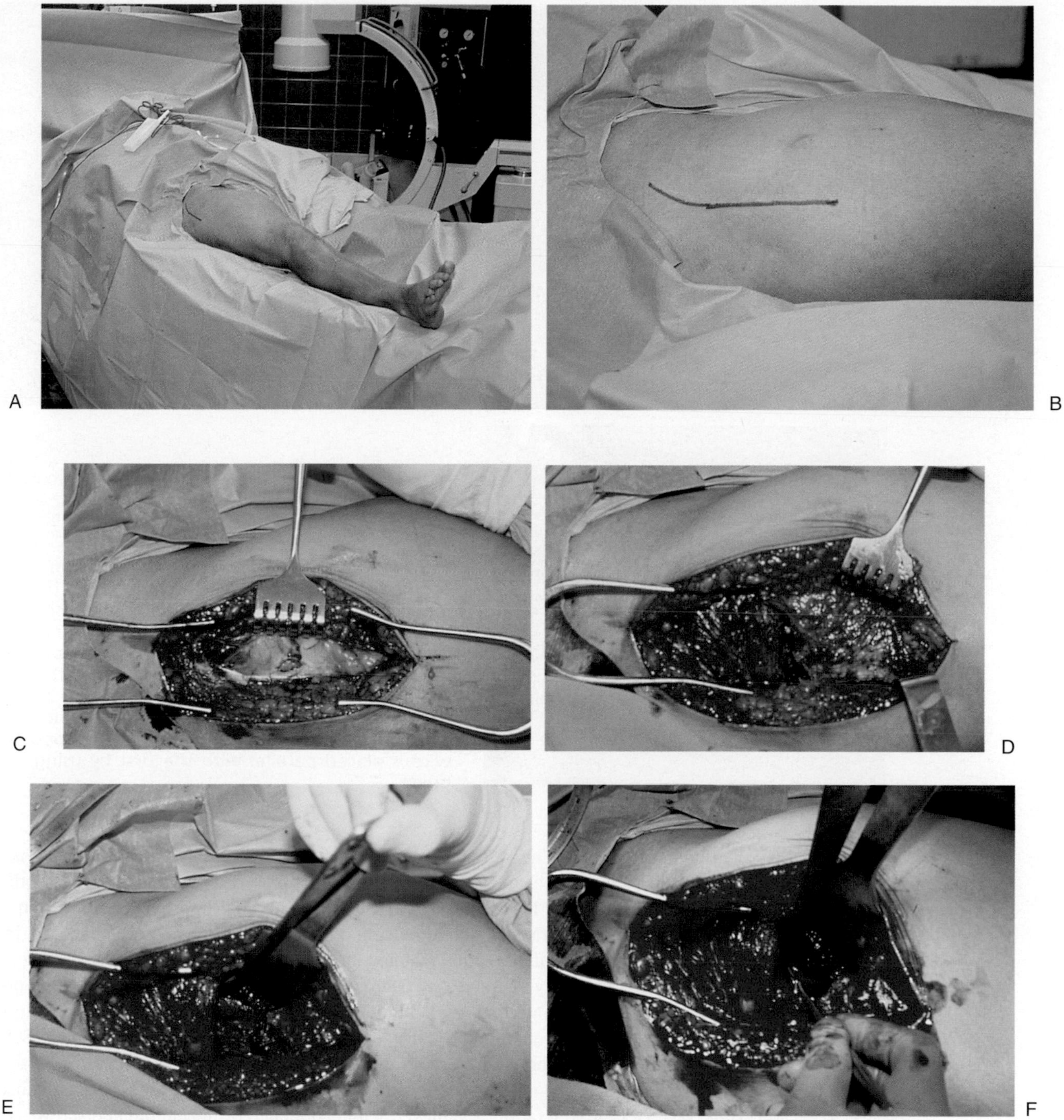

Figure 1. A: The technique of open reduction is illustrated in this markedly displaced femoral neck fracture. Positioning of the patient spine on a radiolucent table; alternatively, a fracture table can be used. **B:** The skin incision is 8 to 10 cm long, centered over the Precter trochanter. This patient's foot is to the readers' right. **C:** After incising the fascia lata, the interval between the tensor and gluteus medius muscles is developed. This is visible in the proximal (left side) portion of the wound. **D, E:** The final exposure of the anterior aspect of the hip fracture is accomplished, first by elevating the vastus lateralis off the intertrochanteric ridge **(D)** and then by sweeping the pericapsular fat medially and inserting a Hohmann retractor along the anterior aspect of the acetabulum **(E)**. **F:** The hip capsule is incised in line with the neck of the femur, evacuating any collected intracapsular hematoma.

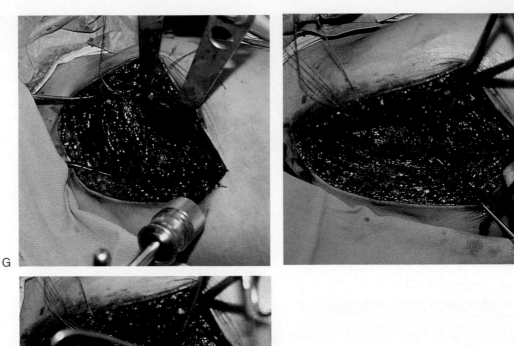

Figure 1. *(continued)* **G:** The reduction maneuver is performed with traction via a Schanz pin in the proximal femur with posterior translation of the shaft relative to the neck with a spiked pusher. The final reduction of the displaced neck fracture is accomplished by internal rotation of the leg by using the Schanz pin. **H:** The first guide wire is inserted after an anatomic reduction is documented with biplanar fluoroscopy and confirmed under direct vision. **I:** A second guide wire is placed parallel with the first by using a drill guide.

ited open technique. When an open reduction of the hip is necessary, the capsule is dissected from the intertrochanteric ridge, and its edges are tagged with no. 1 nonabsorbable suture for retraction. A head lamp is very helpful to provide improved illumination. Another useful technique to aid fracture reduction is placement of a 5-mm Schanz pin in the proximal lateral femur distal to the planned insertion of the cannulated screws (Fig. 1G). The fracture is manually distracted by lateral and distal traction on the pin, and the proximal fragment is lifted anteriorly with a blunt curved instrument. The fracture reduction is completed by internal rotation of the distal fragment and by lifting upward on the Schanz pin and applying a compressive force. Provisional fixation is achieved with three Kirschner wires or cannulated 3.2-mm guide wires placed with the aid of a biplanar image intensifier (Fig. 1H). Definitive fixation is achieved with cannulated or noncannulated screws (Figs. 1I and 2A–E). Several authors (8,11) showed that there is no benefit in using more than three screws when an anatomic reduction is achieved. Furthermore, there is no advantage in terms of postreduction stability comparing similar implants. A sliding hip screw has not been shown to increase mechanical stability when an anatomic reduction has been achieved. However, this device may be of some benefit when the reduction is not anatomic because it relies on the side-plate fixation to resist angular displacement of the fracture rather than the cancellous bone of the femoral head and neck.

In patients with posterior comminution, the reduction can often be improved by aligning the anterior cortices of the femoral neck. I prefer to insert the anterosuperior screw first, which helps to minimize angulating the fracture when more posterior screws are inserted and tightened. A sliding hip screw may also be used when comminution is present to avoid angulation when the fracture is compressed.

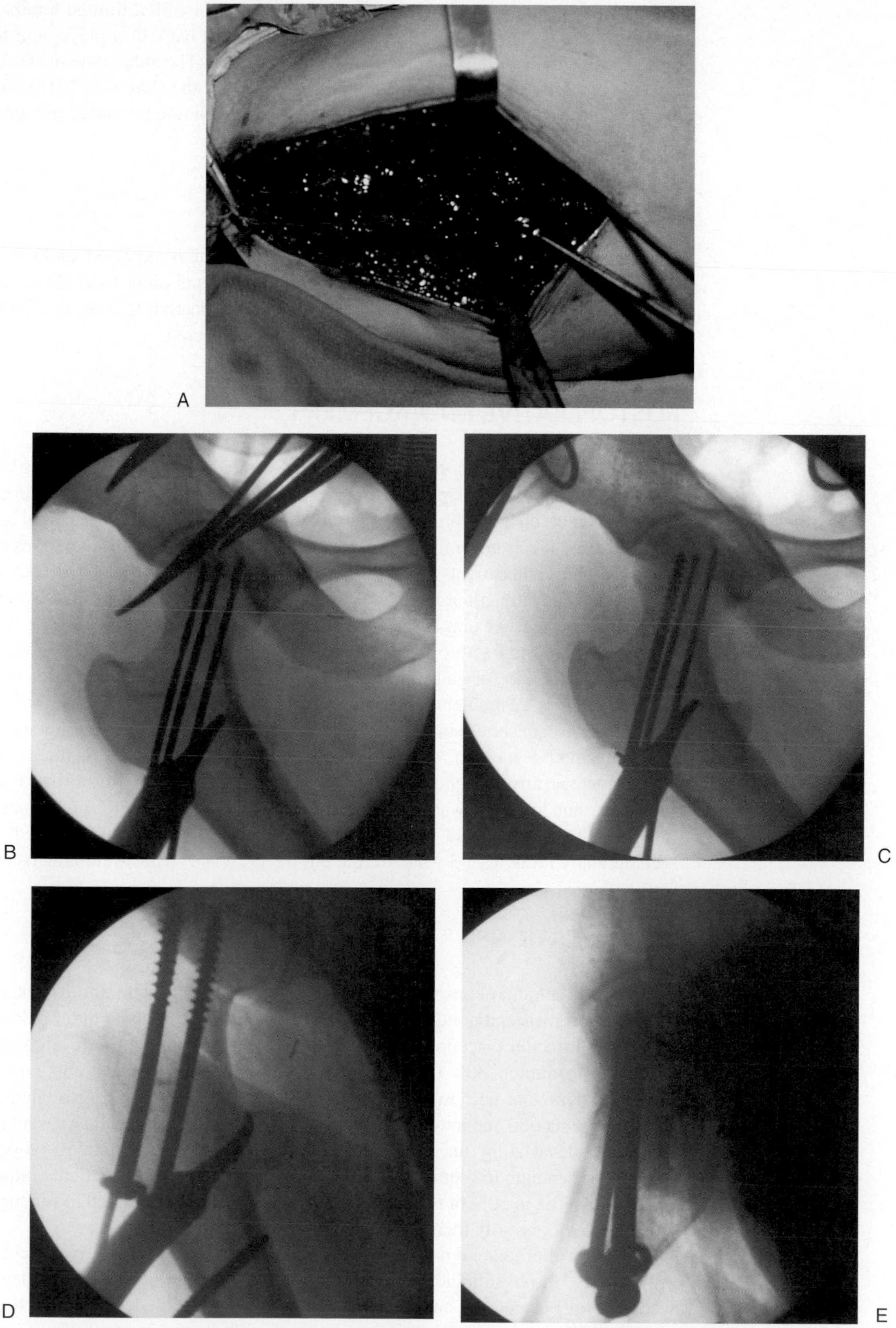

Figure 2. A: The screws are inserted one at a time starting with the anterior-superior screw. **B, C:** The first screw is placed anteriorly and superiorly to generate compression and initial stability opposite the posterior cortex, which may be comminuted and unstable. **D, E:** The final position of the implants and quality of the reduction is confirmed on final fluoroscopic images.

Closure is begun with reapproximation of the capsule with a limited number of nonabsorbable sutures. The vastus lateralis is allowed to fall back into place, and the fascia is closed over a drain with interrupted absorbable sutures. The subcutaneous fat is reapproximated with a limited number of absorbable sutures and the skin with 3-0 nylon or staples. Prophylactic first-generation cephalosporin antibiotics should be started preoperatively and continued for 24 hours postoperatively.

Results

For displaced femoral neck fractures, a 90% union rate is expected, and a there is a 20% to 30% chance of posttraumatic osteonecrosis. In patients older than 65 years, only 70% reach their prefracture functional level. A 12% risk of death related to the fracture (excess of mortality over age-matched controls) should be expected.

POSTOPERATIVE MANAGEMENT

Patients are rapidly mobilized and are instructed in protected weight-bearing with crutches or a walker. Patients who are able to maintain limited weight-bearing (up to 50% of body weight) on the injured limb should continue to do so for 12 weeks. In patients older than 60 years, this is generally accomplished with a walker, whereas younger patients usually use crutches. In patients with upper-extremity injuries or those who do not have enough upper-extremity strength or balance to use crutches or a walker, postoperative care must be individualized. Early excessive weight-bearing has been shown to increase the risk of redisplacement of the fracture and may dictate a period of wheelchair dependency. Physical therapy consultation for gait training is advisable. In some patients, a brief stay in a rehabilitation unit is desirable. Range-of-motion exercises are not generally necessary. The postoperative care should include deep-vein thrombosis (DVT) screening and prophylaxis until the patient is mobile. A Doppler duplex scan is generally obtained within the first 36 hours postoperatively, and weekly until the patient is fully mobilized. Enoxaparin (Lovenox) and low-dose warfarin (Coumadin) are equally efficacious for prophylaxis. Follow-up radiographs should be obtained monthly until the fracture is healed. Patients are seen annually for at least 3 years to rule out the presence of posttraumatic osteonecrosis.

COMPLICATIONS

The most common complications after internal fixation of femoral neck fractures are avascular necrosis and nonunion. The risk of avascular necrosis in older patients with displaced neck fractures, according to a recent meta-analysis of the English literature, is 16%, and that of nonunion, 30% (4). The rate of nonunion in younger patients ranges from 0 to 86%, and avascular necrosis, 20% to 59%. These complications are related primarily to quality of reduction and may be related to timing of fixation as well. Avascular necrosis is not always devastating functionally. Nearly all patients younger than 50 years have symptoms severe enough to require additional surgery, whereas older patients require reoperation in only 30% to 50% of the cases. Symptoms are therefore related to functional demand and can be successfully treated with arthroplasty.

Nonunion after femoral neck fractures can be treated with a corrective osteotomy or joint arthroplasty. In physiologically younger patients, nonunion can be treated with closing-wedge valgus osteotomy and fixation with a 120-degree blade plate. Marti et al. (5) reported on 50 patients who underwent osteotomy, of whom 37 were followed up for a minimum of 7 years and achieved an average Harris hip score of 90. Interestingly, 22 of these patients had radiographic evidence of avascular necrosis, illustrating the point that this complication is not always functionally devastating. Less common complications include infection, DVT, pulmonary embolism (PE), loss of reduction, and subtrochanteric fracture through entry portal in the proximal femur. Loss of reduction is almost always related to

poor bone quality or poor reduction. Loss of reduction should be treated with repeated reduction and internal fixation (usually by switching to a sliding hip screw) if the patient's
bone density is good and with a cemented endoprosthesis if not. Deep infection is managed
with early aggressive surgical debridement, culture-specific antibiotics, and closure over a
drain. Hip motion should be limited until the wound is sealed.

ILLUSTRATIVE CASE FOR TECHNIQUE

A 23-year-old man sustained a markedly displaced femoral neck fracture in a fall from
an 8-foot height (Fig. 3A and B). His medical history was notable for long-term phenytoin
(Dilantin) therapy for a seizure disorder. He was treated with open reduction and screw fixation within 8 hours of injury. Postoperatively, he maintained on crutches for 12 weeks, and
the fracture healed by 7 weeks (Fig. 3C). No signs or symptoms indicated avascular necrosis at the 2-year follow-up. Postoperative technetium 99 methyldiphosphate bone scan obtained at 3 weeks after injury showed marked hyperemia of the femoral head. A 10-year

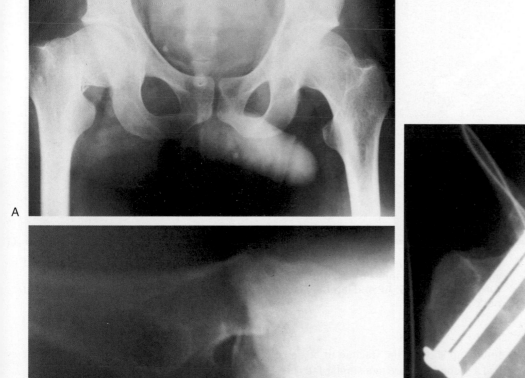

A

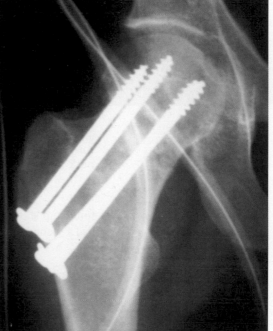

B   C

Figure 3. A, B: Radiographs of the pelvis show a displaced femoral neck fracture in a
23-year-old patient after a fall from a height. **C:** Postoperative anteroposterior (AP)
view of the hip after open reduction. The fracture was placed in valgus because of comminution of the posterior femoral neck.

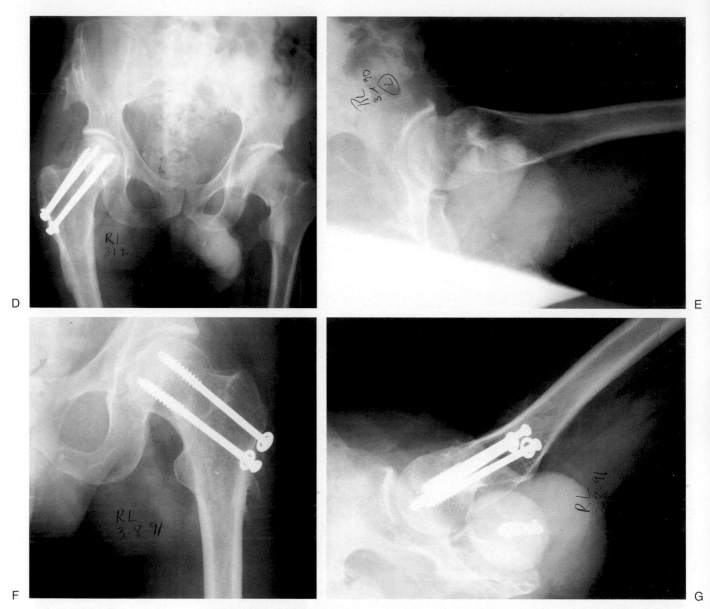

Figure 3. *(continued)* **D:** A 10-year follow-up radiograph of the right hip was obtained when the patient injured his contralateral hip in a fall. **E:** Lateral radiograph of fractured left hip. **F, G:** AP and lateral views 1 year after open reduction of the left femoral neck fracture.

follow-up showed the fracture to be completely healed and remodeled, when the patient had a second fracture in a similar fall (Fig. 3D–G).

RECOMMENDED READING

1. Anderson, G.H., Harper, W.M., Connolly, C.D., Badham, J., Goodrich, N., Gregg, P.J.: Preoperative skin traction for fractures of the proximal femur. *J. Bone Joint Surg. [Br]*, 75:794–796, 1993.
2. Drake, J.K., and Meyers, M.H.: Intracapsular pressure and hemiarthrosis following femoral neck fracture. *Clin. Orthop.*, 182:172–176, 1984.
3. Kenzora, J.E., McCarthy, R.E., Lowell, J.D., Sledge, C.B.: Hip fracture mortality: relation to age, treatment, preoperative illness, time of surgery and complications. *Clin. Orthop.*, 186:45–56, 1984.
4. Lu-Yao, G.L., Keller, R.B., Littenberg, B., Wennberg J.E.: Outcomes after displaced fractures of the femoral neck: a meta-analysis of one hundred and six published reports. *J. Bone Joint Surg. [Am]*, 76:15–25, 1994.

5. Marti, R.K., Schuller, H.M., Raaymakers E.L.F.B.: Intertrochanteric osteotomy for non-union of the femoral neck. *J. Bone Joint Surg. [Br]*, 71:782–787, 1989.

6. Singh, M., Nagarath, A.R., Maini, P.S.: Changes in trabecular pattern of the upper end of the femur as an index of osteoporosis. *J. Bone Joint Surg. [Am]*, 52:457–467, 1970.

7. Speer, K.P., Spritzer, C.E., Harrelson, J.M., Nunley, J.A.: Magnetic resonance imaging of the femoral head after acute intracapsular fracture of the femoral neck. *J. Bone Joint Surg. [Am]*, 72:98–113, 1990.

8. Springer, E.R., Lachiewicz, P.F., Gilbert, J.A.: Internal fixation of femoral neck fractures: a comparative biomechanical study of Knowles pins and 6.5-mm cancellous screws. *Clin. Orthop.*, 267:85–92, 1991.

9. Stromqvist, B.: Femoral head vitality after intracapsular hip fracture: 490 cases studied by intravital tetracycline labeling and Tc-MDP radionuclide imaging. *Acta Orthop. Scand.*, (suppl 2):5–71, 1983.

10. Swiontkowski, M.F.: Intracapsular fractures of the hip. *J. Bone Joint Surg. [Am]*, 76:129–138, 1994.

11. Swiontkowski, M.F., Harrington, R.M., Keller, T.S., VanPatten, P.K.: Torsion and bending analysis of internal fixation techniques for femoral neck fractures: the role of implant design and bone density. *J. Orthop. Res.* 5(3):433–444, 1987.

12. Trueta, J., and Harrison, M.H.M.: The normal vascular anatomy of the femoral head in adult man. *J. Bone Joint Surg. [Br]*, 35:442–461, 1953.

Master Techniques in Orthopaedic Surgery,
FRACTURES, edited by D. A. Wiss,
Lippincott–Raven Publishers, Philadelphia © 1998.

15

Intertrochanteric Hip Fractures: Sliding Hip Screw

Kenneth J. Koval

INDICATIONS/CONTRAINDICATIONS

The primary goal of fracture treatment is to return patients to their prefracture level of function. There is general agreement that in a patient with an intertrochanteric hip fracture, this can best be accomplished operatively. Nonoperative management is appropriate only in patients who are nonambulatory with minimal pain and in selected younger healthy patients with nondisplaced fractures. These patients, however, must be closely monitored to detect any evidence of fracture displacement. Patients who are treated nonoperatively should be rapidly mobilized to avoid the complications of prolonged recumbency.

The most important factor in any classification of intertrochanteric fractures is the stability of the fracture. Stability is enhanced when the posteromedial cortex is intact or restored at the time of surgery. Unstable intertrochanteric fracture patterns include loss of the posteromedial buttress, subtrochanteric extension, and reverse obliquity fracture patterns.

The sliding hip screw remains the implant of choice for most intertrochanteric hip fractures. Intramedullary nail/sliding hip screw devices such as the Gamma nail or Intramedullary Hip Screw also have been used in the treatment of intertrochanteric hip fractures. However, studies comparing these devices with a sliding hip screw have found no statistically significant differences with respect to operating time, blood loss, duration of hospital stay, infection rate or wound complications, implant failure, screw cutout, or screw sliding. However, patients treated with the intramedullary nail have had increased rates of femoral-shaft fractures at the nail tip or the insertion sites of the distal locking bolts.

K. J. Koval, M.D.: Fracture Service, Department of Orthopaedic Surgery, Hospital for Joint Diseases, New York, New York 10003.

PREOPERATIVE PLANNING

Deformity after fracture depends on the degree of displacement and comminution of the fracture. Nondisplaced fractures usually have little or no clinical deformity, whereas patients with displaced comminuted fractures have the classic shortened and externally rotated extremity. Range of motion of the injured hip is invariably painful and should be avoided. Although neurovascular injuries are rare, a careful evaluation should be performed. In patients whose fractures occurred as the result of high-energy trauma, a careful assessment is necessary to rule out associated injuries.

Standard radiographic examination of intertrochanteric fractures should include an anteroposterior (AP) view of the pelvis and an AP and cross-table lateral of the affected hip. The cross-table lateral radiograph helps to define posteromedial comminution. Occasionally, the fracture geometry is not fully appreciated on the standard AP lateral views. In these cases, a 15- to 20-degree internal-rotation view may be helpful. If an intramedullary fixation device is to be used, contralateral radiographs are useful to template the size and angle of the proposed implant.

SURGERY

Surgery is optimally performed with the patient positioned supine on a fracture table with both lower extremities resting in foot holders (Fig. 1). A padded perineal post is placed in the ipsilateral groin, taking care to avoid impingement on the labia or scrotum. The fracture is reduced by using gentle longitudinal traction with the leg externally rotated, followed by internal rotation (Fig. 2A and B). The uninvolved leg is then flexed, abducted, and externally rotated to allow space for C-arm image intensifier (Fig. 3A). Alternatively, the contralateral extremity can be abducted with the hip and knee extended; this maneuver, however, places greater pressure on the perineum from the perineal post (Fig. 3B).

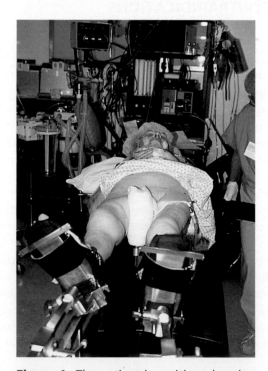

Figure 1. The patient is positioned supine on a fracture table with both lower extremities resting in foot holders. A padded perineal post is placed in the ipsilateral groin, taking care that there is no impingement of the labia or scrotum.

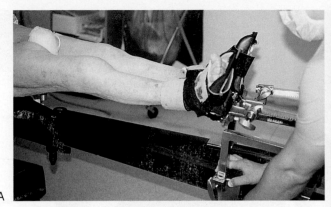

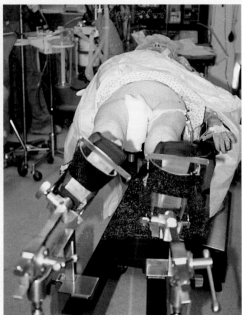

Figure 2. Fracture reduction involves longitudinal traction with the leg externally rotated **(A)** followed by internal rotation **(B)**.

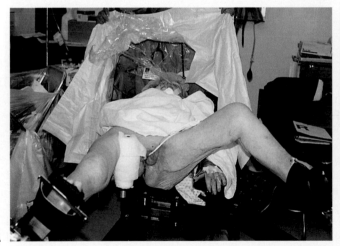

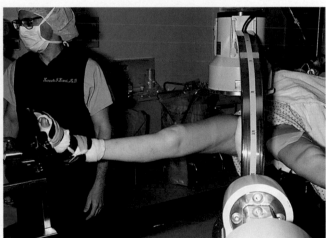

Figure 3. The uninvolved leg is then flexed, abducted, and externally rotated to allow the image intensifier to come around for a lateral view **(A)**. Alternatively, the contralateral extremity can be abducted with the hip and knee extended; this maneuver, however, places greater perineal post pressure on the perineum **(B)**.

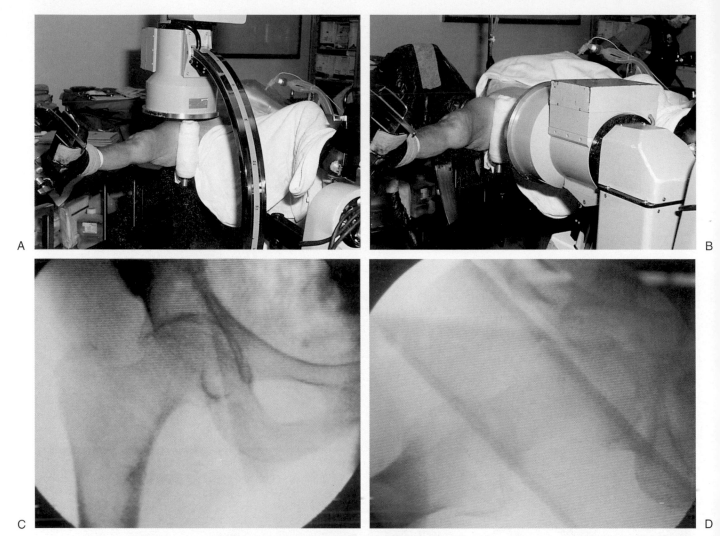

Figure 4. Positioning of the image intensifier for anteroposterior (AP) and lateral radiographic views **(A, B)**. AP and lateral radiographs of a reduced intertrochanteric fracture before patient draping **(C, D)**.

The fracture should be reduced or be reducible before prepping and draping the patient. The image intensifier should provide nonobstructive biplanar radiographic visualization of the entire proximal femur, including the hip joint (Fig. 4A–D). The surgeon must be prepared to deal with residual varus angulation, posterior sag, or malrotation. Residual varus angulation or posterior sag may lead to difficulty centering the lag screw in the femoral neck and head. Varus malalignment can usually be corrected with additional longitudinal traction to disengage the fracture fragments, followed by re-reduction. Posterior sag is usually the result of posterior comminution and requires manual correction using a crutch, bone hook, or periosteal elevator (Fig. 5). Once reduced, the lower extremity is rotated under fluoroscopic control to determine whether the fracture fragments move as a single unit. In patients in whom the femoral shaft moves independent of the proximal fragment, excessive internal rotation of the leg should be avoided. In these cases, we place the lower extremity in neutral rotation. Once the fracture is reduced, the patient is prepped and draped. We prefer an isolation screen (Fig. 6).

Stable Fractures

A straight lateral incision is made from the base of the greater trochanter, extending down the thigh (Fig. 7). The iliotibial band is divided longitudinally, remaining posterior to the insertion of the tensor fascia muscle proximally (Fig. 8). A Hohmann retractor is

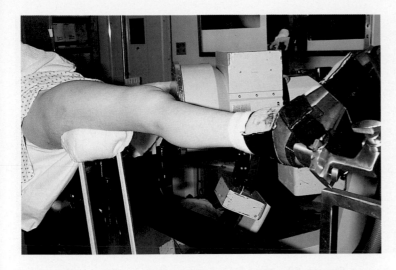

Figure 5. Correction of posterior sag with use of a crutch.

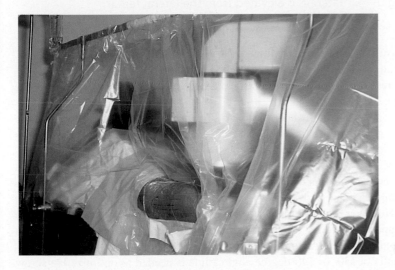

Figure 6. Patient draping with an isolation screen.

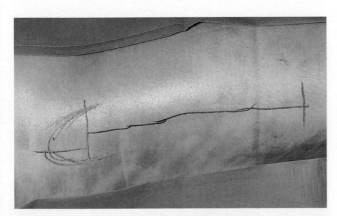

Figure 7. A straight lateral incision is made from the base of the greater trochanter, extending down the thigh.

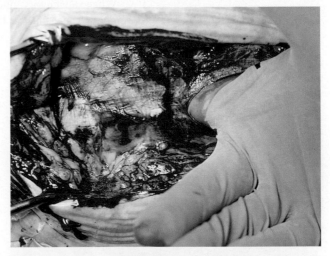

Figure 8. The iliotibial band is incised longitudinally in line with skin incision. A finger is inserted proximally to ensure that one remains posterior to the tensor fascia muscle.

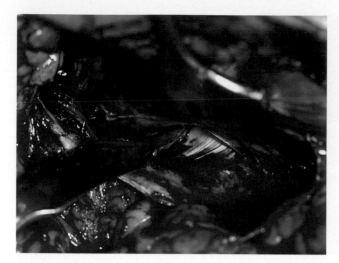

Figure 9. Insertion of a Hohmann retractor under the vastus lateralis, just proximal to the insertion of the gluteus maximus tendon.

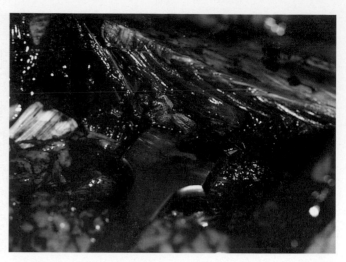

Figure 10. After Hohmann retractor insertion, the vastus lateralis is elevated from the lateral femur.

placed under the vastus lateralis, just proximal to the insertion of the gluteus maximus (Fig. 9). The vastus lateralis is carefully elevated from the lateral intermuscular septum in a posterior-to-anterior direction, taking care to identify and ligate the perforating branches of the femoral artery (Figs. 10–12).

A 3.2-mm drill hole is made in the lateral cortex of the proximal femur at the level of the lesser trochanter. A guide wire is then inserted under image intensification by using the 135-degree guide (Fig. 13A and B). Some surgeons recommend placing a guide wire anterior to the femoral neck to estimate femoral-neck anteversion; however, in our experience, this is usually not necessary. The position of the guide wire is adjusted until it lies in the center of the femoral head and neck (Fig. 14A and B); a slightly posteroinferior position also is acceptable. However, the superoanterior position should be avoided because of the increased risk for superior "cutout." If the guide wire cannot be positioned appropriately in the femoral head and neck, the fracture reduction and neck–shaft angle are critically reassessed. Occasionally, a 130- or 140-degree angle guide is needed to optimize lag-screw position.

When satisfactory guide wire is confirmed, it is advanced to the subchondral bone of the femoral head, and the length of the lag screw determined (Fig. 15). In stable intertro-

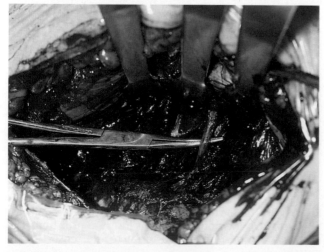

Figure 11. Identification and ligation of the perforating branches of the femoral artery.

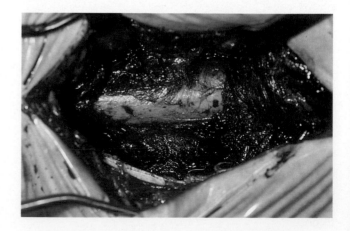

Figure 12. Final exposure of the lateral femur.

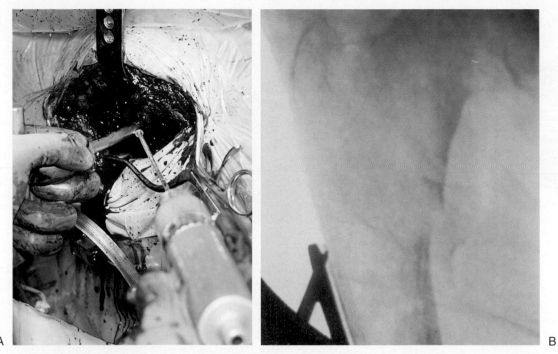

Figure 13. Use of the 135-degree guide **(A, B)** to place a guide wire into the femoral head under image intensification.

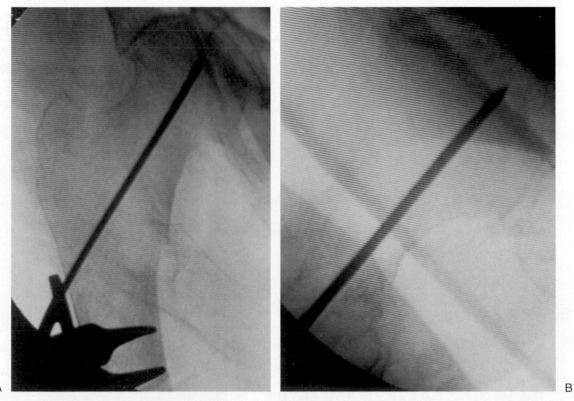

Figure 14. Anteroposterior (AP; **A**) and lateral **(B)** image intensifier radiographs of the fully seated guide wire.

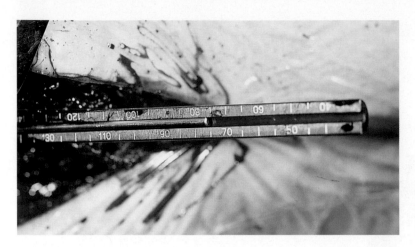

Figure 15. Measurement of the guide wire length. To verify this measurement, use a second, similar-length guide wire and subtract the length of exposed wire.

chanteric fractures, significant impaction is not necessary; therefore a screw length is chosen that maximizes screw–barrel engagement, allows about 5 mm of impaction, and lies within 1 cm of the subchondral bone. For example, if the guide wire measures 100 mm to the subchondral bone, a 90-mm length lag screw would be selected. Once fully seated 5 mm from the subchondral bone, the lag screw would be inset 5 mm into the plate barrel. Reaming is performed under image intensification over the guide wire to 5 mm from the subchondral bone (Fig. 16). The position of the guide wire during reaming should be monitored (Fig. 17) to detect binding of the guide wire within the reamer, which may result in femoral-head penetration. Not infrequently, the guide wire is pulled out during reamer removal.

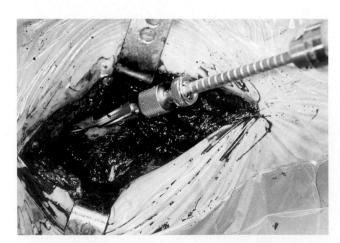

Figure 16. Reaming of the proximal femur.

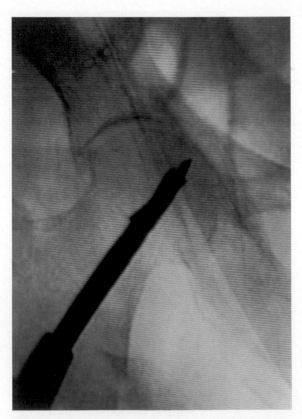

Figure 17. One must monitor the position of the guide wire during reaming to detect binding of the guide wire within the reamer, which may result in femoral-head penetration.

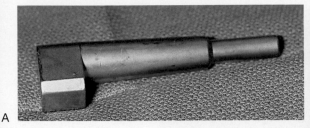

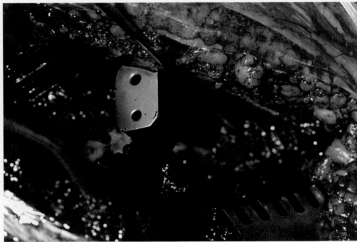

A

B

Figure 18. Use of a guide wire repositioner **(A, B)** to reinsert a guide wire that was lost during reamer removal.

When this happens, the guide wire can be replaced by using either a guide-wire repositioner, which is available on many sliding hip-screw sets (Fig. 18A and B), or a lag screw inserted backward into the reaming channel. The proximal femur is tapped, even in elderly patients, to prevent femoral-head rotation during lag-screw insertion (Fig. 19), and the lag screw then inserted to within 0.5 to 10 mm of the subchondral bone. When the screw is properly positioned within the femoral head, a four-hole, 135-degree plate is inserted over the screw. A "keyed" sliding hip-screw system is preferred to enhance rotational stability; however, the screw must be oriented so that the plate is positioned along the femoral shaft. A short-barrel plate is used if an 80 mm or less lag screw has been inserted (Fig. 20), and a long barrel used for the rest.

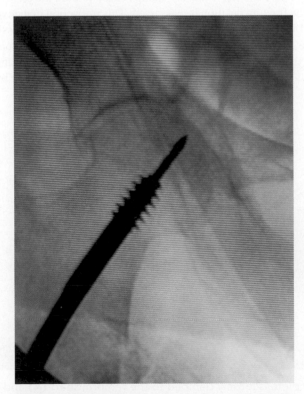

Figure 19. Fracture malreduction caused by femoral-head rotation during lag-screw insertion.

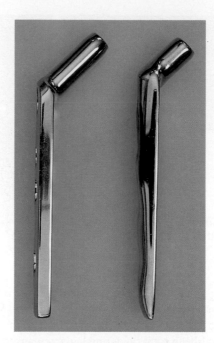

Figure 20. The regular and short-barrel sliding hip screw plates. The short barrel is used only if a lag screw 80 mm or less has been inserted.

The plate is slid over the hip screw and loosely clamped to the femoral shaft. The fracture is impacted by releasing the traction and gently displacing the shaft toward the proximal fragment (Fig. 21A and B). A narrow clamp is used to hold the plate to the bone and is tightened while the fracture position is reassessed. This impaction maneuver improves fracture stability and helps prevent distraction, which might result in excessive shortening in the postoperative period. Three to four fixation screws are inserted through the plate, depending on bone quality. The fracture is manually impacted once again, and the fracture position rechecked. The need for a compression set screw is determined by visualizing the

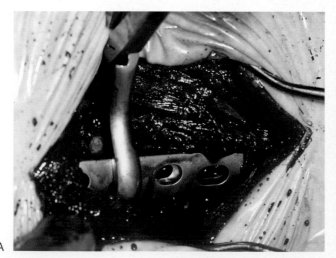
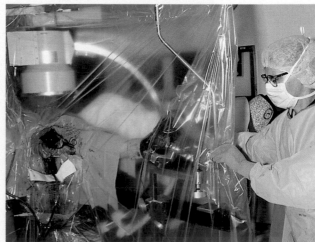

A   B

Figure 21. The plate is loosely clamped to the femoral shaft **(A)** and the fracture impacted by releasing the traction on the leg and gently displacing the shaft toward the proximal fragment **(B)**.

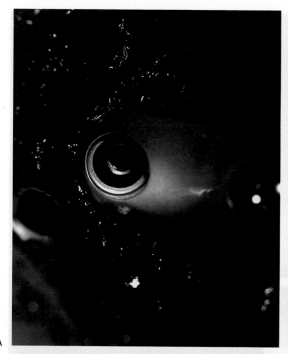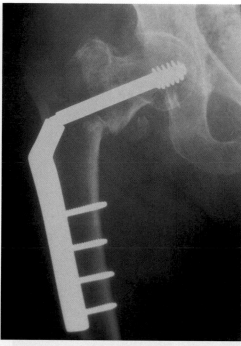

A   B

Figure 22. The need for a compression screw is assessed by visualizing the amount of screw–barrel engagement **(A)**. A compression screw is inserted if there fear of postoperative screw–barrel disengagement **(B)**.

amount of screw–barrel engagement (Fig. 22A); a compression screw is inserted if there is concern about possible postoperative screw–barrel disengagement (Fig. 22B). The wound is closed in layers over suction drains (Fig. 23).

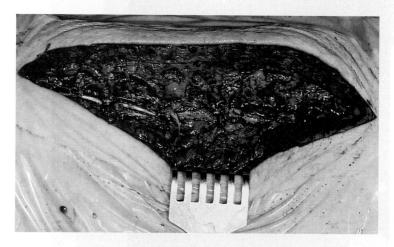

Figure 23. The iliotibial band is reapproximated by using interrupted sutures.

Unstable Fractures

Unstable intertrochanteric fractures are characterized by loss of the posteromedial buttress (Fig. 24). Another type of unstable intertrochanteric fracture is the reverse obliquity pattern, in which the fracture begins just proximal to the lesser trochanter and extends laterally in an oblique orientation (Fig. 25).

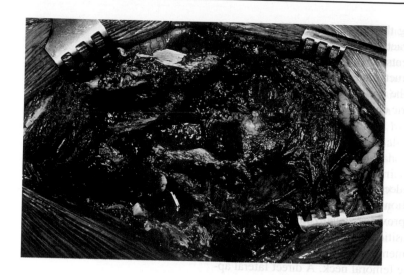

Figure 5. Prereduction exposure of the subtrochanteric fracture. Minimal stripping of individual bone fragments is mandatory to ensure viability of fragments after reduction.

rior edges of the base of the femoral neck provides the surgeon an additional landmark of the orientation of the femoral neck. One finger defines the anterior border of the femoral neck through the anterior edge of the abductor medius muscle. The second finger identifies the posterior border of the neck near the insertion of the short external rotators underneath the posterior border of the gluteus medius muscle (Fig. 8). This technique provides an additional indirect image of the middle of the femoral neck, acting as an additional reference point for seating chisel placement (Figs. 7, 9, and 10).

It is essential to remember that the femoral neck arises from the anterior half of the greater trochanter; therefore, the seating chisel should enter the anterior half of the trochanter just proximal to the lateral trochanteric ridge and not in the anatomic middle of the greater trochanter (Fig. 7). The seating chisel is placed through the insertion guide (which is preset to an angle of 95 degrees) and checked fluoroscopically to verify position. One of the more common errors with the use of this implant is penetration of the anterior femoral-neck cortex with the seating chisel, which will result in the blade-plate malposition and a tendency to external rotation of the fracture when the side plate is reduced to the femoral shaft. This can be avoided by constant fluoroscopic evaluation as the seating chisel is sequentially placed into the femoral head. The weight of the insertion handle has a tendency to fall posteriorly as the chisel is advanced. Constant attention to the angle of insertion, rotation of the chisel, and internal or external torsion in the femur will reduce the inci-

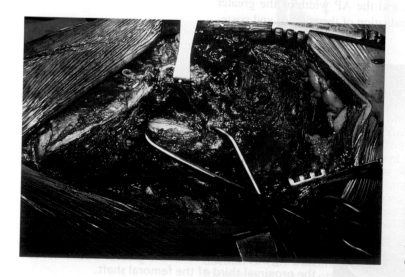

Figure 6. Reduction of the lateral femoral cortex beneath the trochanteric ridge is performed by using large reduction forceps and stabilized with K-wires or lag screws. Lag screws are preferable for definitive fixation. Reduction of fragments three and four to the main proximal neck–trochanteric fragment reconstructs the lateral proximal femoral cortex.

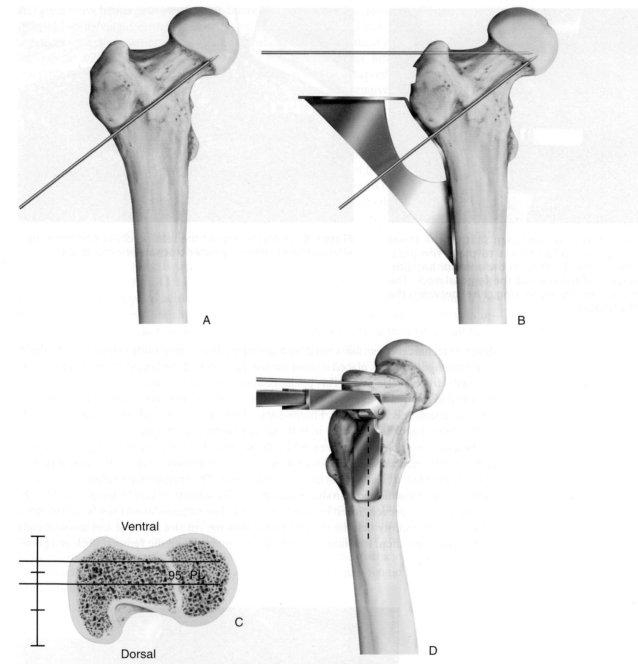

A,B

surgeo
proxin
failed

COM

Bla
any pl
can oc
some
turely
trocha
varus
shorte
compl
penetr
and e>
ously
side-p
plate
ion or
rotate
nated
drillir
comp
fixatic
femor
tratior

Figure 7. Illustrative technique of placement of guiding K-wires to facilitate cutting of the blade slot into the femoral neck. **A:** Anterior femoral-neck guide wire indicating femoral-neck anteversion. **B:** The 95-degree angled guide placing the corresponding guide wire into the proximal portion of the femoral neck. **C:** Relation of the femoral neck to the proximal greater trochanter for insertion of the 95-degree fixed-angle blade plate. Note the central femoral neck corresponds to the anterior half of the greater trochanter at this level. **D:** Anterior lateral view of the seating chisel placement, cutting the blade slot into the base of the femoral head (note the flange of the seating guide is in the midportion of the femoral shaft). Reconstruction of the lateral proximal femoral cortex enhances the correct position of the seating chisel guide.

RECOMMENDED READING

1. Asher, M.A., Tippett, J.W., Rockwood, C.A., Zilber, S.: Compression fixation of subtrochanteric fractures. *Clin. Orthop.,* 117:202–208, 1976.
2. Goldhagen, P.R., O'Connor, D.R., Schwarze, D., Schwartz, E.: A prospective comparative study of the compression hip screw and the gamma nail. *J. Orthop. Trauma,* 8(5):367–372, 1994.
3. Haas, N.P., Schutz, M., Mauch, C., Hoffmann, R., Sudkamp, N.P.: Management of ipsilateral fractures of the femur shaft and proximal femur—therapy overview and current management. *Zentralbl. Chir.,* 120(11):856–861, 1995.
4. Hoffmann, R., Sudkamp, N.P., Schutz, M., Raschke, M., Haas, N.P.: Current status of therapy of subtrochanteric femoral fractures. *Unfallchirurgie* 99(4):240–248, 1996.
5. Kinast, C., Bolhofner, B.R., Mast, J.W., Ganz, R.: Subtrochanteric fractures of the femur: results of treatment with the 95 degrees condylar blade-plate. *Clin. Orthop.,* 238:122–130, 1989.
6. Müller, M.E., Allgöwer, M., Schnieder, R., Willenegger, H.: Angled plates. In *Manual of internal fixation: techniques recommended by the AO-ASIF Group,* 2nd ed. Springer-Verlag: Berlin, 1979, pp. 85–97.
7. Müller, M.E., Allgöwer, M., Schnieder, R., Willenegger, H.: Angled plates. In *Manual of internal fixation: techniques recommended by the AO-ASIF Group,* 3rd ed. Springer-Verlag: Berlin, 1991, pp. 254–265.
8. Nungu, K.S., Olerud, C., Rehnberg, L.: Treatment of subtrochanteric fractures with the AO dynamic condylar screw. *Injury,* 24(2):90–92, 1993.
9. Pai, C.H.: Dynamic condylar screw for subtrochanteric femur fractures with greater trochanteric extension. *J. Orthop. Trauma,* 10(5):317–322, 1996.
10. Radford, P.J., and Howell, C.J.: The AO dynamic condylar screw for fractures of the femur. *Injury,* 23(2):89–93, 1992.
11. Vanderspeeten, K., Verheyen, L., Broos, P.: A review on 161 subtrochanteric fractures—risk factors influencing outcome: age, fracture pattern and fracture level. *Unfallchirurgie* 98(5):265–271, 1995.
12. Warwick, D.J., Crichlow, T.P., Langkamer, V.G., Jackson, M.: The dynamic condylar screw in the management of subtrochanteric fractures of the femur. *Injury,* 26(4):241–244, 1995.
13. Whatley, J.R., Garland, D.E., Whitecloud, T. III, Whickstrom, J.: Subtrochanteric fractures of the femur: treatment with ASIF blade plate fixation. *South. Med. J.,* 71(11):1372–1375, 1978.
14. Wiss, D.A., and Brien, W.W.: Subtrochanteric fractures of the femur: results of treatment by interlocking nailing. *Clin. Orthop.,* 283:231–236, 1992.
15. Wiss, D.A., Fleming, C.H., Matta, J.M., Clark D.: Comminuted and rotationally unstable fractures of the femur treated with an interlocking nail. *Clin. Orthop.,* 212:35–47, 1986.

Master Techniques in Orthopaedic Surgery,
FRACTURES, edited by D. A. Wiss,
Lippincott–Raven Publishers, Philadelphia © 1998.

17

Subtrochanteric Femur Fractures: Reconstruction Nailing

Thomas A. Russell

INDICATIONS/CONTRAINDICATIONS

A reconstruction nail combines a closed antegrade intramedullary nail technique with interlocking screws that permit fixation into the femoral head. Interlocking screws in the distal femur provide rotational and axial stability to the femoral shaft. All reconstruction nails have an anterior bow to facilitate insertion. The nail geometry is altered throughout its length with variations in cross section to maximize its strength and to minimize its stiffness.

A reconstruction interlocking nail is an intramedullary implant with interlocking lag screws, which are inserted diagonally into the femoral head with distal interlocking screws in a transverse orientation (Fig. 1). Mechanically, a statically locked reconstruction nail can be used to stabilize injuries and deformities from the femoral neck to about 4 cm above the knee. A reconstruction nail is frequently used for stabilization of "high" subtrochanteric femur fractures, including pathologic fractures and impending fractures in the intertrochanteric–subtrochanteric region.

Russell and Taylor (1) described a classification for subtrochanteric femur fractures based on the presence or absence of fracture involvement of the lesser trochanter/medial calcar and greater trochanter (piriformis fossa) (Fig. 2). Fractures involving the lesser trochanter but without extension into the greater trochanter (Russell–Taylor I-B), are perhaps the best indication for a reconstruction nail (Fig. 3). Segmental fractures of the femur, in which the proximal fracture extends into the upper femoral metaphysis, are also good indications for reconstruction nails. This implant is also indicated in the treatment of malunions, nonunions, and failed plate fixation of subtrochanteric femur fractures. A reconstruction nail may also be used to manage selected ipsilateral femoral neck and shaft fractures.

A reconstruction nail should not be considered the nail of first choice for diaphyseal fractures of the femur, because of the complexity of targeting and placing screws in the femoral

T. A. Russell, M.D.: Department of Orthopaedic Surgery, University of Tennessee, and Memphis Orthopaedic Group, Inc., Memphis, Tennessee 38104.

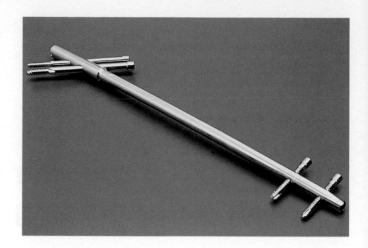

Figure 1. Reconstruction nail (Smith & Nephew, Inc.,)

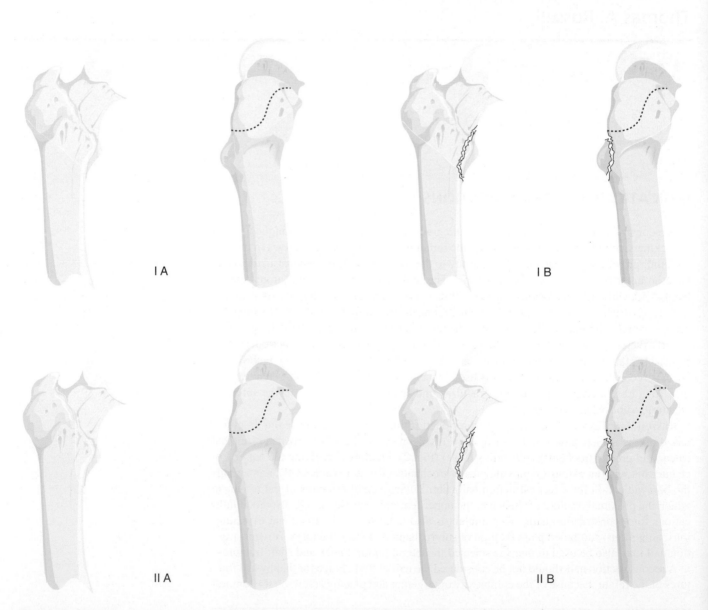

Figure 2. Diagram of components of Russell–Taylor IB subtrochanteric pattern with greater trochanter intact and lesser trochanteric fracture.

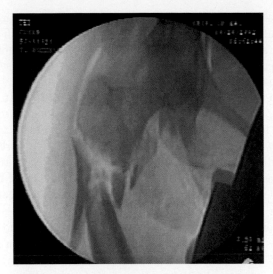

Figure 3. Subtrochanteric fracture with intact greater trochanter and fracture of the lesser trochanter.

head. Reconstruction nailing also is contraindicated in children with open physeal plates. The device may be inserted by using a closed or open technique at the fracture site, although for biologic reasons, a closed technique is preferred.

PREOPERATIVE PLANNING

Subtrochanteric fractures also may be characterized as high-energy and low-energy mechanisms. Low-energy subtrochanteric fractures are more commonly seen in older patients with some degree of osteopenia. High-energy fracture mechanisms are usually seen in younger age groups with associated injuries in up to 50%, as reported in 1987 by Bergman et al. (2). Waddell's (3) retrospective review of 130 patients found surgical lesions in 27 of their patients involving the cranium, thorax, pelvis, spine, viscus, and other large bones (3). Twenty of these 27 patients had more than one other lesion. Open fractures are rare, as are compartment syndromes, but both of these complications increase the morbidity of the injury if rapid assessment and treatment are not instituted.

Patients with subtrochanteric femur fractures invariably have pain referable to the proximal thigh, an external rotation deformity, and possibly angulation in the proximal anterior thigh, if the extremity is unsplinted. Inability to bear weight on the affected extremity usually necessitates transport by ambulance and stretcher. Frequently ecchymosis and swelling of the thigh are apparent, depending on the mechanism and time lapsed since injury. Neurologic or vascular injuries are uncommon with subtrochanteric fractures unless they are the result of penetrating trauma.

Preoperative radiographs should include an anteroposterior (AP) and lateral of the entire femur including the femoral head, neck, and knee. The radiographs should be carefully inspected to rule out intraarticular propagation of fractures or concomitant disease. Preoperative radiographs of the uninjured femur may be used to estimate nail diameter, expected amount of reaming, and final nail length in comminuted fractures. Radiographic templates for preoperative planning for reconstruction nails are available from the implant manufacturer. If surgery is delayed, restoration of length at the fracture site must be obtained with traction before closed nailing. Failure to restore length may lead to excessive intraoperative traction and resultant pudendal or sciatic nerve injuries.

High-quality radiographs must be scrutinized to determine whether there is fracture extension into the greater trochanter and piriformis fossa. In patients with extension of the fracture above the lesser trochanter, a coronal split in the proximal fragment is frequently present. This may result in comminution of the proximal fragment with loss of the entry portal during reaming and nailing. In these cases, nailing may be contraindicated. If the fracture is nailed, an open reduction of the proximal fragment with provisional stabilization of the trochanteric region with reduction forceps is strongly advised.

Most reconstruction nails are available in sizes ranging from 10 to 16 mm in diameter with lengths between 24 and 50 cm. The nails are right- and left-sided, to compensate for the anteversion of the femoral neck in relation to the shaft axis in the coronal plane. The proximal locking screw holes are oriented 8 to 15 degrees anteriorly in relation to the distal screw holes to facilitate screw entry into the femoral head. Reconstruction nails typically use two sliding lag screws proximally to maximize purchase in the femoral head and minimize rotation of the proximal fragment. These lag screws vary between 6.4 and 8.0 mm in diameter.

Precise knowledge of the neck–shaft angle of the screws in relation to the nail, spacing between the proximal screws, and their enclosed diameter are important in implant selection. Nail "neck–shaft" angles vary from 125 to 135 degrees. Higher-angle designs maximize sliding capabilities but are difficult to insert in hips with a relative varus position. Lower-angle designs have higher stresses and less sliding capability but are easier to insert. Most designs are moving toward a compromise of 130 degrees. Reconstruction nails have an effective spread between the two proximal screws of 17 to 21 mm in most designs. Measurement of the preoperative radiographs is necessary to document the patient's neck–shaft angle and plan screw spacing and final nail position. Reconstruction nails are typically enlarged proximally to compensate for the higher stresses in the subtrochanteric region. This must be recognized in preoperative planning because additional reaming of the proximal fragment is necessary. Distal interlocking screws are usually 4.5 to 6.4 mm in diameter and vary from full-threaded to partially-threaded designs.

Nail length and diameter depend on the size of the patient and the extent of femoral comminution. To minimize the risk of nail failure, the largest implant suitable for the patient should be used. The nail should fill the medullary canal at the isthmus to minimize translational deformation even when interlocking is used. Static locking is recommended in acute fractures for maximal stability. The nail tip should extend into the distal femoral metaphysis to avoid stress risers in the diaphyseal area and facilitate distal interlocking. Excessive nail length could result in nail migration into the knee with dynamization.

SURGERY

Patient Positioning

The supine position is recommended for reconstruction nailing, as it is familiar to most surgeons and allows adequate visualization of the hip in both AP and lateral views, which is critical to successful implantation of the device. The lateral decubitus position is helpful with revision nailing, especially in failed nailings with incorrect entry portals because the entry portal is better visualized in this position.

With the patient in the supine position, the unaffected limb and trunk are abducted while the affected extremity is adducted. The affected hip is flexed 15 degrees, with maintenance of the "heel-to-toe" relation (Fig. 4A and B). Traction is applied through the foot holder attached to the fracture table or through a skeletal pin in the distal femur or proximal tibia. Rotational alignment of the proximal fragment is determined with the image intensifier. The distal fragment is rotated to align with the proximal fragment. It is important to remember that femoral-neck anteversion in adults averages 15 degrees in most whites, but may be up to 30 degrees in Asian populations. In the supine position, the leg will usually lie in 0 to 15 degrees of external rotation when the distal fragment is correctly rotated. Always check the uninvolved leg for rotational alignment. If hip motion is restricted preoperatively, the more important correct rotational alignment will be in the postoperative rehabilitation phase.

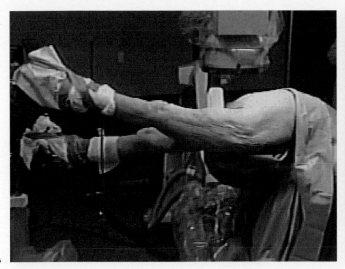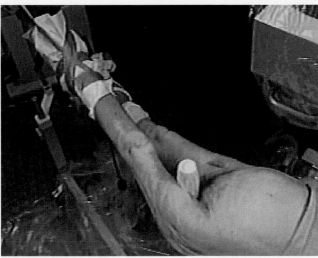

A   B

Figure 4. A, B: Supine position with affected extremity in foot traction, adducted for facilitation of entry portal, flexed approximately 15 degrees at the hip, knee extended.

Patient Preparation

Prep and drape the patient from the iliac crest, including the buttocks and lateral thigh, distally to below the knee. Cover the image-intensifier arm with a sterile isolation drape. A first-generation cephalosporin is administered. Vancomycin or an aminoglycoside is added if the fracture is open. Usually cephazolin, 1 g i.v., is continued for 48 hours after surgery for closed fractures. Reconstruction nailing of open fractures should be performed only after appropriate debridement and irrigation of the open fracture wound. Reprepping and redraping of the extremity are required to minimize cross-contamination at the nail-insertion site.

Surgical Approach

A 10-cm oblique skin incision is made just proximal to the greater trochanter (Fig. 5). The fascia of the gluteus maximus is incised, and the muscle is opened in line with its fibers. The subfascial plane of the gluteus maximus is identified, and the trochanteric or piriformis fossa is palpated.

Femoral Preparation

Establishing the correct portal for nail entry is crucial. Incorrect starting points can lead to angular deformities. For conventional reamed intramedullary nailing, the correct start-

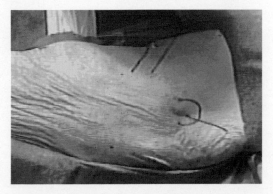

Figure 5. Skin incision.

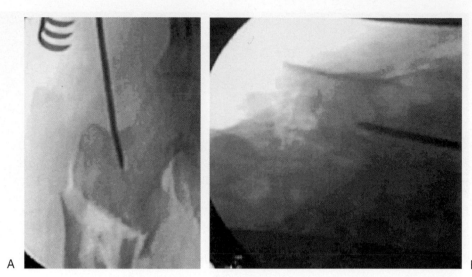

Figure 6. A, B: Tip-threaded guide pin inserted into piriformis fossa, centered on lateral view.

ing point is in the piriformis fossa. However, for reconstruction nailing, the portal of entry is slightly anterior to the fossa. Because the femoral neck arises from the anterior portion of the proximal femur, moving the starting point 3 to 4 mm anteriorly facilitates proximal screw insertion. The entry site is determined by using a 3.2-mm threaded guide pin inserted in the trochanteric fossa, placing the pin in the midplane of the femur in both AP and lateral views (Fig. 6A and B). The entry portal is enlarged with the cannulated reamer over the guide pin (Fig. 7A and B). If the proximal femoral fragment is flexed, externally rotated, and adducted to such a degree that the entry portal cannot be visualized, manipulate the proximal fragment with a pointed reduction forceps or percutaneously inserted Schanz pin into a position that normalizes the AP projection.

To assist in reduction of the shaft fracture, a ball-tipped guide wire, which does not exceed the maximal unreamed diameter of the femur at the isthmus, is bent at its tip. The wire is advanced to the level of the fracture with the curve opposing the medial cortex. Its position is confirmed within the femur in AP and lateral views with the image intensifier (Fig. 8A and B). The proximal fragment is reduced to the distal fragment manually or with an internal fracture-alignment device (Fig. 9A–C). The guide wire is advanced into the center of the distal fragment until its tip reaches the old epiphyseal scar. Containment of the guide wire is verified within the femur by image intensification (Fig. 10).

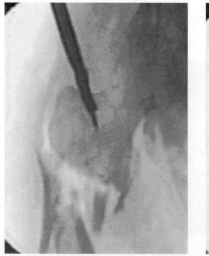
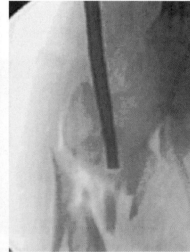

Figure 7. A, B: Overream guide wire with 8-mm cannulated rigid reamer for correct entry portal.

A,B

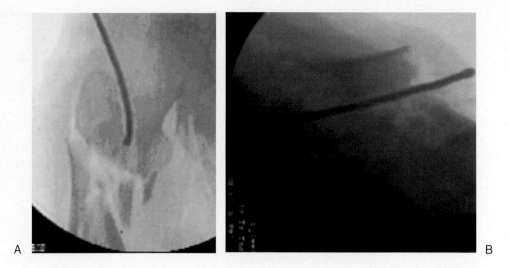

Figure 8. A, B: Insert 3.2-mm guide wire to fracture site. Tip of wire bent to facilitate fracture reduction.

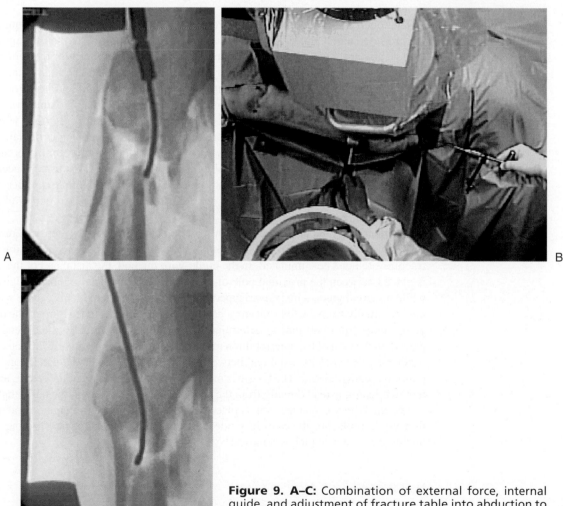

Figure 9. A–C: Combination of external force, internal guide, and adjustment of fracture table into abduction to accomplish fracture reduction.

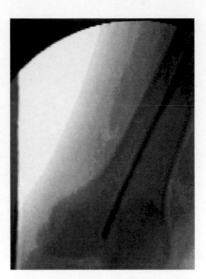

Figure 10. Guide wire inserted to knee for reaming and length determination of nail.

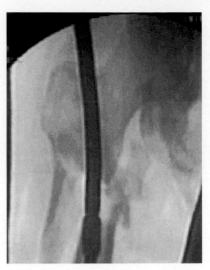

Figure 11. Progressive flexible reamers in 0.5-mm increments, with proximal 8 to 9 mm overreaming for reconstruction nail proximal expansion.

The femur is reamed in 0.5-mm increments from 9.0 mm to at least 1.0 mm more than the proposed nail diameter. In patients with a large anterior bow of their femur, as seen on lateral radiographs, or fracture extension into the distal one fourth of the femur, it is important to overream 1.5 to 2 mm larger than the nail diameter. The final reamer diameter should be verified with the reamer template before nail selection and insertion. Never insert a nail that has a larger diameter than the last reamer used. The proximal 8 cm of the femur is reamed to 15 mm in diameter with progressive reamers, starting with a 9-mm reamer, to accommodate the enlarged proximal end of most reconstruction nails (Fig. 11). Because the proximal fragment must be reamed substantially, it is very important to avoid destruction of the proximal entry portal by eccentric reaming. This usually occurs during insertion of the reamer and during its extraction. Use a slotted hammer or other instrument to direct a medial force on the reamer shaft during insertion and extraction to avoid this complication (Fig. 12A and B).

Verification of the proper nail length may be determined by two separate methods, the guide-wire method or the nail-length gauge. With either method, residual distraction at the fracture site must be eliminated. In the guide-wire method, the distal end of the guide wire is placed between the proximal pole of the patella and the distal femoral epiphyseal scar, while a second guide wire is overlapped to the portion of the reduction guide wire extending proximally from the femoral entry portal. Subtract the length (in mm) of the overlapped guide wires from 900 mm to determine nail length. Alternatively, a nail-length ruler is placed on the skin of the anterior thigh (unaffected femur preoperatively; affected femur intraoperatively) with its distal end between the proximal pole of the patella and the distal femoral epiphyseal scar. The C-arm is moved to the proximal end of the femur, and the correct nail length is read directly from the stamped measurements on the nail-length ruler.

The medullary exchange tube is placed over the guide wire to maintain fracture reduction while replacing the ball-tip guide wire with a non–ball-tip nail-driving wire. The medullary exchange tube is removed.

Nail Insertion

The appropriate nail is attached to the proximal driving/proximal drill guide. When assembled properly, the nail will have an anterior bow, and the orientation of the proximal drill guide points laterally.

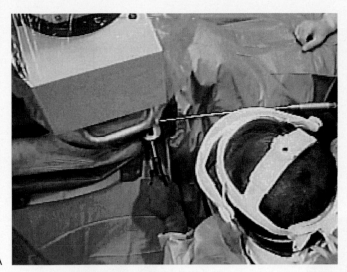
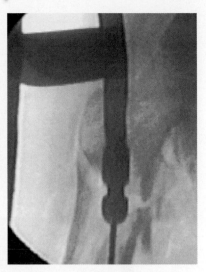

A   B

Figure 12. A, B: Slotted hammer inserts a medial force on the reamer shaft to avoid damage to greater trochanter during reamer head insertion and extraction.

Assemble either the sliding hammer or supine driver to the proximal drill guide and insert the nail over the guide wire. The proximal drill guide acts as a handle to control rotation and aid in insertion of the nail (Fig. 13). It is very important not to strike the proximal drill guide directly, because this may deform the targeting device and compromise proximal interlocking. Once the nail has been inserted, the proximal targeting device should be retightened. The nail is driven under radiographic control to within 1 to 2 cm of its anticipated depth.

Because the anatomy of the proximal femur varies from person to person, a reconstruction nail is inserted to the point where the upper end of the nail will accommodate two proximal screws. Frequently, minor adjustments in nail position, either proximal or distal, are necessary to line up the holes in the nail with the femoral head and neck. External extrapolation for final nail insertion and screw centralization can be initially performed with the nail-length ruler and a radiopaque rule or guide. Its outline is drawn with a skin marker over the femoral head and neck (Figs. 14 and 15). With the nail nearly fully seated, the inferior drill sleeves are placed into the proximal drill guide to extrapolate the eventual location of the inferior screw.

The C-arm is positioned to obtain a true lateral view of the femoral head and neck. The proximal targeting guide is aligned with the C-arm axis by rotating the proximal drill guide in the transverse plane (Fig. 16). If the proximal targeting device is radiopaque, the guide is centralized with respect to the femoral head, bisecting the femoral head in the coronal plane on the true lateral C-arm view. The posterior and anterior portion of the femoral head

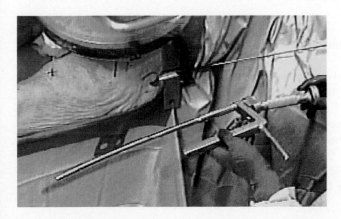

Figure 13. Nail assembly with proximal drill guide.

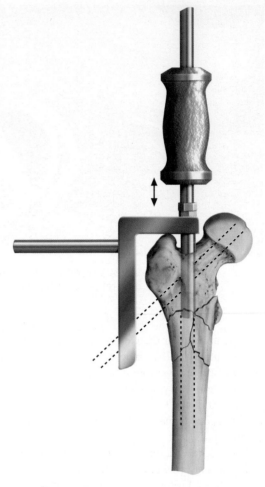

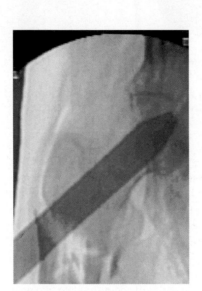

Figure 14. Overlay ruler to access anticipated final screw-insertion zone.

Figure 15. Adjust nail-insertion depth for centering of proximal locking screws.

must be seen in relation to the proximal drill guide to confirm that the screws will be contained within the femoral head (Fig. 17). Further verification of the proximal guide wires, drill bits, and locking screws may be obtained with oblique C-arm views. With a skin marker, a horizontal line is drawn on the lateral thigh as a reference to correct rotation of the proximal drill guide (Fig. 18). The traction is released, and the nail is seated. The intramedullary guide wire is removed from the femur.

Interlocking-Screw Technique

Proximal interlocking involves insertion of large cancellous screws. The proximal interlocking screws should reach the dense subchondral bone of the femoral head for maximal stability. The skin and fascia are incised through the inferior hole of the proximal drill guide. The stacked drill sleeves are inserted through the inferior hole and pushed to bone. The appropriate guide pin is inserted through the drill sleeve and advanced into the femoral head at least 4 mm superior to the calcar, within 5 mm of the subchondral bone of the femoral head. The position of the guide pin within the head is confirmed with AP and oblique lateral views with the C-arm (Fig. 19A and B).

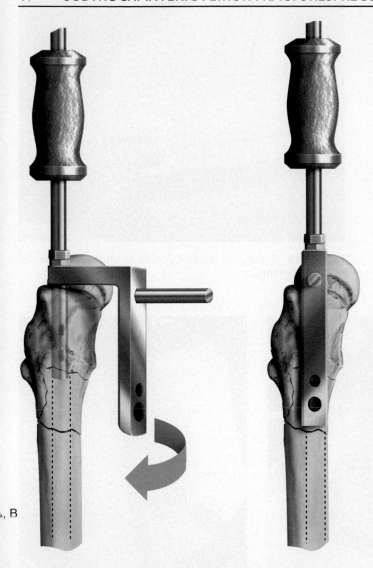

, B

Figure 16. A, B: Rotation of proximal drill guide to center guide for correct anteversion of screws into femoral head; drill guide should bisect the femoral head on the true lateral radiographic view.

If on the true lateral view, the guide pin is obstructed by the proximal drill guide but the femoral head anteriorly and posteriorly is visible, central placement of the pin can be inferred. For further confirmation, the C-arm can be rotated anteriorly and posteriorly from the true lateral position. The second guide pin is placed in the superior hole of the nail, and its location within the femoral head confirmed with the C-arm. The skin and fascia are incised through the superior hole of the proximal drill guide, and the stacked drill sleeves are inserted through the superior hole. The drill sleeves are pushed to bone. The second proximal guide pin is inserted through the drill sleeve and advanced into the femoral head (Fig. 20).

The inferior guide pin and inner drill sleeves are removed if the screw is noncannulated. This leaves a pilot hole to center the large step drill. The appropriate step drill is inserted through the remaining drill sleeve into the femoral head to within 5 mm of subchondral bone. Verify that the drill sleeves are against bone (Fig. 21). Screw-length measurement is determined with calibrated drill bits (Fig. 22). Alternatively, length can be assessed by using a depth gauge. The appropriate lag screw is inserted through the drill sleeve into the femoral head (Fig. 23). The threads of the screws must lie totally within the femoral head and not in the femoral neck to maximize purchase. The remaining drill sleeves are removed.

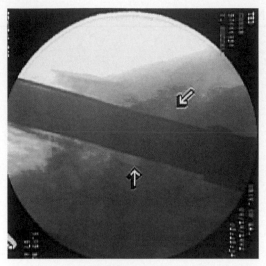

Figure 17. Lateral fluoroscopic view with bi-section of femoral head with drill guide for correct screw position.

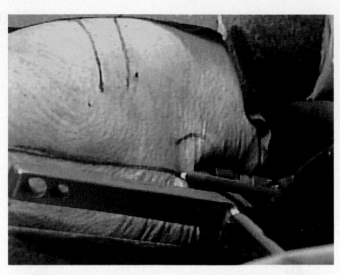

Figure 18. Trace drill guide to serve as visual reminder of correct anteversion.

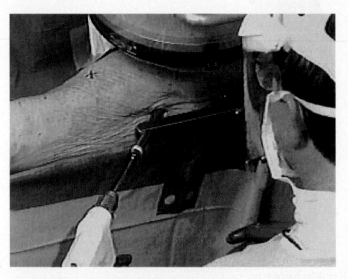

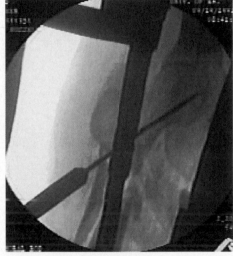

A   B

Figure 19. A, B: Insert inferior guide wire and confirm correct placement to within 5 mm subchondral bone and correct neck–shaft alignment.

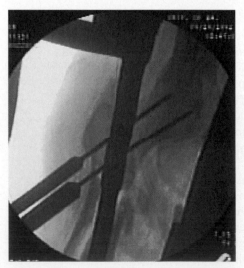

Figure 20. Insert second guide wire for centering and stability of proximal guide.

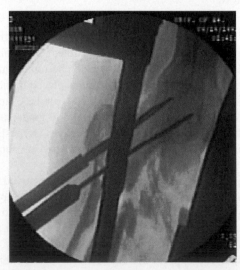

Figure 21. Use step-drill for screw-tract preparation.

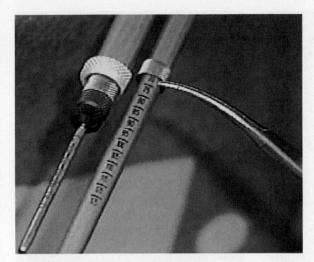

Figure 22. Determine correct screw-length selection from calibrated step-drill.

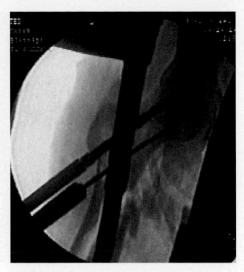

Figure 23. Insert proximal lag screw.

Insert the second proximal screw in a similar fashion, with the superior hole of the drill guide, and a guide pin, if not already in place, is advanced to within 5 mm of subchondral bone. The guide pin and appropriate drill sheaths for noncannulated screws are removed. The step drill is inserted through the drill sleeve into the femoral head to within 5 mm of the subchondral bone. Verify that the drill sleeve is against bone. The screw length is determined at this point by using the calibrated drills or by using a depth gauge. Remove the step drill. Tapping is usually recommended, but in dense bone in young patients, it is required (Fig. 24). The appropriate size proximal screw is inserted into the femoral head. The drill sleeve is removed. Confirm containment of both screws in the femoral head with AP, lateral, and oblique views (Fig. 25). For maximal stability, all threads of the proximal locking screws should be within the femoral head. No screw threads must be passed across any fracture line, to avoid distraction by the threads. Proximal interlocking is now complete.

Insertion of a distal locking screw improves stability and decreases the incidence of malunion. I prefer a freehand technique or use a radiolucent drill guide for distal interlocking screw placement (Fig. 26A–C).

The proximal drill guide is removed from the nail. The entire femur is scanned with the C-arm to confirm correct screw placement, adequacy of reduction, stability at fracture site, and proper nail length. The wounds are irrigated and closed in layers (fascia, subcutaneous, and skin) in the standard fashion. Sterile dressings are applied. If skeletal traction was used, the traction pin is removed, and the wounds covered with sterile dressings.

POSTOPERATIVE MANAGEMENT

In the absence of associated injuries, patients are mobilized from the bed to chair and gait trained with a walker or crutches on the first or second postoperative day. Thromboembolic prophylaxis is usually begun 12 hours after surgery with a low-molecular-weight heparin and continued for 7 to 14 days, depending on the patient's mobility. Weight bearing is restricted to 10 to 15 kg on the affected extremity in comminuted fractures. If cortical contact is restored, and there is good bone quality, weight bearing is permitted as tolerated with crutches or walker. Range-of-motion exercises and straight-leg lifts are started in the first week. Patients are usually discharged to home on the third or fourth postoperative day, when they demonstrate lower-extremity control sufficient for household ambulation with crutches or a walker. Patients are followed up at 3- to 4-week intervals, and radiographs are obtained at each visit. When callus is detected (usually at 4 to 8 weeks), progressive weight

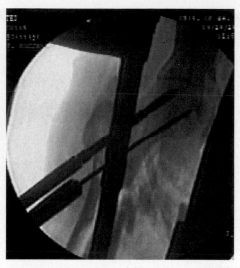

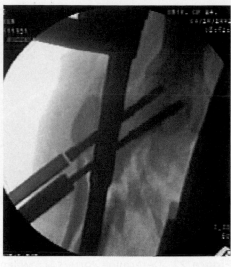

Figure 24. Remove second guide wire and drill with step-drill for second screw; tapping is frequently required in dense bone.

Figure 25. Insert second proximal screw, and confirm seating radiographically.

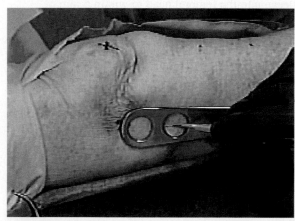

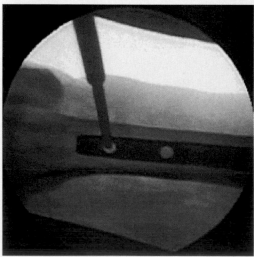

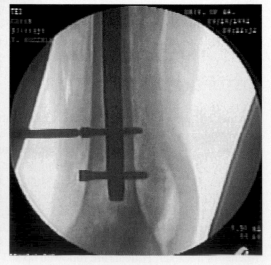

Figure 26. A–C: Freehand technique: locate hole with external marker, and make a stab incision over the hole axis, insert trocar to dimple bone, drill for bicortical fixation, and insert screws.

bearing is allowed. Patients must demonstrate full weight bearing on the affected leg for 60 seconds before crutches are discontinued. A progressive-resistance exercise program is prescribed, and swimming or stationary bicycling is recommended.

Implant removal is not considered until there is mature radiographic callus bridging the fracture site on both the AP and lateral radiographs and rarely before 1 year. A general anesthetic is required and usually a 24-hour hospitalization. Patients use crutches after implant removal until their gait returns to the preimplant-removal status. After implant removal, contact sports are avoided for 3 months.

With isolated fractures, most patients attain community-ambulation status within 6 to 8 weeks with crutches, begin driving motor vehicles at 8 to 16 weeks, and are full weight bearing by 3 to 5 months after injury. Patients can expect functional recovery sufficient to return to their previous occupations in most cases. Union rates after closed reconstruction nailing are 95% to 100% in acute subtrochanteric fractures uncomplicated by other injuries.

There is no current-outcomes research on differing treatments for subtrochanteric femur fractures. It is only over the past 10 years that as surgeons, we have focused on obtaining union with an implant failure rate of less than 10% in these difficult fractures. As with most hip fractures, avoidance of varus and significant leg-length discrepancies are tantamount to a good result for the surgeon and the patient. Most patients return to their previous occupations and recreational activities if functional restoration is achieved. Most persisting problems are related to associated knee or neurologic injuries. Sanders et al. (4) proposed a rating system for subtrochanteric fractures, but no comparative series are yet available with this outcome measure.

COMPLICATIONS

Malreduction

Entry-portal selection for the reconstruction nail is significantly more difficult than for standard femoral nailing. After subtrochanteric fractures, strong muscle pull leads to flexion, external rotation, and varus positioning of the proximal fragment. This increases the difficulty in visualizing the entry portal with the C-arm. This may be solved by either internally rotating the leg and attempting a closed reduction of the hip or by inserting a pin percutaneously into the trochanteric mass and using this as a joystick to rotate the proximal femur into a more anatomically recognizable position. In obese patients, a straight nail driver will tend to offset the nail laterally and force the hip into varus if fracture extension or comminution is present medially. This occurs because of pressure of the driver on the lateral ilium. One may use an offset driver and apply pressure medially through the driver after correct depth insertion of the nail to restore normal hip alignment. Alternatively, nailing in the lateral decubitus position decreases varus malalignment.

Proximal Screw Placement Errors

Gauging the proper depth of insertion of the nail to maximize screw centralization of the femoral head can be surprisingly difficult. Preoperative templates can be helpful in determining the diameter of the femoral neck and aid in selection of the proper implant.

Radiographic visualization of the proximal femur, particularly in the lateral projection, may be difficult. Rotation of the C-arm until a true lateral of the femoral head and neck is the key to successful proximal screw placement. This is facilitated by temporarily rotating the proximal guide anteriorly. Once a true lateral of the femoral neck can be visualized and a reduction confirmed, the handle is rotated posteriorly until the opaque guide bisects the femoral head. This will allow visualization of the femoral head anterior and posterior to the locking guide. When a portion of the femoral head anterior and posterior to the proximal guide handle is visualized, the screws will be contained in the centered position of the femoral head (Fig. 16). I favor screws slightly anterior in the femoral head.

In the supine position, the femoral head is anterior to the shaft of the femur, which requires the proximal drill guide to be rotated below horizontal to prevent posterior screw placement in the femoral head. Anteversion built into the nail compensates for the anterior offset of the femoral neck from the center of the medullary canal. This minimizes the amount of external rotation needed to insert the nail and to optimize distal interlocking so that distal screw insertion is not too posterior at the knee. During insertion of the proximal locking screws, they tend to be placed in retroversion. Even though 8 to 15 degrees of anteversion is built into most reconstruction nails in relation to the distal locking holes, the proximal drill guide should be positioned slightly below the horizontal axis of the limb. Rotational alignment and centralization of the proximal drill guide is confirmed on the lateral C-arm view.

In some patients, there may be difficulty placing two screws within the femoral head. The most common causes for this problem are varus reduction of the proximal fragment, a narrow femoral neck, and preexisting coxa vara in reference to the "neck–shaft" angle of the proximal screws and nail. If the proximal screws transverse an inferior to superior tract in the femoral head or it is the surgeon's perspective that only one screw can be inserted, the fracture is probably in varus. Another common mistake is inadequate depth insertion of the nail. This can be minimized by preoperative planning and referencing the tip of the greater trochanter to the center of the femoral head. The goal is to try to place the inferior screw just above the medial femoral cortex. If the nail is inserted too deep, it will be difficult to insert the screw or the screw will penetrate the cortex. The guide wire should be placed 4 to 5 mm above the medial femoral neck. Alternatively, a K-wire may be inserted percutaneously anterior to the femoral neck into the desired position and the proximal driving guide inserted by using this reference point.

Frequently during proximal screw insertion, the surgeon will note that the proximal locking screw will not advance past the nail into the femoral neck. This is usually because of the partially threaded proximal screw functioning as a bolt. When all of the threads of the bolt become contained within the proximal nail, there are no threads to pull the nail into the bone. At this point, it is frequently helpful just to tap the screw into the femoral head until threads contact bone and start the threading process again.

The proximal screws must provide stable fixation in the operating room. In cases of severe osteoporosis or pathologic lesions in which the screws do not have good fixation, augmentation of the proximal screw fixation with nonpressurized methylmethacrylate is advisable.

Infection

Infection is relatively uncommon with closed nailing techniques and probably occurs at a rate of 1% in closed fractures and slightly higher in open fractures. If the implant is stable, incision and drainage of the acute infection and intravenous antibiotics are recommended. Once the fracture has united, the implant should be removed and the canal debrided. A more difficult problem is loss of fixation accompanied with an occult infection. Depending on the type of organism, debridement and renailing and antibiotics may be successful. If a virulent organism is encountered with loss of nail stability, traction or external fixation or both may be required, with a higher morbidity expected in this situation.

Fixation Disruption

Loss of fixation may occur from failure of screw fixation or nail or screw breakage. Nail breakage usually implies nonunion and fatigue failure. If aseptic, exchange reamed nailing is recommended. Loss of proximal screw fixation acutely reflects pathologic bone (i.e., osteopenia or neoplasia) or poor initial screw placement. Late loss of screw fixation implicates nonunion. Revision nailing and bone grafting are required for successful salvage. Distal screw breakage early is usually the result of premature or excessive weight bearing. Length or rotational loss may occur if distal screws are removed prematurely or if the patient engages in excessive weight bearing.

Nonunion

Aseptic nonunions are biologic failures that may or may not be complicated with implant failure. If the existing implant is loose, it should be revised to the most suitable fixation, usually to a larger reamed interlocking reconstruction nail. In hypertrophic nonunions, exchange nailing is frequently all that will be required. When in doubt or in atrophic nonunions, autologous cancellous iliac bone graft to the nonunion site with a Phemister–Judet technique is advised.

Functional Loss

Functional loss is almost always the result of complications about the hip or knee. Heterotopic ossification is a frequent radiographic finding but rarely symptomatic. Associated patella, periarticular knee fractures, and soft-tissue injuries can result in the loss of motion after subtrochanteric fractures. Neurologic injuries associated with the subtrochanteric fracture are rare, but must be evaluated carefully before nailing. Sciatic and pudendal nerve injuries observed postoperatively are usually caused by excessive traction required for reduction or compartment syndrome. These injuries do not always resolve with time, resulting in significant morbidity.

ILLUSTRATIVE CASE FOR TECHNIQUE

A 49-year-old man had parachute malfunction while jumping. On impact, he had a closed displaced proximal femur fracture (Fig. 27A and B). The patient underwent reamed static reconstruction nailing. His fracture united at 3 months, and he returned to his work without restrictions. This fracture pattern probably represents the ideal indication for a reconstruction nail, that is, a subtrochanteric fracture with loss of medial cortical stability with fracture of the lesser trochanter (Russell–Taylor IB). The fracture does not extend into the piriformis fossa.

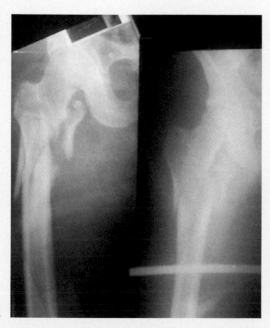 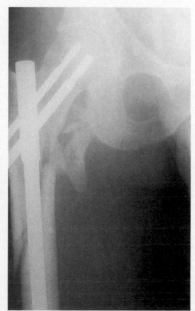

Figure 27. A, B: Subtrochanteric fracture from parachuting accident. Stabilization with Russell–Taylor reconstruction nail, static mode.

RECOMMENDED READING

1. Bergman, G.D., Winquist, R.A., Mayo, K.A., Hansen, S.T., Jr.: Subtrochanteric fracture of the femur: fixation using the Zickel nail. *J. Bone Joint Surg. [Am],* 69:1032–1040, 1987.
2. Charnley, G.J., and Ward, A.J.: Reconstruction femoral nailing for nonunion of subtrochanteric fracture: a revision technique following dynamic condylar screw failure. *Int. Orthop.,* 20:55–57, 1996.
3. Russell, T.A., and Taylor, J.C.: Subtrochanteric fractures. In Browner, B. (ed.): *Skeletal Trauma,* 1993.
4. Sanders, R., Regazzoni, P., Routt, M.L., Jr.: The treatment of subtrochanteric fractures of the femur using the dynamic condylar screw. *J. Orthop. Trauma,* 3:206–213, 1989.
5. Slater, J.C., Russell, T.A., Walker, F.M.: Intramedullary nailing of complex subtrochanteric fracture of the femur. Presented at AAOS Orthopaedic Transactions, 1992.
6. Taylor, D.C., Erpelding, J.M., Whitman, C.S., Kragh, J.R., Jr.: Treatment of comminuted subtrochanteric femoral fractures in a young population with a reconstruction nail. *Mil. Med.,* 161:735–738, 1996.
7. Waddell, J.P.: Subtrochanteric fractures of the femur: a review of 130 patients. *J. Trauma,* 19:585–592, 1979.
8. Wheeler, D.L., Croy, T.J., Well, T.S., Scott, M.D., Senft, D.C., Duwellius, P.J.: Comparisons of reconstruction nails for high subtrochanteric femur fracture fixation. *Clin. Orthop.,* 338:231–239, 1997.
9. Wiss, D.A., and Brien, W.W.: Subtrochanteric fractures of the femur: results of treatment with interlocking nails. *Clin. Orthop.,* 283:231–236, 1992.

Master Techniques in Orthopaedic Surgery,
FRACTURES, edited by D. A. Wiss,
Lippincott–Raven Publishers, Philadelphia © 1998.

18

Femur Fractures: Intramedullary Nailing

Bruce D. Browner, Andrew E. Caputo, and Augustus D. Mazzocca

INDICATIONS/CONTRAINDICATIONS

Intramedullary nailing is the treatment of choice for virtually all diaphyseal femoral fractures in adults. There are two types of locked intramedullary nailing: static and dynamic. Static locking involves placement of proximal and distal locking screws, which prevent malrotation and shortening. Dynamic locking uses locking screws on only one side of the fracture, either proximal or distal. Because static interlocking does not inhibit fracture healing, virtually all diaphyseal femoral fractures should be statically locked. Occasionally, dynamic locking is indicated in short oblique or transverse middiaphyseal fractures without comminution.

Many classification systems have been described for femur fractures. Winquist and Hansen developed a classification based on the amount of comminution (Fig. 1). Type I and II fractures have stable bone contact between the proximal and distal fragments and are considered length stable. Type III and IV comminution results in no contact between the proximal and distal fragments and requires static interlocking to maintain correct limb length and rotation.

Indications for intramedullary nailing of the femur include simple or comminuted fractures below the lesser trochanter extending distally to within 7 cm of the knee joint. Most Grade I and Grade II open femoral-shaft fractures can be treated with reamed intramedullary nails. Isolated Grade III fractures may be better treated with aggressive wound management, skeletal traction, and delayed intramedullary fixation. Patients with multiple injuries including open femur fractures require early skeletal stabilization to prevent pulmonary compromise. In these circumstances, nonreamed intramedullary nailing may be biologically attractive. However, the mechanical benefits of reaming with insertion of a larger nail, providing more stability and strength, are sacrificed.

B. D. Browner, M.D.: Department of Orthopaedic Surgery, University of Connecticut Health Center, John Dempsey Hospital, Farmington, Connecticut 06034-4037.

A. E. Caputo, M.D., and A. D. Mazzocca, M.D.: Department of Orthopaedics, University of Connecticut Health Center, Farmington, Connecticut 06034-4037.

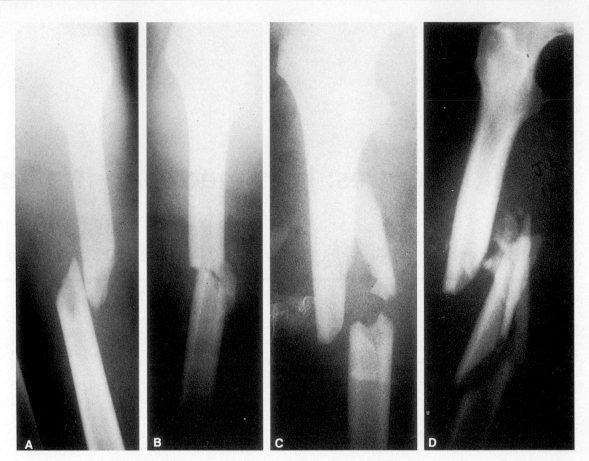

Figure 1. A–D: Winquist–Hansen fracture classification based on the amount of comminution.

Contraindications to intramedullary nailing include active local or systemic infections. Antegrade nailing in adolescents with open growth plates can damage the blood supply to the femoral head, causing osteonecrosis. These fractures may be better treated by using flexible intramedullary nails, which are inserted retrograde, proximal to the distal femoral growth plate. Although there is no definitive scientific support, a higher incidence of infection has been noted if reamed nailing is performed after a prolonged period of initial external fixation. Other contraindications to nailing include patients with very narrow medullary canals or those with preexisting deformities that would preclude closed nailing.

PREOPERATIVE PLANNING

All patients with femur fractures resulting from blunt trauma should be evaluated for other injuries. Trauma evaluation and resuscitation with a multidisciplinary approach is necessary in multiply injured patients. High-quality, full-length anteroposterior (AP) and lateral radiographs of the femur should be obtained to evaluate the fracture (Fig. 2A and B). The fracture location and the degree of comminution should be assessed on plain films. Ipsilateral fractures of the hip or femoral condyles must be ruled out before nailing. Specific hip or knee films are often necessary the better to visualize these fractures. Unrecognized nondisplaced fractures in these areas may displace during nailing. Once recognized, these fractures may be amenable to fixation with percutaneous screws. Osteoarthritis of the hip joint with a flexion contracture may limit hip motion on the traction table and make nailing difficult in the supine position. When severe comminution or segmental defects exist, full-length films of the opposite femur may be helpful in determining appropriate length.

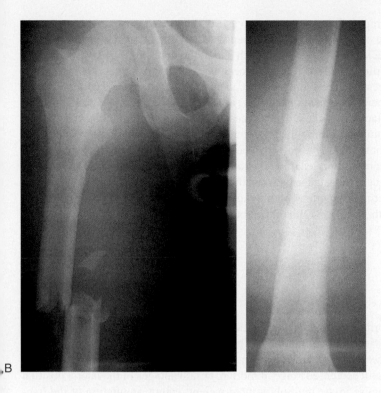

Figure 2. A, B: Anteroposterior radiograph of the right femur showing a transverse middiaphyseal fracture with minimal comminution.

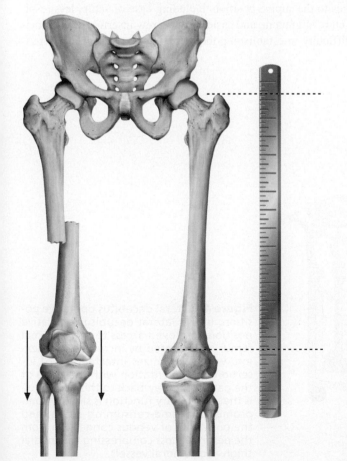

Figure 3. Preoperative evaluation of leg length. For simple fractures with limited comminution, the fracture can usually be reduced with minimal problems to restore the correct limb length. In patients with Winquist III and IV fracture comminution, length is reestablished by using the contralateral intact femur as a reference. The length between the tip of the trochanter and the adductor tubercle is determined. Intraoperatively, the length of the fractured femur is adjusted by using traction to duplicate the correct trochanter–adductor tubercle length. This can be confirmed by using two overlapping guide wires of the same length.

Contralateral radiographs also may be used to assess the medullary canal diameter and the degree of curvature of the intact femur. Patients with extremely small intramedullary canals may require special-sized implants, which should be determined preoperatively to ensure implant availability. The remodeling process associated with aging and osteoporosis often lead to an increase in the diameter of the medullary canal. In these patients, insertion of very-large-diameter nails is not necessary, as stability is better achieved with 12- to 14-mm nails that are statically locked. The increased stiffness of large-diameter nails can cause iatrogenic comminution during insertion into brittle osteoporotic bone; therefore, it is particularly important to match the curve of the implant to the curve of the femur.

Reestablishing the correct limb length and choosing the appropriate-length nail require a reference length. We use the distance between the tip of the greater trochanter and the adductor tubercle to determine length. A radiograph of the intact femur with a radiopaque ruler placed along the thigh (Fig. 3) should be obtained.

SURGERY

Patient Positioning

Nailing can be performed with the patient in the lateral decubitus (Fig. 4) or supine position (Fig. 5) with or without a fracture table. The advantages of the lateral decubitus position are improved access to the piriformis fossa, especially in large patients or those with ipsilateral hip disease with decreased range of motion. Disadvantages of the lateral position are respiratory compromise in the multiply injured patient, valgus angulation of the fracture, difficulty determining proper rotation, venous congestion caused by pressure of the perineal post, and greater difficulty inserting distal locking screws.

There are several advantages to the supine position, including ease of setup, less respiratory compromise, better fracture alignment, and easier distal screw insertion. The principal disadvantage is greater difficulty in establishing the correct starting point in the piriformis fossa.

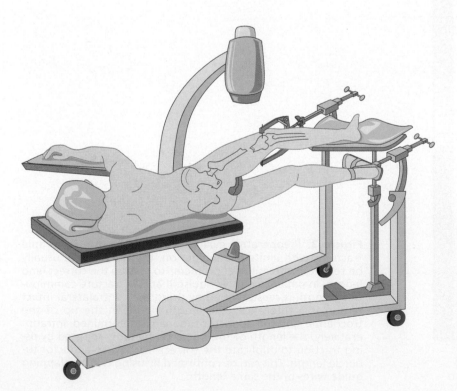

Figure 4. Lateral decubitus operative position. In the lateral decubitus operative position, improved access to the proximal femur is facilitated by increased hip flexion, which minimizes interference of insertion instrumentation with the torso of the patient. A drawback to this technique is that pulmonary function is slightly compromised, a time-consuming setup, and the possibility of venous congestion from the peroneal post compressing the medial thigh and femoral vessels.

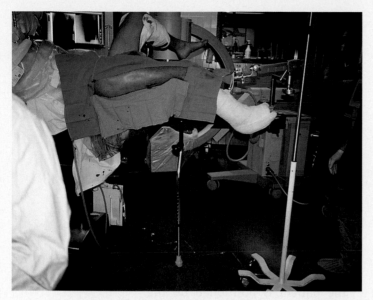

Figure 5. Supine operative position. To gain better access to the proximal femur on the operative side, the patient's arm is positioned above the body, and the torso is shifted away from the injured side. The operative limb is adducted at the hip. Rotational alignment is obtained with the knee flexed and the foot hanging free. Traction should be applied by using a Steinmann pin placed at the level of the tibial tubercle. The attachment points for the traction bow should be placed close to the skin to avoid bending of the Steinmann pin when traction is applied. Bending of the pin dissipates the traction force and produces difficulties in pin removal. The protruding Steinmann pin should be cut close to the bow and the remaining sharp ends covered with tape to avoid injury to health-care personnel.

Classically, intramedullary nailing is done on a fracture table that achieves fracture reduction through sustained longitudinal traction with or without a skeletal pin. A perineal post provides a fulcrum against which traction is applied. The design of most fracture tables allows circumferential access to the extremity for manipulation, surgical exposure, and imaging. Setup time is longer with a fracture table in patients with multiple trauma who require simultaneous or sequential surgical procedures.

Alternatively, intramedullary nailing can be performed on a radiolucent table. Traction can be applied manually or with the use of a femoral distractor. Nailing can be performed through an antegrade or retrograde approach. The technique works best when nailing is

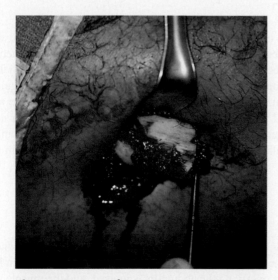

Figure 6. Open fracture management. An open fracture wound should be debrided before nailing. The bone ends should be inspected and carefully cleaned with a curette. Surgical extensions of the incision should be closed, and the original wound left open. At the end of the debridement, all of the instruments, gowns, gloves, and drapes should be changed, and the intramedullary nailing treated as a separate procedure.

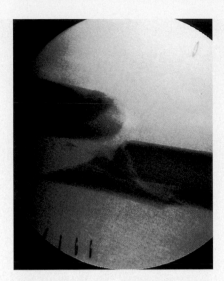

Figure 7. Fracture alignment. Once the patient is positioned on the fracture table, there is posterior displacement of the distal fragment.

done less than 24 hours after injury. Setup time is minimal, and access to the piriformis fossa is improved by adducting the limb. Disadvantages with this technique include difficulty visualizing the hip and proximal femur in the lateral projection, difficulty reducing and holding the fracture alignment, risk to the femoral neurovascular structures, and blockage of the operative field by the femoral distractor (Fig. 6).

Closed Reduction

Closed reduction is performed by traction through the fracture table and external manipulation. An in-line boot, with proximal tibial or distal femoral pin traction, is applied, and the alignment is checked with the image intensifier (Fig. 7). Occasionally manipulation of the leg by the surgeon or a crutch may be useful for reduction of an angulated fracture (Figs. 8 and 9). To minimize the risk of a pudendal nerve palsy, the traction is decreased during the prep, drape, and proximal exposure. Frequently a small-diameter nail may be used in the proximal fragment to reduce a flexed and externally rotated proximal fragment. Alternatively, many implant manufacturers include a small-diameter rod in the nailing sets for this purpose.

Entry Point

The entry point is critical to proper nail placement and fracture reduction. A longitudinal incision 6 to 10 cm in length is made over the greater trochanter in line with the femur (Fig. 10). The fascia overlying the abductors is incised, and the muscle split in line with its fibers down to the piriformis fossa (Fig. 11). A sharp awl is placed in the piriformis fossa and its position confirmed with fluoroscopy. The tip should be centered directly in line with the medullary canal in both the AP and lateral views. Medial portal placement should be avoided, as this may cause a femoral-neck fracture. Portal placement laterally may lead to comminution and varus alignment in proximal fractures. Once the awl is properly positioned in the piriformis fossa and is confirmed fluoroscopically, a pilot hole is created (Fig. 12A–D). Alternatively, a guide wire may be placed in the piriformis fossa and the proximal femur opened with a cannulated drill (Figs. 13–20).

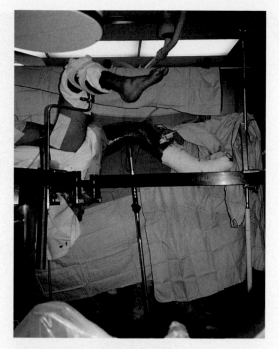

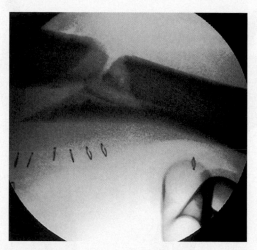

Figure 8. Fracture reduction. A crutch is placed between the floor and the posterior aspect of the leg to assist reduction. This places the distal fragment in a neutral position. Note that use of the push-button expandable crutch allows precise intraoperative adjustment and greater flexibility in reduction.

Figure 9. Fracture reduction. This lateral view shows the fracture after correction of the posterior displacement of the distal fragment with the crutch.

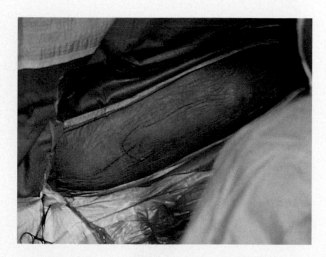

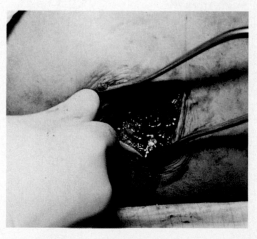

Figure 10. Surgical incision planning. A longitudinal incision is made about 6 to 10 cm in length just proximal to the tip of the greater trochanter. The surgical field must include the distal femur to accommodate distal locking.

Figure 11. Incision and dissection. The incision has been made and the dissection carried through the subcutaneous tissue and the fibers of the gluteus maximus down to the posterior edge of the gluteus medius. The tip of the greater trochanter and the piriformis fossa are localized by digital palpation.

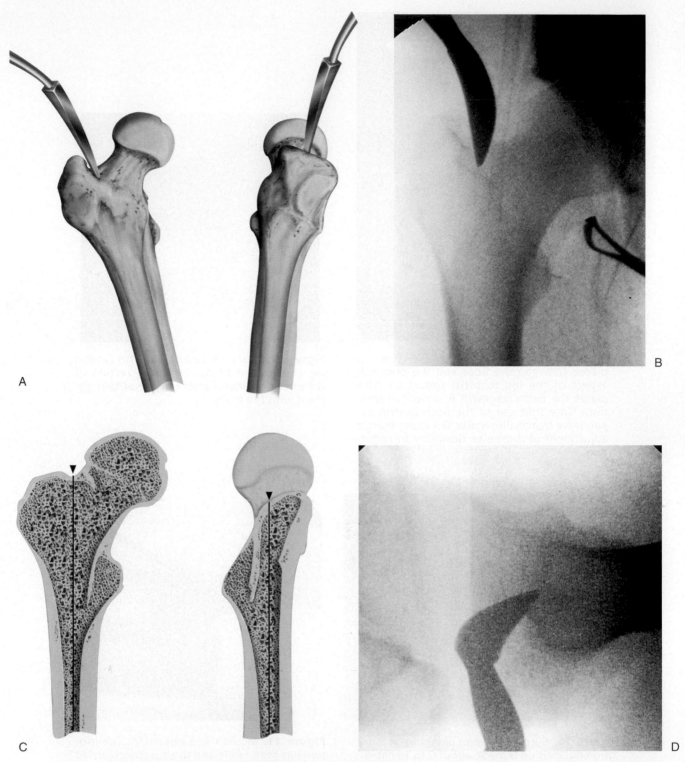

Figure 12. Femoral entry portal establishment with Küntscher awl. One alternative for establishing an entry portal in the proximal femur is the use of the curved awl **(A)**. Initial position of the awl established by digital palpation should be confirmed radiographically with the C-arm on anteroposterior (AP) and lateral views, which includes the greater trochanter, femoral head, and the proximal portion of the medullary canal **(B)**. The surgeon should imagine a line passing down the center of the medullary canal and projecting out the top of the femur **(C)**. The entry portal should be established exactly where this line emerges in the AP view **(D)**.

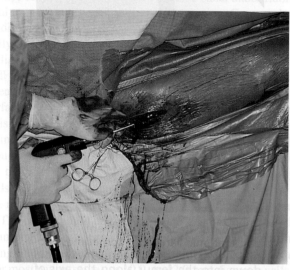

Figure 13. Femoral entry portal establishment with cannulated drill. Alternatively, the entry portal can be established by using a cannulated drill. As shown here, a ⁵⁄₃₂ Steinmann pin is guided radiographically and drilled into the piriformis fossa.

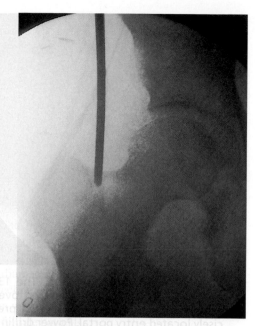

Figure 14. Steinmann-pin placement. The correct position of the Steinmann pin as it enters the top of the femur at a point where the line defining the center of the medullary canal would emerge from the top of the bone.

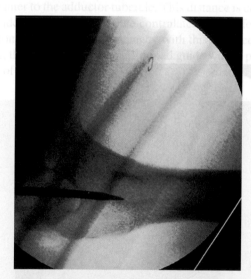

Figure 15. Steinmann-pin placement. As in the anteroposterior (AP) view, the lateral view of the proximal femur shows that the ⁵⁄₃₂ Steinmann pin penetrates the bone exactly at a point where the line defining the center of the medullary canal emerges from the top of the bone.

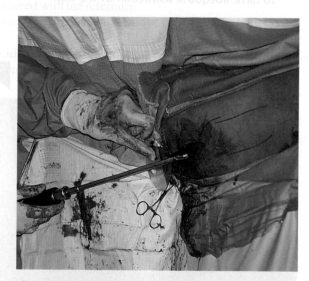

Figure 16. Cannulated drill with reamer. The cannulated drill is inserted with the soft-tissue protector in place over the ⁵⁄₃₂ Steinmann pin.

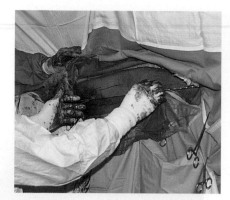

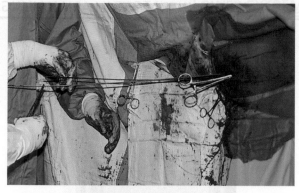

Figure 36

Figure 37

Figures 36 and 37. Ruler measurement. Reestablishing the correct length of the fractured femur and choosing the correct length of the intramedullary nail both require the use of a reference length, which is the distance between the tip of the greater trochanter and the adductor tubercle. This can be measured by using a radiopaque ruler held lateral to the thigh at the level of the femur.

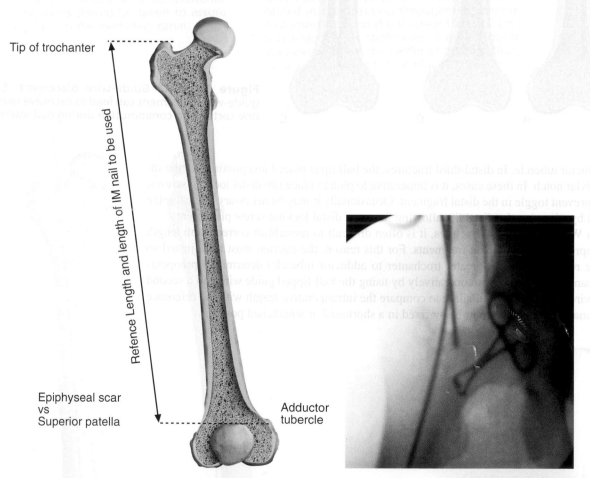

Tip of trochanter

Refence Length and length of IM nail to be used

Epiphyseal scar
vs
Superior patella

Adductor
tubercle

Figure 38

Figure 39

Figures 38 and 39. Wire measurement. A second guide wire equal in length to the ball-tip guide wire is inserted into the wound to the level of the entry portal at the top of the femur. A clamp is placed on the guide wire at the point where it overlaps the tip of the ball-tipped guide wire. The distance between the clamp and the free end of the second guide wire is measured and estimates the distance from the tip of the greater trochanter to the adductor tubercle. This distance is compared with the reference measurement made preoperatively on the contralateral intact femur. Adjustments must be made with traction to correct any discrepancy with this distance.

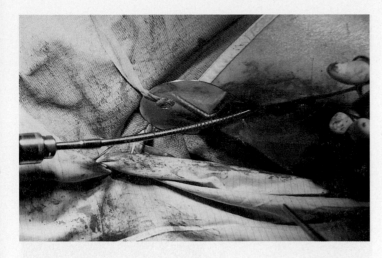

Figure 40. Reaming. The soft-tissue protector should always be used to avoid injury to the skin and muscle from the rotating reamer shaft. A lap-pad strap is tied to the protector to prevent it from falling to the floor. When the reamer is pulled back, a Kocher clamp is used to grasp the guide wire, avoiding its extraction across the fracture site. The initial reamer should be a small end-cutting type to create a path for subsequent reamers.

The ball-tipped guide wire is not designed for nail insertion. The tip of the guide wire is often bent to facilitate cannulation of the distal fragment, and the width of the ball is often wider than the inner diameter of the nail tip. Consequently, the curved ball-tipped guide wire may become trapped if used for nail insertion. Additionally, a larger-diameter guide wire that more completely fills the inner diameter of the nail tip is preferable for nail insertion. If the nail is inserted over a thin guide wire, the larger inner diameter at the nail tip can allow the nail to displace into an eccentric position. This can cause inadvertent incarceration on the cortex of the distal fragment. Therefore, a straight, smooth, large guide wire is necessary. A plastic sheath is used to maintain canal continuity while the ball-tipped guide wire is exchanged for the smooth guide wire (Figs. 43–45).

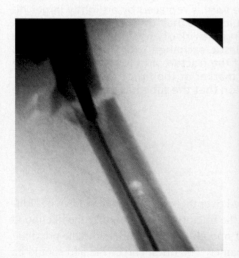
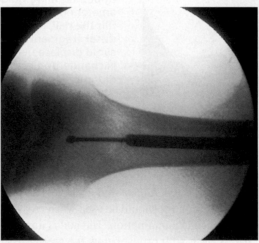

Figure 41   **Figure 42**

Figures 41 and 42. Reaming. To avoid excessive pressure in the medullary canal, reamers should be sharp, have deep flutes, and have a small shaft relative to the diameter of the reamer head. In addition, the reamer should be advanced slowly, and multiple passes should be made with each reamer size. Side-cutting reamers are used to enlarge the canal to 1.0 mm larger than the intended nail diameter. The diameter of the reamers can be increased by 1-mm increments initially. Once the reamers begin to bite into cortical bone, reaming diameter should be increased in 0.5-mm increments. If excessive resistance is encountered with a particular reamer, the last diameter that successfully passed should be reintroduced, and several more passes should be made with this reamer to remove additional bone. Overreaming from 1.0 to 2.0 mm is used when the femur has a significant bow, when the isthmus is long and narrow, or if driving the nail is difficult.

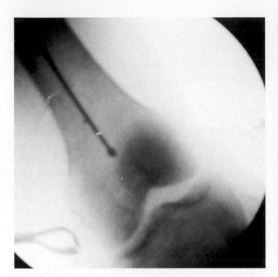

Figure 43

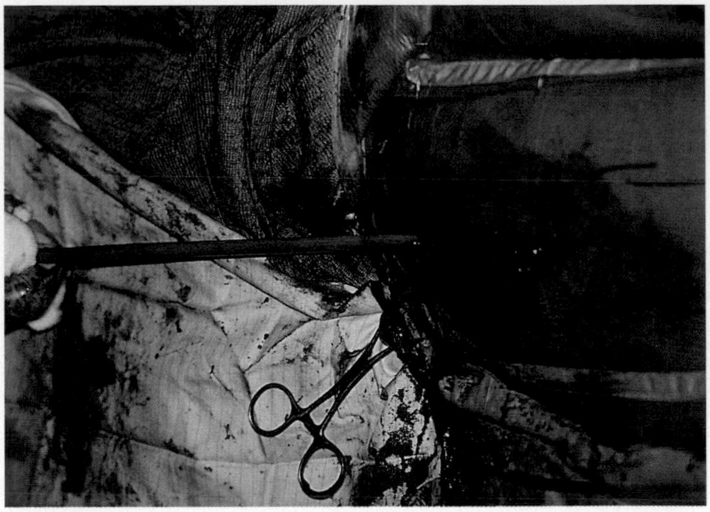

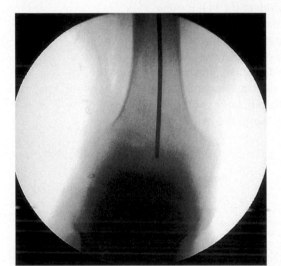

Figure 45

Figure 44

Figures 43, 44, and 45. Guide-wire exchange. The purpose of the spherical end on a ball-tipped guide wire is to assist in extracting an incarcerated reamer. However, because of the ball, this wire should not be used for nail insertion. The ball-tipped reaming guide wire is replaced by a slightly larger diameter nonbeaded guide wire (nail-driving guide wire), which fills the nail, minimizing the risk of engaging the cortex of the distal fragment. A plastic exchange tube should be used to avoid displacement of the fracture and to simplify guide-wire exchange. A metallic marker at the tip of the tube allows radiographic confirmation that the tube has passed the fracture site.

Nail Placement

The nail is assembled onto its driver and placed over the smooth-tipped guide wire. Fluoroscopic control should be used when crossing the fracture site to minimize the likelihood of iatrogenic comminution. The nail is impacted smoothly with a mallet until the proximal nail is flush with or just below the greater trochanter. The distal end of the nail should be inserted to the chosen reference point (adductor tubercle for diaphyseal fractures and adjacent to the intercondylar notch for distal-third fractures; Figs. 46–52). Most nails are designed with transfixion screws in the coronal plane. To achieve proper rotation, the nail must be controlled with the driver/proximal locking device during insertion.

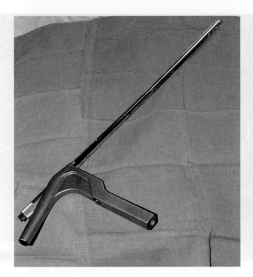

Figure 46

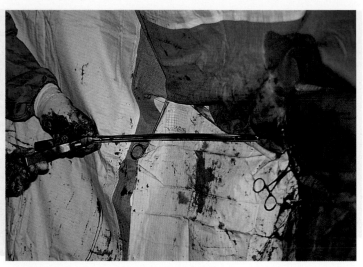

Figure 47

Figures 46 and 47. Intramedullary (IM) nail assembly and insertion. The proximal targeting nail and driving device is secured to the top of the nail. The nail driver can loosen after multiple mallet blows during insertion and should be retightened frequently. The nail is inserted over the guide wire into the femur, with the handle of the targeting device projecting parallel to the floor so that the proximal and distal screw holes will be located in the coronal plane.

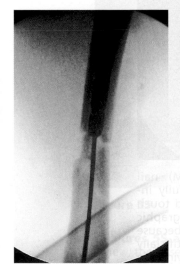

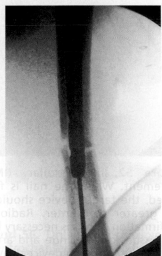

Figures 48 and 49. Intramedullary (IM) nail advancement. To avoid incarcerating comminuted fragments that lie in the path of the nail, the proximal end of the nail is pushed medially into the patient to direct the distal end of the nail laterally away from the fragment. The nail should be advanced slowly under fluoroscopic control.

Figure 48

Figure 49

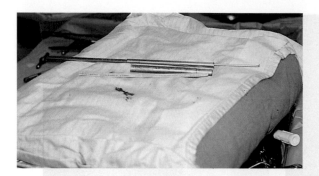

Figure 57. Depth gauge and tissue protector. If there is a problem with measuring and hooking the opposite cortex with a depth gauge, depth can be estimated radiographically. This image shows the difference between the length of the depth gauge and the tissue protector. Note that the tissue protector is 1.0 cm shorter than the sleeve on the depth gauge. To obtain correct measurement, the soft-tissue protector should be removed and the depth gauge used with its own sleeve.

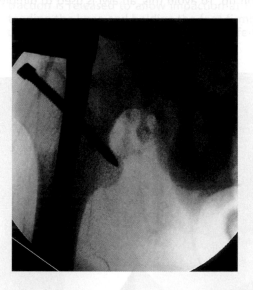

Figure 58. Proximal screw placement. Many patients complain of pain at the trochanter because of prominence of the head of the proximal screw. To decrease this discomfort, the screw head can be partially buried. It is a self-tapping fully threaded screw, and the nail is threaded so the surgeon can countersink the screw effectively.

Distal Locking

A number of different methods have been devised to facilitate distal locking (Figs. 59–69). The flexibility of target devices mounted on the image intensifier caused inaccurate screw insertion. The device, which requires direct attachment to the image intensifier, also lost popularity because of the fear of voiding the warranty of the image intensifier. A number of manufacturers designed target devices for distal locking, which attach to the proximal end of the nail. The tendency for open-section intramedullary nails torsionally to deform on insertion will disturb the alignment between the target device and the distal

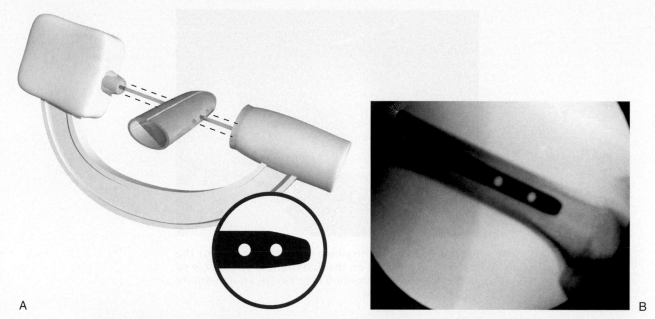

Figure 59. Distal fixation. Correct rotational alignment of the fracture should be confirmed before distal fixation. The C-arm should be positioned to obtain an optimal lateral view of the distal end of the nail. The goal is to pass the beam exactly in line with the axis of the screw holes **(A).** This position has been obtained when the holes appear perfectly round **(B).** An elliptical appearance of the holes suggests malalignment of the beam.

screw holes. The length of these devices makes them subject to displacement and inaccurate screw placement, particularly when used in the supine position. Because of these problems, most surgeons have resorted to the use of hand-held devices and the "freehand" technique. The devices include drill guides, awls, sharp pins, and drill bits. Radiolucent offset drill attachments, which are used in conjunction with standard power drills, have been developed to allow direct drilling under radiographic control.

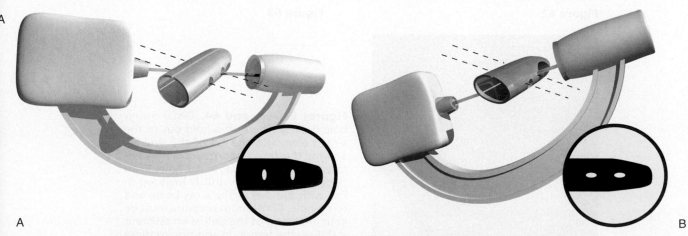

Figure 60. Illustration of oblique distal screw holes resulting from rotation. **A:** Malalignment of the beam in the coronal plane makes the holes appear as vertical ellipses. **B:** While in B, malalignment in sagittal plane makes holes appear as horizontal ellipses.

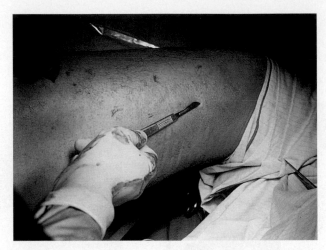

Figure 61. Distal entry-hole targeting. The tip of the scalpel is positioned on the skin over the screw hole so that once correct targeting is achieved, an immediate incision can be made.

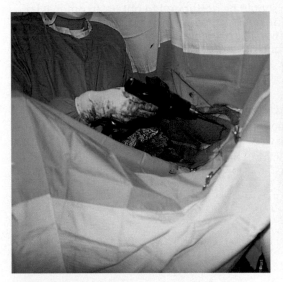

Figure 62

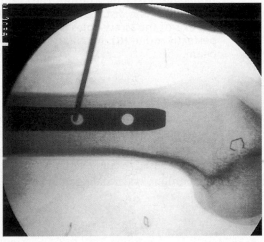

Figure 63

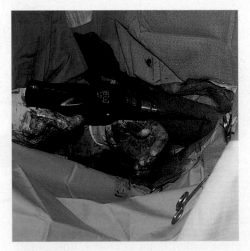

Figure 64

Figures 62, 63, and 64. Distal entry-hole drilling. The drill is held out of the x-ray beam with the tip of the drill bit against the lateral cortex, exactly centered on the proximal screw hole. With fluoroscopy off, the drill is lowered in line with the axis of the x-ray beam and screw hole. Continuous pressure must be kept on the tip of the drill as an assistant stabilizes the femur. In addition to these steps, the use of a sharp-tip drill bit helps avoid migration of the drill bit.

We routinely use a modified freehand technique for distal interlocking. Imperative for success of this technique is proper positioning of the image intensifier directly perpendicular to the femur and centered over the distal screw holes. With proper positioning, the holes in the distal nail should appear as perfect circles and not as ellipses. A long Kirschner wire is placed on the skin in the center of the hole and confirmed fluoroscopically. A 2-cm skin incision is made with blunt dissection to the lateral femoral cortex. The wire is then tapped into the bone in the center of the hole, creating a starting point to facilitate drilling. Fluoroscopic confirmation that the drill bit has successfully traversed the

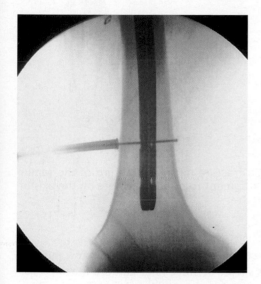

Figure 65. Distal fixation-hole depth measurement. Depth measurement for correct screw-length determination. Five millimeters should be added to the screw length to ensure projection beyond the opposite cortex to facilitate removal if the screws break.

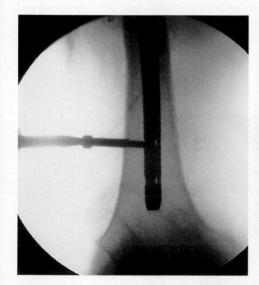

Figure 66

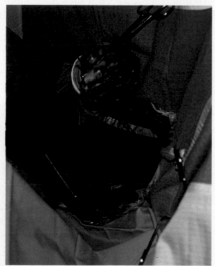

Figure 67

Figures 66 and 67. Distal screw insertion. The screw driver is used to define the axis of the first screw to assist with insertion of the second screw.

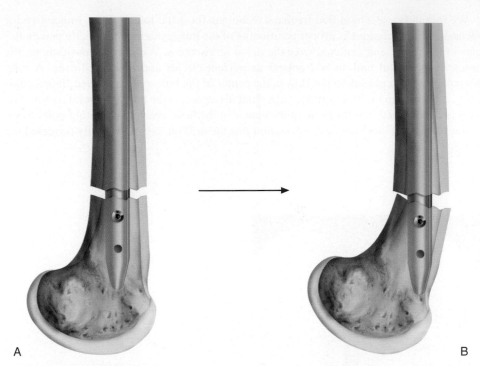

A   B

Figure 68. A and B: Toggle cross-locking a fracture in the distal third of the femur with a single screw permits the short distal fragment to toggle or rotate on the axis of the screw.

nail is essential before drilling the opposite cortex. Similarly the locking screw must be confirmed with the C-arm. Both screw holes should be filled in distal-third fractures, because the diameter of the distal fragment is larger than that of the nail, and fixation with a single screw could lead to rotation of the fragment around the screw and motion at the fracture site. To enhance screw purchase, two distal screws should also be used for any diaphyseal fractures in weak osteoporotic bone. A single distal screw placed in the proximal of the two distal nail holes is sufficient for fractures in the upper and middle thirds if a reamed nail is used. In these cases, the diameter of the medullary canal at the proximal end of the distal fragment is usually similar in size to the diameter of the nail, preventing distal-fragment rotation.

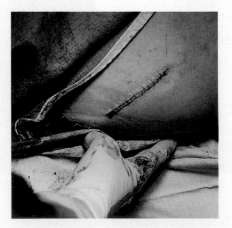

Figure 69. Wound closure.

POSTOPERATIVE MANAGEMENT

Postoperative management depends on the fracture location and amount of comminution, age of patient, preoperative mobility, and extent of coexisting injuries. Early weight bearing is encouraged in the patient with a transverse or short oblique fracture where there is stable contact between the two major fragments so that weight will be transmitted through the bone. When comminution prevents transmission of weight through the bone, 2 to 3 months of partial weight bearing is recommended to permit callus formation. In reality, pain is usually the the patient's limiting factor for weight bearing.

The majority of fractures will heal with the nail in the static locked mode. This is advantageous, even in stable transverse fractures, as it helps to control rotation. Dynamization (the removal of proximal or distal screws from a statically locked nail) may be useful to allow impaction in those few fractures that do not show progressive healing 3 to 4 months after nailing.

Physical therapy including active range of motion, resistive muscle strengthening, gait training, and pool therapy are routinely used to speed rehabilitation, enhance fracture healing, and increase the ultimate level of functional recovery.

Patients are seen in the outpatient office 10 to 14 days after surgery for suture removal and wound inspection. AP and lateral radiographs are obtained to inspect the implant position, fracture alignment, and progress of union immediately after surgery and at 6 weeks, 12 weeks, and 20 to 24 weeks. A final set of radiographs is obtained at 6 months to document adequate healing of the fracture. The average uncomplicated femoral diaphyseal fracture will unite in 3 to 5 months. In the absence of patellar fractures or knee-ligament injuries, patients generally achieve excellent recovery of knee motion. Several months of exercise are required to achieve the ultimate range of knee motion. The speed of recovery and degree of motion are enhanced by early physical therapy.

COMPLICATIONS

Malunion

The routine use of static locking has decreased the incidence of postoperative fracture displacement leading to malunion. The majority of malunions result when fractures are fixed in a position of malalignment. Transverse and short oblique fractures in the isthmus are naturally aligned because of greater endosteal contact with the nail. Fractures above and below the isthmus have a short fragment with a large medullary canal, predisposing the fragment to angular malalignment unless its position is carefully controlled. Intraoperatively, the correct position of the fragment is confirmed by visualizing the fracture site under low magnification (camera close to the limb) and by ensuring that the guide wire is in the center of the fragment on both AP and lateral views. If the short fragment is held in correct position during guide passage, reaming, and nail and screw insertion, malalignment will be prevented. Correct entry-portal placement in the piriformis fossa in line with the medullary canal is important in preventing varus malunions in proximal-third fractures. In addition to avoiding angular malalignment, it is essential that the correct rotational alignment be established before nail insertion. In the supine position, diaphyseal fractures are aligned by allowing the knee to flex with the foot hanging to the floor. Proximal placement of the tibial traction pin at the level of the tibial tubercle will facilitate knee flexion, which improves rotational alignment and transmits greater traction force along the femur. More distal placement of the traction pin causes knee extension when traction is applied. This reduces the force transmitted into the femur, reduces the rotational moment arm of the distal fragment, and results in posterior angulation of the femoral fracture.

Malrotation, if recognized early, may be corrected by removal of the distal screws, deformity correction, and reinsertion of the screws. Angulation of 5 to 7 degrees in any plane is usually well tolerated; however, malalignment of more than 10 degrees usually requires early revision to avoid late symptoms. Increased comminution associated with nailing is not uncommon and is tolerated as long as the comminution is between the static locking screws.

Delayed and Nonunion

The use of a closed technique for the insertion of locked nails results in a 1% to 2% incidence of nonunion. Introduction of the nails at a distance from the fracture site avoids direct dissection and periosteal stripping, thereby preserving the fracture biology. Systemic (poor nutrition, diabetes, steroids, smoking, etc.) and local factors (severe periosteal stripping, infection, or vascular injury) can combine to cause delayed or nonunion. Each of these factors must be taken into consideration, and treatment plans developed accordingly.

Pudendal Nerve Palsy

Pudendal nerve palsies usually result from excessive continuous traction on the perineal post. This complication can usually be avoided if the nailing is performed on the day of injury. Only limited traction is needed during this early phase to achieve excellent reductions. When nailing is delayed, sufficient skeletal traction should be applied to overdistract the fracture slightly. This should be confirmed by a lateral radiograph. The AP view alone should not be used to determine length, as the film is usually taken parallel to the surface of the bed rather than the limb, and can give a false impression of distraction in the presence of overlap. By maintaining overdistraction preoperatively, it is easier to reduce the fracture when nailing occurs without resorting to excessive traction. Pudendal nerve palsies are usually neuropraxias and frequently resolve in 3 to 4 months.

Femoral-Neck Fractures

Most studies on ipsilateral hip and shaft fractures suggest that a femoral-neck fracture more likely represents a missed injury rather than iatrogenic fracture. Radiographs of the hip must be examined carefully to rule out a hip dislocation or femoral-neck fracture. A separate internal rotation AP of the proximal femur can be very helpful in visualizing the femoral neck.

A variety of techniques have been developed to treat these combined fractures including insertion of multiple cannulated screws around an existing nail, reconstruction nail, and multiple cannulated screws with a retrograde locked nail.

Infection

Despite the reaming of the medullary canal and the insertion of an implant that extends the length of the femur, infection after closed intramedullary nailing is surprisingly infrequent. The closed technique, which eliminates dissection at the fracture site, contributes to the low incidence of infection and nonunion. When infection does occur, the extent of involvement can vary. Fortunately, the infection may be confined to the superficial layers of the wound or the hematoma at the entry wound or the fracture site. These infections can be treated by intravenous antibiotics and local drainage. Less frequently, the entire medullary cavity can become infected. The inner half of the thickness of the cortex, devascularized by the reaming, can become an extensive sequestrum. In this circumstance, treatment requires removal of the nail and repeated reaming to debride the endosteal cortex. A new nail or an external fixator may be necessary if the fracture is not united.

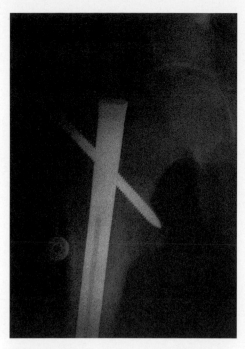

Figure 70. Postoperative radiograph.

ILLUSTRATIVE CASE FOR TECHNIQUE

A 23-year-old man sustained blunt abdominal trauma and a closed right femur fracture as a result of a head-on motor vehicle accident. The patient lost consciousness at the site of the accident and experienced mild retrograde amnesia. On initial examination, there was an obvious closed right midshaft femur deformity. The peripheral pulses were intact, as was the neurologic examination. Cervical spine, chest, and pelvic radiographs were normal. A cranial computed tomography (CT) scan was negative for fracture or intracranial bleed. AP and lateral radiographs of the femur showed a middiaphyseal transverse fracture (Fig. 2A and B). The patient had an abdominal injury that required exploratory laparotomy. At surgery, the patient was found to have a complete jejunal transection that was repaired. Immediately after the laparotomy, a closed intramedullary nailing was performed with a static locked nail. As the fracture was middiaphyseal, a single distal screw was used for fixation (Fig. 70). The patient was mobilized on the second postoperative day. The fracture healed uneventfully in 4 months with excellent restoration of function.

RECOMMENDED READING

1. Browner, B.D.: *The Science and Practice of Intramedullary Nailing,* 2nd ed. Williams & Wilkins, Baltimore, 1996.
2. Brumback, R.J., Reilly, J.P., Poka, A., Lakatos, R.P., Bathon, G.H., Burgess, A.R.: Intramedullary nailing of femoral shaft fractures, Part I: Decision making errors with interlocking fixation. *J. Bone Joint Surg. [Am],* 70:1441–1452, 1988.
3. Brumback, R.J., Stribling, E.P., Poka, A., Lakatos, R., Bathon, G.H., Burgess, A.R.: Intramedullary nailing of open fractures of the femoral shaft. *J. Bone Joint Surg. [Am],* 71:1324–1330, 1989.

Figure 78. Postoperative radiograph.

ILLUSTRATIVE CASE FOR TECHNIQUE

RECOMMENDED READING

Master Techniques in Orthopaedic Surgery,
FRACTURES, edited by D. A. Wiss,
Lippincott–Raven Publishers, Philadelphia © 1998.

19

Supracondylar Femur Fractures: Dynamic Condylar Screw

Roy W. Sanders

INDICATIONS/CONTRAINDICATIONS

In an effort to make the 95-degree blade plate more "user friendly," while maintaining stable fracture fixation, the Dynamic Condylar Screw (DCS) was developed (Synthes, Paoli, PA, U.S.A.). The DCS is a two-piece system consisting of a screw and side plate that are separate, thereby making it easier to insert than a fixed-angle blade device, particularly when long side plates are required. Furthermore, the condylar screw is placed over a guide wire and requires orientation in only two planes for insertion. The condylar screw is key locked to prevent rotation within the barrel and can be tightened against the plate, permitting intracondylar compression, an option not possible with a fixed-angle device. The plate has two round holes, just proximal to the condylar screw barrel, for insertion of 6.5-mm cancellous lag screws, which help prevent distal femoral condylar rotation around the condylar screw. Finally, the plate has dynamic compression holes to facilitate intrafragmentary compression between individual shaft fragments, the condyles, or both.

Indications for use of this device are supracondylar–intracondylar femur fractures in skeletally mature patients in whom a minimum of 4 cm of the medial femoral condyle is intact, so that sufficient bone is available for condylar screw insertion. These fractures are best described by the AO/ASIF fracture classification and include the A_1, A_2, and A_3 fractures, as well as C_1, C_2, and C_3 fractures (Fig. 1).

Contraindications for fixation with this device are related to the amount of comminution of the condyles. When extensive comminution exists, multiple small screws are usually required to fix condylar fragments. When this occurs, it may be impossible to place the condylar screw through its needed path without encountering individual lag screws. Another device, such as a condylar buttress plate or an intramedullary nail, should then be considered. Additionally, an open fracture or an injury in a polytraumatized patient may initially preclude the use of internal fixation. In these instances, a temporary external fixator can be placed until the patient or the wound is better suited for definitive stabilization.

R. W. Sanders, M.D.: Department of Orthopaedics, University of South Florida, Tampa, Florida 33612.

must be planned so as not to interfere with the insertion of the DCS implant, specifically, impingement with the side plate. Therefore, the starting point of the DCS and the width of the side plate should be determined before the lag screw is inserted.

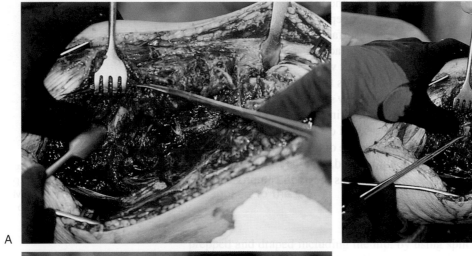

A

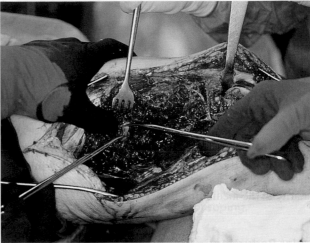

B

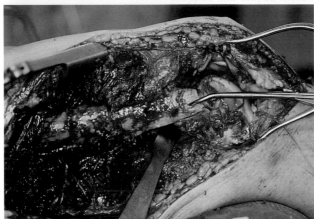

C

Figure 10. A: A rake is used to apply tension to the vastus lateralis, and the periosteal elevator is used gently to cut the muscle. All perforators can be easily found in this way, as white structures traversing perpendicular to the muscle fibers. **B:** Once found, these vessels are clamped, tied, cauterized, or clipped to prevent bleeding. **C:** The lateral surface of the femoral shaft is now exposed. Notice that self-retaining retractors are used. Also important is the fact that the posterior distal shaft, where the condyles meet the shaft, is exposed and restored to its anatomic position (note Hohmann) by replacing comminuted fragments if needed. In this way, the exact position of the condyles and correct placement of the DCS will be assured.

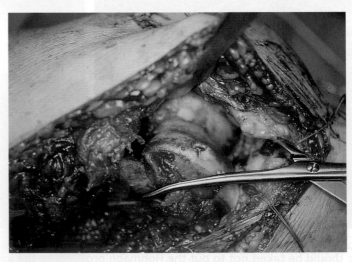

Figure 11. A 3.5-mm lag screw countersunk and buried under cartilage and well away from DCS screw.

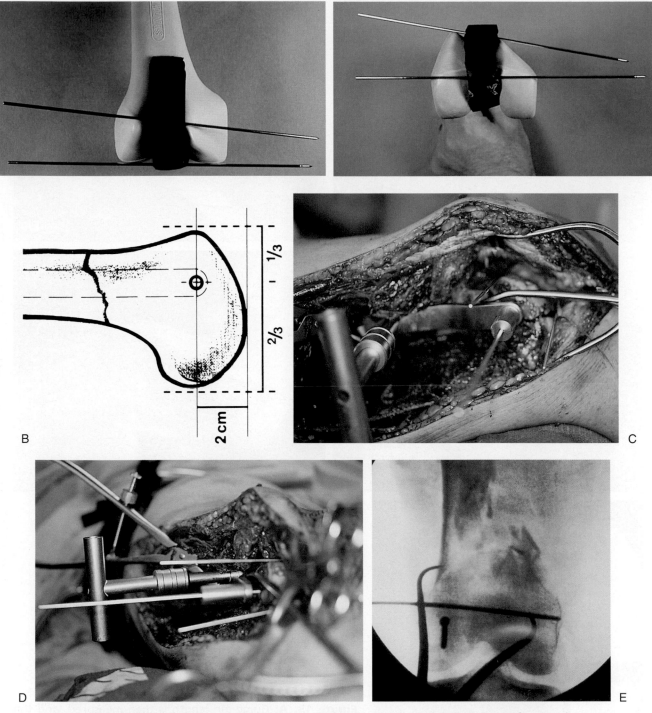

Figure 12. A1, A2: Two guide wires are placed, one along the anterior surface, and one along the distal surface of the condyles. **B:** Schematic representation of the placement of the guide pin for insertion of the condylar screw. **C, D:** "Lateral and AP" view of the distal condyles, by using both guide and alignment wires to ascertain perfect position for the summation guide pin. Note that the summation guide pin is parallel to one of the pins in each view. After the summation guide pin is placed, its position is verified by radiograph. **E:** Placement of the guide wire by using the "jig" and image-intensification control.

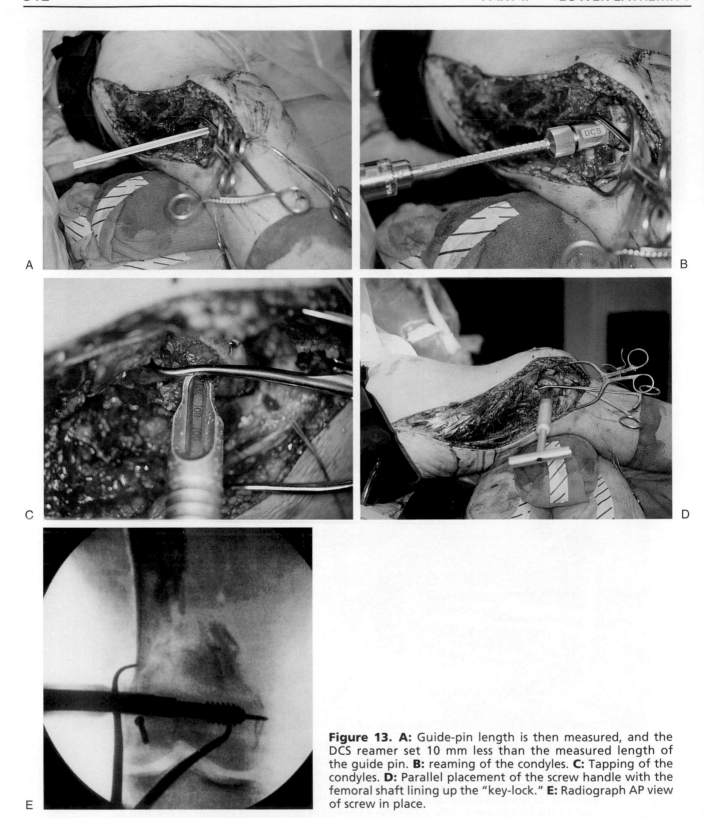

Figure 13. A: Guide-pin length is then measured, and the DCS reamer set 10 mm less than the measured length of the guide pin. **B:** reaming of the condyles. **C:** Tapping of the condyles. **D:** Parallel placement of the screw handle with the femoral shaft lining up the "key-lock." **E:** Radiograph AP view of screw in place.

Dynamic Condylar Screw Insertion

The key to successful insertion of the DCS implant is the proper placement of the guide pin in the distal femur. Visualization of the lateral condyle in its entirety from anterior to posterior, taking care to avoid cutting the lateral collateral ligament, is essential. Proximally, it is only necessary to see the point where the lateral condyle meets the posterior cortex of the shaft; this corner gives positional information about the shaft–plate interface (Fig. 10C). Appreciation of these landmarks allows insertion of the 95-degree device, even in the face of severe distal lateral shaft comminution.

Alignment wires are placed superior and distal to the distal femoral condyles (Fig. 12A). A summation guide pin is drilled into the lateral condyle 2 cm from the joint line, as opposed to 1.5 cm for the blade plate. This accommodates the larger diameter of the condylar screw. The guide pin should enter the middle of the anterior half of the lateral condyle (Fig. 12B). Image intensification should be used to verify that placement of the guide pin is parallel to the knee-joint axis, and that medial protrusion of the K-wire is not present (Fig. 12E). Alternatively, the DCS guide can be placed along the lateral cortex of the distal femur (after anatomic reduction of the distal femur), with the K-wire inserted under radiographic control (Fig. 12C and D). Care must be taken, however, to evaluate the placement of the guide before the K-wire is inserted. If this is not done, the DCS guide may place the guide wire in a suboptimal position.

Guide-pin length is then measured, and the DCS reamer set 10 mm less than the measured length of the guide pin (Fig. 13A). The femoral condyles are reamed (Fig. 13B). If hard cancellous bone is present, the entire length of the hole is tapped (Fig. 13C). During condylar screw insertion, the screw may be inserted an additional 5 mm to increase purchase. In osteopenic bone, tapping is not routinely performed. If bony purchase is still insufficient, the screw is removed and methylmethacrylate inserted into the screw hole. The screw is then inserted so that only the threads engage cement. This permits subsequent intracondylar compression if necessary, while still allowing plate rotation for shaft reduction. The screw should be seated with the handle parallel to the shaft to line up the key-lock mechanism (Fig. 13D and E).

Extraarticular supracondylar fractures are treated without intracondylar compression; condylar screw length should equal the reamer setting. Intracondylar fractures, on the other

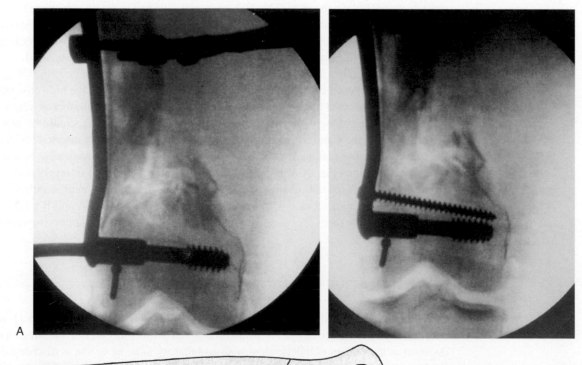

A   B

C

Figure 14. A, B: Side-plate placement. **C:** Schematic showing the position of shorter and longer plates on the femoral shaft. Note that the longer plate needs to be placed posteriorly to stay on bone because of the femoral bow.

hand, require compression. If the condylar screw length equals the reamer setting in this case, when compression is applied, lateral protrusion of the screw shaft may result. This will prevent maximal intracondylar compression when the compression bolt is applied.

Therefore in this case, a condylar screw 5 to 10 mm less in length than the reamer setting is used. The goal in either case is an anatomically reconstructed, stable distal-femoral block that can be then fixed to the shaft.

Shaft-Reduction and Plate Application

The side plate is then threaded over the condylar screw (Fig. 14A). The shaft is yet to be reduced. The plate is lined up with the posterior shaft, at the level at which the condyle meets the shaft. If the shaft fracture extends into the diaphysis, a long side plate will be needed. In this case, the plate should be secured more posteriorly on the shaft to account for the anterior femoral bow (Fig. 14C). Once aligned, one or two 6.5-mm cancellous lag screws are placed in the round holes of the plate (Fig. 14B). Finally the compression screw is placed into the distal hole to lock the condylar screw to the plate.

Once it is secure distally, manual traction is applied. This usually realigns the femur grossly. A no. 3 Verbrugge clamp is placed on the proximal plate and shaft. An articulating tension device (ATD) is inserted in the closed position (green) with a bicortical screw, in line with the plate (Fig. 15A). The Verbrugge clamp prevents translation of the shaft fragments when lengthening with the ATD. If AP fracture buckling is encountered, or if the plate seems to be slipping off the femoral shaft, a standard (lion-jaw) clamp is placed on the bone, so that one arm grabs the apex of the angle made by the fracture fragments and the other grabs the plate. As this is locked, the buckling of the fracture or the shifting of the plate will be prevented. With the socket wrench, the ATD is lengthened so that the fracture fragments are slightly distracted (Fig. 15B). The no. 3 Verbrugge clamp is tightened, and the fracture fragments reduced. The hooked foot of the ATD is then flipped to engage the most proximal hole in the plate. The socket wrench is turned to create compression with the ATD (red) until the fracture is stable and well reduced (Fig. 15F). In cases with extensive comminution medially, this maneuver can still obtain compression on the lateral cortex. When lateral cortical compression is not possible, this technique cannot be used.

Once it is securely reduced, cortical screws are inserted into the plate (Fig. 15C). Typically a screw is placed in the most proximal plate hole, as well as in the hole closest to the fracture. This maximal spread will give maximal purchase. If the number of screw holes left open between these two holes exceeds three, then more screws should be placed as needed. Finally, the distal fragment is secured, and any lag screws are inserted based on the fracture pattern. The clamps are removed, and the hip and knee are maximally flexed to assure stable fixation (Fig. 16A and B). The wounds are then closed in layers over a deep drain (Fig. 16C). Final radiographs are obtained before the conclusion of anesthesia, and a soft dressing and a knee brace with open hinges are applied (Fig. 17A and B). The patient is transferred to the recovery room where the limb is placed into a continuous-passive-motion machine.

POSTOPERATIVE MANAGEMENT

The patient is mobilized out of bed on postoperative day 1 and begins toe-touch weight bearing on postoperative day 2. The drain is removed at this time, and the dressing changed. As soon as the patient is independent with ambulatory aids, he or she is discharged from the hospital, typically on postoperative day 3.

Outpatient physical therapy for strengthening and range of motion is performed over the next 12 weeks. At 8 weeks after surgery, radiographs should show signs of fracture consolidation. Partial weight bearing can be started at this time, if there are clear signs of fracture healing. Weight bearing is advanced, based on the radiographic progression of heal-

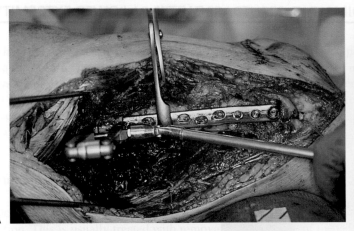

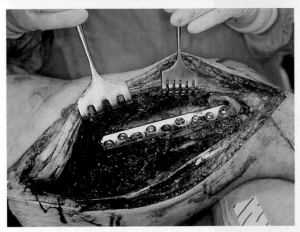

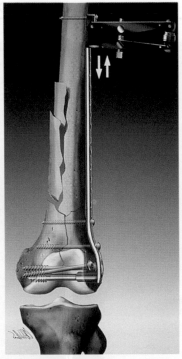

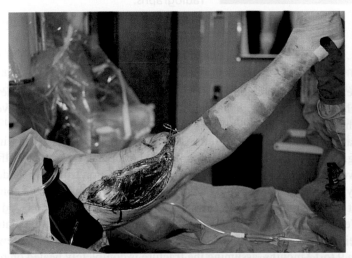

Figure 15. A: The articulating tension device (ATD) and its initial application. **B:** Distraction, reduction, and compression by using the ATD. **C:** Application of cortical screws into the side plate.

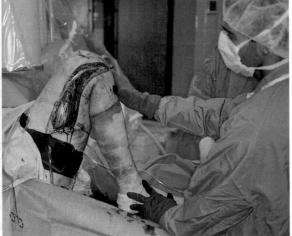

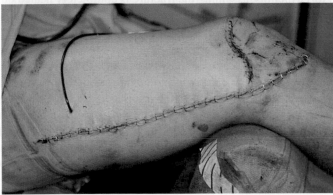

Figure 16. A–C: Intraoperative evaluation of stability and range of motion at the knee.

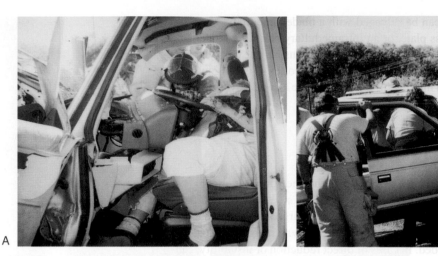

Figure 18. A, B: Photographs at the accident before extrication. Please note the dashboard crushing and trapping his femur and leg.

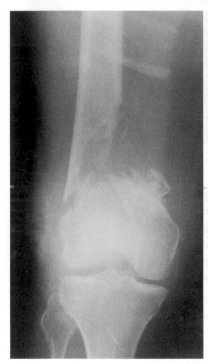

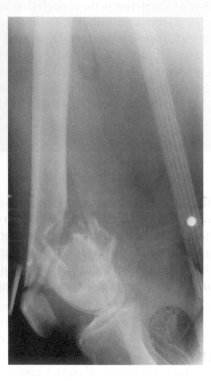

Figure 19. A, B: Anteroposterior (AP) and lateral views of injured distal femur. Please note flexion of distal condyles.

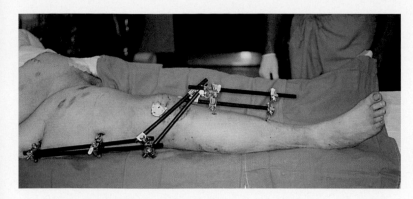

Figure 20. Debrided and stabilized distal femur. Epigard is in place, and a multiplanar external fixator acts as "portable traction," pulling the femur out to length.

RECOMMENDED READING

1. Bolhoffner, B.R., Carmen, B., Clifford, P.: The results of open reduction and internal fixation of distal femur fractures using a biologic (indirect) reduction technique. *J. Orthop. Trauma,* 10:372–377, 1996.
2. Marymont, J.V., and Mizel, M.S.: Fracture of the subtalar joint in springboard divers: a report of two cases. *Am. J. Sports Med.,* 24:123–124, 1996.
3. Mast, J., Jakob, R., Ganz, R.: *Planning and Reduction Technique in Fracture Surgery.* Springer-Verlag, Berlin, 1989.
4. Muller, M.E., Allgower, M., Schneider, R., Willinegger H.: *Manual of Internal Fixation: Techniques Recommended by the AO Group.* Springer-Verlag, Berlin, 1990.
5. Ostrum, R.F., and Geel, C.: Indirect reduction and internal fixation of supracondylar femur fractures without bone graft. *J. Orthop. Trauma,* 9:278–284, 1995.
6. Sanders, R., Regazzoni, P., Ruedi, T.: The treatment of supracondylar-intracondylar fractures of the femur using the dynamic condylar screw. *J. Orthop. Trauma,* 3:214–222, 1989.
7. Schatzker, J., Tile, M.: *The Rationale for Operative Fracture Care.* Springer-Verlag, New York, 1990.
8. Siliski, J.M., Mahring, M., Hofer, H.P.: Supracondylar-intercondylar fractures of the femur: treatment by internal fixation. *J. Bone Joint Surg.,* 71:95–104, 1989.
9. Wiss, D.A., Missakian, M.: Supracondylar fracture of the femur. *Orthopaedics,* 8:921, 1985.

Master Techniques in Orthopaedic Surgery,
FRACTURES, edited by D. A. Wiss,
Lippincott–Raven Publishers, Philadelphia © 1998.

20

Supracondylar Femur Fractures: Intramedullary Nailing

David Seligson

INDICATIONS/CONTRAINDICATIONS

The intramedullary supracondylar nail is an excellent method of treatment for fractures of the distal femur. Supracondylar fractures present as a diverse group of fractures involving bone and cartilage of varying quality. These injuries have been classified as Type A, extraarticular fractures; Type B, unicondylar fractures; and Type C, intraarticular fractures (16). In Type A and C fractures, the articular surface and femoral condyles are separated from the femur shaft and are good indications for retrograde intramedullary nailing (Fig. 1). Type B unicondylar fractures are best treated with screws or plates or both and are not amenable to supracondylar nailing. Of the various techniques available for fixation of the distal femur, the intramedullary supracondylar nail has many advantages. It is easier to perform than an antegrade femoral nail because it eliminates the need for a fracture table and an incision at the hip for nail insertion. The procedure is more biologically favorable than plate osteosynthesis, such as angle blade plates and condylar screws, because an open approach with devascularization of the soft tissues is not necessary, thereby promoting fracture healing. Although external fixateurs are occasionally useful in severe distal-femur fractures, they are cumbersome, may be accompanied by loss of fixation, and have a high incidence of pin-tract complications. Open reduction and internal fixation of comminuted distal-femur fractures can lead to prolonged operative procedures with less than satisfactory anatomic and functional results. For most orthopaedic surgeons, a simple solution to a supracondylar femur fracture, with or without extension into the knee joint, is the intramedullary supracondylar nail. In a patient with significant polytrauma, supracondylar nailing offers many biologic and mechanical advantages (Figs. 2A and B, 3A and B). With Type C fractures, particularly with comminution of the articular surface, open reduction and internal fixation of the joint may be required. Often the nail can be introduced after as-

D. Seligson, M.D.: Department of Orthopaedics, University of Louisville, Louisville, Kentucky 40202; and Ortho Trauma Associates, Louisville, Kentucky 40207.

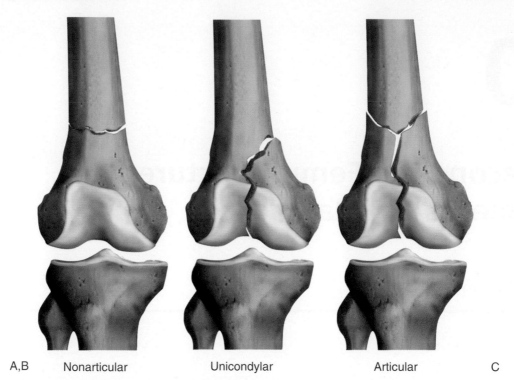

A,B   Nonarticular   Unicondylar   Articular   C

Figure 1. A–C: Fractures of the distal femur: Type A, nonarticular; Type B, unicondylar; Type C, articular (from ref. 16).

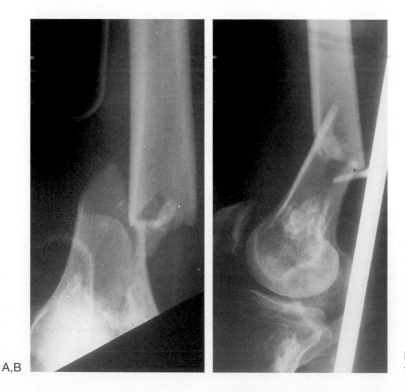

A,B

Figure 2. A, B: Preoperative radiographs in patient with a distal femoral shaft fracture.

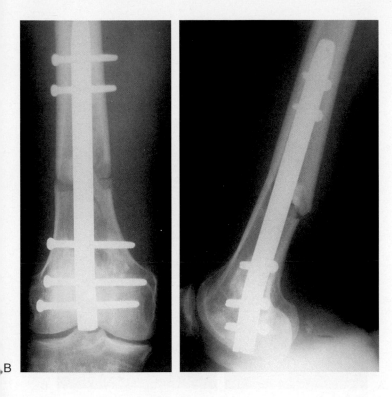

B

Figure 3. A, B: Postoperative radiographs after nailing from the knee.

sembly of the articular mass, and there may be less difficulty achieving correct varus–valgus alignment of the distal femur than with plating techniques.

Extremely distal transcondylar fractures involving the distal 2 to 3 cm of the femur are not amenable to nailing. Here open reduction with direct fracture fixation is necessary. These injury patterns are often associated with fracture–dislocations of the knee in young patients. For corrective osteotomies of the distal femur, I prefer a 95-degree condylar blade plate. Condylar plates can be used with a percutaneous technique for comminuted metaphyseal fractures in young patients. With this biologic method, neither the joint (for an entrance point) nor the periosteum is significantly disturbed.

The intramedullary supracondylar nail is particularly useful in situations in which alterations in femoral geometry preclude other methods of treatment. This includes supracondylar fractures proximal to a knee prosthesis or distal to hip implants, as well as fractures in which the femur cannot be instrumented because of medullary canal malalignment. The supracondylar nail should also be considered for patients with complex problems such as obesity, in which the use of a fracture table for nailing could be awkward.

Supracondylar nailing is more difficult in patients with intraarticular distal-femur fractures (Type C) who may require an open reduction of the joint surface (Figs. 4, 5A and B). It cannot be used when there is a centromedullary implant in the distal-femoral canal such as a centrally stemmed femoral component of a total knee arthroplasty. In addition, intramedullary supracondylar nailing alone will not solve the problem of an established supracondylar pseudarthrosis (11).

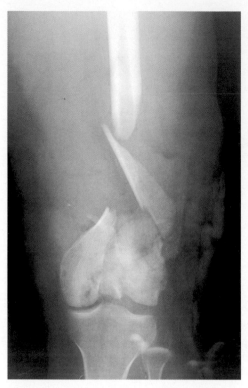

Figure 4. Preoperative radiograph in Type C supracondylar fracture. (Courtesy of William G. DeLong, Jr., M.D., Haddonfield, N.J.)

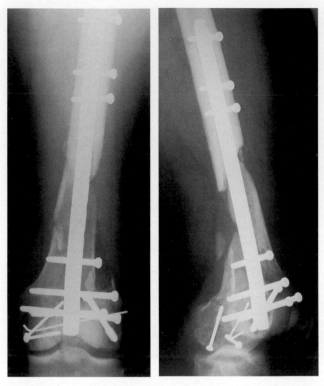

Figure 5. A, B: Radiographs at 6 weeks. An open reduction with joint-surface reconstruction has been performed. (Courtesy of William G. DeLong, Jr., M.D., Haddonfield, N.J.)

PREOPERATIVE PLANNING

In healthy patients with isolated distal-femur fractures, nailing can be performed shortly after injury. The workup includes a history and physical examination, complete blood count (CBC), urinalysis, prothrombin time, and high quality anteroposterior (AP) and lateral radiographs of the knee and distal femur. In addition to routine plain films of the supracondylar area and knee, a radiograph perpendicular to the plane of the knee joint and a tunnel view may also help in identifying intercondylar comminution. Computed tomography (CT) scans have not been used routinely to assess the complexity of the fracture problem. A type and screen should be obtained if an open reduction is planned or appears likely. In patients with multiple injuries or with associated medical comorbidities, the procedure is delayed until the patient's general or local condition has improved. The operation occasionally must be delayed for several days to a week after injury. In patients with minimal fracture displacement, in whom surgery is to be delayed, a bulky dressing with a knee immobilizer is used. However, in patients with comminution or significant displacement of the fracture, skeletal traction with 10 to 20 pounds through a proximal tibial pin and a bulky dressing with supporting rolled towels or sand bags on either side of the knee reduces fracture-site motion and increases patient comfort. Formal skeletal traction with a Thomas splint and Pearson attachment can also be used.

Preoperatively it is important to determine whether nailing can be performed by using a closed technique or if an open method will be required, because open reduction requires more time and equipment. The open method is indicated in Type C fracture patterns in which a satisfactory reduction of the distal femoral articular surface cannot be achieved percutaneously. Unfortunately, the universal fracture classification does not provide this information (16). Some simple C-1 fractures are malrotated and will not reduce with traction, requiring open reduction. Conversely, many comminuted C-3 fractures can be done closed. A preoperative radiograph with the limb in traction may help assess whether an open reduction will be necessary or if the condyles can be reduced and fixed percutaneously. Nail length is estimated preoperatively by using implant templates superimposed on the injury radiographs. If the fracture is confined to the area distal to the metaphyseal flare, shorter nails (150 mm in length) will be sufficient. If the fracture extends proximally into the lower diaphysis of the femur, nails 200 to 250 mm in length will be necessary. With some of the newer digital radiographic imaging systems that reduce image, size templates may lead to errors because they require that the film be taken at a standard distance and not reduced in scale. In thin, elderly patients, distal fractures can usually be managed with an 11×150-mm nail with holes the entire length of the nail. Young, heavy, or high-demand individuals require larger and longer nails that have a central portion without screw holes. However, the greater the nail diameter, the larger the entrance hole in the trochlea, and therefore, the greater the likelihood that the condyles will either be held apart or split apart by the implant. Conical nuts and washers are especially useful in patients with osteopenia to improve fixation in the distal femur. A full set of conventional bone screws, screws for interlocking, and cannulated screws should be available for fixation of sagittal or coronal fractures, which may not be detected until the time of surgery.

Whenever supracondylar nailing is done as an open procedure, the fracture sites should be bone grafted by using autogenous cancellous bone from the ipsilateral iliac crest. If only a small amount of bone is needed, the graft can be obtained from the lateral aspect of the proximal tibia. Significant metaphyseal defects can be filled with synthetic bone substitutes or bank bone. Rarely cortical struts are needed to reconstruct the distal femoral diaphysis; however, I prefer not to use allograft bone in association with supracondylar nailing.

Perioperatively, most patients receive 1 g of cefazolin intravenously just before the incision and every 8 hours for a total of six doses. A proximal thigh tourniquet can be helpful in controlling blood loss in distal fractures. The surgeon should be familiar with the freehand technique for placement of distal interlocking screws. Although an outrigger guide is used to insert interlocking screws, it may be ineffective with longer nails in the proximal portion. Therefore the surgeon should be able, by removing the screw guide, to place screws through the holes in the nail by using the freehand technique.

SURGERY

Intramedullary supracondylar nailing is performed under general or spinal anesthesia with the patient on a radiolucent table with the aid of image intensification. The leg is prepped and draped free. A sterile proximal thigh tourniquet can be useful in distal fracture patterns. A small rolled towel placed beneath the greater trochanter improves the alignment of the leg by preventing external rotation. A folded drape or bolster is placed under the knee to keep the knee in 30 degrees of flexion.

Manual traction is applied to the leg to reduce the fracture. The reduction is verified in two planes by using the image intensifier. The fluoroscopy unit can be arced over or under the table for a lateral view. The surgeon should be certain that the image intensifier is brought in at right angles to the extremity so that true AP and lateral images are obtained during the procedure. If a satisfactory reduction can be achieved closed, then the operation can be done *percutaneously*. It may be possible to manipulate the fracture manually to improve the reduction. The surgeon can push, with his hands, on comminuted fracture fragments or grasp the distal femur and manually improve the reduction. In elderly patients, particularly in the presence of marked metaphyseal comminution, 1 to 2 cm of shortening may be acceptable. Throughout the procedure, it is important to visualize the leg and maintain limb alignment. Up to 5 degrees of varus or valgus angulation is acceptable. Occasionally in an elderly patient with medial-compartment arthrosis, some valgus may help unload the medial compartment. More than 10 degrees of varus or valgus angulation usually leads to postoperative complications and should be avoided. When an acceptable reduction with respect to the patient's expected activity demand and functional status cannot be achieved closed, then the procedure should be performed open. A limited, medial or lateral parapatellar arthrotomy made from a straight vertical skin incision allows direct articular surface reduction or correction of distal metaphyseal displacement.

Pelvic bone-holding clamps can be used to improve fracture reduction by placing them percutaneously and applying a gentle force through the points of the clamps. It is also possible to make limited skin incisions to reduce articular fragments and then hold these in place with large pointed bone-reduction clamps. Once a satisfactory reduction is achieved, temporary fixation with Kirschner wires (K-wires) maintains the reduction. The K-wires used for temporary fixation can serve as guide wires for cannulated screws in later stages of the operation. Whenever possible, it is desirable to pass these temporary fixation wires transversely through the condyles anterior or posterior or both to the planned position of the nail. In general, the distal femoral articular block is wide enough in the anteroposterior direction so that wires passed anterior or posterior to the condyles will not interfere with the placement of the intramedullary supracondylar nail. For definitive fixation of the condyles, 5.5- or 6.5-mm cannulated screws can be passed over the guide wires. Only after the articular surface of the femoral condyles has been reduced and provisionally or definitively fixed should the supracondylar nail be inserted. The intercondylar screws, however, can be inserted before or after placement of the nail. If they are placed before nail insertion, then they are tightened after the placement of the nail to avoid loosening as the distal femur is instrumented.

The optimal portal of entry for the nail is in the intercondylar notch, centered between the condyles in the AP projection and in line with the medullary canal in the lateral view. Incise the skin and patella ligament vertically for 2 to 3 cm to permit entry of the awl. Skin flaps are not developed subcutaneously. The medullary canal is opened under C-arm control with a Küntscher awl. A ball-tipped reamer guide is passed across the fracture, and the reduction is verified in two planes. An alternative method to open the distal femur is with a guide wire and a cannulated hip-screw reamer. When the shaft and condyles do not reduce, a useful trick is to use a femoral distractor with pins temporarily placed in the femoral shaft and the femoral condyles to improve reduction and restore length (Fig. 6). This maneuver is helpful when there is a translation deformity that is difficult to control manually. By using flexible or straight reamers, the medullary canal is reamed 1.5 to 2 mm more than the planned diameter of the nail (Fig. 7). In young patients with narrow canals, the distal-femur shaft will need to be reamed. In elderly patients with wide medullary canals, reaming is needed just in the portal of entry. The ball-tipped guide is exchanged over a plastic tube for the nail-driving guide (Fig. 8). The nail is inserted over a guide wire crossing the fracture by using only manual pressure (Fig. 9). The nail should never be hammered into place. This is an important point in the procedure. *During nail placement, the fracture must*

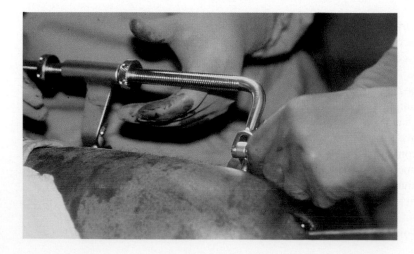

Figure 6. Application of a femoral distractor with placement of pins in the distal femur and lateral condyle. The distractor is used to facilitate fracture reduction and nail placement.

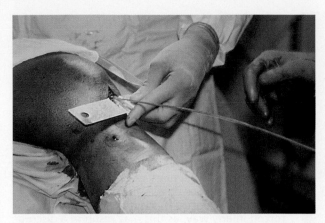

Figure 7. Regular Küntscher guides and reamers are used to open the medullary canal.

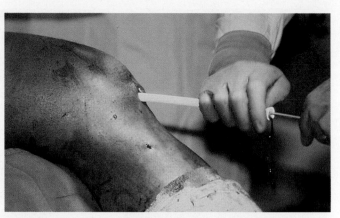

Figure 8. The ball-tip guide for reaming is exchanged for the nail guide for driving. Remember to remove the nail-drawing guide so the screws can be placed.

be reduced and limb alignment restored (Fig. 10). Attention must be paid to avoid varus–valgus malalignment or malrotation of the femoral condyles on the femoral shaft or both. The anterior bow of the distal femur can be restored by moving the bolster or rolled towel supporting the distal femur. The nail is usually placed with the apex (bend) ventral, but if the reduction is better, the apex can be placed dorsally. The bend in the nail allows the implant to be placed in a better position in the distal femur if the entrance point is too anterior or posterior.

As the reduction is achieved, some shortening (1 to 2 cm) may be observed. This may be acceptable, particularly in geriatric patients. It is safer to impact the fracture at the time of surgery than to have the condyles gradually subside with screw- or nail-protrusion problems postoperatively. The surgeon should avoid using the nail as a lever to reduce the fracture, and it is better to manipulate the fracture around the nail. The correct depth of the nail is determined on the lateral C-arm projection. The nail end should be brought flush to the articular surface of the trochlea or countersunk 1 to 2 mm in the distal femur. It is important to realize that the trochlea has a deep groove, so the zone for screw fixation in the distal femur is very narrow.

The guide for the interlocking screws has two positions. The more outboard position is for large limbs. The near position is more accurate because of the reduced distance to the holes in the nail. The guide and the nail with the drill sleeves and drill are checked to be sure they match before inserting the nail. Any slight discrepancy between the nail and the guide can cause the drill to miss the hole in the nail. Common reasons the drill does not pass

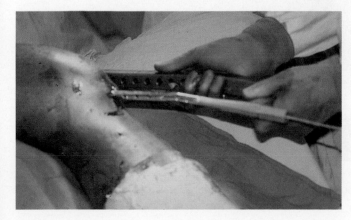

Figure 9. The nail is inserted into the intramedullary canal and across the fracture site.

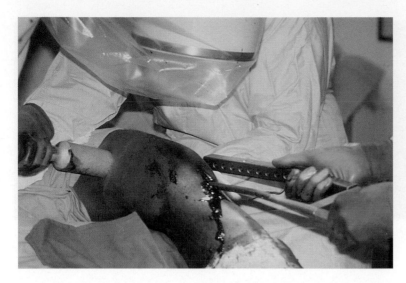

Figure 10. The fracture is reduced and held in alignment. Care is taken to ensure the correct varus–valgus alignment of the knee, as well as proper placement of the distal femur. The nail is positioned gently. It should not be driven or forced in any way, as this may result in a discrepancy between the nail and the screw guide. Correct positioning should be determined from a lateral radiograph.

through the nail include failure to fasten the targeting device securely to the guide, hitting the nail during driving and bending it, wedging either the nail or the target arm against the femur or the thigh, which causes misalignment, failure to use the whole group of stacked sleeves, and bringing the drill into the thigh at a slight angle so it slips off-center on the surface of the femur.

Locking screws are inserted from lateral to medial and from distal to proximal by using two pairs of drill sleeves and drill bits. One drill bit is passed through the guide and sleeves to stabilize the position between the guide and the nail (Fig. 11). The second drill bit and sleeves are used to place one distal and two proximal 5-mm screws through the nail. The drill is removed, and the position of the drill bit is checked on the AP and lateral radiograph projections to verify its position. It is much more difficult to insert interlocking screws correctly if an erroneous drill hole has been made, because the drill has a tendency to find the old hole. Once the first screw has been inserted, the drill bit used to stabilize the guide is removed and replaced with a distal screw. The sequence of screw placement from distal to proximal is important. If screws are placed proximally first, the femoral condyles may piston around the nail, making reduction difficult. Screw length is determined with the aid of the C-arm. Distally 60- to 70-mm screws are generally sufficient. Rotating the C-arm to the

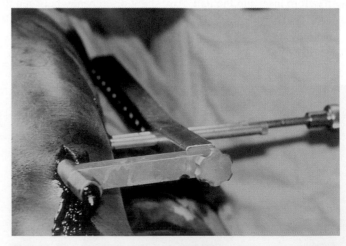

Figure 11. The nail is fixed in the distal femur by a drill bit passed through the guide and sleeves.

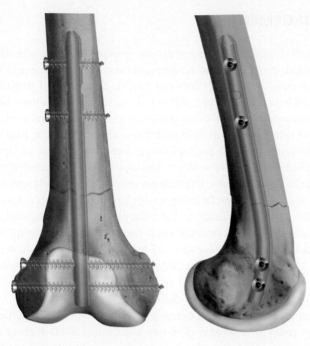

A,B   Anterior - Posterior View   Lateral View

Figure 12. A, B: The configuration of screws proximal and distal to the fracture should be balanced.

oblique projection helps ensure that the tip of the screw is just through the medial femoral cortex and not protruding into the soft tissues.

The number of interlocking screws should be balanced proximal and distal to the fracture (Fig. 12). For most fractures, two screws are placed proximal and two distal to the principal transverse fracture plane. In stable transverse, Type A and simple Type C fractures, the fracture site can be loaded by using a nail with an oval slot (Fig. 13).

Supplemental interfragmentary lag screws can be placed over guide wires used for temporary fixation to complete the osteosynthesis. The incision is closed with simple sutures, and the knee is placed in a bulky dressing with a knee immobilizer (Fig. 14). Final AP and lateral radiographs are obtained before leaving the operating room.

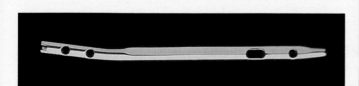

Figure 13. Supracondylar nail with proximal oval compression hole. This allows a stable fracture to compress with weight bearing.

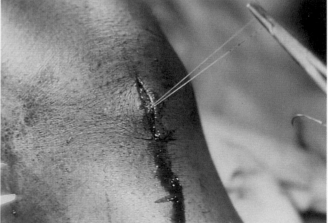

Figure 14. The wound is closed with simple sutures. After closing the wound, the knee will be placed in a bulky dressing and a knee immobilizer.

POSTOPERATIVE MANAGEMENT

Because the supracondylar nail is used in a large and diverse group of patients with different fracture patterns, postoperative management must be individualized if outcome is to be successful. Retrograde supracondylar "nailing" does not provide the degree of stability when compared with an interlocking nail for diaphyseal femur fracture, which allows immediate use of the limb. The supracondylar nail–bone construct will *not* withstand immediate weight bearing. Aggressive range of knee motion with physiotherapy also can lead to failure. The goals of surgery during the first postoperative week are control of limb swelling, quadriceps muscle rehabilitation, and active ankle motion. Thromboembolism prophylaxis is routinely used. In low-risk patients, intermittent venous compression and aspirin are used, whereas in high-risk patients, warfarin (anticoagulation to 1.5 times control, INR, 2.0 to 2.5) is recommended. In special situations, for example, when anticoagulation has to be reversed from another operation, intermittent intravenous heparin (50 mg q12h) is used. The operative dressings are left in place for 48 to 72 hours. Drains are placed if an open reduction was necessary. Drains are removed at 24 to 48 hours when output is minimal. Subsequently the wounds are either left undressed, or a simple dressing is applied. At 5 days, mobile patients are allowed to shower and dry the wound.

In cooperative patients with stable fixation, a continuous-passive-motion machine (CPM) is begun in the recovery room. It is set at a slow rate and limited to 60 degrees of flexion. As the swelling subsides, a quadriceps-reeducation program is instituted through a program of active-assisted knee motion with a defined limit (initially 45 degrees of flexion). Straight-leg raising is *not* prescribed or encouraged. Knee motion is progressed on an individual basis. Alert and cooperative patients are mobilized with the aid of a sliding board. As the patients gain leg control, they are mobilized to a wheelchair. Once the patients have reached 30 to 50 degrees of flexion and can transfer to a wheelchair, they are discharged from the hospital. Knee flexion is progressed to 90 degrees, and isometric quadriceps strengthening and patellar mobilization are emphasized. Cooperative patients with good leg control are gait trained with a walker or crutches, non–weight bearing. Skin sutures are removed between 10 and 14 days. Weight bearing is not allowed until there is good muscle function and radiographic evidence of fracture healing 6 to 8 weeks after surgery. Postoperatively, patients are fitted with long-leg compression stockings 3 to 5 days after surgery. A knee immobilizer is used in bed and for mobilization. A cast brace can be helpful in young patients with unstable fracture patterns, as they begin to load the limb at 6 to 8 weeks.

Physiologically young patients with isolated fractures can return to most types of light work 14 to 16 weeks after injury. We favor intensive conditioning and formal work hardening for an additional 4 to 6 weeks in patients with heavy-demand jobs such as construction work and assembly-line work. Most patients lose some knee motion after surgery and should be warned about the possibility of shortening and arthrosis from articular comminution. Elderly patients usually return to their preinjury level of self-care, shopping, recreational activity, and driving. Most patients reach maximal medical improvement 6 to 8 months after injury.

COMPLICATIONS

Few complications have been noted when this technique is used. One common problem is prominent screws in the distal femur. This is caused by placing screws that are too long. The distal femur is trapezoidal in shape: wider dorsally than ventrally. The appropriate-size interlocking screws are generally 60- to 70-mm long. Screw length can be checked by looking at the oblique fluoroscopic views during surgery. If the screws are too long and cause pain, the screws can be removed or exchanged as an outpatient procedure. Among the few other complications that are known are the following: nonunion, infection, nail breakage

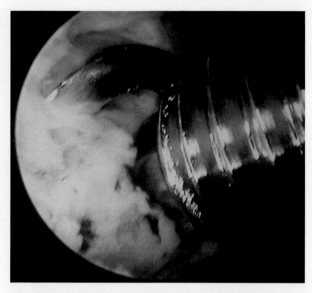

Figure 15. Arthroscopic view showing the nail extractor being threaded into the end of the supracondylar nail.

(reduced by the development of stronger nails with fewer holes), and screw breakage (reduced by the development of stronger screws). Bent screws can usually be taken out through the same incisions they were put in with. To remove a broken screw, first take out the screw head. Then put a 4-mm pin, blunt end first, into the screw hole. Tap on this pin with a mallet to drive the screw tip so it tents the skin on the opposite side, cut down on the screw, and remove it.

Infection represents a serious therapeutic challenge. An early infection can be suppressed by lavage of the knee and continued high-dose antibiotic (oral or intravenous) until the nail can be removed. Infections after fracture healing are treated with nail removal and irrigation of the knee joint. The incidence rate for complications after supracondylar nailing is low, especially considering the difficult indications for which this nail is used. Nail removal is occasionally indicated. It can be done either fluoroscopically or arthroscopically. Under the arthroscope, the nail end can be seen and the extractor placed under direct vision (Fig. 15). At the same time, significant adhesions can be lysed, and the articular surface debrided.

ILLUSTRATIVE CASE FOR TECHNIQUE

A 57-year-old orthopaedic operating room nurse was struck in a head-on collision as she was driving, wearing her seat belt, down Dixie Highway. Her injuries consisted of a compound comminuted fracture of the left distal femur with intraarticular involvement and loss of skin, a nondisplaced left tibial plateau fracture, metatarsal fractures, and other minor lacerations, bruises, and loss of a tooth. Her injury film is shown in Figure 16A.

Her initial treatment consisted of debridement of her compound fracture, placement of antibiotic-impregnated bead chains, and stabilization across the knee joint by using a large-pin external fixateur (Fig. 16B).

Subsequently, a retrograde intramedullary nail was placed with fixation of the distal femoral articular block with bioabsorbable screws and pins, a steel cannulated screw, and one interlocking screw through the nail (Fig. 16C). She was hospitalized for 10 days. By 4 months postoperatively, she was full weight bearing but had knee motion restricted to 75 degrees at flexion. Her knee was stable. She was able to return to work at 6 months as an operating room nurse. Her radiograph at 4 months is shown in Figure 16D.

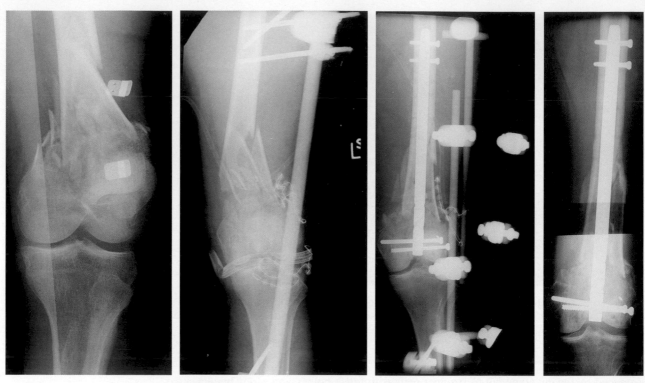

A,B

C

Figure 16. A: Preoperative radiograph showing a compound comminuted fracture of the left distal femur and a nondisplaced tibial plateau fracture. **B:** Radiograph showing the stabilization of the fracture using a large pin external fixateur and the insertion of antibotic impregnated bead chains. **C:** Addition of bioabsorbable screws and pins. A retrograde intermedullary nail, a steel cannulated screw, and an interlocking screw are also used to further fix the fracture sites. **D:** A 4-month postoperative radiograph with removal of the external fixateur.

RECOMMENDED READING

1. David, S.M., Harrow, M.E., Peindl, R.D., Frick, S.L., Kellam, J.F.: Comparative biomechanical analysis of supracondylar femur fracture fixation: locked intramedullary nail vs. 95 degree angled plate. *J. Orthop. Trauma.*, 11:344–350, 1997.

2. DeLong, W.G., Watson, J.T., Born, C.T., Iannacone, W.M.: Treatment of supracondylar and femoral shaft fractures by retrograde nail techniques. Orthopedic Trauma Association 11th Annual Meeting, Tampa, Florida, September 28–October 1, 1995.

3. Green, S.: Distal intramedullary fixation of supracondylar fractures of the femur. *Tech. Orthop.*, 3:71–76, 1988.

4. Guerra, J.J., Della-Valle, C.J., Corcoran, J.A., Duda, J.R.: Arthroscopically assisted placement of a supracondylar intramedullary nail. *Arthroscopy*, 11(2):239–244, 1995.

5. Henry, S.L.: Management of supracondylar fractures proximal to total knee arthroplasty with the GSH supracondylar nail. *Contemp. Orthop.*, 31(4):231–238, 1995.

6. Henry, S.L., Busconi, B., Gold, S., Watson, T., Licht, T., Schaper, L.: Management of supracondylar fractures of the femur with the GSH intramedullary nail: a preliminary report. *Contemp. Orthop.*, 22(6):631–640, 1991.

7. Henry, S.L., Green, S., Trager, S., Seligson, D.: Management of supracondylar femur fractures with the GSH intramedullary nail: a preliminary report. *Contemp. Orthop.*, 22(6):631–640, 1991.

8. Henry, S.L., and Seligson, D.: Management of supracondylar fractures of the femur with the GSH supracondylar nail: the percutaneous technique. *Tech. Orthop.*, 9(3):189–194, 1994.

9. Iannacone, W.M., Bennet, F.S., DeLong, W.G., Born, C.T., Dalsey, R.M.: Initial experience with the supracondylar femoral fractures using the supracondylar intramedullary nail: a preliminary report. *J. Orthop. Trauma*, 8(4):322–327, 1994.

10. Jabozenski, F.F., and Crawford, M.: Retrograde intramedullary nailing of supracondylar femur fractures above total knee arthroplasty: a preliminary report of four cases. *J. Arthroplasty*, 10(1):95–101, 1995.

11. Khalily, C., Voor, M.J., Seligson, D.: Fracture site motion with Ilizarov and hybrid external fixation. *J. Orthop. Trauma*, 12:21–26, 1998.

12. Koval, K.J., Seligson, D., Rosen, H., Fee, K.: Distal femoral nonunion: treatment with a retrograde inserted locked intramedullary nail. *J. Orthop. Trauma,* 9(4):285–291, 1995.
13. Lessen, M.R., Jensen, S., Borris, L.C., Kristensen, K., Nielsen, P.T.: Early experience with retrograde supracondylar intramedullary nailing. *Acta Orthop. Scand.,* 65(suppl 260):75, 1994.
14. Lucas, S.F., Seligson, D., Henry, S.L.: Intramedullary supracondylar nailing of femoral fractures: a preliminary report of the GSH supracondylar nail. *Clin. Orthop.,* 296:200–206, 1993.
15. Moed, B.R., and Watson, J.T.: Retrograde intramedullary nailing, without reaming of fractures of the femoral shaft in multiply injured patients. *J. Bone Joint Surg. [Am],* 77(10):1520–1527, 1995.
16. Müller, M.E., Nazarian, S., Koch, P., Schatzker, J.: *The Comprehensive Classification of Fractures of Long Bones.* Springer-Verlag, Berlin, 1990.
17. Murrel, G.A., and Nunley, J.A.: Interlocked supracondylar intramedullary nails for supracondylar fractures after total knee arthroplasty: a new treatment method. *J. Arthroplasty,* 10(1):37–42, Feb 1995.
18. Ostermann, P.A.W., Hahn, M.P., Ekkernkamp, A., Dávid, A., Muhr, G.: Behandlung einer suprakondylären Femurfraktur proximal einer Kniegelenksendoprothese durch retrograde Verriegelungsnagelung. *Zentrbl. Chir.,* 120:731–733, 1995.
19. Ostermann, P.A.W., Hahn, M.P., Ekkernkamp, A., Muhr, G.: Die retrograde Verriegelungsnagelung distaler Femurfrakturen mit dem GSH-Nagel. *Chirurgie,* 67:1135–1140, 1996.
20. Seligson, D., Been, J.N., Howard, P.A.: Supracondylar fractures: an historical perspective. *Tech. Orthop.,* 9(3):180–188, 1994.
21. Seligson, D., Henry, S.L., Weiss, G.: The intramedullary supracondylar nail. *Unfallchirurgie,* 229:275–278, 1993.
22. Wozasek, G.E., Seligson, D., Durgin, R., Voor, M.: Distal interlocking screw fixation strength in femoral intramedullary nailing: influence of bone quality and supplemental buttress nut. *Osteosyn. Int.,* 2:123–127, 1996.
23. Wurst, C., and Seligson, D.: The treatment of supracondylar fractures of the femur with an interlocking nail: initial case experience. *Osteosyn. Int.,* 3:204–208, 1995.

Master Techniques in Orthopaedic Surgery,
FRACTURES, edited by D. A. Wiss,
Lippincott–Raven Publishers, Philadelphia © 1998.

21

Patellar Fractures: Open Reduction Internal Fixation

John H. Wilber

INDICATIONS/CONTRAINDICATIONS

Operative management is the treatment of choice for the majority of displaced patellar fractures. Surgical options include open reduction and internal fixation, partial or complete patellectomy, with the choice of treatment dependent on the fracture pattern and the amount of displacement. Patellar fractures are classified into two groups and are either nondisplaced or displaced. Within each of these groups, fractures are subdivided into stellate, transverse, and vertical patterns. Transverse fractures usually occur in the central third, although apical and distal transverse fractures do occur. The fractures can be further classified based on the degree of comminution as being noncomminuted, comminuted, or highly comminuted.

The patella is both an integral component of the extensor mechanism of the knee and an articular component of the knee joint. Treatment must achieve anatomic reduction of the articular surface while reestablishing the continuity of the extensor mechanism. Displacement more than 3 mm or articular incongruity of more than 2 mm is considered strong indication for surgical treatment.

Total patellectomy is generally indicated when the patella is so severely comminuted that a well-reduced and stable construct cannot be achieved with open reduction and internal fixation. Partial patellectomy is indicated for cases that have severe comminution of either the inferior or superior pole that is not amenable to open reduction and internal fixation techniques.

Open reduction and internal fixation is indicated for displaced patellar fractures that have fragments large enough to be reduced and stably repaired and is the treatment of choice for the majority of displaced patellar fractures in physiologically young patients. Many comminuted fractures can be salvaged.

J. H. Wilber, M.D.: Department of Orthopaedic Surgery, Case Western Reserve University, University Orthopaedic Associates, Cleveland, Ohio 44106.

Contraindications and relative contraindications to surgical treatment include nondisplaced or minimally displaced stable fracture patterns, contused or injured skin that precludes safe surgical approaches to the fracture, active infection involving the extremity with the patellar fracture, and medical conditions of the patient that would preclude safe surgical intervention.

PREOPERATIVE PLANNING

The first step in preoperative planning includes an accurate history and careful physical examination. The history should include pertinent medical history, current problems, and the activity level of the patient. The mechanism of injury may explain the severity of injury as well as the fracture pattern. It is helpful to know whether the injury occurred as a result of a direct blow (e.g., a fall on the knee) or from resisted flexion of the knee resulting in a traction-type injury.

The physical examination should include a thorough evaluation of the extremity, looking for signs of direct trauma and swelling. The presence of fracture blisters, lacerations, abrasions, and contusions should be documented. It is essential to determine whether the fracture is open. Wounds should be checked and if necessary carefully explored to determine whether they are in continuity with the fracture or the knee joint. In displaced patellar fractures, a visible or palpable defect is often noted between the fragments, although this

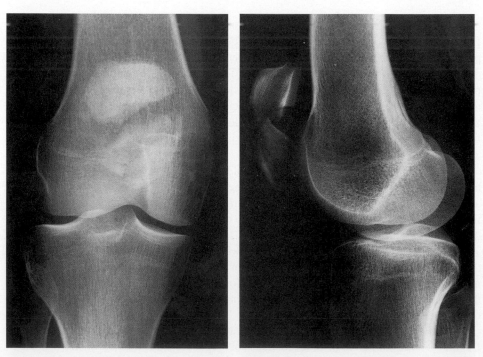

A   B

Figure 1. A, B: Anteroposterior (AP) and lateral radiographs showing a transverse fracture of the patella with comminution of the distal fragment. The lateral view shows significant comminution involving the articular surface in addition to displacement of the proximal and distal pole fragments.

may be masked by significant swelling, which develops rapidly. In some cases, a hemarthrosis is not apparent because of a large retinacular tear that allows blood to dissipate into the surrounding soft tissues. The absence of a hemarthrosis does not rule out a patellar fracture.

The continuity of the quadriceps mechanism is next evaluated. A painful, tense hemarthrosis often complicates this part of the examination. Aspiration of the knee with injection of a local anesthetic usually decreases pain. The patient is asked to contract the quadriceps mechanism and attempt fully to extend the knee. The ability to do this does not rule out a patellar fracture, because the medial and lateral retinacula may still be intact, providing partial continuity of the extensor mechanism. However, the inability to do this usually indicates that a patella fracture that tears the medial and lateral retinaculum exists. Evaluation of knee stability should be carefully performed. Flexion of the knee should be avoided because this may further displace the fracture in addition to causing significant discomfort to the patient. The peripheral pulses, the compartments of the leg, and a neurologic examination should be performed.

After the physical examination, radiographs of the knee should be obtained. The standard radiographic evaluation includes anteroposterior (AP), lateral, and axial views of the patella. A supine AP radiograph is obtained, centered over the patella (Fig. 1). Care should be taken to have the patella centered midline on the femur; this usually requires slight internal rotation of the extremity. The lateral radiograph can be taken as a cross-table lateral, with the knee slightly flexed. For an axial view, a Merchant's view is most easily and safely obtained in the injured patient (Fig. 2). The patient is placed supine on the x-ray table with the knee flexed 45 degrees over the end of the table. The x-ray beam is angled at 30 degrees from the horizontal, and the cassette is placed perpendicular to this x-ray beam 1 foot below the knee. Comparison views of the uninjured knee can be helpful in selected patients (i.e., a bipartite patella). Occasionally in patients with complex fracture patterns, tomography or computerized tomography can be helpful.

Vertical fractures are often missed on both the AP and lateral views and are best visualized on the axial view. Larger displaced fracture lines can be readily seen, although smaller, nondisplaced fracture lines are often obscured because of the superimposition of the patella

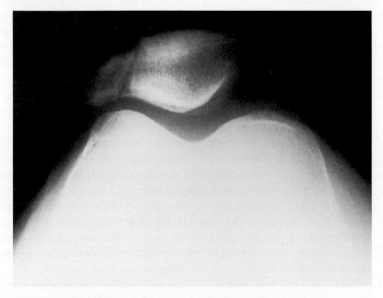

Figure 2. Axial view of the patella showing a vertical fracture of the lateral facet of the patella. There is minimal displacement of the fragments.

on the femur in the AP view. In most cases, the fracture is more comminuted than what is apparent on the radiographic evaluation. Displacement more than 3 mm or articular incongruity more than 2 mm are indications for surgery.

Preoperative drawings should be performed on complex fracture patterns. Make a tracing on both the AP and lateral views of the uninjured contralateral side and then superimpose the fracture lines from the injured side onto this normal template. The fixation should be drawn, and the procedural steps carefully listed. The operating room should be informed of the equipment required, based on the preoperative plan. Equipment needed for surgery usually includes various-sized pointed bone-reduction clamps, small curettes, wire cutters, benders, and wire tighteners, 1.2-mm Kirschner wires (K-wires), and 1-mm wire. Power drills and wire drivers will also be necessary. Small fragment screws and instruments should be available.

Surgery can be undertaken as soon as the patient has been prepared and appropriate preoperative plans completed. If the fracture is open, surgery must be done urgently. Closed fractures should be operated on when the soft-tissue injury and the general condition of the patient permit.

SURGERY

The patient is positioned supine on a standard operating table. Because there is a tendency for the leg externally to rotate, a small bump can be placed under the ipsilateral hip. A tourniquet is placed high on the involved thigh. The procedure can be done under a general or spinal anesthetic. The patient is prepped in a standard fashion, and the leg is draped free by using an extremity drape. The leg is exsanguinated with a sterile Esmarch, and the tourniquet inflated to a pressure appropriate for the size of the leg and the patient's blood pressure. Before inflating the tourniquet, the quadriceps is pulled distally to ensure that it is not trapped under the tourniquet, which can displace the patella proximally, making reduction difficult. When the retinaculum is intact, flexion of the knee will help advance the quadriceps from underneath the tourniquet. If the retinaculum is not intact, the patella can be manually pulled distally, while flexing the knee and then inflating the tourniquet. A sterile bump can be placed behind the knee, which allows the knee to flex 15 to 20 degrees. Appropriate antibiotic prophylaxis should be given before inflating the tourniquet.

The skin incision can be either transverse or longitudinal. A longitudinal incision is preferred when more proximal and distal dissection is necessary for the repair of comminuted fractures, in cases in which wire augmentation may be necessary down to the tibial tubercle, and when later reconstruction procedures are anticipated. Cosmetically, the transverse incision is preferred, and it also avoids potential damage to the saphenous branch of the femoral nerve.

The incision is carried down through the subcutaneous tissue and through the prepatellar bursa. A hematoma is usually encountered as soon as the bursa is opened, which usually leads directly into the fracture site (Fig. 3). Care should be taken to minimize direct dissection of the fracture fragments. The soft tissues surrounding the patella often hold nondisplaced fractures in place, and if this is disrupted, they may displace, creating a more complicated and unstable fracture pattern. The displaced fracture should be exposed. Clot should be removed with a combination of small curettes and the use of a small suction-tip device. Irrigation should be used liberally to help remove the hematoma and small inconsequential comminuted fragments. The extent of the medial and lateral retinacular injuries should be identified and the edges tagged for later repair. The undersurface of the patella, in addition to the patellar groove, should be inspected for evidence of articular damage. The knee joint should be inspected and irrigated to remove any loose fragments.

After the fracture and the knee joint have been thoroughly irrigated, the fracture edges carefully exposed, and the fracture pattern has been thoroughly delineated, a preliminary reduction is performed. The small bump behind the knee will need to be removed at this time, because flexion of the knee will make reduction more difficult. In the case of a simple central transverse fracture, one can proceed directly to the tension-band technique. In

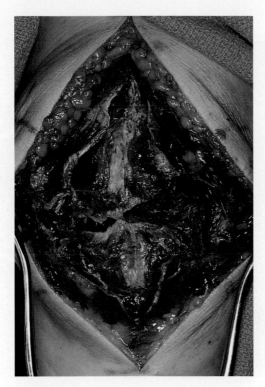

Figure 3. Surgical exposure through a vertical midline incision showing the transverse fracture of the patella with medial and lateral retinaculum tears. The soft tissues have been left intact over the surfaces of the patella.

other more complex fractures, the goal is to try to reduce the fragments to create a transverse fracture pattern that can then be further stabilized with a tension-band technique. An example of this is a transverse fracture pattern that also has a vertical split through either the proximal or distal fragments. The vertical split is first reduced and held temporarily with a large pointed reduction forceps. This is then temporarily stabilized with 1.2-mm K-wires. Definitive stabilization of this fragment depends on its size and can be either with K-wires or small-fragment or mini-fragment screws. Once this has been performed, the tenaculum clamps and the provisional fixation are removed. The goal is to try to convert a complex fracture pattern into a simple transverse pattern.

Once a transverse fracture pattern has been created, a tension-band wire technique is performed. By using a 2-mm drill, two parallel drill holes are placed in a retrograde fashion through the proximal bony fragment. A 1.6- or 1.8-mm K-wire is then advanced through these holes and out through the quadriceps tendon (Fig. 4). They are advanced until the sharp tip of the K-wire is fully within the proximal bony fragment. The two fracture fragments are then reduced and held with a large pointed reduction forceps. Care should be taken to ensure that the articular surface is anatomically reduced by inspecting both the anterior cortical and posterior articular surfaces. The articular surface can be inspected through the preexisting tears in the retinaculum. If there is no significant tear in the retinaculum, a small medial or lateral arthrotomy should be made to allow inspection or palpation of the articular surface. The K-wires are then sequentially attached to the drill and advanced into the distal fragment (Fig. 5). They should be advanced distally at least 1 cm beyond the inferior tip of the patella. Once again, the adequacy of the reduction should be checked. A 30-cm segment of 1-mm wire is passed adjacent to the patella and quadriceps mechanism proximally and distally, passing behind the K-wires and closely approximated to both the proximal and distal poles of the patella. If this is not achieved, the wire will not obtain adequate fixation and may loosen, eventually resulting in loss of fixation and re-

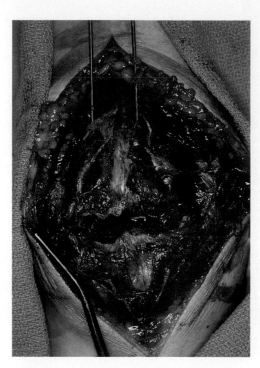

Figure 4. The hematoma has been evacuated, and the joint and fracture lines debrided. The K-wires have been advanced retrograde through the patella, and the patella fragments are now ready to be reduced.

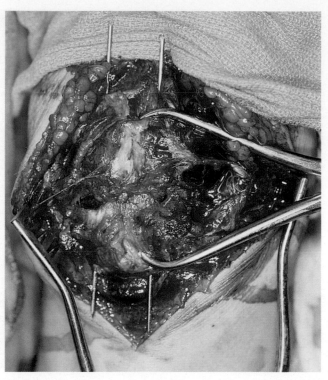

Figure 5. The transverse fracture has been anatomically reduced by using a pointed fracture-reduction clamp, and the K-wires have been advanced antegrade through the distal fragment. The K-wires are parallel to each other.

duction. To facilitate passage of the wire, I pass a 16-gauge angiocath through the quadriceps mechanism, just above the superior pole of the patella and behind the K-wires (Fig. 6). The 1-mm wire is passed through the catheter, which is then removed. The identical technique is performed distally. Because the patella has a flat surface, it is not necessary to place the tension-band wire in a figure-eight fashion. To ensure symmetrical tensioning of

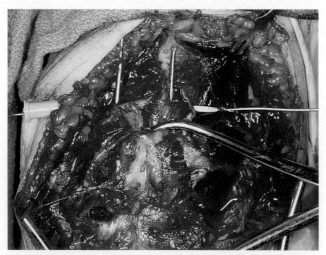

Figure 6. A 16-gauge angiocath is passed through the quadriceps tendon behind the K-wires and just superior to the patella. The cerclage wire is being passed through the angiocath, which will then be removed. An identical procedure is then performed through the distal pole.

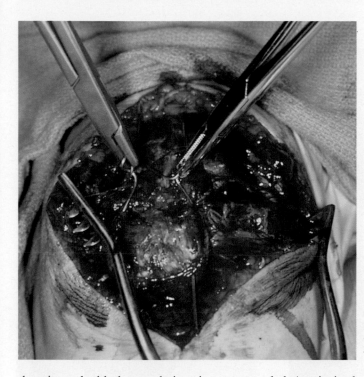

Figure 7. A double-tensioning technique is performed by consecutively tightening each side of the tension-band wire. The fracture gap can be seen to close down with this technique.

the wire, a double-loop technique is recommended. A twist is placed in the wire on its continuous side, and on the contralateral side, the two ends of the wires are hand-tightened and twisted. Excessive wire is removed. By using either a large needle driver or a large clamp specifically designed for wire tightening, the two ends of the wire are sequentially tightened (Fig. 7). The technique of wire tightening is critical. Before twisting, the wire should be tensioned by lifting up on the clamp. The wire is then gently twisted. This will ensure that both wires twist around each other rather than one wire wrapping around the other wire. The wires are sequentially tightened in this manner until adequate compression has been achieved. Once again, the quality of the reduction is checked, and the knee is gently flexed to check the stability of the fixation (Fig. 8). The twisted wire is clipped, and the ends are bent over by using a large needle driver and gently flattened by using a bone tamp and a mallet so they lie close to the superior surface of the bone. The K-wires are bent next. They are bent by stabilizing the wire close to the bone with a needle driver and then using the wire bender, trying to bend it to 110 degrees. The excess wire is then cut. This is then rotated 180 degrees posteriorly and advanced into the quadriceps mechanism. If the wire is not advanced into the quadriceps mechanism, it will cause excessive irritation, in addition to having an increasing chance of backing out. The distal ends of the wires are then cut so they are not excessively prominent within the patellar tendon. The retinacular defects are repaired with figure of eight sutures of 0 polyglactin 910 (Vicryl; Figs. 9 and 10).

The tourniquet is deflated and hemostasis obtained with electrocoagulation. A suction drain is placed in the knee joint. Closure should be meticulous, including closure of the prepatellar bursa as a separate layer by using 2-0 Vicryl. The subcutaneous tissue is closed by using simple inverted 2-0 Vicryl. Skin closure is dependent on the integrity of the skin. Subcuticular closure gives excellent cosmetic results but should be reserved for those cases without skin injuries and only minimal swelling. If there is concern regarding damage to the skin, nylon sutures should be used. A sterile dressing is applied consisting of fluffs, Webril, and an Ace wrap. The patient is placed into either a knee immobilizer or a hinged knee brace with the knee locked in full extension.

Other variations on the tension-band technique include the use of 4-0 cannulated screws with the tension-band wire passed through the cannulated screws and tightened in a standard double-loop technique. In the case of a distal-pole patella fracture, the tension-band wire technique can be used, although the K-wires must be placed closer together so they both

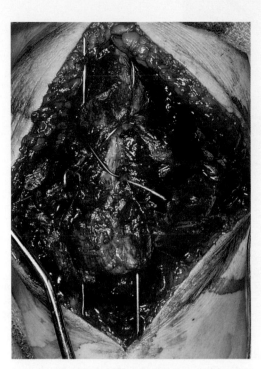

Figure 8. The tension-band wires have been tightened, clipped short, and bent. The K-wires have not yet been shortened, and the retinaculum has not yet been repaired.

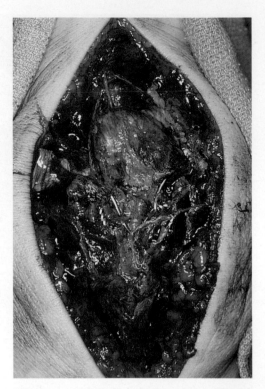

Figure 9. The final tension-band construct with the K-wires cut and bent and buried within the quadriceps and patellar tendon. The retinaculum has been repaired.

capture the distal fragment. An alternative to this is the use of retrograde cannulated or standard 4.0 screws in addition to a tension-band technique. With very small fragments, a single screw can be used. In the case of a stellate fracture, circumferential cerclage wire can be helpful to "bundle" the fracture fragments together (Fig. 11). In stellate fractures, it is critical not to violate the soft tissues around the fragments because this will cause significant disruption of the fracture fragments.

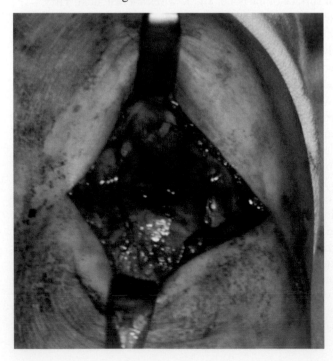

Figure 10. Alternative transverse incision with final construct visualized through the wound.

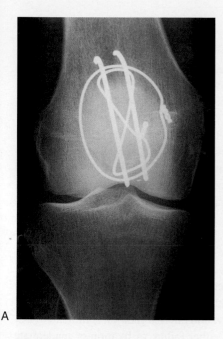 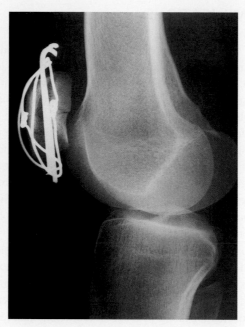

A   B

Figure 11. A, B: Postoperative anteroposterior (AP) and lateral radiographs of a comminuted patellar fracture fixed with a combination tension-band and cerclage-wire technique. The articular surface has been restored anatomically.

POSTOPERATIVE MANAGEMENT

Postoperative care is dependent on the fracture type and the resultant stability after osteosynthesis. In patients with stable fixation, knee motion is begun immediately. The patient is placed into a continuous-passive-motion (CPM) machine in the recovery room. When not in the CPM or receiving therapy, the patient should be protected in either a knee immobilizer or a hinged knee brace with the hinges locked. On the first postoperative day, the patient is mobilized out of bed to ambulate weight bearing as tolerated with the knee locked in full extension. The hinges can either be loosened or the knee immobilizer removed for active range-of-motion exercises. Quadriceps strengthening is started in the immediate postoperative period. The drain is removed at 48 hours, and the patient is usually discharged home shortly thereafter. They are seen in follow-up in approximately 7 to 10 days for a dressing change and suture removal. If the wound is well healed, active extension and straight-leg-raising exercises are begun, and the patient is referred to physical therapy. The patient is seen again at 4 weeks, and radiographs of the patella are obtained out of the brace. If there is radiographic evidence of healing, progressive resistive exercises are started. The patient is progressively weaned from the brace, depending on the motion and strength. Full rehabilitation usually takes 4 to 6 months. If there are any symptoms or signs of loss of fixation during this postoperative period, range of motion is stopped, and the patient is immobilized and followed up closely.

In the case of unstable fracture fixation, early range of motion is not possible. The repair should be protected in either a knee immobilizer or a knee brace with the hinges locked. The braces are removed only for wound checks and extremity cleansing. Quad sets can be initiated, but the repair is protected until there are signs of healing. Range of motion is delayed for 3 to 6 weeks.

COMPLICATIONS

In the immediate postoperative period, the major complications include hemarthrosis and infection. A hemarthrosis can usually be avoided by the use of a postoperative suction drain. If the drain was either not used or was removed prematurely, the hemarthrosis can be aspirated. This is necessary only if a tense hemarthrosis causes significant pain or limits rehabilitation.

Infection is a rare but devastating complication. This can usually be avoided by careful timing of surgery and meticulous surgical techniques. If infection develops, it should be aggressively treated with antibiotics and debridement with drainage. Physical therapy and early range of motion should be stopped while treating the infection. If the infection involves the knee joint, it must be drained and irrigated surgically. Culture-specific intravenous antibiotics should be used for 3 to 6 weeks. Internal fixation in general should not be removed until the fracture has healed.

Loss of fixation and reduction are other possible complications after surgical repair of patella fractures. This is more common in complex fracture patterns, in noncompliant patients, and when therapy is overly aggressive. If there are signs of loss of fixation without significant loss of reduction, this can be treated with immobilization. If there are signs of loss of fixation along with loss of reduction, then revision internal fixation is indicated. Delayed union and nonunion are usually the result of either failure of fixation or inadequate initial reduction. These complications can usually be avoided by good reduction and fixation techniques and close postoperative follow-up. Delayed unions can be treated with repeated cerclage-wire techniques. Significant malunions usually require a patellectomy.

Arthrofibrosis and loss of knee motion are relatively common complications after patella fractures. These complications are more common in severely comminuted fractures and those fractures requiring prolonged immobilization. The majority of patients can be treated with aggressive and persistent physical therapy, although an occasional case will require manipulation under anesthesia. If a patient does not respond to physical therapy and requires manipulation under anesthesia, it is my preference to do an arthroscopic debridement of the arthrofibrosis at the time of the manipulation. This allows inspection of the patellar surface, a direct lysis of the arthrofibrosis involving the suprapatellar pouch and the lateral gutters, in addition to adhesions from the fat pad into the intercondylar notch. Arthroscopic debridement and manipulation should be followed by aggressive physical therapy to maintain motion and increase strength.

Posttraumatic osteoarthritis results from either inadequate reduction of the articular surface or injuries to the articular surface that occur at the time of injury. In the early stages, arthroscopy and patellar debridement can decrease some symptoms. Ultimately in the young patient, a patellectomy may be the treatment of choice. In the elderly patient who also has involvement of the medial and lateral joint space, a total knee replacement may be the treatment of choice.

ILLUSTRATIVE CASE FOR TECHNIQUE

A 58-year-old woman tripped and fell onto her flexed right knee. She had immediate pain and noted inability actively to extend her leg. Radiographs demonstrated a transverse fracture of her patella (Fig. 12). Open reduction and internal fixation by using a tension-band technique was performed. She was managed with early range of motion, but her knee was protected with a knee immobilizer. Her fracture healed uneventfully, and her final range of motion at 1 year postoperative was 0 to 140 degrees with excellent function and no pain (Fig. 13).

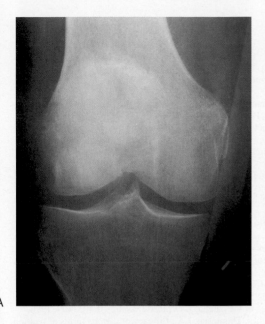
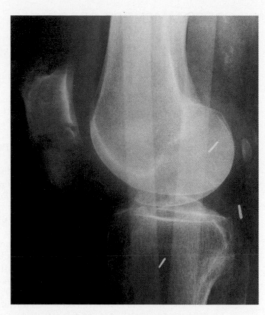

A

B

Figure 12. A, B: Preoperative anteroposterior (AP) and lateral radiograph of a transverse fracture of the patella showing significant displacement and articular incongruity.

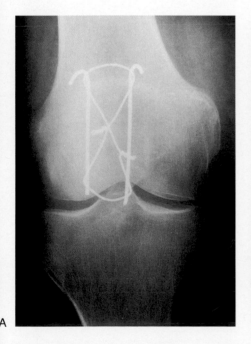
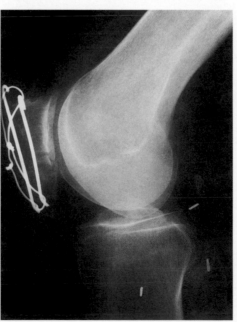

A

B

Figure 13. A, B: Postoperative anteroposterior (AP) and lateral radiographs demonstrating that the fracture has been fixed anatomically with a tension-band technique. The tension-band wire was placed in a figure-of-eight configuration because of a more spherical surface of the patella to avoid slippage of the wires.

RECOMMENDED READING

1. Benjamin, J., Bried, J., Dohm, M., McMurtry, M.: Biomechanical evaluation of various forms of fixation of transverse patellar fractures. *J. Orthop. Trauma,* 1:219–222, 1987.
2. Böstman, O., Kiviluoto, O., Nirhamo, J.: Comminuted displaced fractures of the patella. *Injury,* 13:196–202, 1981.
3. Böstman, O., Kiviluoto, O., Santavirta, S., Nirhamo, J., Wilppula, E.: Fractures of the patella treated by operation. *Arch. Orthop. Trauma Surg.,* 102:78–81, 1983.
4. Carpenter, J.E., Kasman, R., Matthews, L.S.: Fractures of the patella: instructional course lectures. *J. Bone Joint Surg. [Am],* 75:1550–1561, 1993.
5. Edwards, B., Johnell, O., Redlund-Johnell, I.: Patellar fractures: a 30-year follow-up. *Acta Orthop. Scand.,* 60:712–714, 1989.
6. Goodfellow, J., Hungerford, D.S., Zindel, M.: Patello-femoral joint mechanics and pathology: 1. Functional anatomy of the patello-femoral joint. *J. Bone Joint Surg. [Br],* 58:287–290, 1976.
7. Hung, L.K., Chan, K.M., Chow, Y.N., Leung, P.C.: Fractured patella: operative treatment using the tension band principle. *Injury,* 16:343–347, 1985.
8. Levack, B., Flannagan, J.P., Hobbs, S.: Results of surgical treatment of patellar fractures. *J. Bone Joint Surg. [Br],* 67:416–419, 1985.
9. Lotke, P.A., and Ecker, M.L.: Transverse fractures of the patella. *Clin. Orthop.,* 158:180–184, 1981.
10. Muller, M.E., Allgower, M., Schneider, R., Willinegger, H.: *Manual of Internal Fixation: Techniques Recommended by the AO Group.* Springer-Verlag, Berlin, 1991.
11. Smith, S.T., Cramer, K.E., Karges, D.E., Watson, J.T., Moed, B.R.: Early complications in the operative treatment of patella fractures. *J. Orthop. Trauma,* 11:183–187, 1997.
12. Torchia, M.E., and Lewallen, D.G.: Open fractures of the patella. *J. Orthop. Trauma,* 10:403–409, 1996.
13. Weber, M.J., Janecki, C.J., McLeod, P., Nelson, C.L., Thompson, J.A.: Efficacy of various forms of fixation of transverse fractures of the patella. *J. Bone Joint Surg. [Am],* 62:215–220, 1980.

Master Techniques in Orthopaedic Surgery,
FRACTURES, edited by D. A. Wiss,
Lippincott–Raven Publishers, Philadelphia © 1998.

22

Knee Dislocation

John M. Siliski

INDICATIONS/CONTRAINDICATIONS

Immediate operative treatment for knee dislocation is indicated for only a few reasons, including (a) open dislocation, (b) popliteal artery laceration or thrombosis, and (c) an irreducible dislocation.

Early (within 3 weeks) ligament repair and reconstruction is indicated for most knees with multiple ligamentous disruptions. Typically both cruciate, and one or both collateral ligaments, are disrupted in a knee dislocation. Additional injuries that may require surgical treatment are capsular disruptions, tendon avulsions, meniscal tears, and associated intraarticular fractures. Before such complex knee surgery, three prerequisites must be met: (a) the patient must be medically fit for surgery, (b) the limb must have an intact or reconstructed vascular supply, and (c) the soft-tissue coverage over the knee must be in a condition to tolerate surgical incision and dissection. Preoperative planning for ligament repair and reconstruction includes preparation of the patient, limb, and soft- tissue envelope. If the prerequisites cannot be met, ligament repair and reconstruction should be postponed.

Contraindications to ligament repair and reconstruction include the inability during the first few weeks after injury to have the patient, the limb, and the soft tissues acceptable for surgery. In such cases, the knee is best treated by immobilization in a reduced position with slight flexion (~10 degrees) by using a cast, brace, or external fixator. Another contraindication to ligament surgery is an elderly or infirm patient with an anticipated low activity level; extensive knee surgery may have little short- or long-term benefit for such a patient. At the opposite end of the age spectrum is the pediatric patient with open epiphyseal plates. Drilling tunnels about the knee to pass ligament grafts would damage the growth plates. If surgical repair is done in this age group, the techniques used must avoid the growth plates or accept shortening of the limb if the plates are damaged.

J. M. Siliski, M.D.: Department of Orthopaedic Surgery, Massachusetts General Hospital, Harvard Medical School, Boston, Massachusetts 02114.

PREOPERATIVE PLANNING

Evaluation and Preparation

Dislocation of the tibiofemoral joint is an uncommon but severe injury. Although this injury may occur during sports, more commonly it is the result of higher-energy trauma such as a fall from a height or a motor vehicle accident. Consequently, other injuries that may have occurred to the head, chest, and abdomen may take precedence immediately. It is possible therefore for the severity of a knee injury to be overlooked in multiple trauma patients. Because a dislocated knee at the scene of the accident may have been reduced during patient transfer, it is important for those evaluating the patient to identify a grossly unstable knee and to complete the appropriate neurovascular and orthopaedic evaluation of the injured extremity. The knee that has been dislocated, but is first seen in a reduced position, is still at risk for vascular insufficiency of the leg, as much as the knee that is grossly dislocated.

The knee that is grossly dislocated should be reduced and stabilized. The peripheral pulses should be checked. If there are findings on clinical examination of vascular insufficiency, the patient should be taken to the operating room as soon as possible for popliteal artery exploration and saphenous vein bypass grafting by a vascular surgeon. After revascularization, a four-compartment fasciotomy is necessary because of postischemic swelling of the calf. After revascularization, the knee may be stabilized with splints or an external fixator across the knee. When the vascular surgeon is comfortable that the bypass graft will remain open, the soft-tissue injuries of the knee can be repaired and reconstructed at a second procedure, usually at 7 to 10 days after injury.

If the patient has intact pulses in the foot below a knee dislocation, it is still possible that there may be vascular injury such as an intimal tear that may subsequently thrombose. In this scenario, it is safest to obtain an arteriogram. If the arteriogram is negative, the patient may be scheduled for soft-tissue repair at an early and convenient time. If the arteriogram shows an intimal tear, but there is flow through the artery, the patient should be anticoagulated and followed up by a vascular surgeon. If after a week, the popliteal artery has remained open, anticoagulation can be discontinued for surgical repair and reconstruction of the knee.

In addition to popliteal artery injury, peroneal nerve palsies are common associated injuries. In general, these have a poor prognosis and do not respond to surgical decompression. Treatment of the soft-tissue repair around the knee proceeds in a same manner whether or not there is a peroneal nerve injury. The foot should be splinted to prevent an equinus deformity.

Knee dislocations caused by high-energy trauma are frequently open. Open dislocations require emergency irrigation and debridement of the soft-tissue wound and knee joint. Soft-tissue repairs done at the initial debridement should be limited to simple ones done through the irrigation wound and with limited suture material. Extensive dissection and insertion of soft-tissue grafts and hardware should be avoided. It is safer to delay definitive repair for 7 to 21 days to allow soft-tissue healing. If surgery is delayed, the knee can be stabilized in splints or with an external fixator.

The goal in the management of patients with associated problems, such as multiple trauma, popliteal artery injury, and open wounds, is to have the patient and the injured extremity sufficiently improved to permit repair and reconstruction of the knee soft-tissue injuries by 7 to 10 days. If none of these complicating factors exists, then the knee repair and reconstruction can be performed within a day or two of injury.

Knee Examination and Imaging Studies

The most important aspect of preoperative planning is the clinical examination of the knee. An initial examination can be done without anesthesia at the bedside. Ecchymosis,

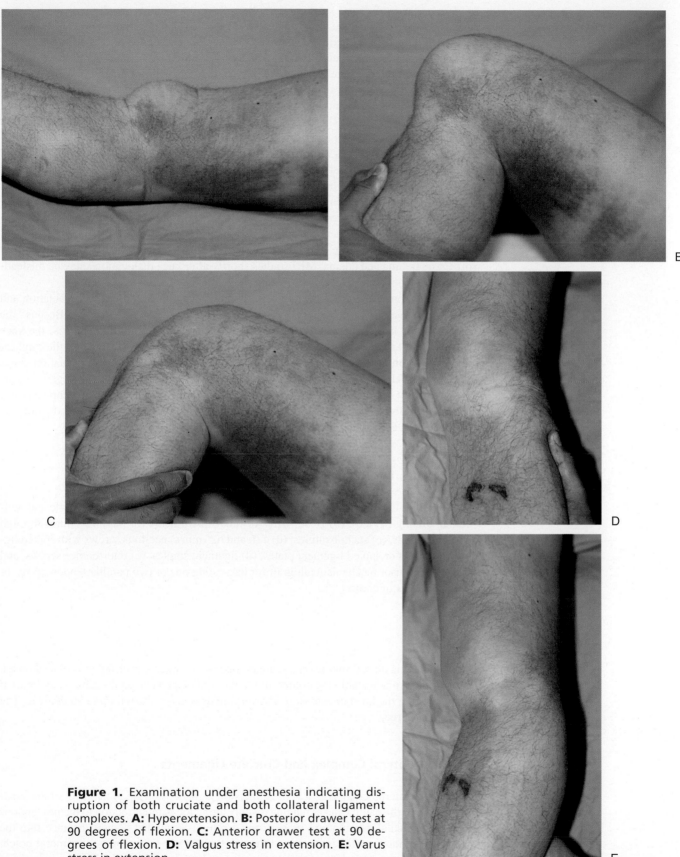

Figure 1. Examination under anesthesia indicating disruption of both cruciate and both collateral ligament complexes. **A:** Hyperextension. **B:** Posterior drawer test at 90 degrees of flexion. **C:** Anterior drawer test at 90 degrees of flexion. **D:** Valgus stress in extension. **E:** Varus stress in extension.

tenderness, and soft-tissue swelling over the collateral ligaments usually indicate injury at those sites. The heel can be slowly elevated off the bed, looking for hyperextension of the knee. At 20 degrees of flexion, opening of the medial and lateral sides of the joint on valgus and varus stress indicate collateral complex disruption. Also at 20 degrees, anteroposterior (AP) instability of the knee indicates cruciate ligament injury. A second examination is performed under anesthesia just before surgical repair. At that time, the knee can be more vigorously examined, including a check of the cruciate ligaments at 90 degrees of flexion (Fig. 1A–E). In most cases, a knee that has been dislocated will have sustained disruption of both the anterior (ACL) and posterior cruciate ligaments (PCL), and the medial or lateral ligament complexes or both.

AP, lateral, tunnel, and sunrise views of the knee should be obtained. Plain radiographs may show no evidence of bony injury, and with the knee reduced and splinted may show only subtle signs of tibiofemoral malalignment or compartment widening. Plain films may also show avulsion fractures from the femur, tibia, and fibula, indicating avulsion at ligament insertion sites. Magnetic resonance imaging (MRI) studies are often helpful in evaluating the menisci, capsule, and ligaments. However, because of the extensive amount of soft-tissue trauma and edema, MRI studies shortly after knee dislocations may be misleading about the degree of soft-tissue disruption.

Although some surgeons have advocated wet or dry arthroscopy in the evaluation and surgical treatment of knee dislocation, there are contraindications to its use. Because the capsule of the knee is usually widely disrupted, arthroscopic fluid pumped into the knee will extravasate into soft tissues, potentially producing massive swelling in the thigh or calf. Evaluation of the knee is best assessed through a combination of examination under anesthesia, MRI, and surgical exploration. Arthroscopy typically adds little. Regarding surgical treatment, many of the soft-tissue repairs cannot be performed arthroscopically but can be completed well only with formal incisions. For these reasons, I do not use arthroscopy in the evaluation or treatment of knee dislocation.

Instruments, Implants, and Grafts

Preparation for surgery should include: (a) ligament guide set, including single and multilumen aiming devices, (b) Beath wires or other instruments for passing sutures through small drill holes, (c) anchor sutures, (d) 4.0- and 6.5-mm cancellous screws with spiked ligament washers or spiked ligament plates, (d) ligament staples, (e) interference screws, and (f) whole extensor mechanism allograft for harvesting one or two patellar tendon grafts, or other allografts of choice.

SURGERY

The patient is placed supine on a standard operating table. A tourniquet is placed on the upper thigh. An adjustable leg holder, or blanket rolls taped across the table, may be used for positioning the knee in extension and varying degrees of flexion up to 90 degrees. The leg is draped free.

Medial Collateral Complex and Cruciate Ligaments

From the anteromedial side, a vertical incision is made, starting at the level of the superior margin of the patella and extending distally along the patellar tendon to the pes tendons (Fig. 2). A medial capsulotomy is performed. This is extended a short distance into the quadriceps tendon, sufficient to retract the patella laterally to examine the femoral notch. The fat pad is elevated off the medial meniscus and retracted laterally. The medial meniscus is carefully preserved. The patellar tendon is checked. In some cases, partial or even complete patellar-tendon disruption occurs, and these should be appropriately repaired.

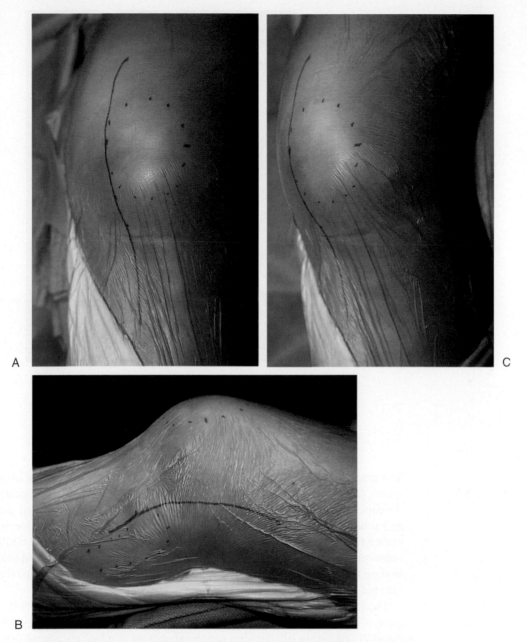

Figure 2. Incisions marked for surgical approaches. **A:** Anterior view showing antero-medial skin incision, just medial to the patella and patellar tendon. **B:** Lateral view showing lateral skin incision, just anterior to the fibula. **C:** Anterolateral view showing wide skin bridge between the two incisions.

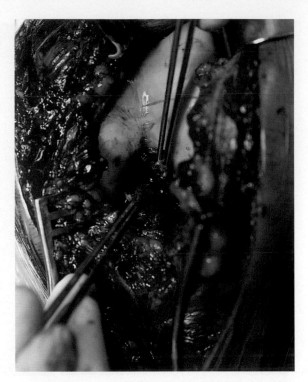

Figure 3. Anterior cruciate ligament torn midsubstance and unrepairable.

The cruciate ligaments are inspected. In most cases, the ACL is torn midsubstance and requires reconstruction as opposed to repair (Fig. 3). With the ligament guides used for endoscopic ACL reconstruction, appropriately sized tunnels can be drilled through the tibia and femur for reconstruction (Fig. 4A–C). An allograft patellar tendon is a reasonable choice for the ACL reconstruction, as it can be prepared on a side table while surgery continues on the knee. Use of an allograft also decreases the additional morbidity of graft harvesting from the injured knee. The ACL graft can then be placed and fixed on the femoral side but left unfixed on the tibial side.

The PCL may be avulsed from the femoral or tibial side of the knee (Fig. 5). If the ligament is avulsed and viable, it may be reattached by using the technique of Marshall (Figs. 6 and 7). Two whip stitches with nonabsorbable no. 5 suture are placed in the avulsed end of the PCL, leaving four free ends at the perimeter of the ligament. At the PCL insertion site on the inner side of the medial femoral condyle, a burr is used to abrade the cortical bone down to a bleeding surface. A ligament guide with multiple holes is used to drill tracks through the medial femoral condyle, exiting at the perimeter of the abraded PCL attachment site in the femoral notch. The sutures in the ends of the PCL are passed through the drill tracks to the medial side of the medial femoral condyle. The four sutures can then be pulled snug to inspect the approximation of the PCL to its insertion site. The sutures are left untied until the end of the surgery.

If the PCL is avulsed from the tibial side, which occurs less commonly, it can be reattached by using a similar technique. The tibia is subluxed forward sufficiently to visualize the posterior insertion site of the PCL. Passing wires are drilled by using a guide from anterior to posterior, out the back of the tibia at the PCL insertion site. The same suturing technique is used in the end of the PCL. Care is taken to prevent any injury to the neurovascular structures during drilling and suture passage.

If the PCL is not reattachable, it may be reconstructed by using allograft or autograft. In the femur, the tunnel is drilled just anterior to the origin of the medial collateral ligament

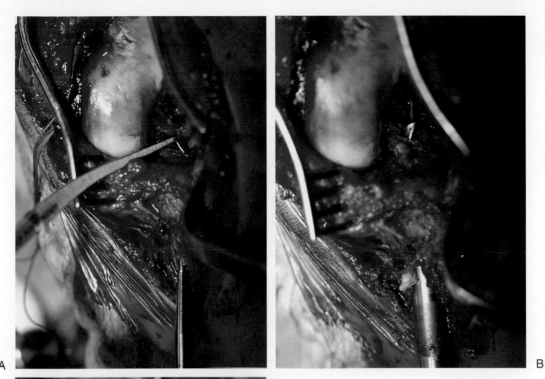

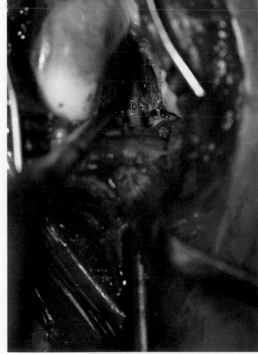

Figure 4. Open anterior cruciate ligament (ACL) reconstruction. **A:** A ligament guide is used to drill a wire through the proximal tibia at a 50-degree angle, entering the knee through the stump of the ACL. **B:** An 11-mm cannulated reamer is used to drill a tunnel in the tibia over the guide wire. **C:** With the knee flexed 90 degrees, a femoral guide is passed through the tibial tunnel, across the notch, and into a 1 o'clock position in the posterior recess of the femoral notch. A wire is drilled 40 mm into the femur through the guide. A cannulated reamer is advanced over the guide wire, through the notch, and 30 mm into the femur, to prepare the femoral tunnel. An allograft extensor mechanism is used to harvest an 11-mm patellar tendon graft with bone pegs of 10×25 mm and 11×40 mm. Leading with the smaller bone peg, the graft is advanced through the tibial tunnel, across the notch, and into the femoral tunnel. On the femoral side, the bone peg is secured with a 7×25-mm interference screw. The tibial bone peg is left unsecured while the lateral structures are repaired.

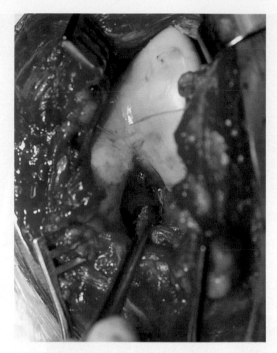

Figure 5. Posterior cruciate ligament (PCL) avulsion from the femur, with a few remaining intact fibers. In this case, the PCL is judged to be repairable.

(MCL) and into the notch at the normal PCL insertion site. In the tibia, the PCL tunnel is drilled distal to the ACL tunnel and through the posterior cortex at the normal PCL insertion site. The ligament reconstruction may be passed and fixed on one side of the knee, but the second fixation is not done until the end of the surgery.

The medial compartment structures are inspected. If the medial meniscus is torn and not repairable, an open partial medial meniscectomy is performed. If the medial meniscus has a repairable bucket-handle tear or peripheral detachment from the capsule, it is sutured (Fig. 8A). If the medial capsule, including the posteromedial corner, is avulsed from the

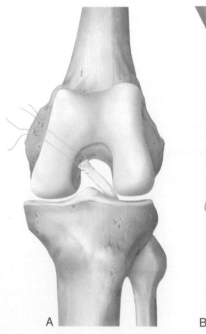
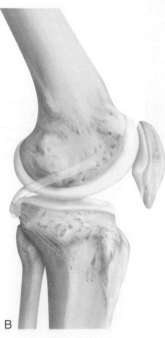

A   B

Figure 6. Posterior cruciate ligament (PCL) reattachment. **A:** To the femur. **B:** To the tibia.

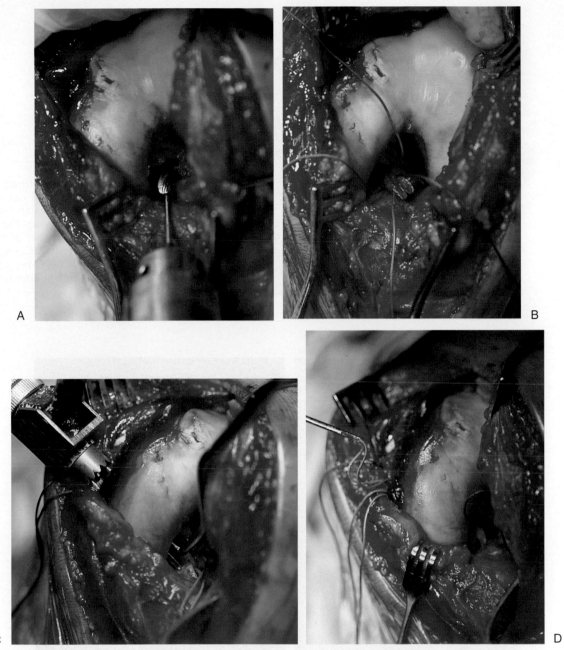

Figure 7. Reattachment of posterior cruciate ligament (PCL) to the femur. **A:** The insertion site is abraded to cancellous bone with a burr. **B:** Two no. 5 nonabsorbable sutures are placed as whip stitches in the PCL, with four free ends left protruding. **C:** A ligament guide is used to drill four holes through the medial femoral condyle, ending at the perimeter of the PCL insertion site. **D:** By using a suture passer, each suture is passed through its matching drill hole to the medial surface of the femoral condyle. The sutures are secured with a clamp but left untied while the other ligaments are repaired.

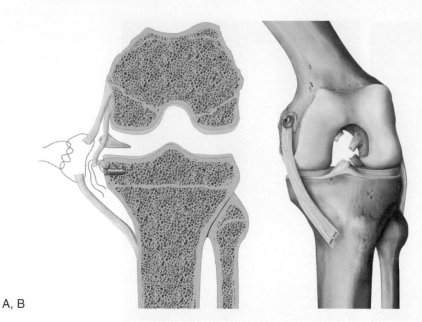

A, B

Figure 8. Types of repairs performed in the medial compartment. **A:** Peripheral detachment of the medial meniscus is sutured to the capsule. Capsular avulsion is reattached to the tibia with anchor sutures. Midsubstance tear of the superficial medial collateral ligament (MCL) is sutured. **B:** Avulsions of the superficial MCL, reattached with either cancellous screw and ligament washer or with ligament staples.

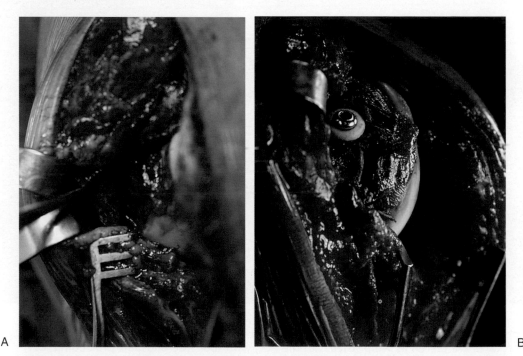

A   B

Figure 9. Medial collateral ligament (MCL) avulsion from the medial epicondyle. **A:** Free end of MCL and its avulsion site. **B:** MCL reattached with large cancellous screw and spiked ligament washer.

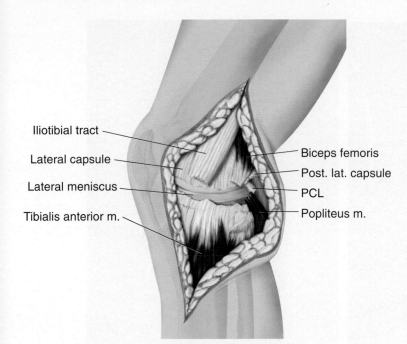

Iliotibial tract

Lateral capsule

Lateral meniscus

Tibialis anterior m.

Biceps femoris

Post. lat. capsule

PCL

Popliteus m.

Figure 10. Structures visualized at the posterolateral side of the knee through a vertical skin incision.

tibia, it may be reattached by using anchor sutures placed along the rim of the tibial plateau. If torn midsubstance, the capsule is sutured. The superficial MCL is inspected (Fig. 8B). If avulsed from the medial epicondyle of the femur, it can usually be reattached with a single large-fragment cancellous screw and a spiked ligament washer (Fig. 9). If torn midsubstance, it may be directly sutured. If avulsed from the tibia, it may be reattached with a number of techniques, including spiked ligament washers or spiked staples.

Posterolateral Repair

If the posterolateral side of the knee is disrupted, a second surgical exposure is performed (Figs. 2B and C). The skin incision is placed just anterior to the proximal fibula and extended distally below the joint by approximately 4 cm and proximally above the joint by approximately 6 cm. A wide skin flap is thereby created between the two incisions. Usually, no further dissection is needed other than a skin incision, because one encounters disrupted deep structures (Fig. 10).

The next step on the lateral side is to identify and tag all of the disrupted structures (Fig. 11A). The peroneal nerve is identified in the posterior portion of the exposure. The posterolateral capsule (arcuate ligament) is identified and tagged (Fig. 11B). It is usually either torn midsubstance or avulsed from the tibia. The gastrocnemius muscle may be completely or partially torn. The popliteus muscle is commonly completely disrupted and not repairable. The lateral capsule is typically either torn midsubstance or avulsed from the tibia (Fig. 11C). If it is torn midsubstance, it may be associated with a capsular detachment of the meniscus. The lateral collateral ligament may be avulsed from the femur or fibula or torn midsubstance (Fig. 11D). The biceps femoris tendon is commonly avulsed from the fibula. Anteriorly, the iliotibial band is commonly avulsed from Gerdy's tubercle.

After identifying and tagging all repairable structures, repair proceeds from deep and posterior to superficial and anterior. The posterior capsule, if torn midsubstance, is sutured, in combination with reattachment of the posterior portion of the lateral meniscus. If it is avulsed from the tibia, anchor sutures are placed along the posterior rim of the lateral tibial plateau and used to reattach the posterolateral capsule (Fig. 12A and B). Repair of the

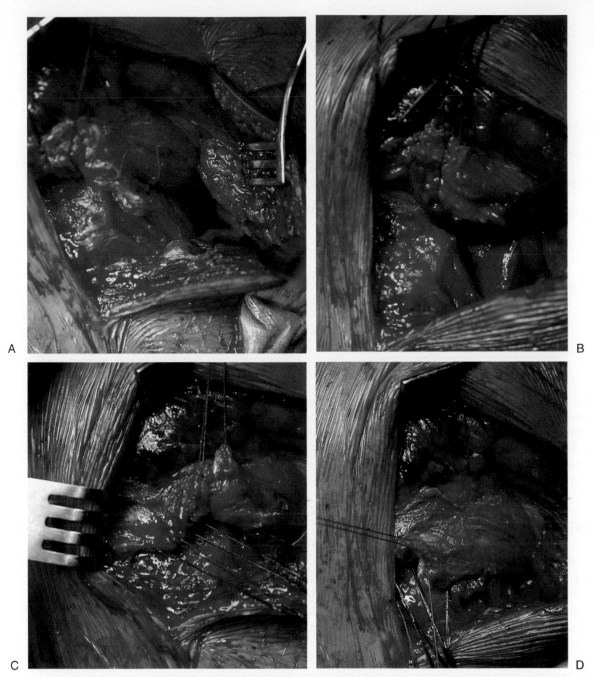

Figure 11. Lateral exposure of the knee. **A:** In this case, the skin incision is the only dissection necessary, as all the deeper structures on the lateral and posterolateral sides of the knee have been disrupted. The next step is to identify each disrupted structure. Peroneal nerve is noted in the posteroinferior recesses. **B:** Avulsion of arcuate ligament from posterolateral tibia. **C:** Avulsion of lateral capsule from the lateral tibia. Underside of lateral meniscus is visible. **D:** Biceps femoris tendon and lateral collateral ligament avulsed from the fibular head.

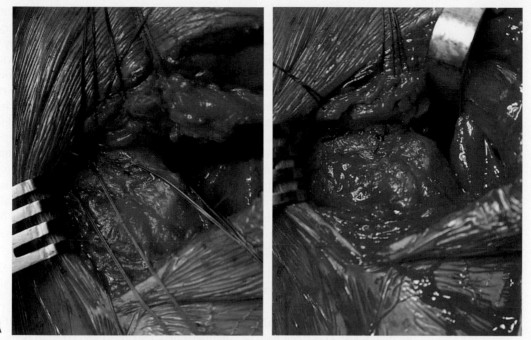

Figure 12. Reattachment of arcuate ligament and lateral capsule. **A:** Anchor sutures are placed along the circumference of the tibia from the posterior cruciate ligament (PCL) to the patellar tendon by using no. 2 nonabsorbable suture. **B:** Sutures are passed through the arcuate ligament and lateral capsule and are tied down, reattaching this deep layer to the tibia.

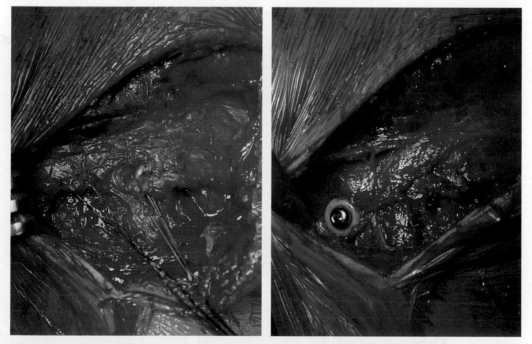

Figure 13. Reattachment of superficial lateral structures. **A:** Whip stitches are placed into the ends of the biceps femoris and lateral collateral ligament. Tagging sutures are placed in the iliotibial band. **B:** The biceps femoris and lateral collateral ligament are reattached to the fibular head by passing their sutures through drill holes. The iliotibial band is reattached to Gerdy's tubercle by using a large cancellous screw and spiked ligament washer.

meniscus and lateral capsule proceeds from posterior to anterior around the circumference of the lateral plateau, proceeding all the way to the patellar tendon if necessary.

The lateral collateral ligament, if torn midsubstance, can be repaired by using whip stitches in both ends of the ligament, pulling the ends together when tying down the sutures. If avulsed from the femur, various reattachment techniques can be used. Commonly, the avulsion includes a small piece of bone and adjacent soft tissue, sufficient to reattach with a cancellous screw and spiked ligament washer. If avulsed from the fibula, but without a bone fragment, the ligament can be reattached by using a whip stitch passed through drill holes in the proximal fibula with no. 5 suture (Fig. 13A).

At times, a sizeable fragment of proximal fibula is avulsed and can be reattached by using a small-fragment cancellous screw, or a tension band with no. 5 suture. The biceps femoris tendon can be reattached to the proximal fibula by using whip stitches passed through drill holes in the fibula or into soft tissue that remains on the proximal fibula (Fig. 13B). The iliotibial band is frequently avulsed from Gerdy's tubercle and can be reattached with a number of techniques. The simplest and quickest is to use a cancellous screw with a spiked ligament washer (Fig. 13B).

Fixation of Cruciate Ligaments

With the medial or lateral structures or both repaired, attention is returned to the cruciate ligaments. These can now be simultaneously tensioned and fixed to bone. If the insertion sites for the cruciate ligaments have been appropriately identified during placement of sutures and grafts, it should make little difference what position of flexion the knee is in while the grafts are tensioned and secured to bone. Before we actually fix the ligaments in place, they can both be tensioned and the knee placed through a range of motion from full extension to 90 degrees or more of flexion. If there is any concern that the ligaments may be too tight in any position, it is probably better to leave them slightly lax, rather than tension them so tightly that knee extension or flexion will be limited. I usually place the knee at 45 degrees of flexion while simultaneously tensioning the ligaments and fixing them in place.

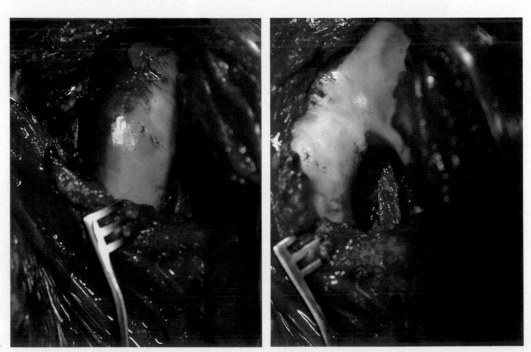

A   B

Figure 14. Cruciate-ligament fixation performed with the knee in partial flexion, and both cruciate ligaments simultaneously tensioned. **A:** Posterior cruciate ligament (PCL) secured to femur by tying down sutures over bone bridges on the medial femoral condyle. **B:** Anterior cruciate ligament (ACL) secured to tibia with an interference screw inserted into the tibial tunnel.

Most commonly the final fixation includes tying down the PCL reattachment sutures over a bone bridge on the medial femoral condyle and inserting an interference screw in the tibial tunnel of the ACL graft (Fig. 14A and B).

Closure

The tourniquet is released before closure. Any bleeding points are identified and cauterized. The anteromedial incision is closed by reapproximating the fat pad and closing the capsular incision. The subcutaneous layer and skin are closed. If a lateral incision also has been used, it is usually only a subcutaneous and skin closure.

POSTOPERATIVE MANAGEMENT

At the conclusion of the surgical procedure, a hinged knee brace is applied. The knee is treated with a continuous-positive-motion (CPM) machine, limiting extension to 10 degrees if the knee hyperextended preoperatively. The amount of flexion is not limited, and the goal is to recover 90 degrees of flexion as early as the patient will tolerate. Varus and valgus stress are avoided to prevent tension on the collateral ligament repairs. Although gentle active assistive range of motion may be used by a physical therapist during the first month, a muscle-strengthening program is not possible until the repair and reconstructions have healed in position. There is no advantage to weight bearing early, and the patient is kept non–weight bearing during the first month and then gradually progressed in a knee brace from partial to full weight bearing during the second month. Between 8 and 12 weeks, patients may become full weight bearing.

There are two contradictory goals in the first postoperative month: protecting the grafts and reconstructions during early healing and recovery of knee motion. In general, stiffness is a greater threat, so I favor early knee motion between 10 and 90 degrees within 1 month of surgery and accept some mild laxity in the knee. After a repaired knee dislocation, most patients will not recover a full range of motion. However, a reasonable goal is full extension and 120 degrees of flexion.

Although some patients achieve an excellent result and return to recreational sports and physically demanding work, most have some permanent symptoms and functional limitations. It is therefore very important for both the patient and surgeon to have realistic expectations for the final outcome of the injury and surgical treatment. Those patients who were most active before their injury are the most likely to require adjustments in their work and sports after their injury.

I often explain my expectations to patients preoperatively in this manner: "Even with surgery, we are unlikely to achieve an A knee. The realistic goal is a B knee, but we may have to settle for a C knee if we have any complications. For me, a B knee has 0 to 120 degrees of motion, no functional instability for light activities, and minimal or no pain." Patients should also be informed that maximal improvement is usually not reached until 1 to 2 years after injury.

COMPLICATIONS

Patients who have a popliteal artery disruption or thrombosis as part of their knee injury are at risk for postischemic contractures in the ankle and foot and even, in some cases, amputation. The quicker revascularization and fasciotomies can be performed, the better the prognosis for the limb.

Infection, particularly after an open knee dislocation, can severely affect the outcome of the joint. Although infection can usually be eradicated by surgical debridement and antibiotics, the joint is at high risk for instability, stiffness, articular cartilage destruction, and early posttraumatic arthritis.

Functional instability is not a frequent problem after a well-performed surgical repair of the soft tissues. However, if at final outcome, some significant functional instability remains, there is the option of secondary reconstruction or brace treatment.

Arthrofibrosis is the most common problem after knee dislocation, treated by surgical repair. If surgical repair is performed, it must be done securely enough that the knee can be moved immediately. Immobilization of a surgically repaired knee dislocation is likely to produce a very stable but very stiff joint. A knee dislocation must be watched closely after surgical repair for progression of motion. If at 2 weeks, there is less than 60 degrees of flexion, I recommend a gentle manipulation under anesthesia before adhesions have become mature. By 6 weeks, if a manipulation is performed for failure to progress beyond 90 degrees of flexion, a more forceful manipulation can be performed with the assumption that the surgical repairs and reconstructions are healing and have some resistance to tension. By 3 months, intraarticular adhesions and extraarticular scarring make recovery of further knee flexion much more difficult. In the worst of cases, heterotopic bone can form, creating structural blocks to flexion. Late efforts to improve motion may start with an "arthroscopic" lysis of adhesions and manipulation but may require open lysis of adhesions and removal of heterotopic bone to recover even modest improvement in flexion.

Although in the past, closed reduction and immobilization for 6 to 8 weeks was argued by some authors to be a preferable form of treatment, with the increased experience in techniques for repair and reconstruction of knee ligament and associated soft tissues, immediate surgical repair of the knee dislocations provides better results than nonoperative treatment.

RECOMMENDED READING

1. Montgomery, T.J., Savoie, F.H., White, J.L., Roberts, T.S., Hughes, J.L.: Orthopaedic management of knee dislocations: comparison of surgical reconstruction and immobilization. *Am. J. Knee Surg.,* 8:97–103, 1995.
2. O'Donnell, T.F., Brewster, D.D., Darling, B.C., Veen, H., Waltman, A.C.: Arterial injuries associated with fractures and/or dislocations of the knee. *J. Trauma,* 17:775–784, 1977.
3. Plancher, K.D., and Siliski, J.M.: Dislocation of the knee. In Siliski, J.M. (ed.): *Traumatic Disorders of the Knee.* Springer-Verlag, New York, 1994, pp. 315–331.
4. Reddy, P.K., Posteraro, R.H., Schenk, R.C.: The role of MRI in evaluation of the cruciate ligaments in knee dislocations. *Orthopedics,* 19:166–170, 1996.
5. Roman, P.D., Hopson, C.N., Zenni, E.J.: Traumatic dislocation of the knee: a report of 30 cases and literature review. *Orthop. Rev.,* 16:33–40, 1987.
6. Seebacher, J.R., Inglis, A.E., Marshall, J.L., Warren, R.F.: The structure of the posterolateral aspect of the knee. *J. Bone Joint Surg. [Am],* 64:536–541, 1982.
7. Shapiro, M.J., and Freedman, E.L.: Allograft reconstruction of the anterior and posterior cruciate ligaments after traumatic knee dislocation. *Am. J. Sports Med.,* 23:580–587, 1995.
8. Shelbourne, K.D., Porter, D.A., Clingman, J.A., McCarroll, J.R., Rettig, A.C.: Low velocity knee dislocations. *Orthop. Rev.,* 20:995–1004, 1991.
9. Sisto, J.D., and Warren, RF.: Complete knee dislocation: a follow-up study of operative treatment. *Clin. Orthop.,* 198:94–101, 1985.
10. Taylor, A.R., Arden, G.P., Rainey, H.A.: Traumatic dislocation of the knee: a report of forty-three cases with special reference to conservative treatment. *J. Bone Joint Surg. [Br],* 54:96–102, 1972.
11. Warren, L.F., and Marshall, J.L.: The supporting structures and layers of the medial side of the knee: an anatomical analysis. *J. Bone Joint Surg. [Am],* 61:56–62, 1979.
12. Wright, D.G., Covey, D.C., Born, C.T., Sadasivan, K.K.: Open dislocation of the knee. *J. Orthop. Trauma,* 9:135–140, 1995.

Master Techniques in Orthopaedic Surgery,
FRACTURES, edited by D. A. Wiss,
Lippincott–Raven Publishers, Philadelphia © 1998.

23

Tibial-Plateau Fractures: Open Reduction Internal Fixation

J. Tracy Watson and Donald A. Wiss

INDICATIONS/CONTRAINDICATIONS

Tibial-plateau fractures are often a challenge to treat effectively. The goals of treatment are to obtain a congruous knee joint that is functionally stable, permitting balanced load transmission across the knee joint.

When considering operative management, the surgeon should individualize treatment with respect to a variety of factors such as patient age, preexisting levels of activity, medical conditions, and the patient's expectations. Injury considerations should include the extent of fracture comminution and joint impaction, associated injuries, and most important, the condition of the soft tissues.

Numerous studies have shown that instability and malalignment of the knee after fracture are the two most important criteria that affect outcome and often dictate surgical management (6,9,10). Instability is usually caused by joint deformity, and less commonly, ligamentous disruption. It is well established that depressed articular fragments cannot reduce by manipulation and traction alone. If fracture displacement is great enough to produce joint instability, then operative management should be selected (1,10).

Absolute indications for surgery include (a) open plateau fractures, (b) fractures with an associated compartment syndrome, and (c) fractures with a vascular injury. Relative indications for surgery include (a) most displaced bicondylar fractures, (b) displaced medial condylar fractures, and (c) lateral plateau fractures that result in joint instability (1,3,10–12).

The most common contraindication to immediate open reduction and internal fixation is a compromised soft-tissue envelope, which can occur in either open or closed fractures. Tibial-plateau fractures that do not result in joint instability or deformity can be treated nonoperatively.

J. T. Watson, M.D.: Division of Orthopaedic Trauma, Wayne State University, Detroit, Michigan 48201.

D. A. Wiss, M.D.: Southern California Orthopedic Institute, Van Nuys, California 91405-3730.

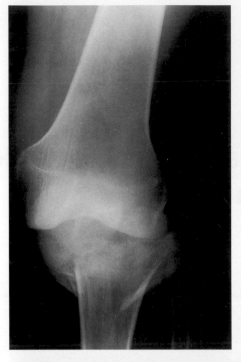
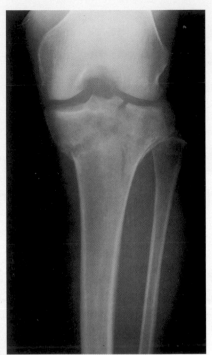

A

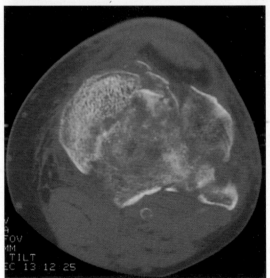

B

Figure 1. A: Anteroposterior (AP) radiograph showing a fracture of the proximal tibia. Because of shortening and displacement, the fracture morphology is not clearly seen. A traction radiograph shows how ligamentotaxis restores length of all fragments. **B:** Traction computed tomography (CT) scan shows greater fracture comminution than the plain films suggest.

PREOPERATIVE PLANNING

History and Physical Examination

Historic information regarding the mechanism of injury is important to elicit, as it is important in determining whether the injury occurred as the result of a high- or low-energy force. This is especially important when considering internal-fixation techniques, as high-energy fractures tend to have more associated soft-tissue injuries. Factors that may compromise early open reduction include fracture blisters, direct skin contusion or necrosis, and compartment syndromes with or without vascular compromise.

The physical examination should focus on the integrity of the soft-tissue envelope in the presence of high-energy injuries with blisters or superficial abrasions. These areas should be avoided if a surgical approach is undertaken. If incisions in compromised skin cannot be avoided, then surgery should be delayed or alternative methods of fracture stabilization should be selected. Additionally, the peripheral pulses and nerve function, as well as the status of the compartments, should be evaluated. Compartment-pressure monitoring should be done in selected patients with high-energy fractures, especially displaced medial-plateau, bicondylar, and plateau fractures with shaft/metaphyseal dissociation. Angiograms should be obtained when the physical examination reveals diminished or absent pulses.

Imaging Studies

Radiographs should include anteroposterior (AP), lateral, and internal and external oblique views. The oblique views often detect subtle degrees of joint impaction or fracture lines not visible on the AP or lateral views. Contemporary surgical techniques using indirect methods of reduction and fixation require precise knowledge of the three-dimensional anatomy of the fracture. Computed tomography (CT) scanning has now replaced linear tomography as the imaging study of choice. CT scans with axial, coronal, and sagittal reconstructions are useful in delineating the extent and location of condylar fracture lines, as well as determining the location and depth of articular comminution and impaction (12).

Recently magnetic resonance imaging (MRI) has been used for preoperative evaluation of tibial-plateau fractures. MRI has been shown to be superior to CT scans in assessing associated soft-tissue injuries such as meniscal and ligamentous disruptions (2). However, MRI may not be widely available immediately in many institutions.

Traction radiographs are an additional (Fig. 1) method used to determine the efficacy of distraction techniques. Traction films may determine if an indirect reduction by using ligamentotaxis is effective and may add useful information in planning surgical incisions.

The development of a preoperative plan and surgical tactic is important to optimize results. The preoperative plan helps to ensure that the proper implants, reduction tools, bone graft or bone graft substitutes, and fluoroscopic equipment are available at the time of surgery. We have found it helpful to stratify tibial-plateau fractures according to the Schatzker classification, which divides these injuries into six distinct subtypes (1). It is important to remember that depressed articular fracture fragments will not reduce by manipulation, traction, or ligamentotaxis techniques alone. If articular defects are sufficient to produce joint instability, the joint surface must be surgically disimpacted, elevated, and supported with bone grafts and fixation hardware.

In many cases, the use of a bone graft, whether autogenous iliac-crest graft, hydroxyapatite substitute, or freeze-dried and processed bone-bank allograft, is required.

SURGERY

The patient is given a general or spinal anesthetic and placed supine on a radiolucent operating table. We prefer a table that has the ability to "break" so the knee can be flexed to 90 degrees (Fig. 2). Alternatively, a large sterile bolster or a beanbag can be used to elevate the operative extremity, allowing flexion to 90 degrees intraoperatively (Fig. 3). A C-arm image intensifier should be brought in from the contralateral side. Before prepping and draping, trial images should be obtained to verify that accurate AP and lateral fluoroscopic images are easily obtainable.

The entire extremity is then prepped and draped. If iliac-crest bone graft is to be used, then the ipsilateral crest is also included in the initial prep, and a sterile tourniquet used.

Because the majority of plateau fractures involve the lateral plateau, a lateral parapatellar incision is most commonly used (Fig. 3). This incision can be extended proximally and distally when more exposure is needed, such as in Schatzker Type V and VI injuries. A medial or posterior medial incision may also be necessary when treating specific fracture patterns. For isolated medial-plateau fractures (Schatzker IV), a medial parapatellar incision is recommended.

Relatively straight incisions are chosen because of their extensile nature, while minimizing damage to the skin flaps.

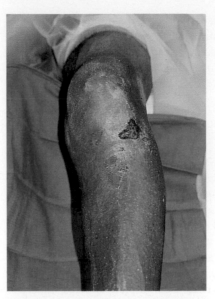

Figure 2. Position in the operating room showing the ability to drop the table and flex the knee to 90 degrees.

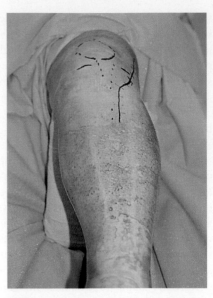

Figure 3. A sterile marker outlines the lateral utility incision. A sterile bump is placed beneath the knee to allow knee flexion intraoperatively.

Treatment of Specific Fracture Types

Type I. The split or wedge fracture (Fig. 4A) of the lateral plateau is often amenable to a percutaneous approach. If the lateral meniscus is intact, as determined by preoperative MRI, it may be possible to perform a closed reduction and percutaneous fixation with cannulated screws. Reduction is achieved by applying longitudinal traction with a varus force manually, or alternatively, by using a laterally based femoral distractor. If an acceptable reduction can be obtained, the fracture is compressed with a large pointed reduction forceps placed percutaneously. Fixation is accomplished with two or three large cannulated screws placed through small stab incisions (5,8). The inclination of these screws should be determined preoperatively based on the MRI scan. If the preoperative MRI scan shows a pe-

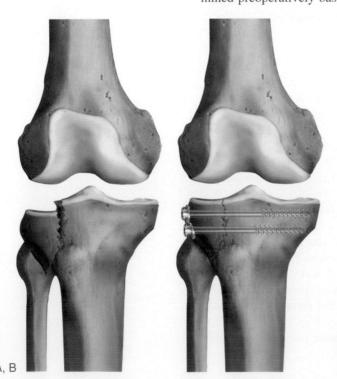

Figure 4. A: Schatzker Type I. Split lateral tibial-condyle fracture without articular impaction. **B:** Fixation with a lateral buttress plate. Alternatively, if no comminution is present, cancellous lag screws may be used.

A, B

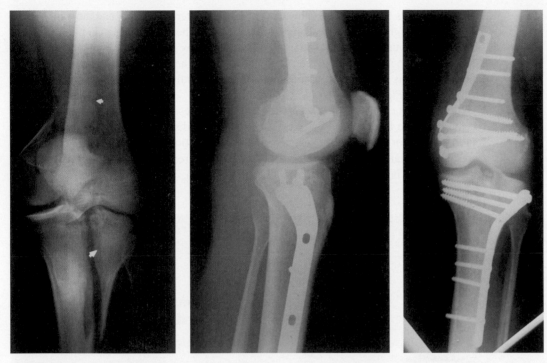

Figure 5. Pre- and postoperative views of a Schatzker I injury. The large lateral condylar fragment required a buttress plate to maintain the reduction.

ripheral meniscal tear or incarceration of the meniscus within the fracture, or if a closed reduction fails adequately to reduce the fracture, an open reduction is indicated. If the fracture fragment is unusually large or comminuted, a lateral buttress plate should be used instead of multiple lag screws (Figs. 4B and C and 5).

Type II. Type II injuries involve the combination of a lateral condyle fracture with depression of its articular surface (Fig. 6A). Preoperative imaging studies are crucial to determine the extent and location of the impacted articular surface.

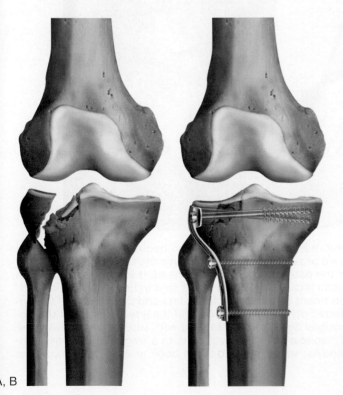

Figure 6. A: Schatzker Type II. Comminution and impaction of the lateral articular surface occurs with a large wedge fracture of the lateral plateau. **B:** The surgical tactic involves disimpaction and elevation of the articular surface. The articular surface must be supported with a combination of bone-graft material and fixation hardware. The most common construct includes cancellous lag screws as well as a lateral antiglide or buttress plate.

A, B

The fracture is best approached by using a standard lateral incision, and the joint surface visualized through a submeniscal approach (Fig. 7A). The lateral meniscal tibial ligament is incised transversely with elevation of the meniscus by using several small traction sutures or small angled retractors. The condylar fracture line is visualized at the level of the joint through this submeniscal approach and traced distally along the lateral aspect of the proximal tibia (Fig. 7A–C).

With the joint exposed, the knee is flexed to 90 degrees. This facilitates visualization of the joint surface by allowing the weight of the leg to distract the joint. Alternatively, a femoral distractor can be used to enhance joint visualization through sustained distraction. Impacted articular fragments can be reduced by two different techniques. In one, the condylar fracture line is wedged open like a book (Fig. 7D–H). The articular depression is eval-

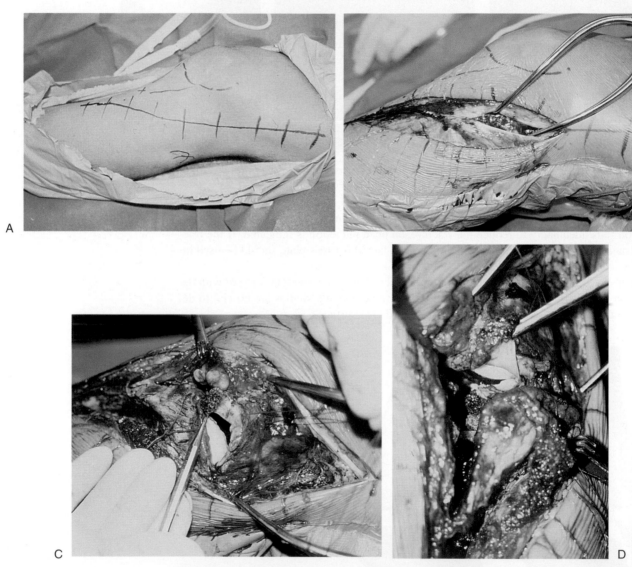

Figure 7. A: Standard lateral utility incision. The incision begins 1.5 to 2.0 cm lateral to the tibial shaft and is carried proximally over Gerdy's tubercle to a point midway between the lateral border of the patella and the fibular head. It extends proximally in line with the fibers of the fascia lata. **B:** The fascia lata is split in line with the skin incision, as is the anterior-compartment fascia. **C:** The fascia lata and the muscles of the anterior compartment are reflected off Gerdy's tubercle and the lateral border of the tibial shaft. The lateral meniscotibial ligaments are tagged with sutures. In this case, the anterior horn of the lateral meniscus has been avulsed with a fragment of bone (dental probe). **D:** The lateral condylar split is opened like a book and articular impaction visualized.

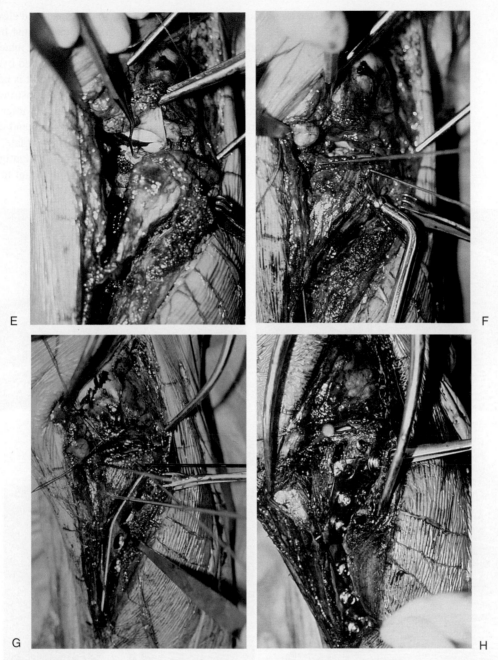

Figure 7. *(continued)* **E:** A dental probe or impactor is used to elevate the impacted articular surface, and bone graft is placed beneath the surface to support it. **F:** After bone grafting, the condyle is reduced by using large percutaneous reduction forceps. Kirschner wires or Steinmann pins are used as an additional tool to augment the re- duction. **G:** Guide wires for cannulated screws are inserted under fluoroscopic control, and the lateral tibial buttress plate is contoured and placed along the shaft. **H:** Final screws are placed into the lateral buttress plate after placement of the more proximally based cannulated condylar lag screws.

uated directly, and an impactor is inserted from below to disimpact and elevate the fracture fragments. To support the articular fragment, bone-graft material must be used. The osteoarticular fragments should be elevated "en masse" by placing graft material beneath the fragment. In this fashion, the pressure from the impactor is distributed over a larger area, preventing fragmentation or splitting of the articular surface. As graft is packed below the articular fragment, the joint surface is slowly and progressively reconstructed. Provisional Kirschner wire (K-wire) fixation can be useful in stabilizing the joint after elevation.

Once the joint has been reconstructed, the split condyle is reduced and held with a large reduction forceps. Fixation of the condyle is achieved with a buttress plate, or if the condylar fracture is minimally comminuted, lag screws with or without an antiglide plate. Care should be taken to repair the meniscotibial ligament. This is important to ensure that the

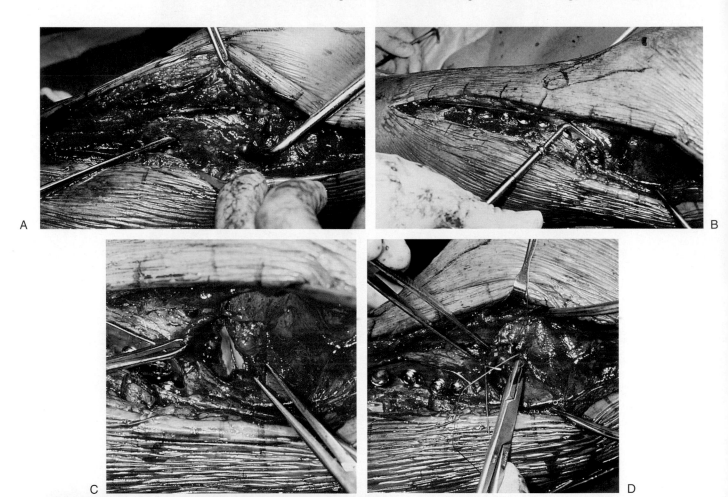

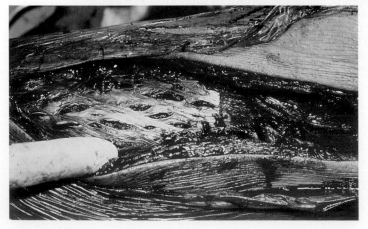

Figure 8. A: The large split condyle is reduced first and tentatively held by using large reduction forceps. A cortical window is fashioned, and a bone impactor is used to elevate the impacted articular surface. (Note impactor through distal cortical window.) **B:** After articular reduction, a lateral tibial buttress plate is positioned, and screws are placed. **C:** The articular reduction can be visualized through the submeniscal exposure. Atraumatic clamps hold either side of the incised meniscotibial ligament. **D:** Meniscotibial ligament is repaired by using nonabsorbable suture. **E:** The fascia lata is closed in line with the skin incision. The overlying anterior-compartment fascia is "pie crusted," by using small incisions in the fascia, minimizing the risk of a postoperative compartment syndrome.

function of the meniscus in transmitting and distributing forces across the lateral joint line is preserved.

Alternatively, if the condylar fracture line extends beyond the surgical exposure, then the condyle should be reduced first and held with a large pointed reduction forceps. Four or five 2-mm drill holes are placed in a 1-cm rectangle or square in the metaphyseal flare. These are connected by using a small osteotome to produce a cortical window. The window is impacted directly into the metaphysis by using a small curved impactor. Additional bone graft is placed through the cortical window into the metaphyseal defect, and the articular fragment is gradually elevated as more graft is applied. The adequacy of reduction is visualized directly through the submeniscal window, as well as indirectly by using the image intensifier (Fig. 8A–E). This technique minimizes stripping of the tibial condyle and proximal tibia.

Type III. This injury usually occurs in an older age group with osteoporotic bone after a low-energy valgus stress. The articular surface of the lateral plateau is impacted without an associated lateral condylar fracture. Imaging studies will specifically locate the area of impaction (Fig. 9A and B).

Treatment of this injury has evolved recently and is less invasive. Traditionally, a standard submeniscal exposure was necessary to visualize and elevate the impacted fragments. This fracture is now treated with small incisions using an image intensifier or arthroscope to visualize the lateral joint surface. A small lateral incision is made over the metaphyseal region of the lateral condyle. Exposure is limited only to gain access to develop a small metaphyseal cortical window. The window must be of sufficient size to allow grafting and elevation of the fragment from below (4,5). Once reduction of the joint is confirmed by arthroscopy or fluoroscopy, the graft is stabilized by percutaneous cannulated screws in a subchondral location (Fig. 10A and B).

Type IV. Fractures of the medial plateau are usually caused by high-energy trauma and are often associated with neurovascular injuries and significant fracture displacement. They often occur with other injuries, specifically knee dislocations with ligamentous disruption. A high index of suspicion is necessary to avoid overlooking a limb-threatening injury with this fracture pattern. In fractures with little or no comminution or displacement, closed reduction can be attempted with large reduction forceps. If successful, fixation by using mul-

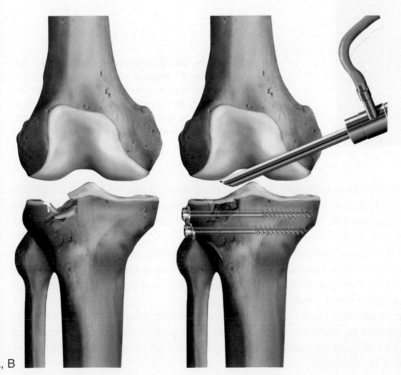

A, B

Figure 9. A: Schatzker Type III. This injury involves impaction and comminution of the lateral articular surface only. The condyle remains intact. **B:** Typical Schatzker III injury after joint elevation and fixation with cancellous screws.

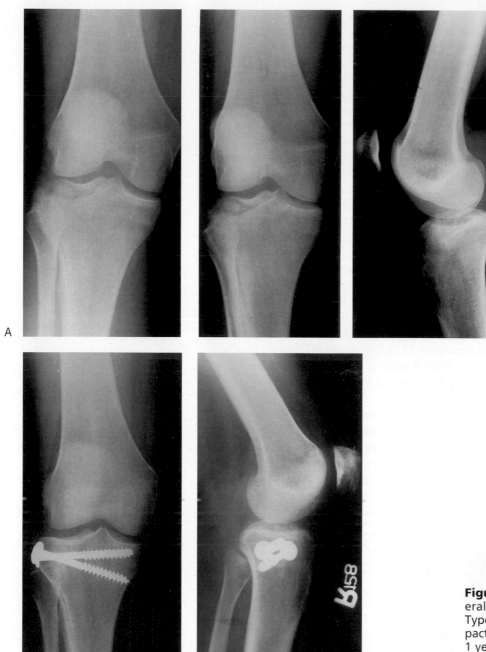

Figure 10. A: Anteroposterior (AP), lateral, and oblique views of a Schatzker Type III injury showing solitary joint impaction. **B:** Postoperative radiographs at 1 year show restoration of articular surface and fixation with solitary cancellous lag screws.

tiple cannulated screws is usually sufficient. However, most medial-plateau fractures are grossly unstable, with comminution in the region of the intracondylar eminence. Often the anterior cruciate ligament (ACL) is avulsed with a piece of bone in this region. These factors preclude percutaneous treatment (Fig. 11A and B).

Where indicated, a medial parapatellar approach is recommended, with direct reduction of the fracture fragments. If an intercondylar fracture is present, it should be repaired. If the ACL is avulsed, it also should be repaired with a small screw or wire suture placed through drill holes in the anterior tibial cortex.

Fixation of the medial tibial condyle is accomplished with a buttress plate by elevating the entire pes anserinus in continuity with the superficial portion of the medial collateral ligament. In this way, the plate contacts the entire medial metaphyseal surface without soft-tissue entrapment (Fig. 12A–C).

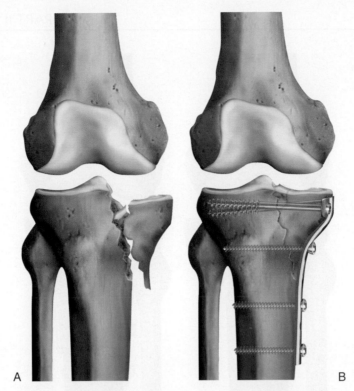

A

B

Figure 11. A: Schatzker Type IV. The medial-condyle fracture is often associated with intracondylar comminution and fragmentation. **B:** The severity of these injuries usually requires fixation with a medial buttress plate.

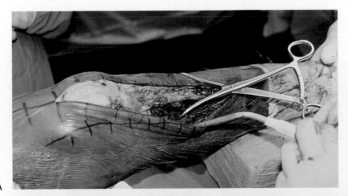

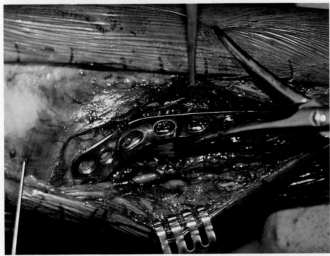

A

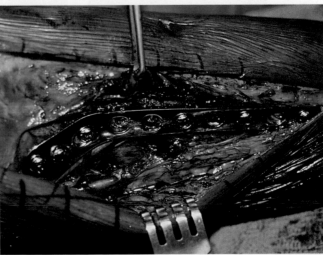

B

C

Figure 12. A: Medial parapatellar exposure of Schatzker IV plateau injury after reduction and temporary fixation with a large reduction clamp. **B:** Note subperiosteal elevation of the entire pes anserinus to allow placement of the plate along the medial surface of the tibia. **C:** Removal of the reduction forceps after placement of all fixation screws. Note the extensile nature of the medial approach.

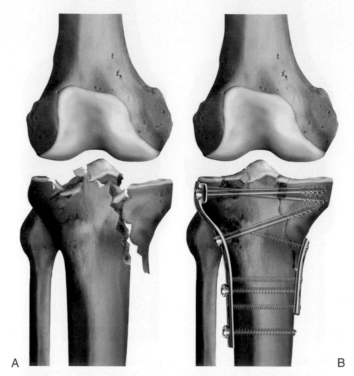

Figure 13. A: Schatzker Type V tibial fracture. This fracture usually involves both condyles with extensive lateral and medial joint comminution and impaction. **B:** Fixation with a lateral buttress plate and a medial buttress antiglide plate.

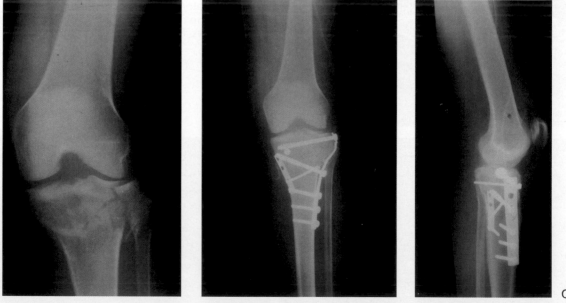

Figure 14. A–C: Bicondylar fracture treated primarily through a lateral exposure. A cannulated screw was used to lag the two condyles together. A laterally based buttress plate was then applied to attach the condyles to the shaft component. A second antiglide plate was positioned through a limited posterior medial approach. This smaller plate was used to buttress the medial plateau.

Types V and VI. These complex plateau injuries are usually the result of high-energy forces and are often associated with compromise of the surrounding soft tissues. In these cases, extensile exposure of the upper tibia with subperiosteal placement of large implants should be avoided. This approach has been associated with an increased risk of wound dehiscence and infection (Fig. 13A and B).

Fractures involving both condyles are frequently comminuted, and there may be dissociation of the shaft from the metaphysis. Many of these fractures are better treated with some type of external fixation. However, if plate fixation is chosen, an indirect reduction technique with one or two femoral distractors is recommended. Distraction often improves alignment of the condyles by ligamentotaxis. Large percutaneously applied reduction forceps may reduce or improve the position of the intercondylar fractures. Definitive fixation of the fracture is approached through a lateral parapatellar approach (3,7). Based on preoperative imaging studies, articular impaction is elevated by using cortical windows placed either medially or laterally.

Cannulated or conventional screws are used first to secure the condylar reduction, after which the condyles must be attached to the tibial shaft (Fig. 14). A buttress plate or stronger tibial condyle plate is placed extraperiosteally along the lateral aspect of the shaft if the soft tissue will allow this dissection. The stronger tibial condylar plates are used for Type VI fractures to "bridge" the zone of comminution that is often found at the metaphyseal/diaphyseal junction. It is important to restore the correct mechanical axis in these injuries (Fig. 15A and B).

If the condylar fracture fragments are not comminuted and the fracture is well reduced, the medial condyle can often be controlled with a laterally based plate and screws. However, in most cases, the medial condyle will require support to prevent late varus deformity. This is accomplished by placement of an extraperiosteal one-third tubular or 3.5-mm dynamic-compression plate. The implant is placed most commonly on the posteromedial or direct medial tibial surface at the apex of the medial metaphyseal fracture line. Care should be taken to limit dissection through this second incision and avoid development of large skin flaps. Lag screws can be placed percutaneously through the skin into the plate (Fig. 16A and B).

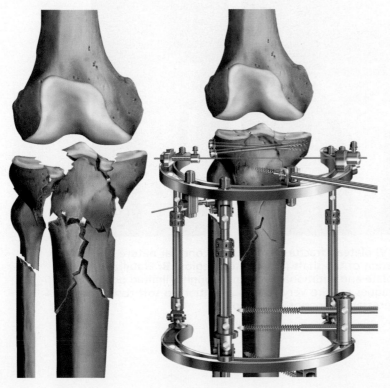

, B

Figure 15. A: Schatzker Type VI plateau fracture. This involves a fracture between the lateral and medial tibial condyles, as well as complete dissociation of the metaphyseal region from the tibial shaft. **B:** Treatment requires placement of a strong lateral buttress plate. This plate must be strong enough to withstand bending forces at the metaphyseal–diaphyseal junction. In many cases, this area is severely comminuted and will require delayed bone grafting to prevent nonunion. Often a limited posteromedial incision is necessary to place a smaller antiglide or buttress plate in an effort to bolster the fractured medial-condylar component.

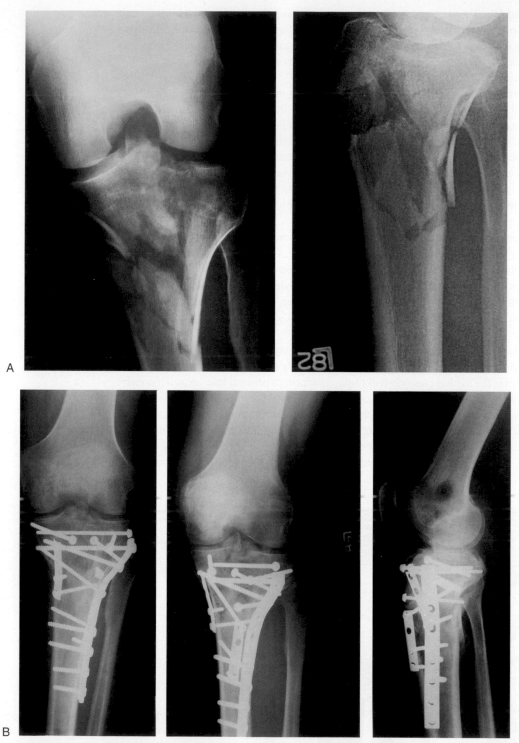

Figure 16. A: A severe Schatzker VI plateau fracture. Note the bicondylar nature of the fracture and complete dissociation of the shaft metaphyseal region. **B:** Stabilization with a dynamic-compression plate and additional fixation through a limited posterior medial incision. These techniques require very careful attention to soft-tissue handling in an effort to avoid unnecessary subperiosteal stripping.

If extensive comminution or soft-tissue injury is present, additional incisions are con-traindicated to avoid wound problems. The medial plate is abandoned in favor of a simple half-pin external fixator. One or two medial half pins are placed percutaneously proximally into the medial condylar fragment parallel to the joint surface. A simple medial monolat-eral frame is constructed and attached to one or two distal pins placed well below the frac-ture site in the tibial shaft. It cannot be overemphasized that when extreme soft-tissue com-promise is present, formal open reduction and plate osteosynthesis should be abandoned in favor of small tensioned wire or hybrid external fixation.

POSTOPERATIVE MANAGEMENT

Postoperatively, the limb is placed into a bulky Jones dressing from the toes to groin. A cephalosporin antibiotic is administered for 24 to 48 hours after surgery. A suction drain is maintained for at least 24 hours or until drainage is less than 30 ml per 8-hour interval.

If the soft-tissue envelope was not significantly damaged at the time of injury and wound closure was achieved without tension, a continuous-passive-motion (CPM) machine is rec-ommended. If significant swelling or tension on the suture line is present, the CPM is de-layed until the swelling has subsided. The bulky dressing is removed at 48 hours, and the limb is placed into a hinged knee brace that allows gradual increase in the range of knee motion.

Physical therapy is initiated early to begin quadriceps strengthening, as well as gait train-ing with crutches or a walker, non–weight bearing. Patients are seen at 2 weeks for suture removal and at monthly intervals thereafter. AP and lateral radiographs are obtained, and weight bearing is advanced as fracture healing progresses. Patients are maintained non–weight bearing for approximately 6 to 8 weeks for all fracture patterns. Once the wound is healed, active and active-assisted range of motion is initiated. The goal is to achieve 90 degrees of knee flexion by the fourth week after surgery. Weight bearing up to 50% of body weight is initiated at 6 to 8 weeks, depending on radiographic evidence of fracture consolidation. In the higher-energy Type V and VI injuries, weight bearing must often be delayed for 10 to 12 weeks. In most low-energy injuries, patients can bear full weight by 12 to 14 weeks. Most patients can expect to resume most simple activities be-tween 4 to 6 months. Running and vigorous athletics may require up to 1 year of rehabili-tation. Patient and surgeon alike can expect a good functional outcome from most low-en-ergy, Schatzker I, II, and III injuries.

Because of comminution at the metaphyseal–diaphyseal junction in Type V and VI in-juries, this area is often slow to consolidate. If union is not progressing, the area should be bone grafted before initiation of weight bearing. Grafting should be planned when the soft tissues have adequately healed, usually by 8 to 10 weeks after injury. These higher-grade injuries often take 12 to 18 months before patients are able to resume many routine daily activities. The functional outcome for these severe injuries is guarded. Patients rarely re-sume competitive athletics. The goals of the surgeon and patient must take into account the degree of articular damage and the extent of soft-tissue injury. Functional range of motion with painless ambulation and resumption of daily activities should be the goal.

COMPLICATIONS

Poorly timed surgical incisions through traumatized soft tissues with extensive soft-tis-sue dissection often contributes to early wound breakdown and infection. These complica-tions can be minimized by careful timing of surgery, limiting the extent of skin flaps, ex-traperiosteal dissection of fracture fragments, and minimizing the soft-tissue stripping at the fracture site.

CT-guided incisions directed at the fracture site, in concert with indirect reduction tech-niques by using a femoral distractor, large percutaneous reduction forceps, and cannulated screws, all help to decrease additional damage to the soft-tissue envelope.

If wound breakdown occurs, immediate surgical intervention is indicated. Irrigation and debridement of all devitalized skin, muscle, and bone is mandatory. If the wound can be closed without tension, then closure over suction drains is recommended.

If a deep infection with pus is encountered, the wound should be packed open and redebrided within 48 hours. When a culture-negative wound has been obtained, secondary wound closure should be accomplished. In most instances, this will require a lateral or medial gastrocnemius rotational flap. Occasionally, a free tissue transfer is necessary.

Hardware should be retained if it provides stability at the fracture site. If the hardware is loose, it should be removed and the limb stabilized with a joint-spanning external fixator. This often results in a knee fusion, as severe intraarticular sepsis combined with instability results in rapid chondrolysis with destruction of the knee joint.

Aseptic nonunion occasionally occurs in the Schatzker Type V and VI fractures at the junction of the metaphysis and diaphysis. These should be bone grafted early. Revision fixation also may be necessary. Malunion can occur in these injuries with late collapse of the articular surface or deformation of the metaphyseal–diaphyseal junction. If the mechanical axis is affected, then a corrective osteotomy may be required. If the patient is older, revision to a total knee arthroplasty may be appropriate.

Knee stiffness often occurs in severe fractures or when range of motion has been delayed. Arthroscopic lysis of adhesions combined with gentle manipulation under anesthesia may be helpful in those patients who fail to achieve 90 degrees of knee flexion within the first 4 weeks after surgery.

ILLUSTRATIVE CASE FOR TECHNIQUE

A 25-year-old man was involved in a motorcycle accident in which he sustained multiple injuries including a Schatzker VI bicondylar tibial-plateau fracture (Fig. 17). AP and lateral radiographs reveal a bicondylar fracture, as well as metaphyseal–diaphyseal disso-

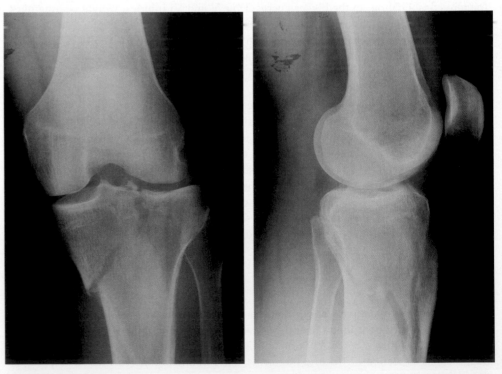

A   B

Figure 17. A: Schatzker VI injury showing the bicondylar nature of the injury with complete metaphyseal–diaphyseal dissociation. **B:** Lateral radiograph of Schatzker VI plateau fracture. Note the anterior extension of the distal fracture lines. This area will require a second plate.

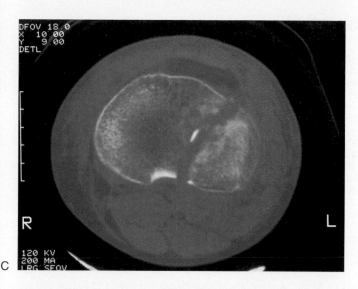

Figure 17. (*continued*) **C:** Computed tomography (CT) scan reveals minimal articular impaction but demonstrates wide separation of lateral and medial condyles.

ciation. The CT scan demonstrated minimal articular depression; however, significant separation between the lateral and medial condyles was apparent.

An extensile lateral parapatellar approach was used. After incision of the anterior compartment fascia and iliotibial band, the large lateral fragment was encountered. The meniscotibial ligament was divided and the knee flexed to 90 degrees to visualize the intraarticular component as well as the major lateral condylar fracture line. By using large percutaneous reduction forceps, the intercondylar split and shaft fracture was reduced. The fracture was stabilized by using a tibial condylar buttress plate, which spanned the shaft/metaphyseal region. Because of the unstable nature of the anteromedial condyle, a percutaneously placed lag screw and anterior antiglide plate were used to buttress this region. The final construct shows restoration of articular congruency as well as maintenance of the mechanical axis at 9 months postoperatively (Fig. 18A and B). The patient returned to his activities of daily living but was not able to resume sporting activities.

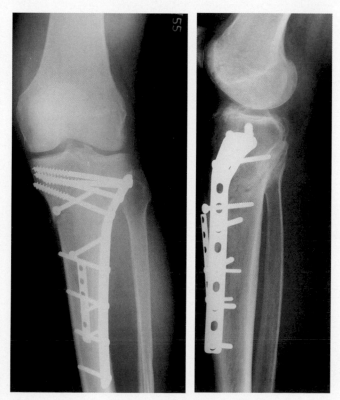

Figure 18. A, B: Radiographs at 9 months after surgery demonstrate consolidation across all fracture lines. No loss of shaft reduction has occurred, and the lateral joint line has been maintained.

RECOMMENDED READING

1. Apley, G.: Fractures of the tibial plateau. *Orthop. Clin. North Am.,* 10:61–76, 1979.
2. Barrow, B.A., Fajiman, W.A., Parker, L.M., Albert, M.J., Divaric, D.M., Hudson, T.M.: Tibial plateau fractures: evaluation with MR imaging. *Radiographics,* 14(3):553–559, 1994.
3. Benirschke, S.K., Agnew, S.G., Mayo, K.A., et al.: Open reduction internal fixation of complex proximal tibial fractures. *J. Orthop. Trauma,* 5:236, 1991.
4. Holzach, P., Matter, P., Minter, J.: Arthroscopically assisted treatment of lateral plateau fractures in skiers: use of a cannulated reduction system. *J. Orthop. Trauma,* 8(4):273–281, 1994.
5. Koval, K.T., Sanders, R., Borrelli, J., et al: Indirect reduction and percutaneous screw fixation of displaced tibial plateau fractures. *J. Orthop. Trauma,* 6:340–351, 1992.
6. Lansinger, O., Bergman, B., Courmaer, L., et al.: Tibial condylar fractures: a 20 year follow-up. *J. Bone Joint Surg. [Am],* 68:13–18, 1986.
7. Mast, J., Ganz, R., Jacob, R.: *Planning and Reduction Techniques in Fracture Surgery.* Springer-Verlag, Berlin, 1989.
8. Rangitsch, M.R., Duwelius, P.J., Colville, M.R.: Limited internal fixation of tibial plateau fractures. *J. Orthop. Trauma,* 7:168–169, 1993.
9. Rasmussen, P.: Tibial condylar fractures: impairment of knee joint stability as an indicator for surgical treatment. *J. Bone Joint Surg. [Am],* 55:1331–1350, 1973.
10. Schatzker, J., and McBroom, R.: Tibial plateau fractures: the Toronto experience 1968-1975. *Clin. Orthop.,* 138:94–104, 1979.
11. Waddell, A.P., Johnston, D.W.C., Meidre, A.: Fractures of tibial plateau: a review of 95 patients and comparison of treatment methods. *J. Trauma,* 2:376–381, 1981.
12. Watson, J.T.: High energy fractures of the tibial plateau. *Orthop. Clin. North Am.,* 25:4723–4752, 1994.

Master Techniques in Orthopaedic Surgery,
FRACTURES, edited by D. A. Wiss,
Lippincott–Raven Publishers, Philadelphia © 1998.

24

Tibial-Plateau Fractures: Ring and Hybrid Frames

Fred F. Behrens

INDICATIONS/CONTRAINDICATIONS

The surgical treatment of tibial-plateau fractures with ring or hybrid frames (1) is an accepted alternative to nonoperative options or internal fixation (2,8,10,11). Periarticular fractures of the proximal tibia ("bumper injuries"; 3) and bicondylar plateau fractures are the most common indications for this method of treatment (Fig. 1). Both fracture patterns have been associated with a high incidence of soft-tissue problems, caused by the severity of the initial injury or the extensive operative dissection that is needed with plate osteosynthesis (3,9,11). Other considerations that favor the use of ring or hybrid frames include osteopenia (7), minimal to moderate articular displacement, extensive metaphyseal or diaphyseal comminution, and the need for early weight bearing (i.e., patients who are debilitated or have bilateral lower-extremity injuries; 2).

Unicondylar and bicondylar plateau fractures in young patients with good bone stock and a few well-defined articular fragments do well with modern reduction and internal fixation techniques (2,5). For the osteopenic elderly with a bicondylar plateau fracture or the patient who is unable to provide adequate pin care, a cast brace (4), possibly followed by a total knee arthroplasty, may be preferable (1).

F. F. Behrens, M.D.: Department of Orthopaedics, New Jersey Medical School, Newark, New Jersey 07103-2499.

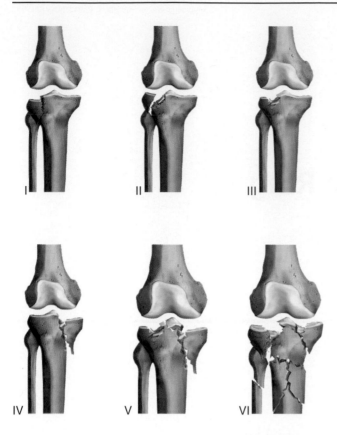

Figure 1. Schatzker's classification of tibial-plateau fractures.

PREOPERATIVE PLANNING

Because many tibial-plateau fractures are caused by high-energy trauma, initial attention must focus on resuscitation and treatment of life- or limb-threatening injuries. The injured extremity is carefully examined for open wounds, abrasions, neurovascular compromise,

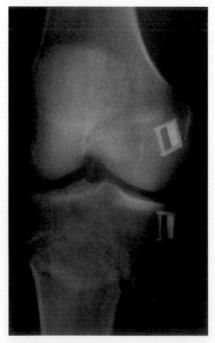

Figure 2. Anteroposterior (AP) radiograph of bicondylar tibial-plateau fracture with minimal displacement of joint surface.

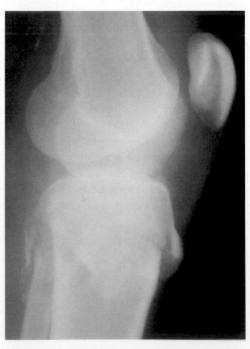

Figure 3. Lateral radiograph showing anterior angulation of proximal fragment and minimal metaphyseal comminution.

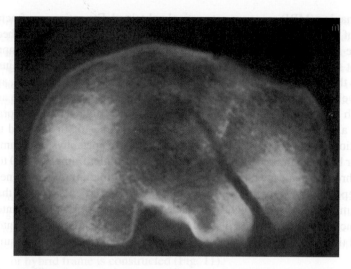

Figure 4. Computed tomography (CT) scan just below joint surface showing principal fracture line in an antero-

and ligamentous injuries. Diminished to absent distal pulses and delayed capillary refill are indications for an urgent angiographic evaluation. Compartment pressure should be obtained in patients who are intoxicated, have a central nervous system lesion, have diminished peripheral sensation, or have pronounced pain on passive plantar- and dorsiflection of the toes.

The radiographic workup includes anteroposterior (AP) and lateral views of the involved tibia/fibula, and a knee series consisting of a true AP plateau view (x-ray tube 10 degrees inclined caudally) and a lateral of the knee (Figs. 2 and 3). In addition, an AP view of the opposite knee on a large film is obtained to document the normal tibiofemoral angle. A computed tomography (CT) scan from the distal femur to the most distal tibial fracture extension, with coronal and sagittal reconstructions, has at most centers replaced tomography (Figs. 4–6). CT scans tend to cause less discomfort to the patient, and the cross-sectional views have become a prerequisite for optimal wire and screw placement. As injuries to the collateral ligaments and the menisci are rare in bicondylar tibial-plateau fractures, magnetic

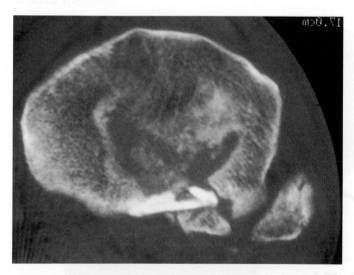

Figure 5. Computed tomography (CT) scan just above metaphyseal fracture showing additional posterior comminution.

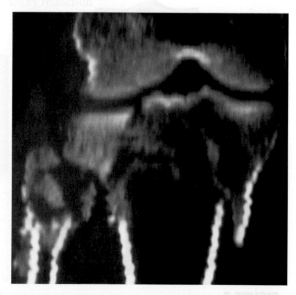

Figure 6. Computed tomography (CT) scan. Sagittal reconstruction showing minimal depression of lateral tibial fragment and extensive comminution of fibular head.

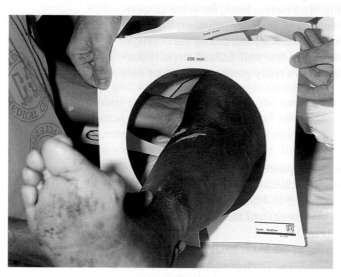

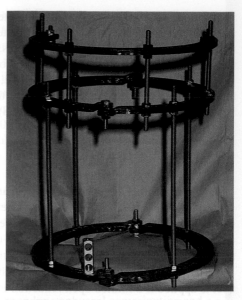

Figure 10. Determination of optimal ring size by using template.

Figure 11. Preassembled ring fixator with wide pin spread in distal fragment and capability for gradual alignment adjustment between proximal and distal fragments.

If the articular fragments are displaced less than 2 to 3 mm, they are percutaneously stabilized with two or more medium-size holding wires of about 2 mm in diameter (Figs. 15 and 16). These holding wires keep the articular fragments reduced and prevent secondary displacement during screw fixation.

Screw fixation of the articular surface is the next step. Because of their ease of use, cannulated screws inserted over guide wires are preferred. The numbers of directions of the screws used are determined by the location and direction of the principal fracture lines as

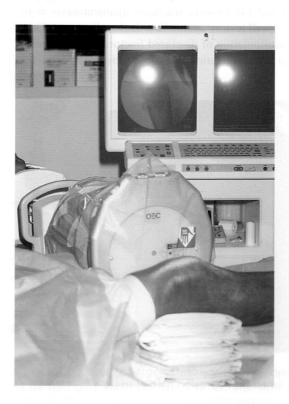

Figure 12. Operating room setup with knee elevated 10 to 15 degrees to permit true anteroposterior (AP) views of the tibial plateau and unencumbered transverse imaging.

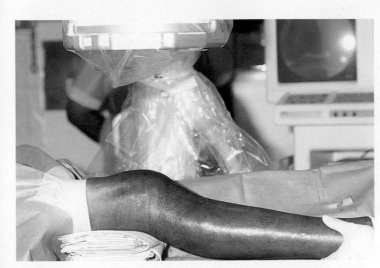

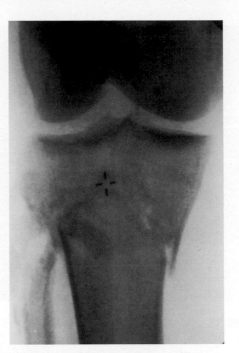

Figure 13. Applying traction to assess fragment reduction and alignment.

Figure 14. Image while applying traction.

seen on CT scan. The appropriate guide wires are then placed within a centimeter of the articular surface, and the cannulated screws are inserted (Figs. 17 and 18). If the holding wires are necessary to secure a stable articular construct, they are cut flush with the outer bony surface; otherwise, they are removed (Figs. 19 and 20). Screws with thread diameters between 6.5 and 7.3 mm are most commonly used.

At the end of this initial part of the procedure, a stable proximal construct of at least 2 to 3 cm in length has been obtained. This reconstructed fragment then serves as the proximal anchor for the external frame.

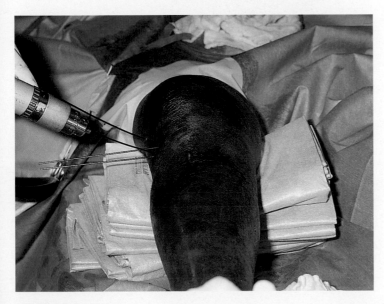

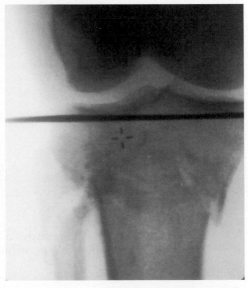

FIGURE 15

FIGURE 16

Figures 15 and 16. Placement of subchondral holding wires.

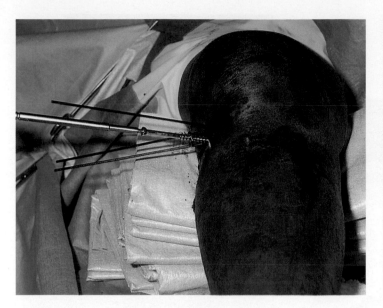

FIGURE 17

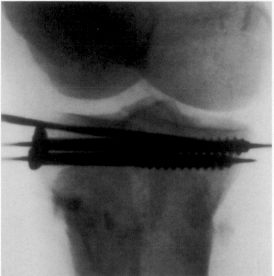

FIGURE 18

Figures 17 and 18. Screw fixation of lateral-plateau fracture by using cannulated screws inserted in anterolateral– posteromedial direction.

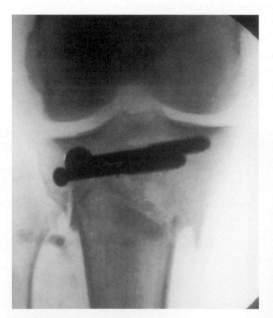

FIGURE 19

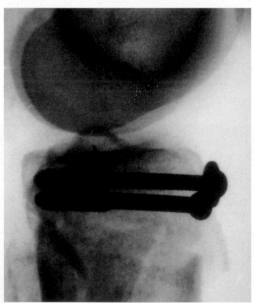

FIGURE 20

Figures 19 and 20. Anteroposterior (AP) and lateral images after screw fixation of intraarticular fragments. Holding wires have been removed.

Tibial Alignment and Stability

Conceptually, the hybrid or ring frame can be applied as a simple or as a clamp fixator (1). With the former method, placement of a wire into the proximal fragment is followed by inserting a wire or a pin into the distal part of the lower fragment. The frame is then anchored on those two implants, assuring proper limb alignment before the remaining wires and pins are inserted. However, because most hybrid frames contain easily adjustable longitudinal connections, the pins and wires in each fragment can be separately inserted. The ring or hybrid frame is then applied as the last step.

To facilitate frame application, the limb is supported proximal to the knee and at the ankle (Fig. 21). Olive wires are preferred, as they provide additional stability and diminish the risk of fragment displacement on the wires. Because synovial reflections of the knee joint can overlap the tibial plateau by up to 14 mm, none of the proximal wires should be placed closer to the articular surface (6). The first wire is inserted from a posterolateral to an anteromedial direction. Because about 10% of patients have a direct connection between the proximal tibiofibular and the knee joint, it is recommended that this wire be placed not through the fibula but just anterior to it into the lateral plateau wall. Once this wire is connected to the proximal ring, it is properly centered and then tensioned to about 60 to 90 lb. This facilitates insertion of the second olive wire from posteromedial to anterolateral. Care must be taken that this wire is started anterior to the gastrocnemius muscle; this will avoid undue pain with knee motion. Both wires are then tightened simultaneously to somewhere between 90 and 130 lb (Fig. 22).

In most circumstances, the distal tibial fragment is stabilized with two half-pins inserted close to the sagittal plane (Fig. 23). The larger the pin diameter and the farther the longitudinal pin spread, the more stable the construct. Before the first pin (the one closest to the ankle joint) is inserted, leg length and overall limb alignment are reassessed. For a quick check of limb alignment, the electrocautery cord is strung taut between a point just medial to the anterior superior iliac spine and the middle of the ankle joint (Figs. 24 and 25). When crossing the knee, the cord should pass close to the intercondylar spine, as seen on the image intensifier. If a ring frame is used, the leg is centered in the most distal ring before the respective pins or wires are inserted. After placing these implants, limb and frame alignment are again evaluated. The remaining pins or wires are then inserted.

A ring or hybrid frame applied in this manner often lacks sufficient stability in the sagit-

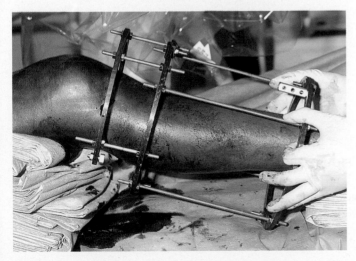

Figure 21. Positioning of preassembled ring frame allowing two finger breadths of space between leg and rings.

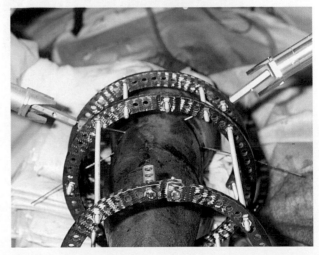

Figure 22. Simultaneous tightening of the two initial olive wires in the proximal fragment.

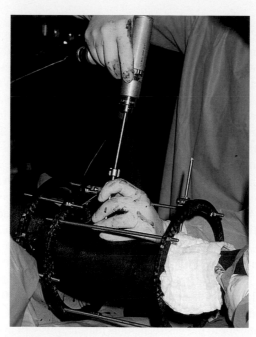

Figure 23. Predrilling of proximal pin in distal fragment.

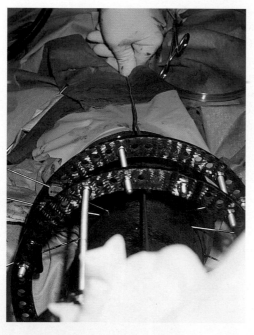

FIGURE 24

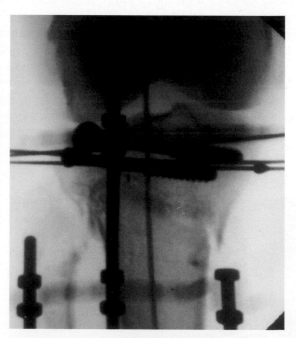

FIGURE 25

Figures 24 and 25. Alignment check by using cord of electrocautery. Image shows cord passing through intercondylar spines.

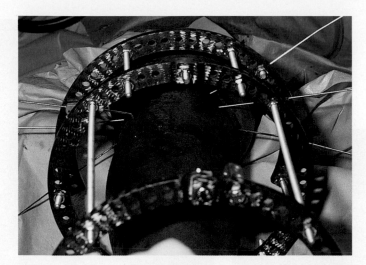

Figure 26. Knee region after placement of third wire into proximal fragment. This is done to reduce sagittal displace-

tal plane because of the pull of the quadriceps mechanism. For this reason, a third or fourth wire may be placed into this fragment (Fig. 26). If the fragment is large enough, a sagittal half-pin anchored on the most proximal ring provides an even more stable construct (Figs. 27 and 28).

At the end of the procedure, but before the conclusion of anesthesia, AP and lateral radiographs of the involved tibia and an AP film centered on the knee are obtained (Figs. 29–32). The latter film is compared for proper femorotibial alignment with the preoperative radiographs obtained of the opposite knee. Alignment corrections, if necessary, are carried out before the patient leaves the operating room.

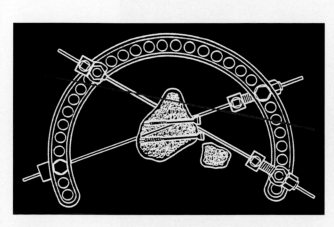

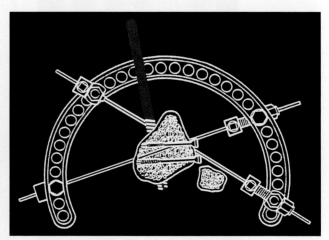

FIGURE 27   **FIGURE 28**

Figures 27 and 28. Placement of additional wire or sagittal pin into proximal fragment to prevent rotation in sagittal plane.

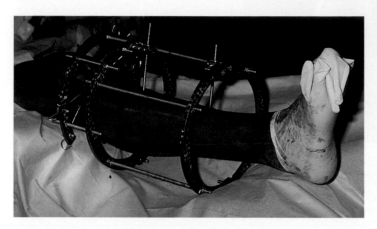

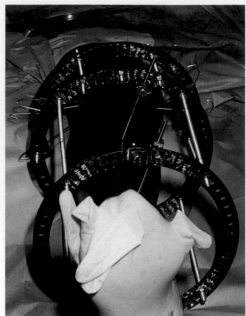

FIGURE 29

FIGURE 30

Figures 29 and 30. Lateral and anterior view of assembled ring frame.

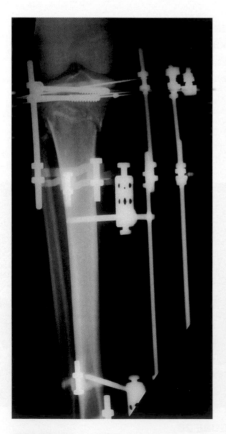

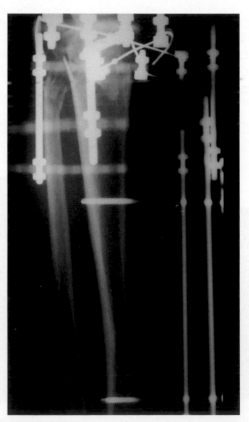

FIGURE 31

FIGURE 32

Figures 31 and 32. Anteroposterior (AP) and lateral radiographs after completed reduction and application of ring frame.

POSTOPERATIVE MANAGEMENT

Even if all wires and pins have been placed below the synovial reflections of the knee joint, bacterial seeding of the joint along the wire tracts and through cracks in the articular fragments is still possible for up to about 4 weeks. For this reason, the proximal pin and wire sites are initially covered with gauze sponges soaked in povidone–iodine (Betadine) and held in place with a Kerlix bandage. These dressings are changed about twice a week for 4 weeks. If the patient has sufficient control and balance, mobilization is started with crutches on postoperative days 1 or 2. Toe touching (10 to 20 lb) is encouraged. Active range-of-motion exercise of knee and ankle are initiated at the same time. Routine pin and wire care consist of washing the leg and the pin-entry sites with soap and water once a day.

After discharge from the hospital, the patient is seen at 3-week intervals in the office, where AP and lateral radiographs of the tibia and the knee are obtained. If there are concerns about alignment changes, AP views of both knees on a large film are added. Alignment corrections can be carried out in the office without the need for anesthesia. Depending on the severity of the comminution and the degree of osteopenia, full weight bearing is permitted within 4 to 8 weeks after surgery. At that time, most patients have attained an active range of motion from about 5 to 90 degrees. On average, the frames can be removed 4 months after the injury. When the healing process is delayed, the fixators are dynamized at about 3.5 months by loosening the connections between the tibial pins and the frame to allow 5 to 10 mm of motion. Two weeks after "dynamization" of the frame, fracture alignment is reassessed on standard films. If there has been no axis deviation, the patient continues to walk on the dynamized frame until the fracture is healed. After the fixator has been removed, the patient is enrolled in a short physical therapy program that focuses on restoring full range of knee motion as well as strength and endurance in the involved extremity. If the fracture is not healed, the frame is retightened, possibly compressed, and the patient is encouraged to continue with full weight bearing until the fracture is healed and the frame can be removed.

The ultimate functional outcome of a bicondylar tibial-plateau fracture treated in a ring fixator appears to be very similar to that seen after internal fixation, with the exception that secondary fixation failures, soft-tissue necrosis, and deep infections are less common (9). Most younger patients are able to return to their preinjury occupations and most of their recreational endeavors. Older patients employed in occupations with high physical demands may have to change their jobs.

COMPLICATIONS

There are few reports in the literature of tibial-plateau fractures managed with ring or hybrid frames, and no series presents follow-up information exceeding 3 years (8,10,11). The available information indicates that most plateau fractures treated with this method are healed within 3 to 5 months. The average range of knee motion is between 105 and 120 degrees, and most patients return to full weight bearing without support. Hospital for Special Surgery knee scores generally range between 82 and 90 (8,10,11). Some pin or wire drainage will occur in about 30% to 50% of all patients. It responds quickly to improved local wound care or a short course of oral antibiotics. The most severe problems have been deep wound infections, in particular, pyarthrosis, which has occurred in 5% to 15%. Although these usually resolve with open or arthroscopic irrigation and drainage, they can lead to permanent knee-flexion contractures. Placing the proximal wires farther than 15 mm distal to the articular surface of the knee and enhanced pin and wire care have largely eliminated this serious complication. Nonunions occur in about 4%; consolidation tends to occur quickly after local bone grafting. Malunions, mostly valgus deformities from 8 to 15 degrees, occur occasionally, but corrective osteotomies are rarely needed.

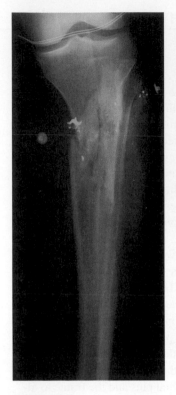

FIGURE 33

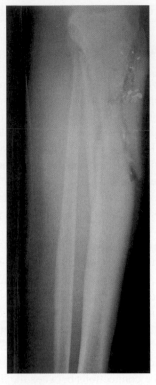

FIGURE 34

Figures 33 and 34. Anteroposterior (AP) and lateral radiographs of proximal tibial fracture adjacent to the tibial plateau.

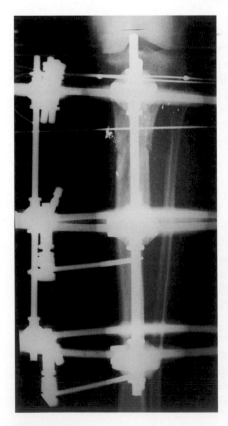

FIGURE 35

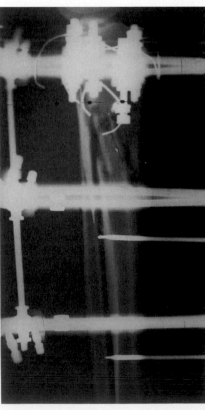

FIGURE 36

Figures 35 and 36. Anteroposterior (AP) and lateral views after stabilization with ring fixator.

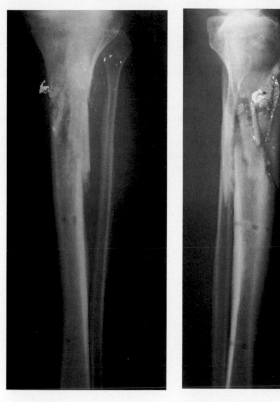

FIGURE 37   **FIGURE 38**

Figures 37 and 38. Anteroposterior (AP) and lateral views at 3.5 months after fixator removal. Although some original fracture lines are still visible, the patient is fully weight bearing without support.

ILLUSTRATIVE CASE FOR TECHNIQUE

A 51-year-old man sustained a gunshot wound to his left proximal tibia (Figs. 33 and 34) and his right middle femur. Both fractures were comminuted. The right femur was stabilized with a locking nail. We elected to use a ring fixator for the periarticular tibial fracture because it could secure, at once, good alignment and sufficient stability to allow early weight bearing—an option that would not have been available with the use of a tibial nail (Figs. 35 and 36).

Two weeks after the injury, the patient was fully weight bearing on the left and toe touching on the right (20 lb). After an additional 4 weeks, the patient had regained a full range of motion in his left knee. The external fixator was removed 3.5 months after the injury when both the right femur and the left periarticular tibial fractures were healed (Figs. 37 and 38).

RECOMMENDED READING

1. Behrens, F.F.: General theory and principles of external fixation. *Clin. Orthop.*, 241:15–23, 1989.
2. Behrens, F.F.: Knee and leg: bone trauma. In Frymoyer, J. (ed.): *Orthopaedic Knowledge Update-4. Home study syllabus.* Academy of Orthopaedic Surgeons, Rosemont, IL 1993, pp. 579–592.
3. Burgess, A.R., Poka, A., Brumback, R.J., Flagle, C.L., Loeb, P.E., Ebraheim, N.A.: Pedestrian tibial injuries. *J. Trauma,* 27:596–600, 1987.
4. DeCoster, T.A., Nepola, J.V., El-Khoury, G.Y.: Cast brace treatment of proximal tibia fractures: a ten-year follow-up study. *Clin. Orthop.*, 231:196–204, 1988.

5. Lansinger, O., Bergman, B., Korner, L., et al.: Tibial condylar fractures: a twenty-year follow-up. *J. Bone Joint Surg. [Am]*, 68:13–19, 1986.
6. Reid, J.S., Vanslyke, M., Moulton, M.J.R., Mann, T.A.: Safe placement of proximal tibial transfixation wires with respect to intracapsular penetration. 1995 Annual Meeting of the Orthopaedic Trauma Association, Tampa, Florida, Sept. 29 to Oct. 1, 1995.
7. Schatzker, J., McBroom, R., Bruce, D.: The tibial plateau fractures: the Toronto experience 1968-1975. *Clin. Orthop.*, 138:94–104, 1979.
8. Stamer, D., Schenk, R., Staggers, B., Aurori, K., Aurori, B., Behrens, F.: Bicondylar tibial plateau fractures treated with a hybrid ring external fixator: a preliminary study. *J. Orthop. Trauma,* 8(6):455–461, 1994.
9. Wagner, H.E., and Jakob, R.P.: Zur Problematik der Plattenosteosynthese bei den bikondylären Tibiakopf-frakturen. *Unfallchirurgie*, 89:304–311, 1986.
10. Watson, J.T.: High-energy fractures of the tibial plateau. *Orthop. Clin. North. Am.*, 25:723–752, 1994.
11. Weiner, L.S., Kelley, M., Yang, E., et al.: The use of combination internal fixation and hybrid external fixation in severe proximal tibia fractures. *J. Orthop. Trauma,* 9(3):244–250, 1995.

Master Techniques in Orthopaedic Surgery,
FRACTURES, edited by D. A. Wiss,
Lippincott–Raven Publishers, Philadelphia © 1998.

25

Tibial-Shaft Fractures: Open Reduction Internal Fixation

Brett R. Bolhofner

INDICATIONS/CONTRAINDICATIONS

Open reduction internal fixation by using plates and screws may be carried out for virtually any fracture of the tibia that has satisfactory soft-tissue conditions. Although intramedullary interlocking nails have become popular for the treatment of many tibial-shaft fractures, plating remains a viable alternative (4). Compared with an intramedullary implant, plating of the tibia requires greater attention to the condition of the soft tissues, more preoperative planning, and greater attention to surgical detail during the procedure.

Strong indications for plate osteosynthesis of tibial-shaft fractures are the presence of compartment syndrome, neurovascular injury, compromised medullary canal, or compromised access to the medullary canal due to associated injury (2,6).

Relative indications for open reduction internal fixation include the following: polytraumatized patients, open fractures, late loss of reduction with closed treatment, segmental injury, fractures that extend into either the knee or ankle joints, fractures of the proximal and distal one third of the shaft, and fractures in patients whose livelihood or recreational habits demand perfect restoration of length and rotation (2,6).

Relative contraindications to plate osteosynthesis include isolated displaced diaphyseal fractures, which may be better treated with a locked intramedullary nail. Grossly contaminated open fractures, which will require serial debridements, are best treated with an external fixator rather than plate osteosynthesis.

A careful assessment of the soft-tissue envelope at the time of injury and at the time of surgery is essential, as it influences the timing of the surgical procedure. Grading the soft-tissue injury according to the Tscherne classification may be helpful in evaluating and assessing the soft-tissue injury associated with a particular fracture pattern (3). In patients whose soft tissue does not permit early internal fixation because of swelling, abrasions, or blisters, a

---

B. R. Bolhofner, M.D.: All Florida Orthopedic Associates, St. Petersburg, Florida 33702.

period of waiting, perhaps as long as 10 to 14 days, is indicated. The skin should have a very fine wrinkled texture or appearance before proceeding with plate osteosynthesis.

When soft-tissue conditions are satisfactory, the tibia is well suited to plate fixation, as it has a large subcutaneous surface that may be used for stabilization without the necessity of muscle stripping.

PREOPERATIVE PLANNING

The initial assessment of the soft tissues and the radiographic pattern of the fracture is carried out immediately. Attention to the neurovascular status as well as the status of the muscle compartments is mandatory. The presence of soft-tissue contusion, skin necrosis, swelling, compartment syndrome, skin abrasion, or any wounds is carefully documented. Anteroposterior (AP) and lateral views of the tibia, to include both knee and ankle joint, must be obtained (Fig. 1).

The timing of the internal fixation is based primarily on the condition of the soft tissues. Open reduction internal fixation of the tibia should only be carried out when satisfactory skin and wound conditions permit a tension-free soft-tissue closure at the conclusion of the procedure. If these conditions do not exist, then internal fixation should be postponed. The extremity should be splinted, casted, or a temporary spanning external fixator applied until more favorable conditions exist. If surgery is delayed, it is necessary that the limb be elevated to help swelling resolve. Necrotic soft tissue should be well demarcated and excised at the time of surgery. In the case of proximal tibia fractures, this may require a gastrocnemius rotational muscle flap at the time of surgery. In the distal tibia, this may necessitate a free tissue transfer or a fasciocutaneous rotational flap. When satisfactory soft-tissue conditions are present, the procedure may be carried out based on a well-conceived preoperative plan and a surgical tactic.

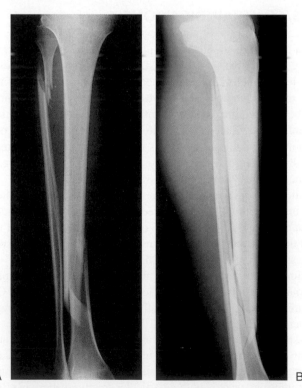

A   B

Figure 1. Anteroposterior (AP; **A**) and lateral (**B**) radiographs of the tibia and fibula show a distal one-third fracture of the tibia with an undisplaced posteromedial butterfly. Radiographs include the joint above and below the fracture.

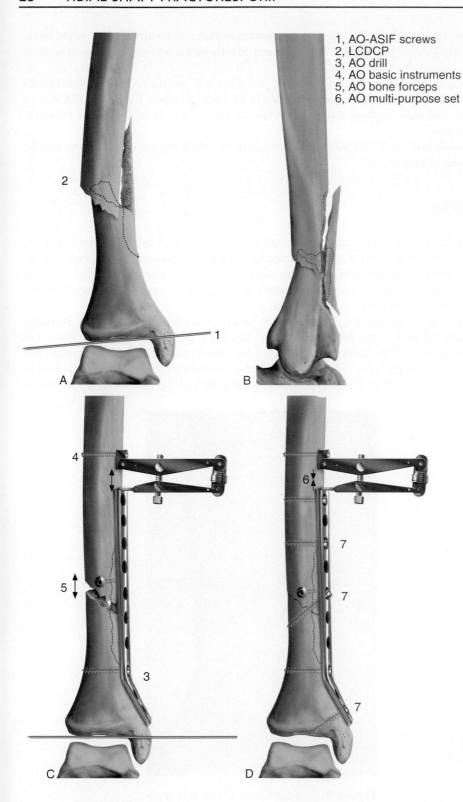

1, AO-ASIF screws
2, LCDCP
3, AO drill
4, AO basic instruments
5, AO bone forceps
6, AO multi-purpose set

Figure 2. A–D: Anteroposterior (AP) and lateral preoperative drawings illustrating the preoperative plan for fracture fixation and the step-by-step procedure to be carried out in numeric order.

AP and lateral radiographs of the injured extremity should be obtained. If the fracture is complex or if there is significant deformity, it may be helpful for preoperative planning to obtain an AP and lateral radiograph of the unaffected side or an AP and lateral radiograph of the affected extremity in traction the better to conceptualize the fracture pattern. The preoperative drawings, which need not be of artistic quality, should be fashioned so that a step-by-step procedure is outlined from start to finish in a simple fashion (Fig. 2A–D). Because the preoperative plans are displayed in the operating room at the time of the surgery, it is quite helpful to indicate directly on the preoperative plan any equipment that might be required. The steps of the procedure are indicated directly on the preoperative plan in numeric order.

The equipment required to carry out the procedure will be AO/ASIF screws and plates (limited-contact dynamic compression plate or LCDCP; Synthes, Paoli, PA, U.S.A.), an AO drill, and basic instruments, bone forceps, and associated small soft-tissue retractors and elevators.

Assumption of basic AO technique is required, including the use of lag screws and the contouring of plates (2).

SURGERY

When the soft tissues are satisfactory, and a preoperative plan has been established, the procedure may be initiated (Fig. 3). It should be noted that, in contrast to preoperative planning for trauma reconstruction such as an osteotomy, intraoperative findings such as undisplaced fracture lines or unrecognized comminution may be present, which may occasionally alter the order of the preoperative plan.

The patient is placed in the supine position on a regular operating room table. A tourniquet is not required for the procedure but may be used if desired. Use of either general or spinal anesthesia is satisfactory. The entire leg from the toes to the groin or proximal thigh is carried out. Prophylactic intravenous antibiotics, usually a single preoperative dose of cephalosporin, is recommended. The location and length of the incision is drawn on the

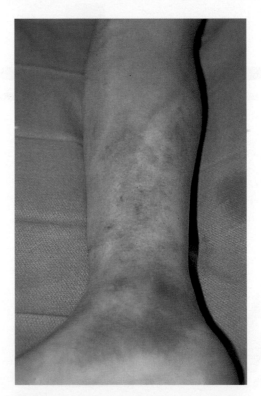

Figure 3. The condition of the skin is ascertained before undertaking an open reduction internal fixation. In this case, there is ecchymosis from the injury; however, there are no obvious areas of skin necrosis or significant abrasion. The edema has resolved sufficiently so that the anterior crest can be seen proximally, and the medial malleolus can be identified distally.

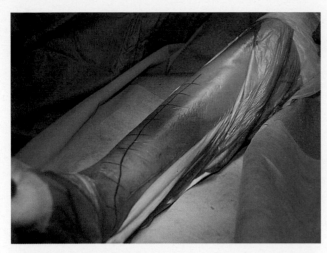

Figure 4. Planned surgical incision indicated on the skin with a marker to assist in surgical approach as well as wound closure. The operative area is draped with adhesive ioband.

skin before application of an adhesive iodine impregnated drape (Fig. 4). I prefer to carry out the procedure in the seated position at the foot of the table, with the surgical assistant also seated.

Surgical Approach

The surgical approach for this procedure is a long anterior incision placed 1 cm lateral to the tibial crest and corresponding to Langer's lines (Fig. 5; 5). The incision is curved gently at its distal portion at the level of the metaphyseal flare in the supramalleolar region. A long surgical incision is preferred to allow satisfactory exposure of the tibia and to avoid unnecessary vigorous skin retraction, particularly on the medial skin flap (Fig. 6A). It is not necessary to sacrifice the saphenous vein or nerves in the distal portion of the incision, as the plate may be placed beneath these structures, leaving them completely intact (Fig. 6B). They should be dissected only enough to allow passage of the plate beneath them. Additionally, it is not necessary to enter the sheath of the tibialis anterior tendon.

The skin and subcutaneous flap are then raised in a medial direction, just enough to allow exposure of the posteromedial border of the tibia and the butterfly fragment, which are seen after removal of the fracture hematoma. The dissection remains extraperiosteal. The periosteum is frequently noted to be stripped at the fracture edges, as a result of fracture displacement. If any additional periosteal elevation is necessary to evaluate reduction, then not more than 1 or 2 mm at the immediate fracture edge should be elevated. The remainder of the procedure should be carried out entirely extraperiosteally (Fig. 7; 5).

Internal Fixation

Once the surgical approach has been completed and satisfactory exposure of the fracture site and the medial surface of the tibia is achieved, then the preoperative plan is followed in order, for reduction and fixation of the fracture (Fig. 2A–D).

The ankle-joint axis is initially marked with a reference Kirschner wire placed by hand into the soft tissues at the level of the ankle joint (step 1, Fig. 2B).

Because the posteromedial butterfly fragment is minimally displaced, it can be directly reduced by using standard reduction forceps without periosteal stripping or damage (step 2, Fig. 2B, and Fig. 8). If significant displacement of the butterfly fragment exists, an indirect reduction technique is preferable rather than risking devascularization of the fragment by stripping of the soft tissues with direct manual manipulation.

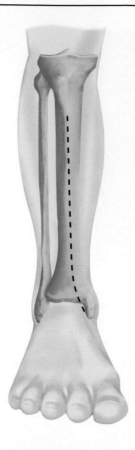

Figure 5. The surgical incision is anterior and curvilinear, beginning 1 cm lateral to the tibial crest and curving medially in the distal portion.

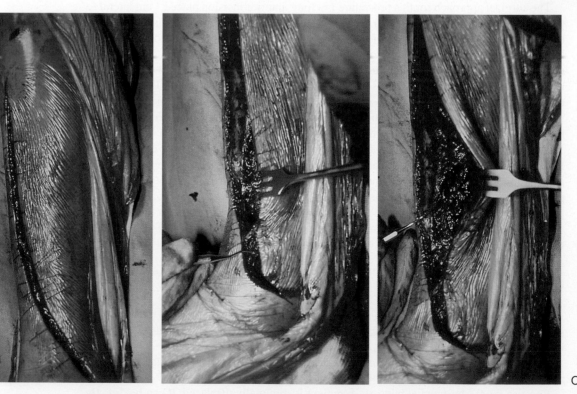

A, B   C

Figure 6. A: The surgical incision carried through the skin and subcutaneous tissue. **B:** The small dental instrument indicates the location of the distal saphenous structures that are preserved during the surgical approach and the procedure. **C:** The small dental instrument indicates the presence of fracture hematoma, which is removed for exposure of the fracture.

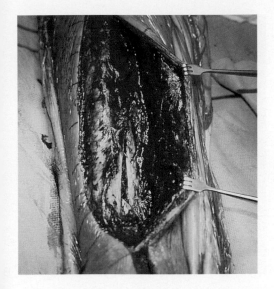

Figure 7. After evacuation of the fracture hematoma, the fracture, including the minimally displaced posteromedial butterfly, can be seen. The edges of the fracture are noted to be white as compared with the surrounding hemorrhagic periosteum. This indicates the amount of periosteum that was stripped by the injury itself. As noted, there is sufficient visualization of the fracture edges by the stripping done only by the injury to allow visualization for reduction. No further periosteal stripping should be necessary for reduction and fixation of this fracture. The periosteum is hemorrhagic because of the injury and also because no tourniquet is used.

With the butterfly fragment reduced and held with an extraperiosteally applied bone forceps, it is fixed with a 4.5-mm cortical lag screw by using standard AO technique (Fig. 9A and B). This is the direct reduction portion of the case. Fixation of the remainder of the fracture is achieved with a 4.5-mm LCDCP tibial plate. The bone or undersurface of this particular plate has small undulations so that plate contacts the bone or periosteum only at intermittent alternating points, allowing preservation of the periosteal circulation. However, standard stainless steel plates without the limited-contact feature also are satisfactory. The plate is contoured to match the naturally occurring contours of the distal medial tibia (Fig. 10). With experience, bending and twisting of the plate is carried out during the procedure. For less experienced surgeons, the plate can be precontoured by using a bone model or skeleton before the procedure and then sterilized. The plate does not have to be absolutely perfectly contoured, and slight undercontouring can be quite helpful, particularly during the reduction portion of the procedure. The LCDCP, in particular, is quite forgiving, particularly in hard bone. The plate is secured to the distal fragment with a single screw in any of the distal screw holes (step 3, Fig. 2C).

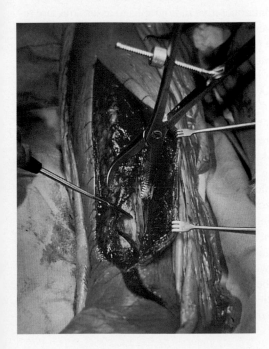

Figure 8. The posteromedial butterfly is directly reduced with bone forceps. Even though the butterfly is directly reduced, the bone forceps is applied extraperiosteally, and no soft-tissue stripping is necessary to accomplish this. The small elevator indicates the location of the posteromedial butterfly fragment.

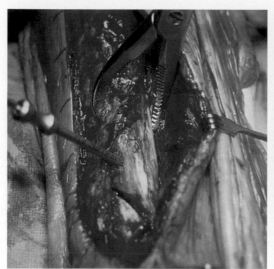
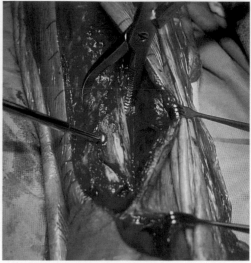

Figure 9. **A:** Lag-screw fixation is then carried out of the butterfly fragment with standard AO technique. The near cortex has been overdrilled, and the drill sleeve is used to drill the far cortex. **B:** The lag screw has been placed without additional soft-tissue stripping. Note also that the medial flap is tethered somewhat distally by the saphenous structures, which remain intact.

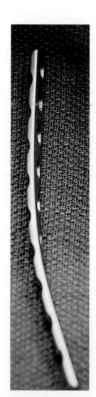

Figure 10. A 4.5-mm tibial plate, limited-contact dynamic compression plate (LCDCP), is contoured for the distal tibial medial surface with a distal bend and a proximal medial twist.

A push–pull screw is then inserted 1 or 2 cm proximal to the plate. The AO articulating tension device is then applied at the proximal end of the plate and distracted (step 4, Fig. 2C). If the plate is properly contoured, it is not necessary to clamp the plate to the shaft proximally. However, clamp application may be carried out carefully, if necessary, by making a small incision to allow the bone clamp to be placed laterally with minimal stripping of soft tissue.

The fracture is then distracted (step 5, Fig. 2D), and reduction is adjusted for angulation and rotation with small position changes in the extremity, or with reduction clamps placed extraperiosteally (Fig. 11A and B). This is the indirect reduction portion of the case (1).

Once the fracture has been reduced, the articulating tension device is placed in the compression mode and compressed to approximately 60 kPa (step 6, Fig. 2D; 2). This construct, with only one screw and the articulating tension device, is usually quite stable, and this is often a good point in the case for obtaining intraoperative radiographs to assess fracture reduction and alignment. I prefer standard overhead films to C-arm images, as they allow a better assessment of overall axial alignment (Fig. 12). At this point in the procedure, virtually no bridges have been burned, and any step is easily reversed.

If the reduction is satisfactory, then the major fragments should be secured with lag screws placed through or outside the plate. Additional screws are inserted into the plate to enhance stability (Fig. 13A and B and step 7, Fig. 2D). The exact number of screws is not precisely known, but an attempt is made to "balance" the fixation with fairly equally dispersed screws on either side of the plate. Intraoperative radiographs are obtained, and final fixation adjustments are carried out (Fig. 14 A and B). The final radiograph should correspond closely with the preoperative drawing.

The wound is irrigated with antibiotic solution and closed over a small drain. The skin itself is approximated with interrupted horizontal mattress sutures of 4-0 nylon. No tension should be present at the skin edges at the time of closure (Fig. 15). If tension-free closure cannot be obtained after osteosynthesis, then I prefer to make multiple small relaxing incisions or "pie-crusting" with a no. 10 blade on both sides of the surgical incision, which frequently allows closure without tension. If wound closure without tension is not possible, then only the portion of the wound that can be closed without tension is carried out, and the remainder of the wound is left open. The patient may then be returned to the operating room in several days for delayed primary closure or flap coverage, if necessary.

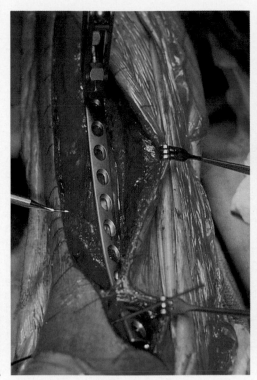
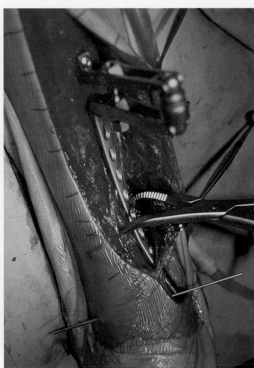

A   B

Figure 11. A: Application of the limited-contact dynamic compression plate (LCDCP) by a single screw distally. The plate has been placed beneath the saphenous vein and nerve. The articulating tension device is in the distraction mode, and the dental instrument indicates a small amount of distraction being carried out at the fracture site, which is still not anatomically reduced. **B:** The reduction is fine-tuned by the application of a reduction clamp, once again extraperiosteally, with the articulating tension device still in distraction mode. Note also the free Kirschner wire at the level of the ankle joint, which is helpful in identifying the location of the ankle joint intraoperatively.

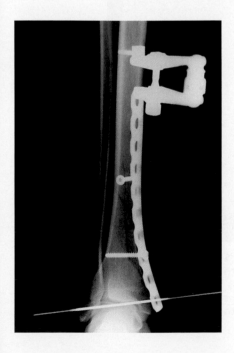

Figure 12. Anteroposterior (AP) intraoperative radiograph showing the contoured tibial plate applied with a single distal screw. The articulating tension device is now in compression, and the construct is stable.

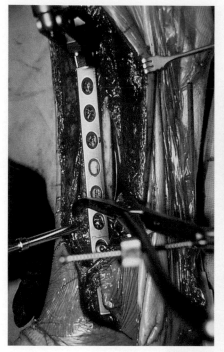
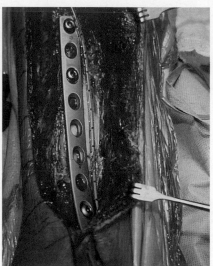

A, B

Figure 13. **A:** Additional lag-screw fixation of the two major fracture fragments. In contrast to the anticipated lag-screw placement through the plate, based on the preoperative plan, it was decided intraoperatively to place this lag screw outside the plate, which was done without any additional stripping of soft tissue. **B:** Placement of the additional screws in the plate and removal of the articulating tension device. Note that the plate is beneath the saphenous structures distally; these are preserved throughout the entire case. A single surgical drain has been placed adjacent to the plate before wound closure.

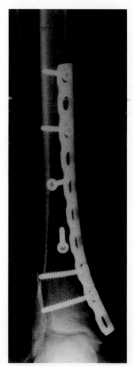
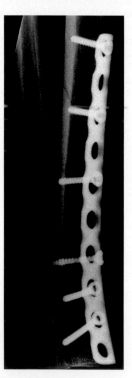
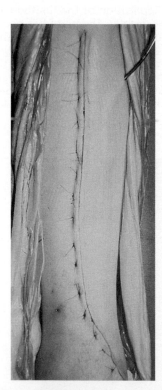

A, B

Figure 14. Anteroposterior (AP; **A**) and lateral **(B)** radiographs of the final osteosynthesis are made at the conclusion of the case. Any adjustments in screw length or position can be made easily at this point.

Figure 15. Skin closure is carried out with interrupted horizontal mattress sutures of 4-0 nylon. No tension should be present in the skin at the time of closure.

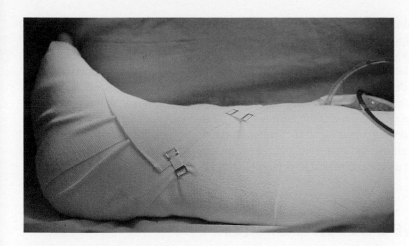

Figure 16. Bulky soft-tissue dressing is applied at the conclusion of the operation.

A sterile nonadhesive dressing is applied over the wound, followed by application of a bulky Jones-type dressing. A splint may be incorporated into the Jones dressing if desired, particularly if there are more distal injuries (Fig. 16). This also helps to prevent equinus deformity. Postoperatively, the limb is elevated on a Bohler–Braun frame for 1 to 3 days.

Diaphyseal tibial fractures are frequently accompanied by an associated fibular fracture, which usually does not require repair. However, if the tibia fracture is proximal or distal, plate osteosynthesis may be carried out at the time of tibial stabilization to enhance fracture stability. If there is excessive shortening due to fracture, it may additionally be helpful to carry out the fibular osteosynthesis before the tibial osteosynthesis. Care must be taken in preoperative planning to allow satisfactory skin bridges between the tibial and fibular incisions, which should be a minimum of 8 cm.

POSTOPERATIVE CARE

The patient is mobilized on the first postoperative day with partial weight bearing (20 kg) on the affected side if his overall condition permits.

The drain is usually removed between 2 and 4 days after surgery, followed by removal of the surgical dressing the next day. Active and active-assisted range of motion of the ankle, hip, and knee is then initiated. A light dry dressing may be required for several days for any subsequent wound drainage. Any portion of the postoperative regimen may be carried out on an outpatient basis, depending on the clinical situation.

The patient is followed up at 4-week intervals with clinical examination and radiographs. Weight bearing is advanced based on the clinical examination of discomfort or localized tenderness and the radiographic appearance of the fracture at follow-up. Typically, weight bearing will be advanced to partial (50 kg) by 6 to 8 weeks and to full by 8 to 12 weeks.

COMPLICATIONS

Of primary concern after open reduction internal fixation of a tibial fracture is that the incision heals uneventfully. Even with the utmost care, there may on occasion be minimal skin and wound-edge necrosis of 1 to 2 mm, which usually requires nothing more than observation. More extended skin and wound-edge necrosis may require surgical excision with irrigation, debridement, and reclosure of the wound, occasionally with flap advancement. Significant loss of skin and soft tissue in the postoperative period may require flap coverage.

Deep infection, occurring in the first 6 to 8 weeks after open reduction internal fixation, should be treated with wound irrigation and reclosure over drains with or without antibiotic beads if the fixation remains intact and secure. Late infection in the presence of loosened hardware will require irrigation, debridement, and removal of the hardware and external fixation of the tibia until satisfactory wound and soft-tissue conditions can be obtained.

Treatment of delayed union and nonunion of a tibial shaft fracture after open reduction internal fixation depends on whether the hardware remains intact or has failed, either by loosening or breakage. If the fixation remains intact and the soft-tissue conditions are satisfactory, then delayed union or nonunion may be treated with bone grafting and maintenance of protected weight bearing. If the internal fixation shows signs of failure, then it will be necessary to remove the hardware and repeat the internal fixation with the addition of bone graft and an additional period of protected weight-bearing ambulation.

ILLUSTRATIVE CASE FOR TECHNIQUE

A 31-year-old man had an isolated fracture of the distal third of his tibia in a domestic altercation. The patient was not seen for examination until 24 hours after his injury. At that time, examination revealed a painful, swollen lower extremity with intact pulses. The muscle compartments in the extremity were soft, and a mild external-rotation deformity of the extremity with mild shortening was noted. Because of the swelling, the extremity was initially immobilized in a bulky Robert–Jones type dressing with the support of a posterior splint, and the extremity was elevated for 10 days on an outpatient basis. Subsequent examination revealed satisfactory resolution of soft-tissue swelling, although posttraumatic ecchymosis remained.

The osteosynthesis was planned as presented earlier. The planning and procedure were as illustrated, and follow-up radiographs are shown here at 12 weeks after full weight bearing for the previous 4 weeks (Fig. 17A and B). Additionally, his soft tissue and wound are shown at the 12-week interval (Fig. 18). This implanted hardware will typically be removed at approximately 18 months after fracture healing.

A, B

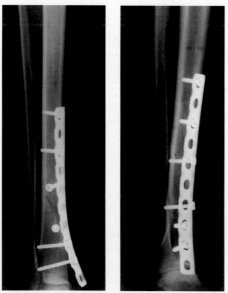

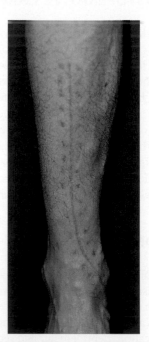

Figure 17. Anteroposterior (AP; **A**) and lateral **(B)** radiographs of the osteosynthesis at 12 weeks. The patient has been full weight bearing for 4 weeks at this point.

Figure 18. The appearance of the surgical scar and the patient's skin and soft tissue at 12 weeks.

RECOMMENDED READING

1. Mast, J., Jakob, R., Ganz, R.: *Planning and Reduction Technique in Fracture Surgery.* Springer-Verlag, Berlin, 1989.
2. Muller, M.R., Allgower, M., Schneider, R., Willenegger, H.: *Manual of Internal Fixation*, 2nd ed. Springer-Verlag, New York, 1979.
3. Oestern, H.J., Tscherne, H.: Pathophysiology and classification of soft tissue injuries associated with fractures. In Tscherne, H., Gotzen, L. (eds.): *Fractures with Soft Tissue Injuries.* Springer-Verlag, Berlin, 1984.
4. Perren, S.M.: Physical and biological aspects of fracture healing with special reference to internal fixation. *Clin. Orthop.,* 138:175–196, 1979.
5. Ruedi, T., von Huchstetter, A., Schlumpf, R.: *Surgical Approaches for Internal Fixation.* Springer-Verlag, Berlin, 1984.
6. Ruedi, T., Webb, J.K., Allgower, M.: Experience with the dynamic compression plate (DCP) in 418 recent fractures of the tibial shaft. *Injury,* 7:252–265, 1976.

Master Techniques in Orthopaedic Surgery,
FRACTURES, edited by D. A. Wiss,
Lippincott–Raven Publishers, Philadelphia © 1998.

26

Tibial-Shaft Fractures: Reamed Intramedullary Nailing

Robert A. Winquist

Fractures of the tibial shaft are associated with more complications than are any other long-bone injury. Nonoperative treatment with casts or braces, while minimizing the risk of infection, often result in unacceptable shortening, malrotation, or angulation. Operative treatment, although it improves alignment and function, is associated with increased rates of infection and nonunion. Plate osteosynthesis of high-energy open or closed tibial-shaft fractures has the highest complication rate, particularly infection. Alternatively, stabilization with an external fixator, although it decreases the infection rate, is associated with poor patient acceptance, repeated surgeries, and angulation after fixator removal. In an effort to improve the overall outcome, many trauma specialists recommend static interlocked intramedullary nailing for unstable displaced closed and open tibial fractures.

There are many variables in defining tibial fractures. The most valuable classifications at this time are the Gustilo Classification for Soft-Tissue Injuries and the OTA Classification for Long Bone Fractures (Fig. 1).

There is no consensus among experts whether the tibia should be minimally reamed or unreamed before nailing. Advantages of intramedullary reaming include placement of a larger nail and screws, which improve alignment and reduce hardware failure rates. Disadvantages include increased endosteal vascular damage (which usually recovers in 6 to 12 weeks), an increased infection rate, risk of thermal necrosis of the bone, and an increased rate of compartment syndrome. Despite these risks, reamed intramedullary nailing is the treatment of choice for unstable closed tibial fractures. In Gustilo Grades I, II, and IIIA open tibial fractures, the predominant method of treatment is a minimally reamed statically locked intramedullary nail (Figs. 2–4). In Grade IIIB and IIIC fractures, treatment is with unreamed statically locked nails or an external fixator.

R. A. Winquist, M.D.: Orthopedic Physician Associates, Seattle, Washington 98104.

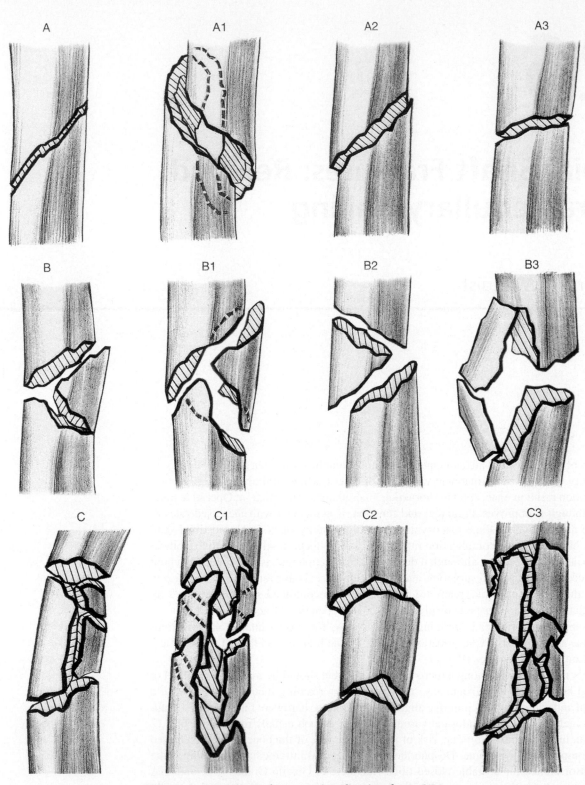

Figure 1. Long-bone fracture classification from OTA.

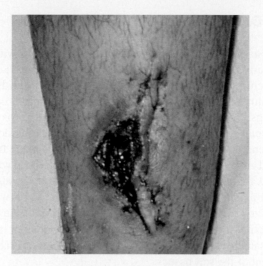

Figure 2. Skin wound of Grade IIIA open fracture.

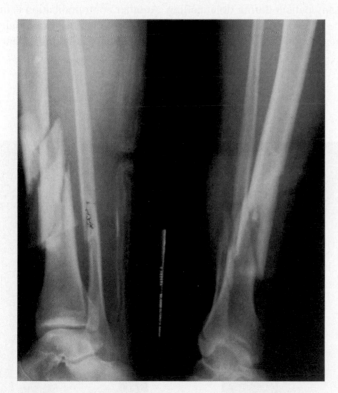

Figure 3. Anteroposterior (AP) and lateral radiographs of comminuted unstable Grade IIIA open fracture.

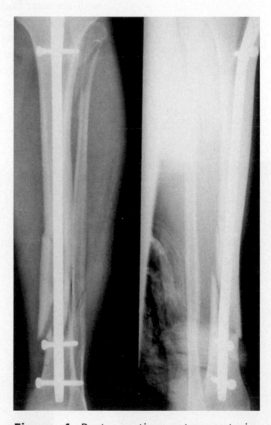

Figure 4. Postoperative anteroposterior (AP) and lateral radiograph with minimally reamed statically interlocked nail.

INDICATIONS/CONTRAINDICATIONS

Stabilization of the tibia is indicated in patients with multiple injuries; an ipsilateral fracture of the femur, ankle, or foot; a vascular injury; compartment syndrome; and bilateral fractures. Fractures located in the middle two-thirds of the tibia, which are amenable to nailing, include transverse, short oblique, spiral, comminuted, and segmental fractures (Figs. 5–8). Indications for nailing may extend proximally or distally, particularly in segmental fractures. Unstable fractures with high-grade soft-tissue injury, whether closed or open, require operative stabilization. Unacceptable fracture position after closed reduction and casting is also an indication for nailing. Those with shortening more than 1.5 to 2.0 cm and angulation in excess of 5 degrees of varus or valgus or 10 degrees of anterior or posterior angulation may be candidates. Tibial fractures with an intact fibula should only be stabilized if there is displacement or angulation of the tibial fracture (Figs. 9 and 10). If the fracture is a minimally or nondisplaced oblique or spiral fracture, nonoperative treatment is satisfactory. Nearly all open fractures require stabilization to allow improved management of the soft tissues.

Contraindications to nailing include immature patients with open epiphyses and a tibial tubercle apophysis. Damage to the apophysis may lead to hyperextension in this group. A lateral radiograph should be carefully inspected, and patients with very small medullary canals may present a hazard in nailing (Fig. 11). If one elects to go ahead with nailing, a small-diameter Ender nail can be placed, or it will be important to have 5-mm-diameter reamers to start the reaming process carefully and not burn bone. A tourniquet should not be used for reaming in any patient during tibial nailing. Another contraindication is infection. Nailing in the face of infection at the wound site carries a high risk for chronic osteomyelitis and decreased union. These patients are better handled with debridement and external fixators.

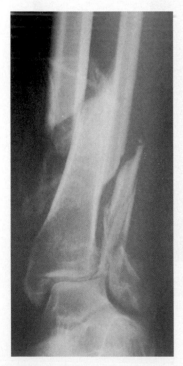

Figure 5. Anteroposterior (AP) radiograph of Grade I open distal tibial fracture and ankle fracture.

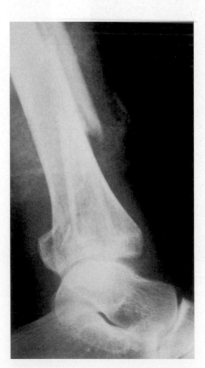

Figure 6. Lateral radiograph showing posterior malleolar fracture.

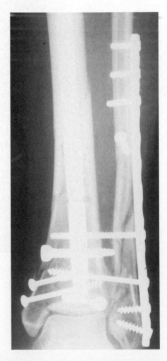

Figure 7. Postoperative anteroposterior (AP) radiograph showing lag screws for ankle fracture and interlocking nail for tibial fracture.

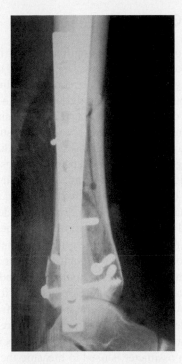

Figure 8. Lateral radiograph showing reduction of posterior malleolus.

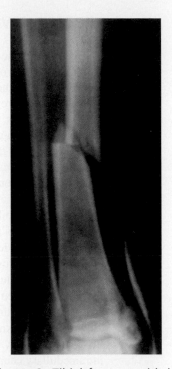

Figure 9. Tibial fracture with intact fibula. Varus angulation and translation indicates operative treatment.

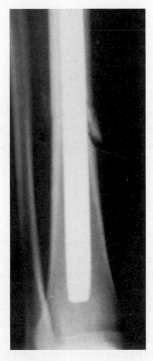

Figure 10. Postoperative anteroposterior (AP) radiograph with nonlocked intramedullary (IM) nail in a stable fracture.

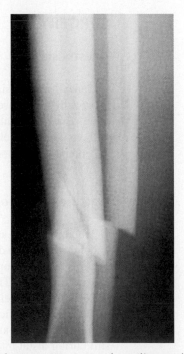

Figure 11. Lateral radiograph demonstrating an extremely small medullary canal. Reaming should be avoided or carried out with very small reamers, starting at 5 mm.

PREOPERATIVE PLANNING

A careful physical examination of the patient is required to look for other injuries. Examination for neurovascular compromise is important. The degree of swelling and any fracture blisters, whether serous or sanguinous, should be recorded. Palpation of the compartment at the fracture site is important to determine the tightness of the compartment. Active motion of the toes, as well as pain on passive stretch and hypesthesia, should be noted. If there is a question of a compartment syndrome, then pressure measurements are of value. It does not appear necessary to delay surgery in patients with a pending compartment syndrome. The intramedullary nailing causes only a transient increase in pressure, which should return to normal rapidly. With careful monitoring, any patient who develops a compartment syndrome preoperatively or postoperatively will still need a release of the compartments and stabilization with a nail. If stabilization of the tibia is delayed, a debridement of open wounds is still necessary. Patients with both closed and open fractures should be splinted in a long-leg splint during the interval between injury and intramedullary nailing.

Patients with closed fractures should be given a cephalosporin for 24 hours surrounding the nailing procedure. Patients with open fractures should be treated with cephalosporins or, in contaminated fractures, cephalosporins and aminoglycosides for 48 hours.

A preoperative anteroposterior (AP) and lateral radiograph of the fractured extremity, including both the knee and the ankle, is critical to define the fracture and geometry of the tibia and the injury. The lateral radiograph should be carefully inspected and the size of the intramedullary canal measured. An ossimeter is used to measure the tibia to establish the length and diameter of the nail required. Positive nail-design features include static and dynamic interlocking holes, oblique holes for proximal fractures, clustered distal holes for distal fractures, and cannulation for ease of placement over a guide wire, as well as for removal if the nail breaks.

SURGERY

Anesthesia

General anesthesia is preferred for tibial nailing. If a spinal is used, it should be very short-acting, because evaluation of the neurologic status and pain level is very important after surgery. A continuous epidural should be avoided in the treatment of tibial fractures. Although it may well benefit the patient from the standpoint of pain relief, it makes clinical compartment monitoring difficult.

Fracture Reduction

Tibial reduction and nailing can be achieved by using a fracture table, a sterile bolster under the knee, or a distractor. A bolster under the knee is the simplest technique and is particularly useful in open fractures that require debridement and reprepping before nailing (Figs. 12 and 13). The knee is flexed over a radiolucent pad, which permits access to the proximal tibia as well as visualization of the starting point. The disadvantage to this method of treatment is difficulty in obtaining and maintaining fracture length in addition to controlling angulation and rotation. It is also difficult for the assistant to hold the leg perfectly still during distal interlocking. The bolster under the knee works best with stable fracture patterns.

A fracture table is more complex to set up but is more effective in maintaining length and rotation. With the fracture table, the knee is flexed 90 degrees over a post, which is placed proximal to the popliteal fossa to prevent compression of the vessels or peroneal nerve (Fig. 14). Tape is placed around the leg to prevent external rotation of the extremity. A fracture table works best in patients with isolated closed injuries of the tibia and is more difficult in patients with multiple traumas or open fractures.

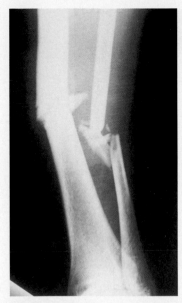

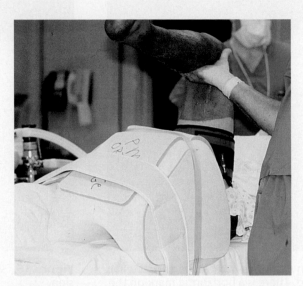

Figure 12. Anteroposterior (AP) radiograph of Grade II open fracture with tibial and fibular fracture at same level.

Figure 13. Foam shoulder immobilizer used for a bolster under the knee.

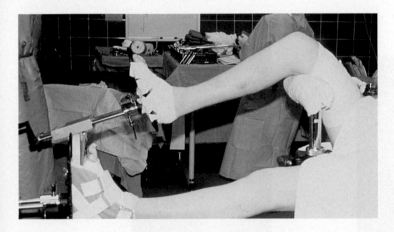

Figure 14. Fracture table with knee flexed 90 degrees and peroneal post against distal thigh, rather than popliteal fossa.

A distractor can be used with a pin placed proximally in the posterior tibia and distally just above the ankle joint. In acute fractures, a unilateral frame is usually adequate. After 10 days to 2 weeks, it becomes more difficult to reobtain length, and a unilateral frame may lead to angulation. Therefore, through-and-through proximal and distal tibial pins are used with a bilateral frame with simultaneous medial and lateral distraction. Compared with a bolster, this method takes longer and is more complex, but it provides good alignment and stability during nailing and interlocking.

Incision and Starting Point

The joint is palpated and marked on the knee. The incision starts at the joint line and extends proximally (Fig. 15). There is no need for an incision that goes distally down to the tibial tubercle. For fractures of the midshaft or below, the incision and starting point is just medial to the patellar tendon. The joint is palpated, and the awl is inserted where the ante-

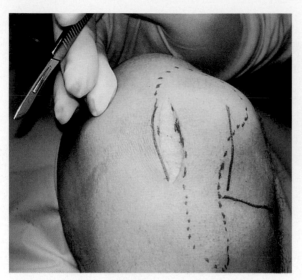

Figure 15. Skin marking with patella and patellar tendon outlined. There is a horizontal mark on the lateral joint line and a longitudinal mark on the lateral border of the patellar tendon, with a medial incision over the medial border of the patellar tendon. The incision starts at the joint line and proceeds proximally.

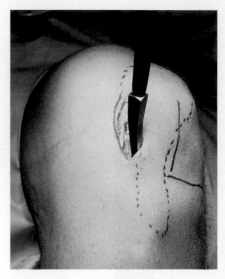

Figure 16. Sharp awl inserted in incision.

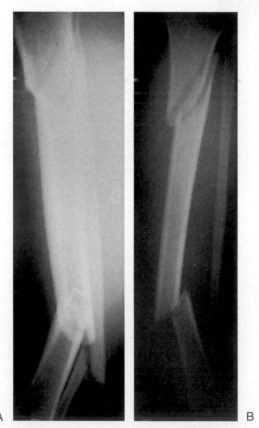

Figure 17. A, B: Segmental tibial fracture.

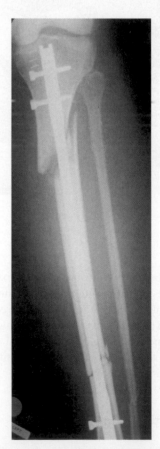

Figure 18. Malalignment of proximal component of segmental fracture with surgical starting point too far medial.

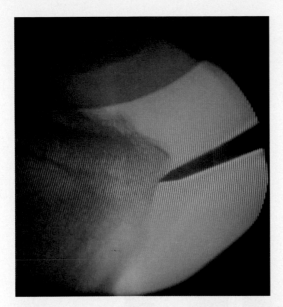

Figure 19. Lateral radiograph with awl slightly inferior to correct starting point.

rior tibia reaches the joint (Fig. 16). It is important to stay extraarticular, because backout of the nail may impinge on the femoral condyle. It is equally important not to enter down at the tibial tubercle, as this leads to a more oblique anterior-to-posterior starting angle with a greater risk of penetration of the posterior cortex with the nail. In proximal fractures, the incision and starting point is just lateral to the patellar tendon (Figs. 17 and 18). It is important to use a sharp, curved tibial awl and to check its position in both the AP and lateral planes with an image intensifier before portal placement. On the lateral radiograph, the point of the awl should be just inferior to the joint line (Fig. 19). On the AP view, it should be in line with the long axis of the tibia (Fig. 20). In proximal fractures, it is helpful to stay a little more lateral and to run the nail abutting against the lateral cortex, to help prevent both translation and angulation. The Synthes (Synthes, Paoli, PA) unreamed nail has been a particular problem in proximal tibial fractures because of its long and distal curve in the nail, which can lead to both translation and angulation of the fracture site (Fig. 21). In proximal fractures, temporary stabilization with a clamp or small plate is sometimes necessary.

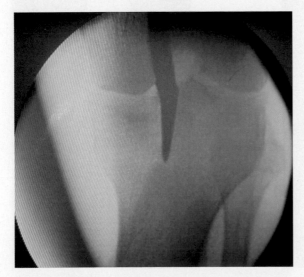

Figure 20. Anteroposterior (AP) radiograph showing the awl is slightly medial.

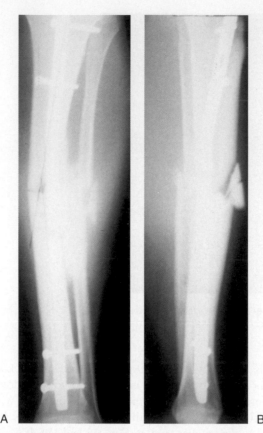

A   B

Figure 21. A, B: Postoperative radiograph of comminuted proximal tibial
fracture with AO nail. The long Herzog
curve with some external rotation of the
nail has created a deformity.

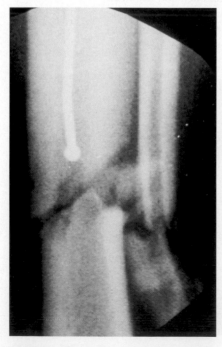

Figure 22. Bulb tip approaching
fracture site.

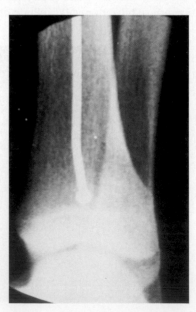

Figure 23. Bulb tip down to
subchondral bone.

Bulb-Tip Guide

A bulb-tip guide wire is inserted down the canal. It is helpful to place a small bend in the guide wire 2 cm from the tip. This often facilitates passing of the wire across the fracture site. A T-handle, which is used to control the bulb-tip guide, is placed in the midportion of the guide. The bulb tip is initially aimed posteriorly to enter the tibia and then immediately turned anteriorly and passed down to the fracture site, avoiding penetration of the posterior cortex proximally or exiting through the fracture site posteriorly. The guide wire is advanced to the fracture site and, under biplanar image intensification, passed into the distal fragment (Fig. 22). It is impacted into the subchondral bone above the ankle to stabilize the bulb tip and to aid in determining length (Fig. 23). A second bulb tip, of identical length, is placed at the joint line, and a long ruler is used to determine nail length. Another method to determine the nail length is to measure the tibia externally with a long ruler, with hatch marks, and confirm it with the image intensifier.

Reaming

Reaming is a critical part of the surgical technique and must be done well to avoid complications (Figs. 24 and 25). Reaming must be done with sharp cutting reamers that dissipate heat and pressure. To prevent soft-tissue damage around the incision, a skin protector should be used. A tourniquet should be avoided. Because the risk of heat necrosis increases during reaming, it should be carried out at a low torque with sharp reamers that dissipate heat (Fig. 26). The surgeon should start with a small-diameter reamer and increase in half-millimeter increments until cortical contact is reached. For closed fractures, reaming one additional millimeter is usually all that is necessary. The fracture must be reduced as the

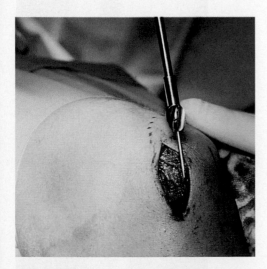

Figure 24. Reamer inserted over bulb tip.

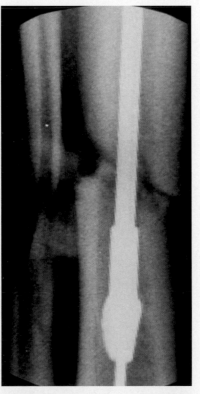

Figure 25. Reamer passed across fracture to metaphyseal flare. Minimal reaming in Grade I open fracture.

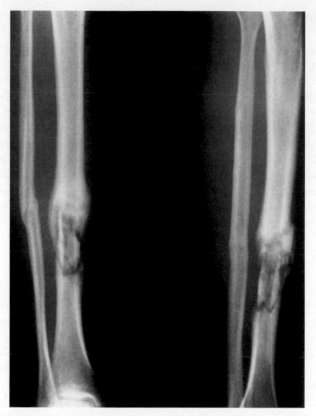

Figure 26. Heat necrosis of tibia.

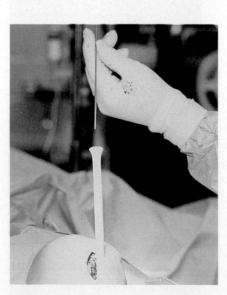

Figure 27. Exchange tube with nail-driving guide.

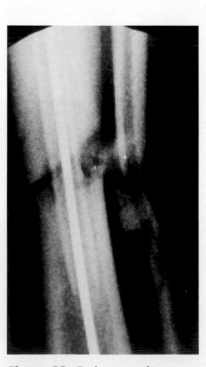

Figure 28. Exchange tube on radiograph seen crossing the fracture site.

reamer passes (aided by the bulb-tip guide). If the canal diameter permits, it is mechanically beneficial to place a nail that is 10 mm in diameter or larger. Excessive reaming should not be done to achieve this, particularly in open fractures. If necessary, an 8- or 9-mm nail may be used. However, with smaller nails, the patient's postoperative management must be modified. The patient should be kept non–weight bearing until there is evidence of healing and, if healing is slow, considered for dynamization or nail exchange. Several investigators suggested that reaming can increase the possibility of a compartment syndrome. At the conclusion of nailing, the compartments should be palpated, and if any concern exists, the compartment pressure can be measured again and over the next 48 hours.

Exchange Tube

Before nail insertion, a plastic exchange tube is passed over the bulb tip and across the fracture site (Figs. 27 and 28). Once the bulb tip is removed, a non–bulb-tip nail-driving guide is inserted, and the plastic tube is removed. The nail is driven over this guide wire. Because the reduction can be maintained with this guide, it is important to use cannulated nails. Rarely does the fracture site have to be open to pass the nail. Solid nails offer no mechanical advantage nor do they decrease the risk of infection compared with cannulated nails. However, in my experience, solid nails make the passage of the nail less predictable and the removal of a broken nail extremely difficult.

Nail Insertion

Insert the nail over the guide wire. It is important to push posteriorly on the proximal end of the nail to minimize penetration of the posterior cortex (Fig. 29). A lateral image should be used while driving the nail in the upper one third of the tibia. As the nail approaches the fracture, the fracture must be aligned in two planes (Fig. 30). The nail must be inserted in slight external rotation. If the nail is allowed to rotate internally, interlocking will take place on the posteromedial cortex proximally and distally, which is much more difficult than if

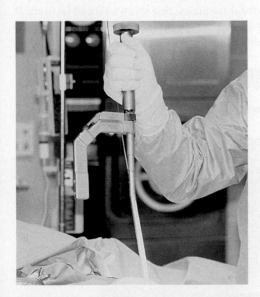

Figure 29. Nail inserted into the proximal tibia with hand pulling the nail posteriorly, to push the tip of the nail anteriorly.

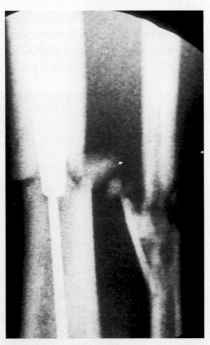

Figure 30. Nail crossing the fracture site.

carried out on the flat surface of the tibia. Therefore to make targeting an easier process, the nail should be externally rotated approximately 10 degrees in relation to the long axis of the tibia.

As the nail crosses the fracture site, it is important to avoid distraction. Overreaming by 1 mm is helpful. In stable fracture patterns, traction should be released when the tip of the nail is 1 cm past the fracture. This should then allow impaction and avoid distraction. Distal counterpressure may be necessary as the nail crosses the fracture, to prevent distraction. Because tibial nails are small and the screw diameters are small, the application of a distal screw with the back-slap technique carries a risk of early fatigue of the distal locking screws. As the nail is driven down the tibia, it is important to reassess the accuracy of its length. The tibia should be inspected proximally and distally. If the nail is too short or too long, then it should be removed and replaced with another nail. In distal fractures, the nail should reach the subchondral bone. The nail should not be countersunk into the proximal tibia for more than 2 to 3 mm, or later extraction will be difficult. Howmedica and Zimmer nails have nail extenders, which can be beneficial for making small adjustments in length.

Insertion of Proximal Screws

Targeting devices that attach to the intramedullary nail are very successful in placing the proximal tibial locking screws (Fig. 31). Anterior–posterior screws have a slight risk of injury to vascular structures and should be avoided if possible (Fig. 32). Oblique screws for proximal fractures are safer. Only one proximal screw is necessary for fractures in the midshaft and below (Fig. 33). For proximal fractures, two screws are necessary in the proximal end of the nail. For stable transverse or short oblique tibial fractures, the use of a dynamic slot at the proximal end of the nail is beneficial to allow impaction of the fracture. If there is any sign of comminution or a spiral component to the fracture, the nail should be statically locked.

Distal Screw Insertion

I prefer the freehand technique of distal screw insertion because none of the other guides is consistently helpful. For fractures in the middle to the proximal half of the tibia, only a single distal screw is necessary, whereas in distal fractures, two screws should be used. It is possible to use a medial–lateral screw and an anterior–posterior screw, but the latter requires attention to both the anterior tibial tendon and posterior vascular structures.

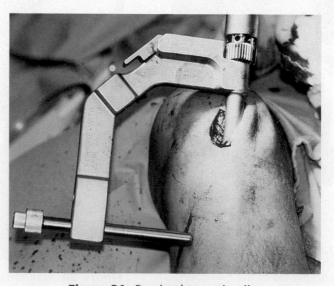

Figure 31. Proximal targeting jig.

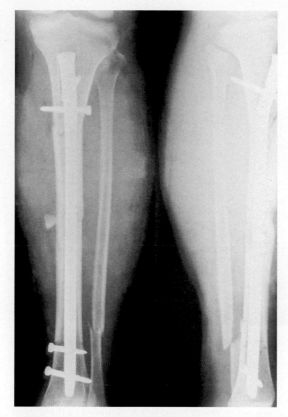

Figure 32. Anterior-to-posterior screw with risk of vascular injury.

It should be emphasized that the nail should be externally rotated 10 degrees to allow targeting on a flat surface. The freehand technique requires, first, targeting of the skin incision. The image intensifier is lined up with the nail and tilted and rotated until a perfectly round hole is visualized. It is best to use an image intensifier that can magnify the hole 2 times its normal size. It is helpful also to move the C-arm head away from the tibia to in-

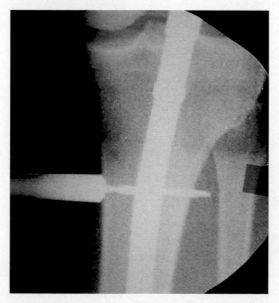

Figure 33. Depth gauge to measure screw length.

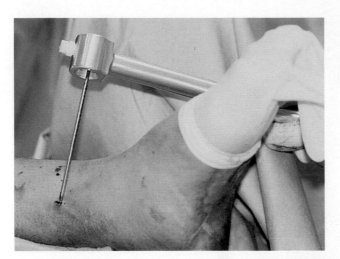

Figure 34. Sharp trochar to mark skin incision.

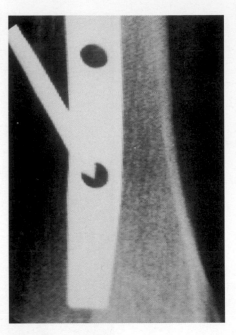

Figure 35. Trochar in center of inter-locking hole.

crease the working space and aid in magnification of the hole. The sharp point of the trochar-tipped pin is placed on the skin until it is centered in the hole (Fig. 34). A 1-cm stab wound is made directly over the hole on the medial aspect of the tibia. Because the saphenous vein is very close to the targeted area, laceration is possible. The sharp point guide is again placed on the bone until it is centered in the hole (Fig. 35). It is brought into the longitudinal axis and checked with fluoroscopy to ensure that it is centered in all planes (Fig.

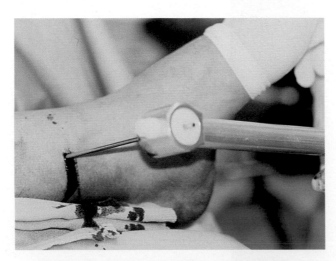

Figure 36. Trochar brought in axis of the hole.

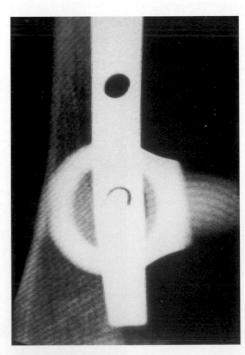

Figure 37. Fluoroscopy to be certain that trochar is centered.

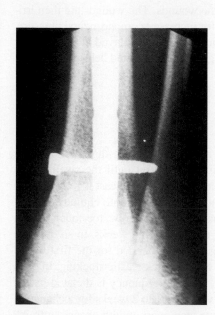

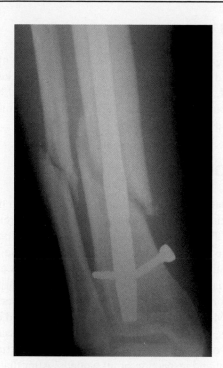

Figure 38. Screw, 5 mm, in case of future breakage.

Figure 39. Broken screw.

36); a halo should be evident around the guide (Fig. 37). The sharp point is then passed into the tibia with a mallet and then removed. The drill bit is then placed freehand through the hole and through the nail. The AP view is checked, and the lateral tibia is drilled and measured for placement of the screw. It is important to use a screw that is 5 mm too long, as this will make removal of a broken screw easier (Fig. 38). The screw should protrude through the cortex; if the screw is not prominent, then it will be very difficult to retrieve if breakage occurs (Fig. 39). A lateral radiograph should be checked again, to be absolutely certain the screw is in the nail and has not moved anteriorly or posteriorly (Fig. 40).

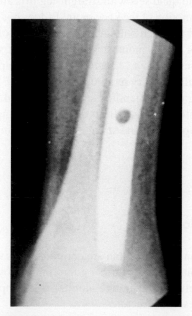

Figure 40. Lateral radiograph, to be certain that distal screw is centered in the hole.

Wound Closure

A long-acting local anesthetic is injected into all the wounds. The wounds are then irrigated and closed. If necessary, the patient is checked for increased compartmental pressure. Grades I, II, and IIIA fractures are left open and brought back for delayed closure. Grade IIIB fractures are scheduled for return to the operating room for repeated debridements and early flap coverage.

POSTOPERATIVE MANAGEMENT

The patient is placed in a posterior splint with the ankle neutral or in slight dorsiflexion to prevent an equinus deformity. The patient remains in a splint until the swelling decreases. This may take as little as 1 week or as long as 6 weeks. If the cast is removed too early, the patient tends to be more uncomfortable, and the foot drops into equinus. In a reliable patient with a stable fracture pattern and a dynamic locking screw, toe-touch weight bearing is desirable with progressive weight bearing over the first 4 weeks. In an unstable pattern or an unreliable patient, non–weight bearing is recommended for the first 6 to 8 weeks. Mild swelling of the leg can be controlled by using a thick elastic stocking. In open fractures, continued wound monitoring is necessary, and the frequency is dictated by the severity of the wound. The first postoperative office visit is in 1 to 2 weeks for a change of the splint and inspection of all wounds. After that, one visit every month occurs, with AP and lateral radiographs taken until the fracture is healed. If there is a question of healing after 2 to 4 months, oblique radiographs may be necessary the better to ascertain the healing. Weight bearing is usually started at 2 months if callus is evident. In addition to looking for callus, it is important to look also for broken screws or broken nails. These signify instability and require a change in treatment. If a screw is broken in a fairly stable fracture pattern, this may lead to healing, and no further treatment will be necessary. If screw breakage occurs in an unstable fracture pattern, shortening will result, as well as a high possibility for a nonunion. The treatment should be changed in that patient population.

Healing is slow in the tibia, and patients should be informed of the length of the process. They rarely have realistic expectations because of lack of realistic knowledge. Postoperative knee pain is almost universal and calms down over 4 to 6 months. Physical therapy is required for gait training and quad sets with straight-leg lifts and active range of motion of the ankle. Passive range of motion of the knee or ankle does not appear to be beneficial, and resistive range of motion of the knee only increases the patellofemoral pain. Most patients require external support for 2 to 4 months. Walking without support gradually increases over 4 to 6 months after injury, with a very gradual loss of limp. Return to running usually requires 6 to 12 months. Full recovery requires a minimum of 1.5 to 2 years. Patients may return to activity according to their comfort levels. In general, they should return slowly, because they are osteoporotic and weak from disuse. Bicycling and swimming are gentle forms of exercise to build up muscle and strength before moving into more difficult sports.

COMPLICATIONS

Delayed Union/Nonunion

Delayed union and nonunion of the tibia are common. This is related to the poor vascular envelope around the tibia, which is further compromised by the injury. Implant failure is common. Therefore careful postoperative monitoring is important, and further surgical procedures are expected in severe fractures.

Dynamization is an excellent choice of treatment for fractures that are slow to heal at 2 or 3 months and have stable fracture patterns that will not lead to excessive shortening or rotation. If callus is not evident at 2 to 3 months in this group, then removal of screws at the end of the nail farthest from the fracture is beneficial. Bone grafting is used in patients with a defect. This is most effective when done in a delayed manner. Six to 8 weeks appears to be an ideal time. Because these are unstable fractures and will shorten, a static nail should be left in place. Exchange nailing also is used in these patients. Its ideal indication is for patients who were initially stabilized with small-diameter nails and screws. Two to 3 months after injury, when the soft tissues are well healed, a new exchange nail is placed with a larger diameter and may or may not be statically locked, depending on the fracture pattern.

Hardware Failure

Screw failure occurs in 10% to 40% of statically locked tibial nails. Weaker screws are those with smaller diameter and those made of titanium. If screw failure occurs in a stable pattern, then no surgery is required, and the fracture will go on to heal. In unstable fracture patterns, including distal fractures, screw breakage is frequently stage I, before nail breakage. In these patients, the broken screws should be removed, and larger nails should be inserted, with larger screws in either a static or dynamic mode. Nail breakage occurs in 5% to 10% of the fractures. This generally occurs after 3 to 4 months. Broken nails should be exchanged. In cannulated nails with a large diameter, a hook can be used for removal. In small-diameter cannulated nails, a bulb-tip guide with a smooth guide rod alongside it can be used to remove the distal fragment. In solid nails, removal of the distal fragment is extremely difficult, and I would advise against the insertion of solid nails in the femur or the tibia.

Infection

Infection after nailing should be subclassified into acute and chronic. In acute infections within a week of surgery, debridement and drainage is the treatment of choice. The nail can be left in place, and 6 weeks of parenteral antibiotics is used. If the infection settles down, the nail is left in place, and the patient is allowed to go on to healing. If healing is slow, posterolateral bone grafting may be necessary.

If the infection is chronic, then there is usually a segmental sequestrum. In these patients, the nail frequently has to be removed and a segment of tibia removed to eradicate the infection. These patients are then placed in external fixators and require cancellous bone grafting for small defects and segmental transport for large defects. Antibiotics are once again necessary and should be parenteral for at least 6 weeks.

Compartment Syndrome

Compartment syndromes are always difficult to diagnose. They generally occur within the first 48 hours of injury but can be seen as late as 5 days after injury. Frequent physical examination in the awake patient is the most reliable diagnostic technique, and pressure measurements in the comatose and uncooperative patient are the best diagnostic technique. Multiple pressure measurements are particularly beneficial to see whether there is a trend. In institutions with frequent monitoring capabilities, the compartment pressure can increase to within 30 mm Hg of diastolic pressure before a compartment release is done. In situations in which coverage is not as good at night or on the weekends, then release of compartment at lower pressure and with early findings is advised. A four-compartment fasciotomy can be performed through either a single lateral incision or a lateral and posteromedial incision. The posteromedial incision is particularly important for distal injuries.

ILLUSTRATIVE CASE FOR TECHNIQUE

This 38-year-old man was involved in a ski accident. He suffered a high proximal oblique metaphyseal tibial fracture and an oblique distal tibial fracture at the junction of the middle and distal one thirds (Fig. 41). The distal fracture was a Gustilo Grade IIIA open, which did not require a flap. He was treated with primary debridement of the open fracture with temporary stabilization by using an external fixator and a primary plate and screw fixation of the proximal tibial fracture (Fig. 42). The wound was allowed to heal and the soft tissue swelling to decrease. Five weeks after injury, the external fixator was removed, and there was a 1-week delay before nailing the tibia, to try to prevent infection. The proximal plate was then removed, and both the proximal and distal fractures were fixed by using a metaphyseal–diaphyseal (MD) nail without distal interlocking. At that time, it was believed that shortening and rotation would not be a problem. The proximal fracture, however, was stabilized with two oblique proximal screws that fit high in the tibia and are ideal for this fracture (Fig. 43). Both fractures went on to excellent healing without infection, and the patient has a full range of motion of the ankle and knee with only minimal aching in the tibia. Another treatment option is primary nailing on the day of injury. Proper reduction of the proximal fracture is always difficult, and reamed versus unreamed nailing of the distal tibial open fracture remains controversial.

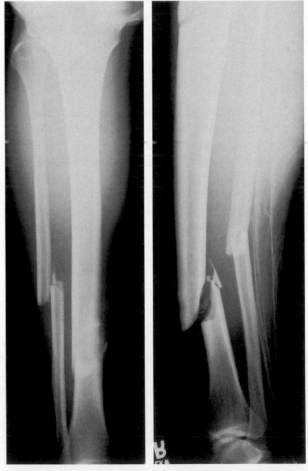

Figure 41. A, B: Anteroposterior (AP) and lateral radiographs of the tibia on the day of injury. This shows displacement of the distal fracture representing soft-tissue injury and a very high, slightly oblique proximal fracture.

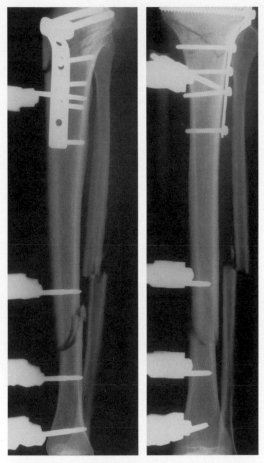

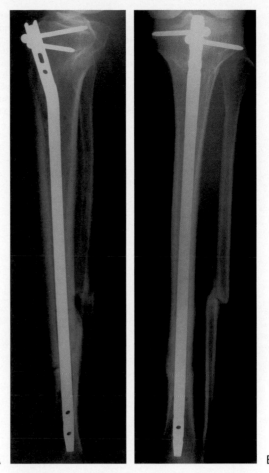

Figure 42. A, B: Postoperative anteroposterior (AP) and lateral radiographs on the day of injury. A proximal tibial T-plate is in position with an external fixator for the distal open fracture.

Figure 43. A, B: Six months after injury, there is complete healing on the anteroposterior (AP) and partial healing on the lateral radiographs. The nail has stabilized both fractures.

RECOMMENDED READING

1. Blick, S.S., Brumback, R.J., Lakatos, R., Poka, A., Burgess, A.R.: Early prophylactic bone grafting of high-energy tibial fractures. *Clin. Orthop.,* 240(3):21–41, 1989.
2. Bone, L.B., and Johnson, K.D.: Treatment of tibia fractures by reaming and intramedullary nailing. *J. Bone Joint Surg. [Am],* 68(6):877–887, 1986.
3. Browner, B.D.: Pitfalls, errors and complications in the use of locking Kuntscher nails. *Clin. Orthop.,* 212:192–208, 1986.
4. Carr, J.B.: Use of the reamed nail in tibial shaft fractures. In Cardea, J.A. (ed.): *Operative Techniques in Orthopaedics.* WB Saunders, Philadelphia, 1991, pp. 319–325.
5. Collins, D.N., Pearce, C.E., McAndrew, M.P.: Successful use of reaming and intramedullary nailing of the tibia. *J. Orthop. Trauma,* 4:315–322, 1990.
6. Court-Brown, D.M.: The clinical results of reamed intramedullary nailing. *Tech. Orthop.,* 11(1):79–85, 1996.
7. Gustilo, R.B., Mendoza, R.M., Williams, D.N.: Problems in the management of type III (severe) open fractures: a new classification of type III open fractures. *J. Trauma,* 24:742, 1984.
8. Henley, M.B.: Intramedullary devices for tibial fracture stabilization. *Clin. Orthop.,* 240:87–96, 1989.
9. Henley, M.B., Champman, J.R., Agel, J., Swiontkowski, M.F., Whorton, A.M.: Treatment of type II, IIIA and IIIB open fractures of the tibial shaft: a randomized prospective comparison of unreamed interlocking nails and half-pin external fixators. *J. Orthop. Trauma,* 12:1–7, 1998.
10. Leunig, M., and Hertel, R.: Thermal necrosis after tibial reaming for intramedullary nail fixation. *J. Bone Joint Surg. [Br],* 78(4):584–587, 1996.
11. McQueen, M.M.: Intramedullary reaming and compartment pressure. *Tech. Orthop.,* 11(1):41–44, 1996.
12. Muller, C., McIff, T., Rahn, B.A., Pfister, U., Weller, S.: Intramedullary pressure strain on the diaphysis and increase in cortical temperature when reaming. *Injury Suppl,* 3:31, 1993.
13. Rhinelander, F.W.: Tibial blood supply in relation to fracture healing. *Clin. Orthop.,* 105:34, 1974.
14. Schendelmaier, P., Kettek, P., Tscherne, H.: Biomechanical study of nine different tibial locking nails. *J. Orthop. Trauma,* 10(1):37–44, 1996.

15. Swiontkowski, M.F.: Tibial shaft fractures. In Hansen, S.T., Swiontkowski, M.F. (eds.): *Orthopaedic Trauma Protocols.* Raven Press, New York, 1993.

16. Tornetta, P., III, Berman, M., Watnik, N., Berkowitz, G., Steuer, J.: Treatment of grade IIIB open tibial fractures. *J. Bone Joint Surg. [Br],* 76(1):13–19, 1994.

17. Trafton, P.G.: Tibial shaft fractures. In Browner, B.D., Jupiter, J.B., Levine, A.M., Trafton, P.G. (eds.): *Skeletal Trauma.* Saunders, Philadelphia, 1992, pp. 1809–1821.

18. Whittle, A.P., Russell, T.A., Taylor, J.C., Lavelle, D.G.: Treatment of open fractures of the tibial shaft with the use of interlocking nailing without reaming. *J. Bone Joint Surg. [Am],* 74(8):1162–1171, 1992.

19. Wiss, D.A.: Flexible medullary nailing of acute tibial shaft fractures. *Clin. Orthop.,* 212:122–132, 1986.

Master Techniques in Orthopaedic Surgery,
FRACTURES, edited by D. A. Wiss,
Lippincott–Raven Publishers, Philadelphia © 1998.

27

Tibial-Shaft Fractures: Small-Diameter Tibial Nailing

Kenneth D. Johnson

INDICATIONS/CONTRAINDICATIONS

Tibial nailing with or without minimal reaming is a surgical technique that has been available to orthopedic surgeons since the early 1950s. Flexible Ender nails (Fig. 1A), originating in Austria, and the semirigid Lottes nails (Fig. 1B), originating in the United States, became popular in the treatment of open tibial-shaft fractures beginning in the late 1970s and early 1980s. At that time, external fixation was considered the treatment of choice or "gold standard" for open tibial-shaft fractures. However, it was not until the early 1980s, with the development of small-diameter intramedullary nails with locking capabilities, that tibial nailing gained widespread acceptance. With information developed by Lottes, Velasco, Holbrook, and others, tremendous interest soon developed regarding the use of small-diameter intramedullary nails in open tibial fractures (5,9,13,14).

Intramedullary nailing of high-energy tibial fractures, although attractive from a mechanical perspective, has many biological weaknesses. Studies using reamed intramedullary nails in open tibial-shaft fractures showed a significant risk of infection (1). This is likely due to the additional tissue damage incurred by repeated reaming, which causes heat generation, compromise of the bone and soft-tissue blood supply, and impaction of the Haversian canals with the products of reaming, thereby slowing revascularization. Therefore in a limb that has already sustained significant injury (the open fracture), the additional insult of reaming compounds tissue damage. The consequences of intramedullary reaming may be enough to overcome the local immune system and prevent it from eliminating bacteria that remain in the open wound. In a normal-size adult, small-diameter tibial nailing can be done with the minimum of reaming. Penetrating the intramedullary canal with a single pass of a reamer, sound, or nail appears to cause the same basic insult to the endosteal blood supply (12). The damage caused by repeated passage of

K.D. Johnson, M.D.: Department of Orthopaedic Surgery, Vanderbilt University Medical Center, Nashville, Tennessee 37212.

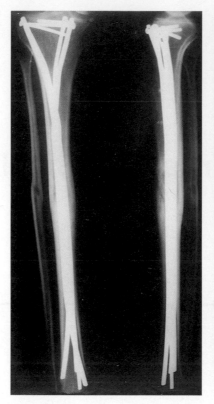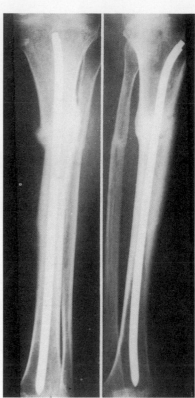

Figure 1. A: Ender nail radiograph. **B:** Lottes nail radiograph.

A,

the reamer as it enlarges the endosteal bone diameter causes the additional insult, predisposing the open tibia fracture to infection (10).

The prime indication for a small-diameter intramedullary nail in the tibia is in the treatment of open tibial-shaft fractures. The technique is most effective when applied to Grades I, II, and IIIA open tibial-shaft fractures (Fig. 2A–C). Tibial nailing should be used with great reservation in Grades IIIB and IIIC open tibial-shaft fractures because of the risk of complications, particularly infection (Fig. 2D; 3). The procedure has been compared with external fixation, both prospectively and retrospectively (4,5,9,11,13,17).

Small-diameter tibial nailing is indicated also for stabilization of tibial-shaft fractures associated with compartment syndromes (15). Immediate fracture stabilization facilitates management of the fasciotomy wounds, minimizing additional pain and disability. Unreamed or small-diameter tibial nails are occasionally indicated in closed tibial fractures with high-grade soft-tissue injuries (Tscherne C-4), in which reaming may be unattractive (7).

Another good indication for small-diameter tibial nailing is in the management of distal-third tibia fractures with extension of the fracture into or near the ankle (Fig. 3A). If the ankle fracture is minimally displaced and there is no joint impaction, a small-diameter intramedullary nail may be an excellent option for treatment (Fig. 3B). This often requires either percutaneous or open reduction of the periarticular fracture to prevent displacement during nail insertion. The use of this device may simplify a difficult and complex treatment problem (Fig. 3C and D).

Small-diameter intramedullary nails also have been effective in managing tibial fractures in patients with small skeletons. The small skeleton is common in certain ethnic groups (Asians, Hispanics), in occasional neurologic disorders (after poliomyelitis), and in some female patients (Fig. 4).

There are multiple contraindications to the use of small-diameter/unreamed tibial nails. These relate mostly to their diminished mechanical strength. Because of their smaller diameter (both the nail and cross-locking bolts), they are more prone to fatigue failure than

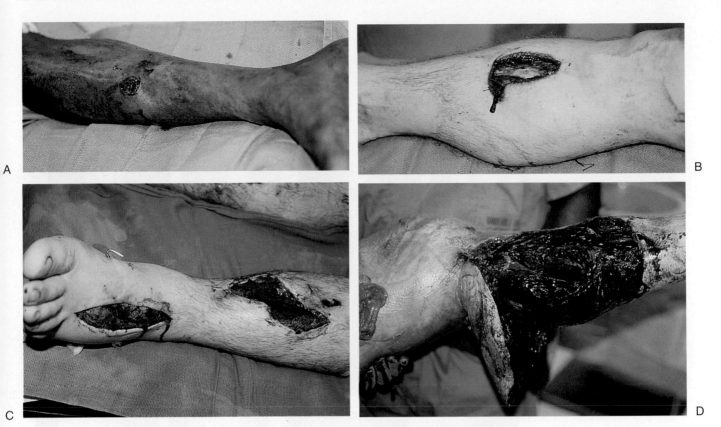

Figure 2. Open tibial-shaft fractures. **A:** Grade I. **B:** Grade II. **C:** Grade IIIA. **D:** Grade IIIB.

are larger nails with larger bolts after reamed nailing (6,18). Therefore these nails are not recommended when nailing displaced closed tibial-shaft fractures because they require additional support (casts, braces, or non–weight bearing) to prevent hardware failure (Fig. 5). By far the most commonly encountered pattern of hardware failure is bolt or screw breakage, either proximally, distally, or both (2,4,11,17). To facilitate removal in the event that they break, the cross-locking bolts should be inserted penetrating the opposite cortex by 2 to 4 mm. Nail breakage is a far greater problem. Removal of a broken intramedullary nail from the tibia can be an extremely difficult task, particularly if this nail is solid.

Another contraindication to the use of tibial nails is in skeletally immature individuals. Adolescents with an open proximal tibial epiphysis and tubercle apophysis may develop leg-length discrepancies or angular deformities, particularly recurvatum, after nailing if the proximal tibial growth center is injured. The proximal tibial apophysis is essentially the starting point for the nail.

The most common and certainly the most controversial contraindication to the use of an intramedullary implant is high-grade open tibial-shaft fractures (1,2,14). Not enough scientific studies have proven the efficacy of tibial nails in Grade IIIB open tibial-shaft fractures, particularly those that require repeated debridements to assure a clean wound with eventual flap coverage. Grade IIIC open tibial-shaft fractures are probably best treated initially with an external fixator or immediate amputation. In successfully revascularized limbs, there is increasing evidence to show that temporary external fixation for a period of 7 to 10 days may be an excellent way to manage these complex injuries before conversion to a small-diameter intramedullary nail. This technique, although promising, is unproven and awaits further clinical trials.

A small-diameter tibial nail should not be used for large segmental defects in the tibia. If an open tibial fracture has a defect greater than 4 cm, the bone grafting and prolonged incorporation will delay recovery and increase the potential for hardware failure. Alternative methods of treatment should be selected, such as external fixation and bone transport. Small-diameter nails can be used for cortical defects and small segmental defects of less

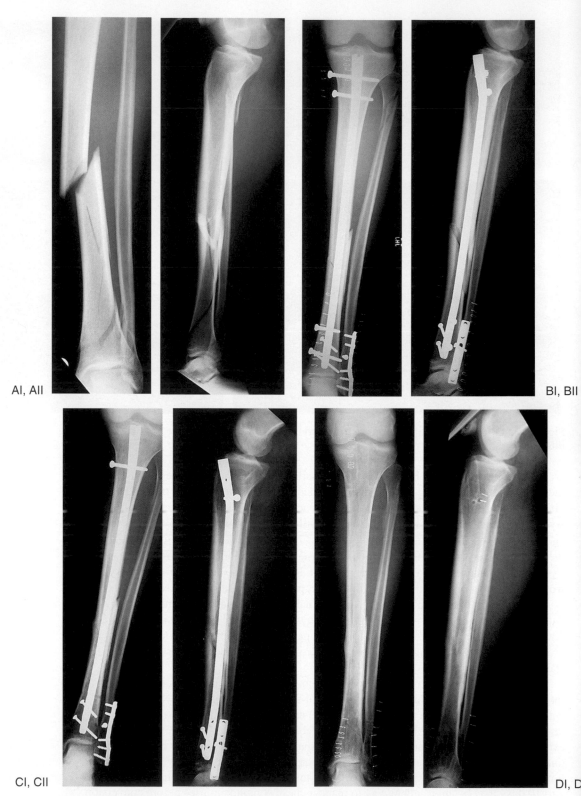

AI, AII

BI, BII

CI, CII

DI, D

Figure 3. A 30-year-old man struck by an automobile sustaining a Grade IIIA open tibial-shaft fracture. **AI, AII:** Anteroposterior (AP) and lateral radiograph of acute fracture. **BI, BII:** Radiographs of postoperative reconstruction. **CI, CII:** Early healing after removal of distal locking bolts. **DI, DII:** Radiographs after hardware removal.

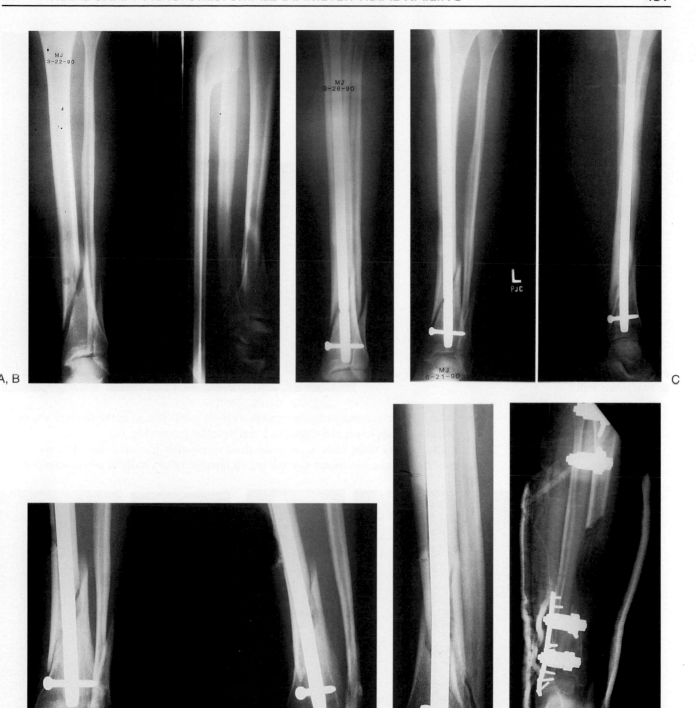

Figure 4. A 55-year-old woman after poliomyelitis who fractured her left tibia while skiing. **A:** Acute fracture, anteroposterior (AP) and lateral (note 5- to 6-mm canal diameter on lateral radiograph). **B:** After a difficult reamed intramedullary nailing, a 9-mm intramedullary nail has been installed. **C:** Three months after injury with necrotic ulcer over tibia, necrotic bone at fracture site, and no evidence of healing. **DI, DII:** Note ulcer just proximal to fracture at 4 months after injury. **E:** After segmental resection.

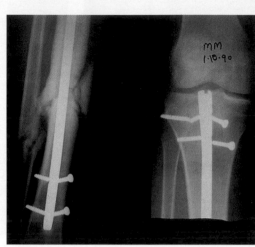

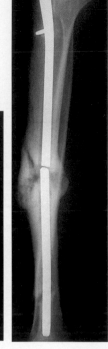

Figure 5. Hardware failure. **A:** Fractured bolts. **B:** Fractured nail.

than 4 cm. These generally require cancellous bone grafts placed at the fracture site or by a posterolateral approach at 6 weeks to 3 months after injury (Fig. 6).

Small-diameter tibial nails in proximal-third tibial-shaft fractures should be used with caution. Experience has shown that the use of intramedullary nails of any diameter in the

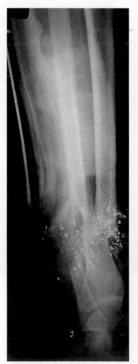
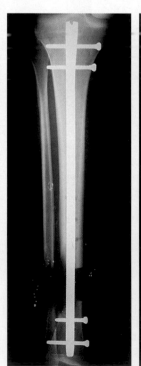
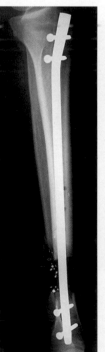
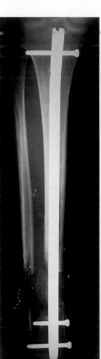
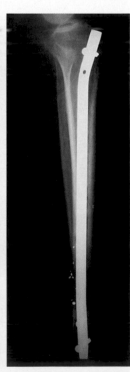

A, BI, BII

Figure 6. A 26-year-old man with an open tibial fracture due to close-range (6 to 10 feet) handgun injury to the distal third of his tibia. **A:** Lateral radiograph of acute injury. **BI, BII:** Postoperative reconstruction of tibia after appropriate bone and soft-tissue debridement. **CI, CII:** After cancellous bone graft to segmental defect 5 months after injury and soft-tissue coverage.

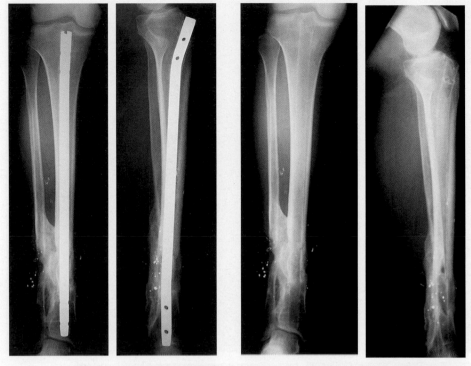

1, DII   EI, EII

Figure 6. *(continued.)* **DI, DII:** Repeated bone graft (posterolateral approach) and exchange nail (larger diameter) at 1 year after injury. **EI, EII:** Healed tibia after hardware removal at 16 months after injury.

proximal-third shaft of the tibia is difficult because of malalignment resulting from a poor portal of entry or muscle imbalance. In several studies, the complication rate with the use of a small-diameter nail in proximal tibial fractures was substantially higher than that with routine tibial-shaft fractures (8). If a nail is to be used, an open nailing with anatomic reduction of the proximal fracture may be indicated.

PREOPERATIVE PLANNING

Preoperative planning should include a careful evaluation of the patient in the emergency room. Radiographs should include an anteroposterior (AP) and lateral view of the tibia, as well as radiographs of the knee or ankle, to determine presence or absence of extension of the fracture proximally or distally. If fracture comminution leads to difficulty in determining overall length (Fig. 7), it may be helpful to obtain a radiograph of the contralateral intact tibia with a radiopaque marking device (Fig. 7C). From a practical point of view, it is easier clinically to measure length in the intact tibia. Regardless of the method used, it is important to consider how length will be determined before surgery, particularly in the comminuted tibial-shaft fracture.

Open fractures should be carefully evaluated and the fracture wound classified according to Gustilo and Anderson (3). If the wound is grossly contaminated and will require repeated debridements to obtain clean, healthy viable tissue margins, small-diameter nailing may be contraindicated. The neurovascular status of the leg should be carefully documented as well. Canal diameter in both AP and lateral projections should be measured preoperatively by using ossimeters that account for magnification (Fig. 4). Excessive power reaming that may be required to fit a nail that is significantly too large can be a disaster.

When scheduling the case with the operating room, the same instrumentation and technique as that used with reamed tibial nailing is necessary. Small-diameter sharp intramedullary reamers should also be available. If the fractures is open, instruments necessary for debridement, specifically pulsatile lavage, are essential. If an open reduction or

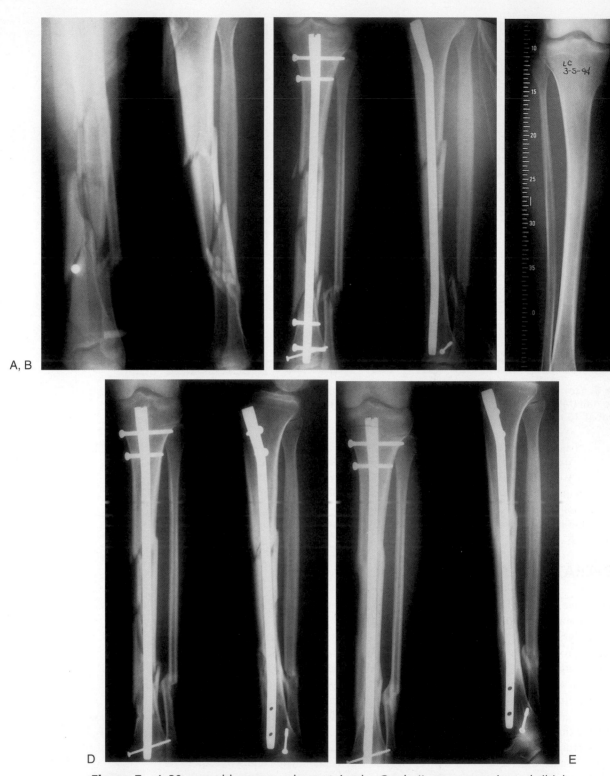

Figure 7. A 20-year-old woman who sustained a Grade II open comminuted tibial-shaft fracture in a motor vehicle accident. **A:** Initial anteroposterior (AP) and lateral radiographs of injury (note minimally displaced fracture of medial malleolus). **B:** Postoperative radiograph demonstrating reconstruction with small-diameter nail and small screw. **C:** Radiographic example of intact tibia with radiopaque marking device used to determine appropriate length of tibia. **D:** Radiograph after removal of distal locking bolts at 4 months after injury. **E:** Fracture union at 7 months after injury.

percutaneous screw fixation of a metaphyseal fracture might be necessary, then cannulated screws, small fragment set, bone clamps, and smooth Kirschner wires (K-wires) should be requested. I prefer to use a radiolucent extension table and a mobile C-arm image intensifier for all tibial nailing, avoiding the need for intraoperative traction.

SURGERY

The patient is brought to the operating room and given a general anesthetic. The use of spinal anesthesia is not recommended for tibial fractures because the lasting effect of the anesthesia can mask a potential compartment syndrome postoperatively, which can be devastating if missed.

The patient is placed supine on a radiolucent operating table (Fig. 8). The radiolucent table extension must allow visualization from the foot to just above the knee with the image intensifier. Many operating tables are radiolucent but have metal sidebars and brackets at the end of the table, which interfere with the x-ray picture and commonly block total visualization. Inexpensive radiolucent pillows (Fig. 9) are placed under the sterile drapes to allow better positioning of the lower extremity during the surgical procedure. A tourniquet is applied above the knee, and the leg is prepped and draped.

If the fracture is open, the traumatic wounds are irrigated and debrided. The wound margins are commonly extended to improve exposure and visualization. All nonviable cortical fragments are removed, as well as any foreign bodies or necrotic tissue (subcutaneous tissue and muscle). The debridement must be orderly, sequential, and complete to render the wound sterile in preparation for the nailing that follows. The fracture ends are carefully inspected and cleaned to ensure that there is no foreign debris in the intramedullary canal proximally or distally. If the degree of contamination is high and the wound cannot be rendered essentially clean and sterile, external fixation may be preferable to a small-diameter tibial nail. The traumatic wound is thoroughly irrigated with 9 to 12 L of normal saline by

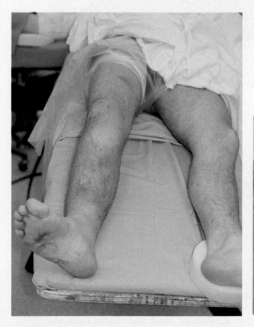

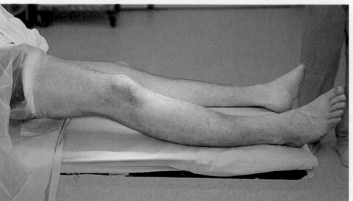

A   B

Figure 8.   A, B: Patient on radiolucent extension table in operating room prepared for intramedullary nailing of the tibia.

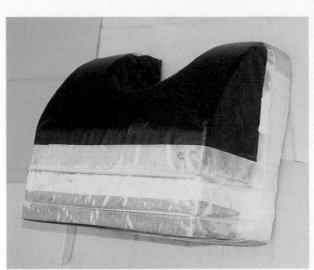

AI

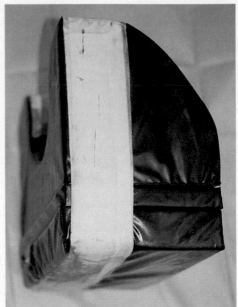

AII

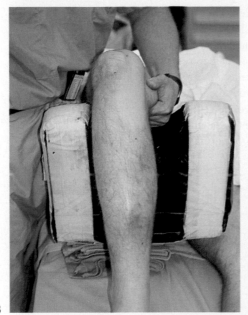

B

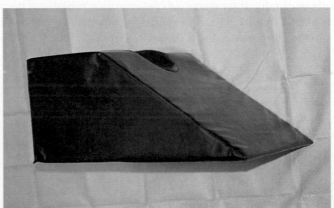

C

D

Figure 9. AI, AII: Pillow used for tibial nail insertion. **B:** Patient leg draped over pillow. **C:** Pillow used for distal bolt insertion. **D:** Patient leg lying on pillow.

using pulsed lavage (Fig. 10). We use a lavage that allows a powered stream of normal saline with suction through the same apparatus.

After irrigation and debridement, attention is turned to skeletal stabilization. A large pillow, mentioned previously, is placed beneath the sterile drapes under the distal femur with sterile towels often placed in the U portion to allow flexion of the knee to 60 to 80 degrees (Fig. 9B). In our institution, we change the outer gloves for this portion of the procedure but do not routinely regown. An incision is made over the anterior aspect of the knee, extending from the midportion of the patella to the tibial tubercle 1 cm medial to the tendon (Fig. 11A and B). Dissection is carried through skin and subcutaneous tissue, carefully defining the medial margin of the patellar tendon. The fascia overlying the patellar tendon, from the inferior margin of the patella to the area of the tibial tubercle, is incised. The skin over the inferior half of the patella is opened to prevent skin damage during the nailing procedure itself. The patellar tendon is retracted laterally, and the prepatellar fat pad is incised to allow access into the proximal tibial metaphysis. A short metallic object (forceps) is

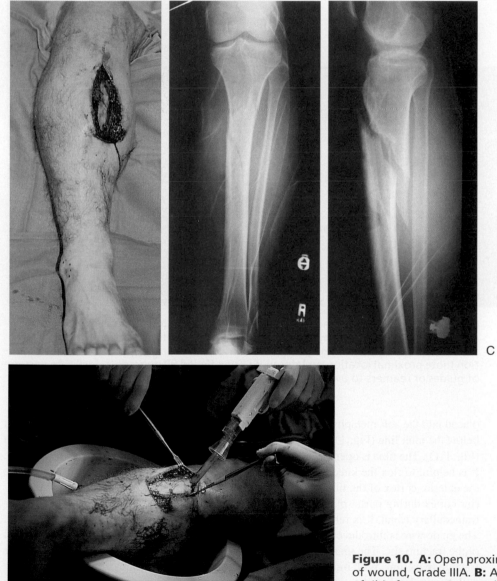

B   C

D

Figure 10. A: Open proximal tibial-shaft fracture, picture of wound, Grade IIIA. **B:** Anteroposterior (AP) radiograph of tibia fracture. **C:** Lateral radiograph of tibia fracture. **D:** Pulsatile lavage of open fracture after careful debridement.

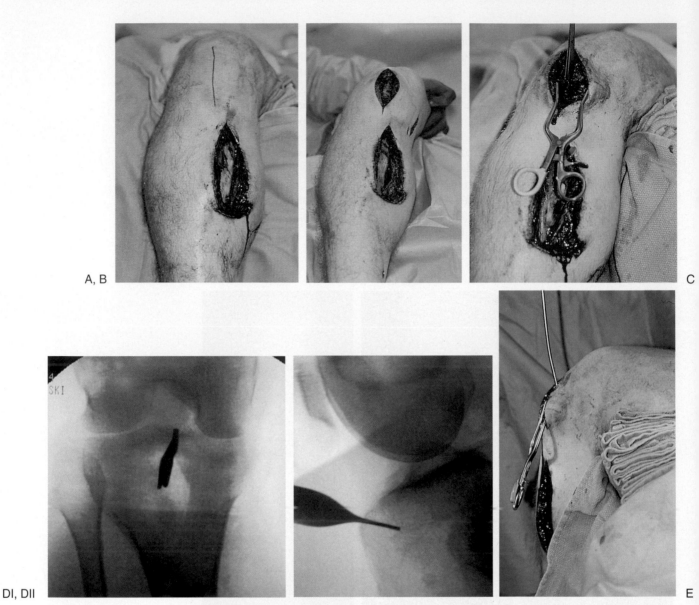

A, B

C

DI, DII

E

Figure 11. A: Drawing of incision for intramedullary nailing. **B:** Incision. **C:** Adson forceps placed into soft metaphyseal bone to determine starting position. **DI, DII:** Anteroposterior (AP) and lateral image of Adson forceps locating appropriate starting position (note proximal location on lateral). **E:** Knee flexed 90 degrees to facilitate passage of guides or reamers to avoid posterior penetration.

placed into the soft metaphyseal bone in the midline of the proximal tibial metaphysis just below the joint line (Fig. 11C). An AP image is used to verify the correct starting position (Fig. 11D). The tibia is opened with a sharp T-handled awl, 6 to 7 mm in diameter (Fig. 12). It is helpful to flex the knee further (90 to 100 degrees) to direct the T-handled awl along the anterior cortex of the tibia (Fig. 11E). It is important to avoid penetration of the posterior cortex during portal placement. Once the sharp T-handled awl has penetrated the intramedullary canal, it is removed and exchanged for a curved ball-tipped reaming guide. The guide wire is introduced through the previously created tract and advanced to the level of the fracture site. The image intensifier is brought into the operative field to visualize the fracture reduction. With most open tibial-shaft fractures, the fracture can be reduced easily with longitudinal traction and held manually or maintained with a pointed reduction clamp if necessary. Usually, simple manipulation of the fracture allows the ball-tipped guide to cross the fracture site into the distal fragment, which is verified by using image intensifi-

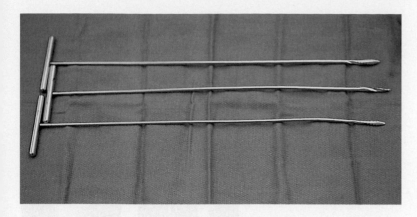

Figure 12. Sharp T-handled hand reamers (6, 7, and 8 mm diameter).

cation. The ball-tipped guide is then impacted into the distal tibial metaphysis at the level of the distal tibial epiphyseal scar. Length is determined by using an equal-length wire to confirm the length that was determined preoperatively.

Some surgeons pass a sound before or after fracture reduction to help determine canal diameter. I prefer to pass a 9-mm end-cutting reamer to open the intramedullary canal to a consistent size and to allow smooth, easy passage of a small-diameter intramedullary nail. Experience has shown that this technique significantly streamlines the operative procedure by preventing excessive force during nail insertion and appears to cause no additional long-term complication. If this reamer passes with significant difficulty, then a smaller-size reamer should be used. As a general rule, I would first try the 6-, 7-, and 8-mm sharp T-handled hand reamers (Fig. 12). Occasionally we use small-diameter power reamers that begin at 5 mm in diameter and increase in size by 0.5-mm increments. These are often necessary for extremely small-diameter tibial canals in adolescents and teenagers, in Asian patients, or certain diseases (osteogenesis imperfecta and after poliomyelitis). It is worth emphasizing that any device passed down the intramedullary canal should pass without difficulty. This includes guides, reamers, and nails. If significant resistance is encountered, its cause must be determined and corrected. A smooth, steady progression of the instruments and the nail is essential.

Once the canal diameter has been determined and reaming is complete, the 3-mm ball-tipped reaming guide is exchanged for a 3-mm non–ball-tipped nail-driving guide. The appropriate length nail is assembled on the driving and proximal targeting device to allow insertion of proximal locking bolts from medial to lateral. I favor cannulated intramedullary nails, which make insertion over a guide wire easy and simple, streamlining the operative procedure. Solid, noncannulated intramedullary nails also are available, but I do not recommend them.

The nail is inserted into the tibia over the 3-mm nail guide wire. Once again, care is taken to flex the knee to at least 90 degrees to facilitate nail insertion. Usually the nail can be "pushed" to near midshaft with simple manual pressure. As the nail approaches the fracture site, care must be taken to maintain the fracture reduction before nail passage. The nail is then carefully driven across the fracture site and into the distal fragment. Once the nail is firmly located in the distal fragment, the guide wire is removed. The nail is then completely seated within the intramedullary canal and driven to the level previously measured in the distal tibial metaphysis. At this point, image intensification is used to visualize the distal and proximal tibia as well as the fracture site. It is not uncommon for some distraction to occur at the fracture site (Fig. 13). This develops because the narrow distal fragment tightly grips the nail and is pushed distally with insertion of the nail. Besides length and alignment, attention should be directed toward correction of rotation, both of the nail within the tibia and the overall alignment of the tibia. If small amounts of distraction are present at the fracture site, these can often be corrected with manual impaction on the plantar aspect of the foot. If distraction persists, the technique of backslapping should be used.

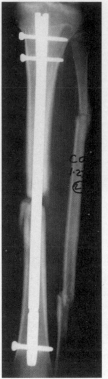
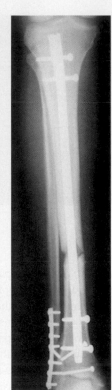

A

Figure 13. A,B: Radiographs of tibial fracture with nail in place and distraction at the fracture site.

Backslapping begins by countersinking the nail 5 to 10 mm deep within the tibia. With the technique of backslapping, distal locking bolts are inserted before insertion of the proximal locking bolts (7). This is opposite to the usual technique of insertion of proximal bolts first. The knee is extended. The lower leg is placed on either a stack of sterile surgical towels or on a previously positioned pillow, either of which will elevate the operative leg higher than the nonoperative leg (Fig. 14A). The image intensifier is brought into the area of the distal tibia and placed perpendicular to the longitudinal axis of the leg. A lateral image is obtained, and perfectly round holes are identified on the image-intensifier screen (Fig. 14B). If the hole is flat on the proximal or distal portion of the hole, a more perpendicular placement of the machine or the leg is required (Fig. 14C). If the hole is flat on either the anterior or posterior portion, rotational changes in either the leg or the machine are required to correct the alignment (Fig. 14D). Once a perfectly round hole has been identified (Fig. 14E), the size of the hole is magnified by moving the beam closer to the lateral aspect of the leg, which also allows more working room between the image and the leg. Many image intensifiers have the ability to magnify the image as well. A stab incision is made in the skin directly over the perfectly round hole, and the soft tissues are bluntly dissected to the subcutaneous border of the tibia. A sharp, pointed instrument is inserted through the stab incision and laid directly on the shaft of the tibia (Fig. 15A). The tibia is approached from anterior to posterior, not parallel to the nail. I prefer a sharp Steinmann pin in a cannulated adjustable T-handled chuck for this portion of the procedure. Once the tip of the pin has been located within the perfectly round hole on the image-intensifier screen, the pin is placed parallel to the image beam, and an indentation or hole is made in the near cortex by gentle tapping of a mallet on the end of the pin (Fig. 15B). This indentation of the cortical surface prevents the drill bit from "walking" on the curved tibial cortex. The sharp Steinmann pin is removed, and the appropriate-size drill bit is placed into the previously created indentation. The image intensifier is again used to check the correct position of the drill bit within the perfectly round circle (Fig. 15C). With the drill parallel to the x-ray beam, the drill bit is advanced through the near cortex, through the hole in the nail, and then through the far cortex (Fig. 15D). Once the near cortex has been penetrated, if obstruction to further passage of the drill bit occurs, the direction of the drill bit should

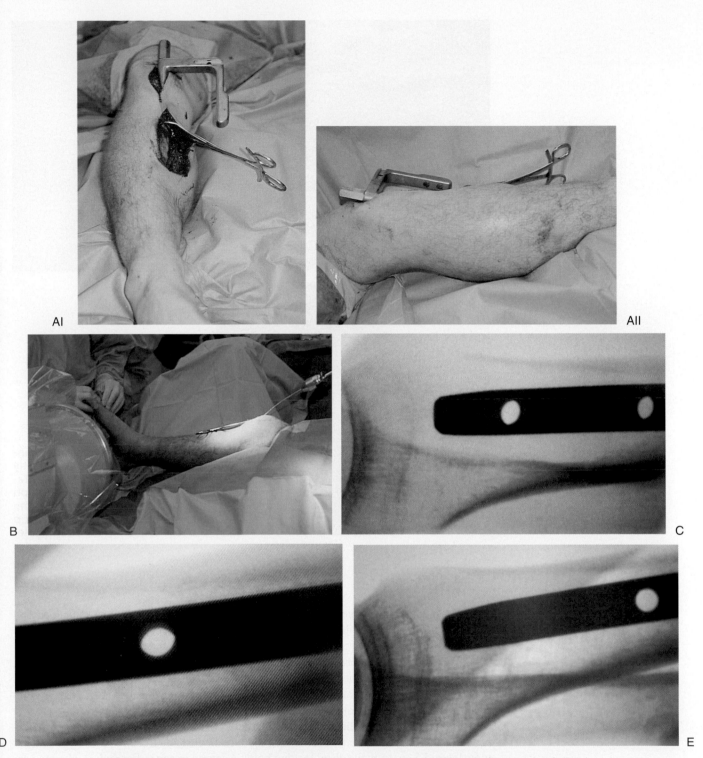

Figure 14. AI, AII: Leg extended and elevated in preparation of placement of distal locking bolt. **B:** Image intensifier in position to view perfectly round holes. **C:** Radiograph with a flat proximal and distal edge to a hole. **D:** Radiograph with a flat anterior and posterior edge to a hole. **E:** Perfectly round hole noted by appropriate correction.

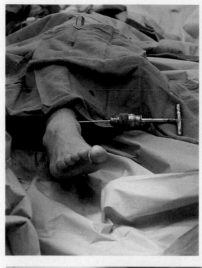

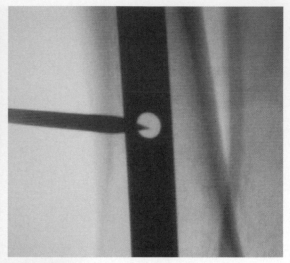

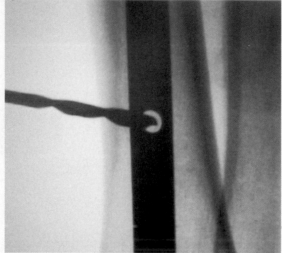

Figure 15. A: Sharp, pointed instrument centered in a perfectly round hole to create an indentation in the cortex. **B:** Radiograph of pointed instrument in the round hole. **C:** Radiograph of tip of the drill bit in the round hole.

be rechecked by using image intensification. Minor corrections in direction can then be easily performed. Once the drill bit has penetrated the far cortex, the drill is removed. The image intensifier is then used to verify that the drill bit lies within the locking hole in the nail (Fig. 15E). The image intensifier is then rotated into an AP view (Fig. 16A), and by using the center drill guide for the proximal targeting device, the length of the potential locking screw is then read directly off of the drill bit without using a depth gauge (Fig. 16B). At this point, the correct length locking bolt is inserted by using image-intensification control in a manner similar to that outlined (Fig. 14C and D). A second distal locking bolt can be inserted if necessary. We use two distal locking bolts in unstable fracture patterns or in fractures located 5 cm from the distal locking bolts. A lateral image radiograph is taken to verify that bolts lie within the hole. This is verified by bolt obliteration of the hole in the nail (Fig. 16C). A slap hammer is attached to the proximal targeting device on the intramedullary nail (Fig. 17A), and under image-intensification control, the fracture site is compressed or impacted by backslapping with the hammer (Fig. 17B). Persistent distraction at the fracture site is associated with an increased incidence of tibial nonunion. Once the fracture site is compressed (Fig. 18A), rotational alignment is reevaluated, and a transverse or oblique proximal locking bolt is placed (Fig. 17D). In the majority of instances, only one transverse or oblique proximal locking bolt is used. Occasionally when fractures occur near the proximal third of the tibia, two transverse locking bolts are placed.

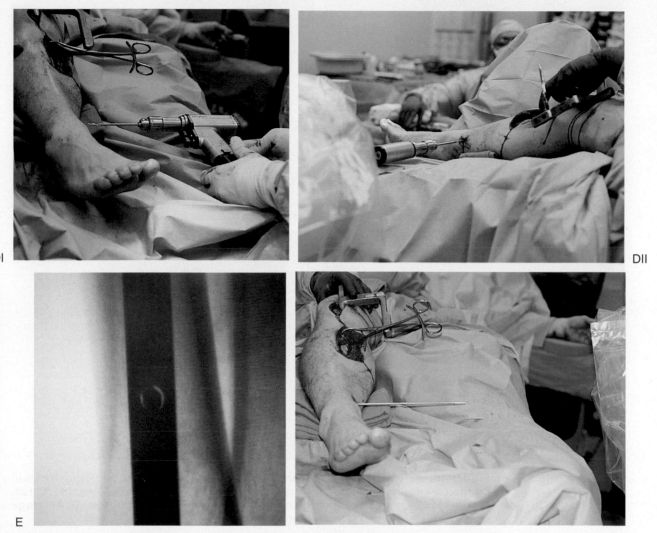

DI

DII

E

Figure 15. *(continued)* **DI, DII:** Drill bit placed in the indentation and drilled parallel to the x-ray beam. **E:** Radiograph of drill bit *(left)* after drilling through the hole, verifying correct placement *(right)*.

Before completion of the operative procedure, the image intensifier is used to check the overall alignment of the tibia. The proximal targeting device is removed only when the surgeon is satisfied that length, alignment, and rotation are satisfactory. It is nearly impossible to reattach a proximal locking device to an intramedullary nail that is well seated within the tibia. After removal of the proximal targeting device, the upper end of the nail, the proximal locking bolts (Fig. 18A and B), the fracture site, and the distal aspect of the nail and locking bolts (Fig. 18C) are evaluated in both AP and lateral views. Care should be taken to ensure that all bolts engage the holes in the intramedullary nail. The tibial nail should lie at or within the proximal tibial cortical bone (Fig. 18D). Permanent copies printed off the image intensifier or intraoperative plain films should be obtained.

The traumatic wounds are carefully reevaluated. Simple wounds (Grades I and II) are commonly closed primarily. If a tension-free wound closure can be accomplished in a Grade IIIA open tibia, this is also performed (Fig. 19A). Otherwise, the wound is covered with Epiguard (Clinipad Corp., Norwich, CT) sterile synthetic skin. If flap coverage is deemed necessary, a plastic surgical consultation is obtained at the time of initial surgery or at a second debridement within 48 hours. Not infrequently, skin grafting is done at 48 to 96 hours by the orthopaedic or plastic surgical service. We routinely use a 1/8-inch

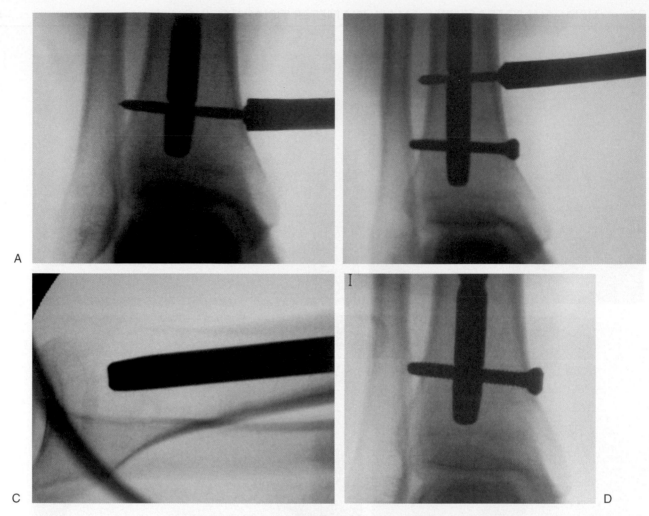

Figure 16. **A:** Image intensifier in anteroposterior (AP) position. **B:** Radiograph of drill bit placed through near and far cortex during length check for screw selection. **C:** Lateral image of screw placed through nail, completely obliterating the hole. **D:** AP image of appropriately placed screw (approximately 2 mm outside bone cortex).

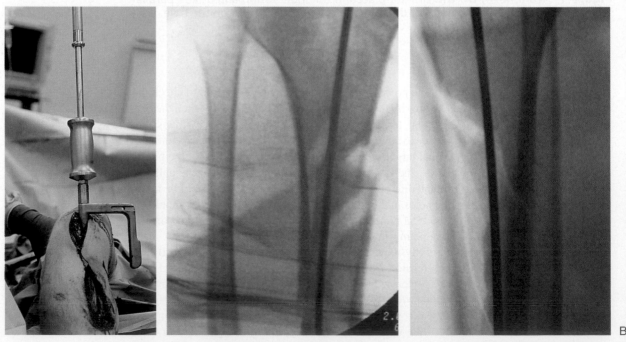

Figure 17. **A:** A slap hammer is attached to proximal targeting device before the backslap maneuver. **BI, BII:** Radiograph of distracted fracture before backslap maneuver.

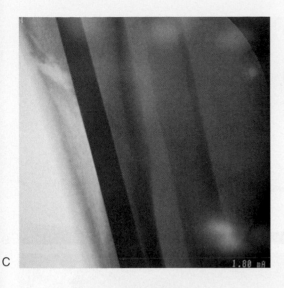

C

Figure 17. *(continued)* **C:** Radiograph of fracture after backslap maneuver with proximal locking bolts in place.

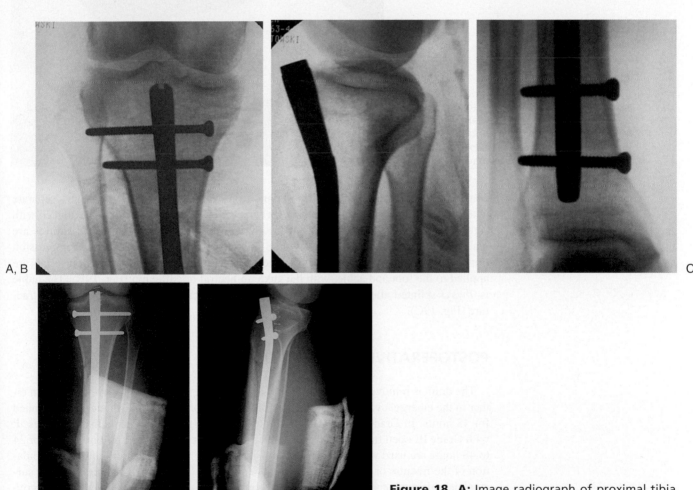

A, B   C

DI, DII

Figure 18. A: Image radiograph of proximal tibia after intramedullary nailing [anteroposterior (AP)]. **B:** Image radiograph of proximal tibia after intramedullary nailing (lateral). **C:** Image radiograph of distal tibia after locking. **DI, DII:** Permanent radiographs of fracture and nail (AP and lateral). Note proximal nail is not ideally placed (5 mm outside proximal cortex).

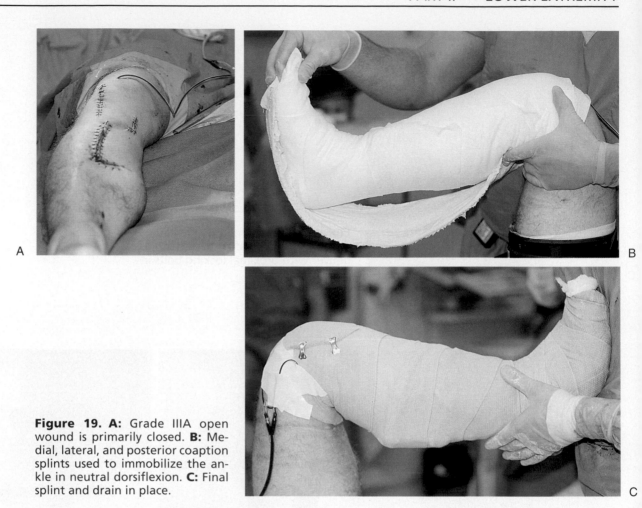

Figure 19. A: Grade IIIA open wound is primarily closed. **B:** Medial, lateral, and posterior coaption splints used to immobilize the ankle in neutral dorsiflexion. **C:** Final splint and drain in place.

hemovac suction drain for the nail-portal incision, which is brought out through a separate anterolateral stab incision. The fascia overlying the patellar tendon is reapproximated with figure-of-eight interrupted absorbable sutures. Small-diameter absorbable sutures are placed in the subcutaneous tissue, and the skin closed with staples. A sterile compression dressing is applied to the lower leg, and medial, lateral, and posterior coaptation splints are applied to the foot and ankle, with the ankle in neutral dorsiflexion (Fig. 19B). The ankle is *always* splinted after insertion of an intramedullary nail to prevent an equinus contracture (Fig. 19C).

POSTOPERATIVE MANAGEMENT

The drain is removed at 24 to 48 hours. Perioperative antibiotics, which were begun either in the emergency room or at the time of induction of general anesthetic, are continued for 48 hours. In Grades I and II open fractures, a first-generation cephalosporin is used; with Grade III open fractures, an aminoglycoside is added. Perioperative antibiotics for 24 to 48 hours are used whenever the patient is returned to the operating room for manipulation of the fracture or debridement of the open wound. Severe open fractures require surgical debridement at 48-hour intervals until final wound coverage is obtained. Wound coverage is accomplished by either delayed primary closure or skin grafting, or local or free-flap coverage by the plastic surgical service. Open wounds that have been primarily closed are not redebrided as a matter of routine. Postoperatively, the patient is gait trained with foot-flat weight bearing (15 to 20 pounds) by using crutches or a walker. Quadriceps- and hamstring-strengthening exercises are instituted on the first postoperative day, particularly by means of quad sets. Range-of-motion exercises of the knee are begun immediately as well. The postoperative splint is usually left in place until the first postoperative

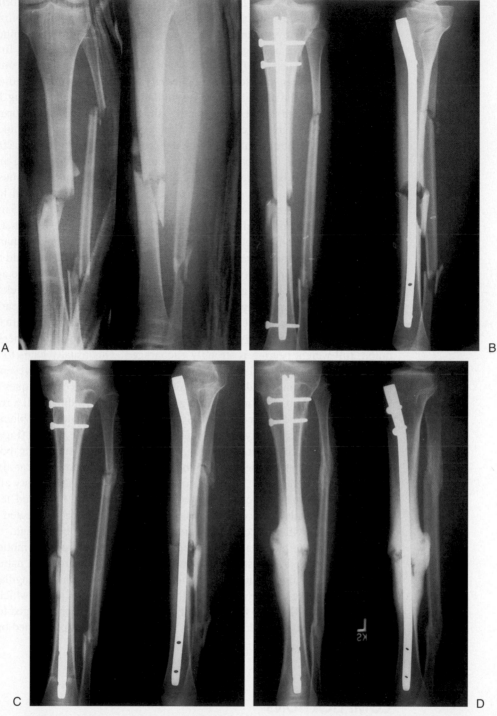

Figure 20. A 15-year-old girl struck by a car, with bilateral open tibia fractures. The left tibia is Grade IIIB open. **A:** Radiograph of acute injury [anteroposterior (AP) and lateral] of left tibia. **B:** Postoperative radiograph after irrigation and debridement, intramedullary nailing, and delayed local flap plus skin graft coverage (two separate operative procedures). Note distraction at fracture site. **C:** Radiograph after removal of distal locking bolts at 3 months after injury performed under local anesthesia in the clinic. Note nail bolt holes now 5 to 10 mm distal to bone bolt holes, indicating shortening at primary fracture site. **D:** Healing at 6 months after injury.

visit (10 days to 2 weeks). This splint is removed at 2 weeks, and no further immobilization is required unless ipsilateral foot or ankle injuries require immobilization. Once the splint has been removed, range-of-motion exercises for the ankle and hindfoot are begun, and foot-flat weight bearing (15 to 20 pounds) is encouraged. On the first postoperative visit, the wound is inspected, and sutures are removed, but radiographs are not obtained.

The patient is seen at 4- to 6-week intervals for wound check and radiographic evaluation. Most often, the patient is kept on limited foot-flat weight bearing for a total of 12 weeks (Fig. 20A and B). At the 3-month visit, early periosteal callus formation should be observed on radiographs. If callus formation is absent, consideration should be given to dynamization of the intramedullary device in a length-stable fracture (Fig. 20C). This is done by removal of distal or proximal locking bolts in the clinic under local anesthesia. In patients in whom the bolts are not easily palpable, or in extremely anxious patients, intravenous sedation or a short general anesthetic may be required. Distal locking bolts are rarely removed before the 3-month visit and are usually removed at 4 to 5 months after nailing if delayed fracture healing is apparent on radiograph in a length-stable fracture. If length stability is not present, such as when a cortical defect of greater than 50% of the circumference of the tibia is present at the fracture site, consideration should be given to early bone grafting. With defect-type fractures, cancellous bone graft may be applied by an anterolateral or posterolateral approach. Grafting is recommended at 6 weeks to 3 months after initial injury to speed fracture healing and promote early weight bearing. Full weight bearing is not allowed on these small-diameter nails until signs of fracture healing are seen, 3 to 4 months postoperatively. If dynamization is necessary to promote healing of a delayed union, full weight bearing is strongly encouraged. This usually leads to fracture healing (Fig. 20D). If fracture healing or periosteal callus formation is not present 6 months after injury, consideration should be given to other, more aggressive techniques to promote healing. In this scenario, I favor an exchange intramedullary nailing with a reamed implant if the traumatic wounds healed and there is no history of infection. Supplemental cancellous bone graft is necessary only if significant cortical defects are present (Fig. 6).

Because of its subcutaneous location, tibial nails can be symptomatic, both over the locking bolts sites and at the knee. If symptomatic, hardware removal 1 year after fracture healing may be indicated (Fig. 7). No postoperative protection is necessary after hardware removal. It is not uncommon to remove transverse locking bolts and leave well-seated intramedullary nails in place. Studies have shown that if the nail is seated beneath the cortex, its removal will not necessarily cure knee pain that may be present.

After healing of the tibia, most patients regain a normal range of motion of their knee, with excellent quadriceps strength. If the nailing was done properly, patients should have shortening of no more than 1 cm and no evidence of rotational or angular malalignment. Occasionally there is some stiffness at the ankle and subtalar joints, which is of little clinical significance. Once the fracture has healed, the patient is encouraged to resume full activities. Hardware removal is discussed with the patient and performed only if symptoms warrant.

COMPLICATIONS

The most feared complication after tibial nailing, particularly in open fractures, is infection (1,11). The infection rate has been relatively low and is equal to or less than that with external fixation for Grades I, II, and IIIA open fractures. In my experience, infection has occurred more commonly at the time of exchange nailing for nonunion than it has with the initial operative treatment (2). In our series of 87 patients, infection occurred in 9% of cases. Six of eight infections occurred after exchange nailing, and only two of eight infections occurred after initial small-diameter nailing. The best way to prevent infection is by performing a thorough and radical irrigation and debridement at the time of the initial procedure and by using appropriate perioperative antibiotics. Wound coverage as soon as is reasonably possible should be encouraged as well.

Hardware failure is another serious potential complication. These nails are less mechanically sound than are larger reamed tibial nails (4,6,17,18). There is little difference in strength between most 8-, 9-, and 10-mm intramedullary nails. I most often use 9-mm nails. Screw breakage is the most common means of hardware failure (Figs. 5, 21F, and 22). Screws with a core diameter of 3.5 mm or less are prone to failure, which occurs at approximately a 20% to 30% rate. Therefore to minimize screw breakage, transverse locking screws that are larger than 3.5 mm in diameter (3.8 mm or more) are recommended. Even with 3.8-mm locking screws, care should be taken to avoid stress on nails and bolts until early fracture healing occurs. If fracture healing is delayed, attempts should be made to decrease stress on the hardware (dynamization) to encourage fracture healing. Because screw breakage is common, it is important to leave the locking screws proud on the far cortex (2 to 4 mm) to facilitate removal if they break (Fig. 18C). Screw breakage may not have an untoward effect on fracture healing, and in fact may be viewed as a form of dynamization (the patient's own attempt at fracture healing; Fig. 21). This may be a problem in patients if hardware removal is contemplated.

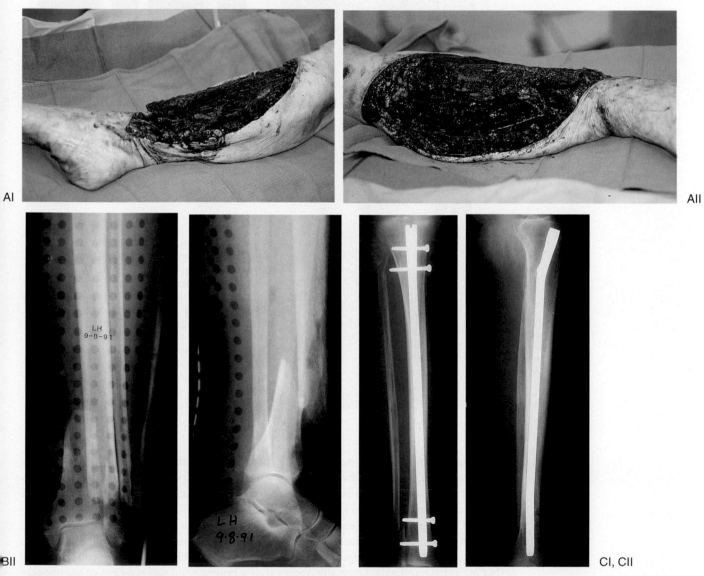

Figure 21. Open distal-third tibia fracture in 77-year-old woman caused by motor vehicle accident. **AI, AII:** Grade IIIA open degloving injury from just below knee to ankle. **BI, BII:** Preoperative anteroposterior (AP) and lateral radiographs. **CI, CII:** Postoperative radiographs after irrigation and debridement, small-diameter intramedullary nailing, and primary wound closure.

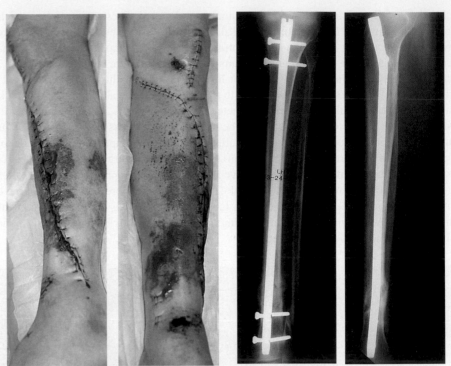

DI, DII   EI, E

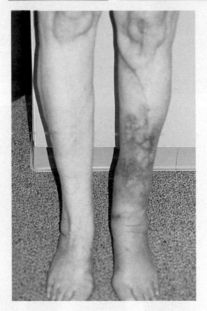

Figure 21. *(continued)* **DI, DII:** Skin at 1 week after surgery with significant epidermolysis. The wound was closely monitored by orthopaedic and plastic surgeons. **EI, EII:** Fracture healing with no further surgery at 6 months after injury with self-dynamization (distal screw breakage) of the intramedullary nail. Weight bearing was allowed at 6 to 8 weeks after injury with this 77-year-old woman. **F:** Status of skin at 6 months. Note only one operative procedure was performed in this patient.

F

A broken intramedullary nail is a major complication. If the broken nail is cannulated, it can usually be removed. Obviously, the broken proximal portion of the nail is easily removed. The proximal tibia is then reamed to 12 mm. Specially designed intramedullary hooks or clamps are used to hook the distal fragment of the broken nail, and the nail is removed by tapping it out. Reaming the intramedullary canal proximal to the broken distal portion of the nail greatly facilitates removing a broken nail. Unfortunately, broken solid-diameter nails are nearly impossible to remove (Fig. 22A). Extractors have been developed but are often unreliable. Generally, removal of a broken solid nail requires either opening the fracture site itself or pushing the broken piece of nail into an unused portion of the tibia (posterior malleolus) where it can be removed through a posterior approach at the ankle or simply left in place (Fig. 22B and C). A broken intramedullary nail invariably occurs in the presence of a delayed union or nonunion that has been unrecognized, or with premature

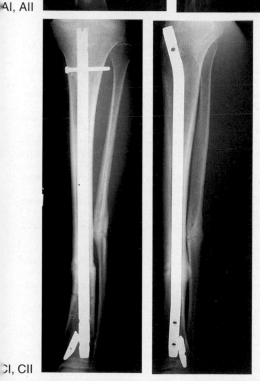

AI, AII

BI, BII

CI, CII

Figure 22. An 18-year-old man referred from outside institution with hardware failure and absent fracture healing at 8 months after internal fixation of a Grade I open tibia fracture with a small-diameter, solid tibial intramedullary nail. **AI, AII:** Anteroposterior (AP) and lateral radiographs at presentation, 8 months after injury. Weight bearing was allowed at 6 weeks, and nail breakage occurred at 3 months. **BI, BII:** AP and lateral radiographs after removal of failed hardware (nail and bolts) and exchange intramedullary nail with large-diameter nail. The broken tip of the solid nail could not be retrieved without opening the wound and osteotomizing the tibia. This debris was simply pushed aside. Full weight bearing was allowed immediately after surgery. **CI, CII:** Healed fracture at 10 weeks after surgery. Hardware removal has not been performed 3 years later.

weight bearing on an unhealed fracture. It should be noted that if the fracture is not healed 6 months after injury and the patient is weight bearing, plans should be developed for treatment of the unhealed fracture. The routine fatigue life for these nails is probably somewhere between 6 months and 1 year, and breakage without fracture healing can be expected.

Delayed union or nonunion are common complications after open tibial-shaft fractures. Nonunion occurs in 10% to 30% of patients with open tibial fractures and increases with the severity of the fracture. Generally, between 3 and 5 months after injury, a decision must be made whether the fracture is progressing reasonably toward "union" or not. In length-stable delayed unions, the fracture should be dynamized by removal of distal locking bolts and rarely by removal of proximal locking bolts (this predisposes to increased symptoms at the knee). Dynamization usually leads to fracture union. Furthermore, it allows full weight bearing and decreases any residual slight distraction that might be present at the fracture site (Fig. 20). Cortical defects greater than half of the circumference of the tibia should undergo early (6-week) cancellous bone grafting. This can speed union and decrease hardware failure. If union has not occurred more than 6 months after injury, the patient has a nonunion and should be a candidate for exchange intramedullary nailing with or without bone graft (14; Fig. 6).

It is uncommon to have a total failure with this technique. Total failure after nailing generally is the result of a poor indication for the procedure in the first place. Failure may occur due to infection that is impossible to control. This usually requires nail removal and application of an external fixator to control the infection. A nonunion can occur if a large defect exists after intramedullary nailing. Large segmental defects (more than 4 cm) are best treated with external fixation and bone transport primarily. In our experience, proximal-third fractures have most often caused failures from malalignment and nonunion (8).

Small amounts of shortening (1 to 1.5 cm) are common with the technique and rarely cause symptoms or impair function. Angulation and rotation are technique related and should be carefully evaluated by the treating surgeon at the time of surgery.

RECOMMENDED READING

1. Bone, L.B., Johnson, K.D.: Treatment of tibial fractures by reaming and intramedullary nailing. *J. Bone Joint Surg. [Am]*, 68:877–887, 1987.
2. Cole, J.D., Ansel, L.J., Schwartzberg, R.: A sequential protocol for management of severe open tibial fractures. *Clin. Orthop.*, 315:84–103, 1995.
3. Gustillo, R.B., Mendoza, R.M., Williams, D.N.: Problems in the management of type III (severe) open fractures: a new classification of type III open fractures. *J. Trauma*, 24:742–746, 1984.
4. Henley, M.B., Mayo, K.: Prospective comparison of unreamed interlocking intramedullary nails and half-pin external fixation for grade II and III open tibia fractures. *J. Orthop. Trauma*, 4:233–234, 1990.
5. Holbrook, J.L., Swiontkowski, M.F., Sanders, R.: Treatment of open fractures of the tibial shaft: Ender nailing versus external fixation: a randomized prospective comparison. *J. Bone Joint Surg. [Am]*, 71:1231–1238, 1989.
6. Hutson, J.J., Zych, G.A., Cole, J.D., et al.: Mechanical failures of intramedullary tibial nails applied without reaming. *Clin. Orthop.*, 315:129–137, 1995.
7. Krettek, C., Schandelmaier, P., Tscherne, H.: Nonreamed interlocking nailing of closed tibial fractures with severe soft tissue injury. *Clin. Orthop.*, 315:34–47, 1995.
8. Lang, G.J., Cohen, B.E., Bosse, M.J., Kellam, J.F.: Proximal third tibial shaft fractures: should they be nailed? *Clin. Orthop.*, 315:64–74, 1995.
9. Lottes, J.O.: Medullary nailing of the tibia with the triflange nail. *Clin. Orthop.*, 105:253–266, 1974.
10. Rhinelander, F.W.: Effects of medullary nailing on the normal blood supply of the diaphyseal cortex. *Instr Course Lect*, 22:161–187, 1973.
11. Singer, R.W., Kellam, J.F.: Open tibial diaphyseal fractures: results of unreamed locked intramedullary nailing. *Clin. Orthop.*, 315:114–118, 1995.
12. Sitter, T., Wilson, J., Browner, B.: The effect of reamed versus unreamed nailing on intramedullary blood supply and cortical viability. *J. Orthop. Trauma*, 4:232–233, 1990.
13. Swanson, T.V., Spiegel, J.D., Sutherland, T.B., Bray, T.J., Chapman, M.W.: A prospective, comparison study of the Lottes nail versus external fixation in 100 open tibial fractures. *Orthop. Trans.*, 14:716–717, 1990.
14. Templeman, D., Thomas, M., Varecka, T., Kyle, R.: Exchange reamed intramedullary nailing for delayed union and nonunion of the tibia. *Clin. Orthop.*, 315:169–175, 1995.
15. Turen, C.H., Burgess, A.R., Vanco, B.: Skeletal stabilization for tibial fractures associated with acute compartment syndrome. *Clin. Orthop.*, 315:163–168, 1995.
16. Velazco, A., Whitesides, T.E., Fleming, L.L.: Open fractures of the tibia treated with the Lottes nail. *J. Bone Joint Surg. [Am]*, 65:879–884, 1983.
17. Whittle, A.P., Russell, T.A., Taylor, J.C., Lavelle, D.G.: Treatment of open fractures of the tibial shaft with the use of interlocking nailing without reaming. *J. Bone Joint Surg. [Am]*, 74:1162–1171, 1992.
18. Whittle, A.P., Wester, W., Russell, T.A.: Fatigue failure in small diameter tibial nails. *Clin. Orthop.*, 315:119–128, 1995.

Master Techniques in Orthopaedic Surgery,
FRACTURES, edited by D. A. Wiss,
Lippincott–Raven Publishers, Philadelphia © 1998.

28

Tibial-Pilon Fractures: Open Reduction Internal Fixation

James A. Goulet

INDICATIONS/CONTRAINDICATIONS

The treatment of tibial-pilon fractures is dictated by the amount of displacement of the articular fragments, the magnitude of fracture comminution, and the extent of soft-tissue damage. Pilon fractures with less than 2 mm of articular incongruity and without significant displacement of the metaphysis do not require surgical treatment. However, numerous studies have shown that the best outcome for displaced fractures is obtained when reconstructable fractures are anatomically reduced and surgically stabilized to allow early ankle motion. This method of treatment also carries the greatest risk of complications, primarily wound infections. It is very important yet difficult to recognize patients with unreconstructable injuries. However, if anatomic reduction without soft-tissue compromise cannot be predicted preoperatively, consideration should be given to alternative types of treatment such as external fixation.

The indications for open reduction and internal fixation of pilon fractures are those injuries with more than 2 mm of articular displacement, a reconstructable fracture, and an adequate soft-tissue envelope. A reconstructable fracture is one in which the subchondral landmarks are recognizable radiographically and the joint fragments are large enough to hold small fragment screws. Generally, if the articular fracture fragments cannot be outlined on tracing paper, the fracture is not reconstructable. On the other hand, metaphyseal comminution can usually be spanned by "bridge-plating" techniques and is not a contraindication to surgery if the joint can be anatomically reconstructed.

The skin and subcutaneous tissues overlying the ankle are thin and easily damaged. This makes open reduction and internal fixation vulnerable to wound complications. Several studies on pilon fractures treated with open reduction and internal fixation have reported high wound-complication rates. Therefore, soft-tissue assessment is critical but highly subjective. Soft-tissue findings that suggest a delay in internal fixation, or using another form

J. A. Goulet, M.D.: Department of Orthopaedic Surgery, University of Michigan Hospitals and Health Center, Ann Arbor, Michigan 48109-0328.

of treatment, include significant swelling relative to the lower leg, ankle, and foot; skin abrasions; fracture blisters and skin discoloration associated with bruising; and closed degloving injuries. In these cases, a simple temporary joint-spanning fixator, or placement of a calcaneal skeletal traction pin, can be used until the soft tissues have improved. Casts and splints should be avoided, as they result in shortening at the fracture site and block access to care of the skin. Once the fracture blisters have resolved and swelling has subsided enough to allow the skin to wrinkle, surgical intervention can be undertaken. Immediate fixation is possible in selected fractures arising from low-energy injuries and in trauma centers skilled in early management. For most pilon fractures in which open reduction and internal fixation is contemplated, temporizing measures are initially used, and the definitive procedure is delayed for a period of 5 to 14 days. Even more time may be required in severe cases.

PREOPERATIVE PLANNING

Although the focus of preoperative planning for most fractures is based on the radiographic examination of the fracture, the clinical assessment of the limb in a patient with a pilon fracture may be the most important element of the preoperative plan. Contraindications to early surgery using plate osteosynthesis include massive swelling, skin abrasions, fracture blisters, and extensive bruising. While waiting for these associated injuries to subside, careful and thorough preoperative planning may proceed.

Radiographic assessment of pilon fractures includes anterior/posterior, lateral, mortise, and oblique views of the distal tibia (Figs. 1 and 2), and may be the only imaging studies required for fractures with little or no comminution. For comminuted fractures, traction radiographs allow a more precise identification of the fracture morphology and may facilitate preoperative planning. If plain films have not fully delineated the fracture geometry or if operative intervention is planned, computed tomography (CT scan) is indicated. CT scans are helpful in determining the precise amount of articular and rotatory displacement of the fracture fragments (Fig. 3).

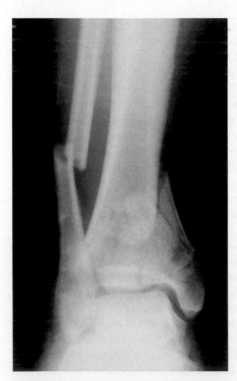

Figure 1. Anteroposterior (AP) radiographs of a closed tibial-pilon fracture with extension of the fracture into the articular surface and an associated fibular fracture.

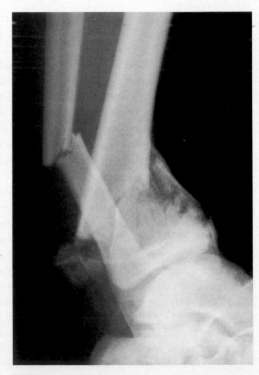

Figure 2. Lateral view of the fracture shows apex posterior angulation. There is an associated calcaneal fracture.

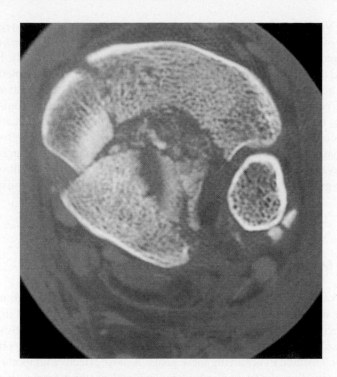

Figure 3. Computerized tomography (CT) of the fracture shown in Figures 1 and 2. A series of consecutive CT images may be used to assess the rotation of displaced fractures and the presence of bony debris between fragments, as shown in this view.

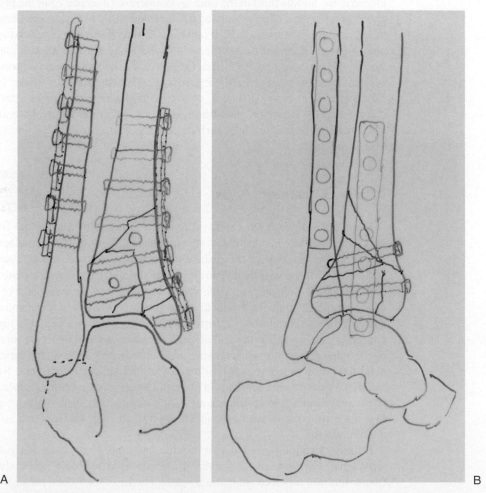

A   B

Figure 4. A, B: Preoperative plan for fracture fixation. A tracing of the contralateral distal tibia is used as a template for reassembling the fracture fragments.

Comparison views of the opposite ankle are used to form a planning template upon which tracings of the fracture on the injured side can be superimposed. This better defines the fragments present and permits development of a surgical tactic (Fig. 4). Preoperative planning should also include patient positioning, placement of incision(s), methods and instruments required for fracture reduction, and the implants necessary for fixation. Instruments that are frequently required include a femoral distractor, articulated compression distraction device, bone spreaders, and an assortment of tissue-sparing reduction forceps. Whenever possible, planning should encompass the setup for the operating room. For example, if an image intensifier is planned as part of the procedure, a radiolucent operating table must be available, as well as a room large enough to accommodate all of the equipment. If a bone graft is likely, the iliac crest bone should be prepped and draped.

SURGERY

Temporizing Measures

If internal fixation must be delayed for more than 6 or 8 hours, the limb must be supported in a safe and effective manner. Temporizing measures are aimed at improving the reduction, restoring length, achieving relative stabilization, and allowing elevation of the leg to hasten resolution of swelling. Calcaneal pin traction with elevation on a Bohler frame is a time-honored method of achieving these goals. A more effective temporary method of treatment is construction of a triangular bridging external fixator incorporating a calcaneal pin to serve as a portable form of calcaneal traction. The proximal-half pins should be placed in the middle third of the tibia, a considerable distance from the projected medial incision site. Fixation of an associated fibular fracture, by using a posterolateral incision, may be accomplished at the time of fixator application if this improves reduction of the distal tibial fracture. External fixation instead of calcaneal pin traction has the advantage of allowing the patient to be mobilized. Occasionally the surgeon may choose against further surgical intervention if an acceptable reduction is achieved after fibular fixation and application of a tibial external fixator, or if contraindications to further internal fixation arise (Figs. 5 and 6). However, joint-bridging external fixation is unable to adequately correct axial malalignment or articular surface malreduction, and definitive internal fixation of the tibia is necessary.

Definitive Treatment

Reudi and Allgower (8) described four sequential steps for internal fixation of a tibial-pilon fracture. First is open reduction and internal fixation of the fibula; second, anatomic reduction and fixation of the distal tibial articular surface; third, attachment of the reassembled distal tibial articular surface to the tibial diaphysis with a plate; and fourth, bone grafting. These steps are still followed in contemporary management of tibial-pilon fractures, but the techniques of reduction and fixation have changed substantially since Reudi and Allgower (8) promulgated them in 1979. Because of unacceptably high rates of wound complications, most fracture authorities have switched the priority from rigid anatomic reduction and fixation of all fragments to anatomic reduction of the articular surface with maximal preservation of soft tissue and vascular supply to the bone fragments. Current techniques use 3.5-mm implants in place of larger, bulkier 4.5-mm implants for many fractures and use plates to span large areas of comminution. Soft-tissue stripping of the fracture site is minimized, with exposure limited to articular surfaces and adjacent portions of the fracture site.

If fibular fixation is needed, two incisions are used—one posterolateral and the other anteromedial. Exposure of the fracture fragments is critical to a successful procedure. The fibular incision is placed along the posterior border of the fibula, rather than directly lateral over the subcutaneous surface, as might be used for ankle-fracture fixation (Fig. 7). A skin

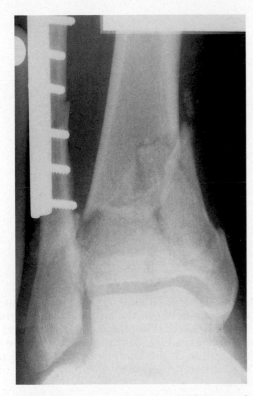

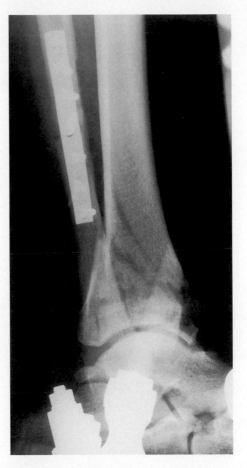

Figure 5. Anteroposterior (AP) view of the fracture after fibular plating and application of an external fixator. Although there is no apparent articular surface step-off, the fracture is in varus, and the impacted articular fragment shown in Figure 3 remains displaced.

Figure 6. Lateral view of the fracture after stabilization of the fibula with a plate and application of an external fixator. The recurvatum deformity apparent in Figure 2 has been corrected. The reduction of the articular surface appears adequate.

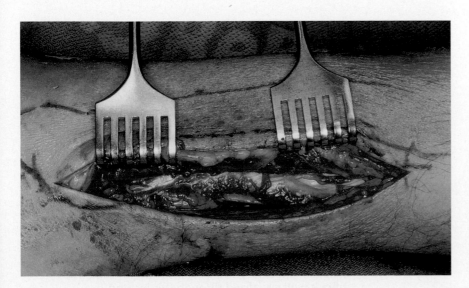

Figure 7. Intraoperative view of the posterolateral approach to the fibula. The surface anatomy of the anterior and posterior fibular borders has been marked with a blue marking pen. The subcutaneous tissues are minimally retracted anteriorly to expose the border between the peroneal tendons and the fibula. Placement of the fibular incision this far posteriorly allows an adequate skin bridge to be created between the two incisions.

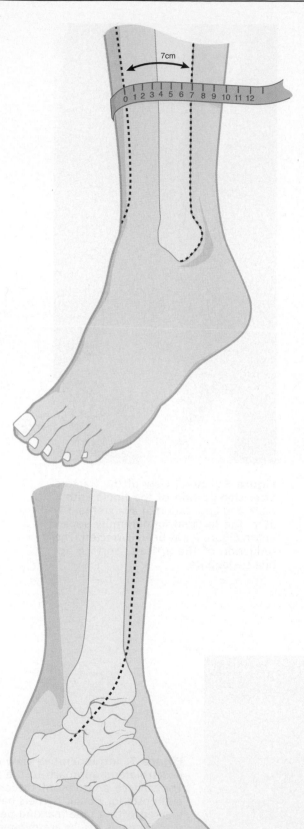

Figure 8. Schematic view demonstrating the 7-cm skin bridge between the anterior and posterior incisions. A wider skin bridge is desirable, and 9-cm skin bridges can frequently be achieved. Note again the position of the lateral incision over the posterior border rather than the midportion of the fibula.

Figure 9. Schematic view demonstrating the anteromedial incision. The incision has a gentle curve medially toward a point just distal to the tip of the medial malleolus. The articular surface of the distal tibia is well visualized through this incision.

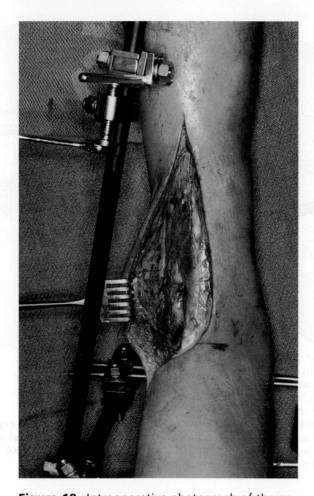

Figure 10. Intraoperative photograph of the anteromedial incision. The extensor tendon sheath has been preserved. A deep incision just medial to the tendon sheaths and over the joint will expose the articular surface. Note the presence of the radiolucent external fixator tube on the medial side, part of a triangular frame placed as a temporizing maneuver at the time of injury. A wrench is applied to a distractor on the fixator to achieve further medial distraction. A flap has been raised medially, just above the periosteum, to allow medial plate placement.

bridge of no less than 7 cm between the incisions must be preserved (Fig. 8). A wider skin bridge is desirable, and a 9-cm skin bridge is frequently possible with adequate planning. The anteromedial incision is started just lateral to the tibial crest proximally and curves toward the medial malleolus at the level of the ankle mortise (Fig. 9). Care is taken to avoid entering the extensor tendon sheaths, particularly the tibialis anterior (Fig. 10). The incisions are made directly to but not through the periosteum, without substantial dissection of the subcutaneous tissues.

Fracture fragments are exposed by elevating the periosteum along the fracture lines. The soft tissue is dissected 2 to 3 mm away from the fracture lines, and the fragments are hinged open to expose the fracture sites (Figs. 11 and 12). A plane of dissection between the periosteum and the subcutaneous layer is developed if necessary for placement of the plate. Self-retaining retractors are avoided.

The single most important factor in avoiding devitalization of the fracture fragments is distraction. Initial distraction may be achieved with a femoral distractor or an external fixator with pins placed in the proximal tibia and the medial calcaneus. If an external fixator

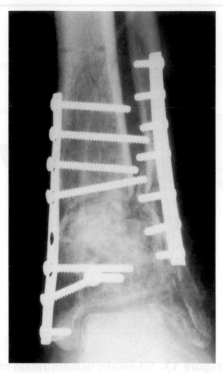

Figure 14. Anteroposterior (AP) view of the fixation construct.

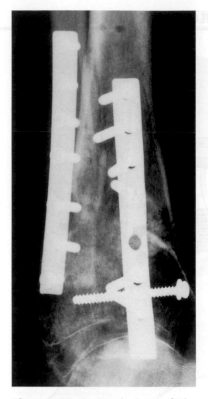

Figure 15. Lateral view of the fracture.

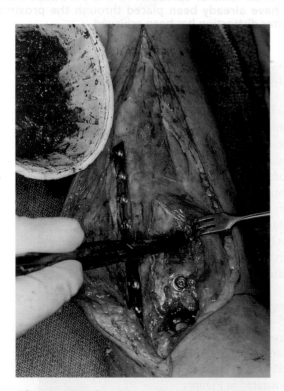

Figure 16. Placement of autogenous bone graft into osseous defect. Most defects are present adjacent to subchondral bone and at the intersection of fracture lines. The periosteal flap will be closed over the graft-recipient site.

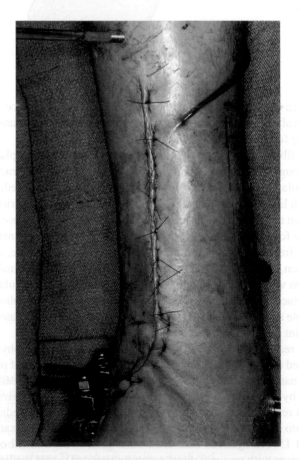

Figure 17. Atraumatic skin sutures have achieved closure without tension. A small suction drain has been placed proximally, with care to avoid violation of either the medial flap or the lateral skin bridge.

of both incisions cannot be obtained, the lateral skin incision is left open. This incision may be closed by delayed primary closure during the first week. A skin graft is rarely needed.

POSTOPERATIVE MANAGEMENT

Strict limb elevation is observed for 24 to 48 hours. A posterior splint is initially applied after surgery. Patients are routinely seen for suture removal 2 weeks after fracture fixation and at monthly intervals thereafter. Radiographs are obtained at monthly intervals and include mortise and lateral views of the ankle and anteroposterior (AP) and lateral views of the tibia if an external fixator was used. If a bridging external fixator was applied in conjunction with limited internal fixation, when bridging callus at the fracture appears, the fixator may be removed. This usually occurs 6 to 8 weeks after surgery. Minimal or no callus 8 weeks or longer after surgery, or the development of axial malalignment at any time, requires further evaluation with tomograms and consideration of further surgery.

Most patients treated with open reduction and internal fixation are fitted with a removable cam-walker and are allowed 30 to 40 pounds of weight bearing (as measured on a bathroom scale). Active and active-assisted motion are encouraged out of the brace as soon as adequate wound healing has been assured. Physical therapy is used during hospitalization for instruction in crutch training but is not routinely used for outpatient treatments. As fracture healing progresses, weight bearing in the cam-walker is advanced. The use of a stationary bicycle is helpful in many patients at 8 to 6 weeks to regain strength and improve ankle motion.

Full weight bearing is allowed in most patients between 3 and 4 months postoperatively. Activity out of the brace is then allowed, and patients are encouraged to resume activities of daily living. Recovery of daily activities including stair climbing, bending, squatting, and stooping can usually be accomplished within 4 to 5 months of surgery, depending on the degree of recovery of ankle motion. Return to recreational activities also depends on the degree of recovery of ankle motion. Most patients are capable of cycling, golf, and other light recreational activities within 6 months of injury. Return to tennis, skiing, and other more vigorous recreational activities is allowed between 6 and 12 months. However, in complex fractures, sports participation is frequently impaired by loss of ankle motion or poor endurance. Although full recovery may not be possible in these patients, gradual improvement can occur up to 18 months after surgery.

COMPLICATIONS

The most feared complication after open reduction and internal fixation of pilon fractures is infection. In one large series, infection occurred in 14% of cases (6). Despite contemporary techniques of soft-tissue management, infection associated with internal fixation of pilon fractures still remains considerably higher than the 1% rate usually associated with elective orthopaedic surgery. Appropriate management of a wound infection after internal fixation of pilon fractures is aggressive surgical debridement, intravenous antibiotics, and placement of a free vascularized muscle flap over the wound if there is a soft-tissue defect. Failure to manage wound infections aggressively may lead to a prolonged course of treatment and may lead to amputation.

Other problems that occur with some frequency after pilon fractures include nonunion, malunion, and osteoarthritis of the ankle. Nonunion after open reduction and internal fixation of pilon fractures occurs in 3% of cases, usually in the metaphyseal region. High-energy, severely comminuted fractures have a much higher rate of nonunion, up to 25% in one series (1). Treatment may be complex but most often involves placement of a bone graft with revision internal fixation of the fracture. Malunion and osteoarthrosis of the ankle joint requiring arthrodesis are the next most common complications after this type of surgery.

The frequency of complications can be predicted by the severity of the injury and by the development of postoperative wound problems. Thorough preoperative assessment and careful patient selection provide the best means of minimizing complications.

ILLUSTRATIVE CASE FOR TECHNIQUE

A 34-year-old man fell 20 feet from a roof, sustaining an isolated intraarticular fracture of the distal tibia and fibula (Fig. 18). The tibial fracture was closed, with moderate soft-tissue swelling, and no fracture blisters. A clean 2-cm laceration was present laterally over the fibular fracture. In the operating room, the traumatic wound was irrigated and minimally debrided. Provisional fixation was obtained with a fibular plate, leading to improved reduction of the distal tibial articular surface (Figs. 19 and 20), and the lateral skin incision was left open. The leg was elevated, and the patient was returned to the operating room 8 days later for definitive fixation of the tibia and closure of the lateral incision. The fracture healed uneventfully (Fig. 21), and the patient returned to full weight bearing 3 months after fracture.

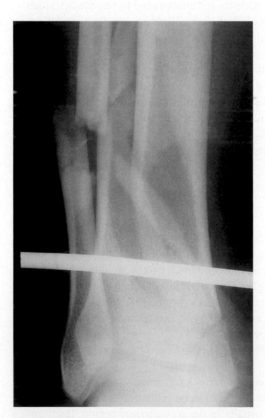

Figure 18. Anteroposterior (AP) view of a distal tibial fracture with an associated fibular fracture. The fracture extends to the tibial articular surface.

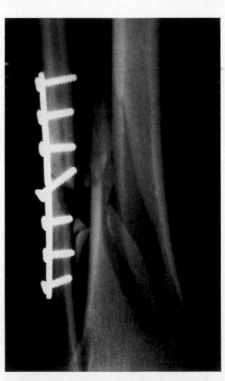

Figure 19. Anteroposterior (AP) view of the fracture after fibular stabilization. The articular surface is well reduced, with residual displacement in the metaphyseal and diaphyseal areas.

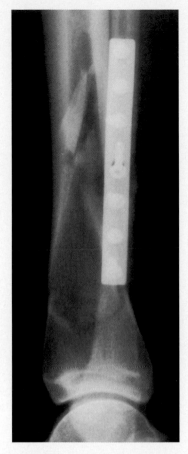

Figure 20. Lateral view after irrigation and debridement. The fibular fracture has been reduced with a 1/3 tubular plate, achieving nearly anatomic reduction in this view.

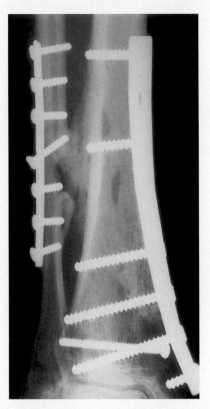

Figure 21. A narrow dynamic-compression plate has been applied medially to maintain the fracture reduction. The plate was precontoured to fit the distal tibia by using a skeletal model. Fracture healing has occurred with formation of a synostosis where the syndesmosis had been disrupted at the fibular fracture site.

RECOMMENDED READING

1. Bourne, R.B., Rorabeck, C.H., Macnab, J.: Intra-articular fractures of the distal tibia: the pilon fracture. *J. Trauma,* 23:591–596, 1983.
2. Carr, J.B., Hansen, S.T., Benirschke, S.K.: Surgical treatment of foot and ankle trauma: use of indirect reduction techniques. *Foot Ankle,* 9:176–178, 1989.
3. Helfet, D.L., Koval, K., Pappas, J., Sanders, R.W., DiPasquale, T.: Intraarticular pilon fractures of the tibia. *Clin. Orthop.,* 298:221–228, 1994.
4. Mast, J., Jakob, R., Ganz, R.: *Planning and reduction technique in fracture surgery.* Springer-Verlag, New York, 1989.
5. Mast, J.W., Spiegel, P.G., Pappas, J.N.: Fractures of the tibial pilon. *Clin Orthop,* 230:68–82, 1988.
6. McFerran, M.A., Smith, S.W., Boulas, H.J., Schwartz, H.S.: Complications encountered in the treatment of pilon fractures. *J. Orthop. Trauma,* 6(2):195–200, 1992.
7. Ovadia, D.N., Beals, R.K.: Fractures of the tibial plafond. *J. Bone Joint Surg. [Am],* 68:543, 1986.
8. Ruedi, T., Allgower, M.: The operative treatment of intra-articular fractures of the lower end of the tibia. *Clin. Orthop.,* 138:105–110, 1979.
9. Teeny, S., Wiss, D.A.: Open reduction and internal fixation of tibial plafond fractures: variables contributing to poor results and complications. *Clin. Orthop.,* 292:108–117, 1993.
10. Tornetta, P. III., Gorup, J.: Axial computed tomography of pilon fractures. *Clin. Orthop.* 323:273, 1996.
11. Tornetta, P. III., Weiner, L., Bergman, M., et al: Pilon fractures: treatment with combined internal and external fixation. *J. Orthop. Trauma,* 7:489–496, 1993.
12. Vander Griend, R., Michelson, J.D., Bone, L.B.: Fractures of the ankle and the distal part of the tibia. *J. Bone Joint Surg. [Am],* 78:1772–1783, 1996.
13. Wyrsch, B., McFerran, M.A., McAndrew, M., et al.: Operative treatment of fractures of the tibial plafond. *J. Bone Joint Surg. [Am],* 78:1646–1657, 1996.

Master Techniques in Orthopaedic Surgery,
FRACTURES, edited by D. A. Wiss,
Lippincott–Raven Publishers, Philadelphia © 1998.

29

Pilon Fractures: Hybrid External Fixation

Lon S. Weiner

INDICATIONS/CONTRAINDICATIONS

Pilon fractures are some of the most challenging injuries to treat effectively because they combine disruption of an articular surface with variable metaphyseal comminution, often in the presence of compromised soft tissues. In the past 10 years, the treatment of pilon fractures has changed dramatically. Whereas in the past, open reduction internal fixation was used for nearly all displaced fractures, hybrid external fixation has now become the treatment of choice for many severe pilon fractures. The impetus for this change was the high rates of complications, particularly wound dehiscence, deep infection, osteomyelitis, and hardware failure, seen after plate osteosynthesis of these fractures. The rationale for hybrid external fixation is to limit incisions and soft-tissue dissection to joint reconstruction, thereby avoiding long incisions through contused and uncooperative soft tissues. Instead of large plates, the fixator maintains length and alignment.

The AO classification divides pilon fractures into three broad types and three subcategories in increasing degrees of severity (Fig. 1). There are extraarticular (Type A), partial articular (Type B), and total articular (Type C) patterns. The method of treatment is guided by the fracture type, configuration, and the magnitude of the soft-tissue injury. The majority of A1 and A2 fractures and virtually all B fractures are best treated either nonoperatively or with classic internal fixation. On the other hand, many A3 and the majority of Type C fractures are better treated with hybrid external fixation (Fig. 2). However, external fixation should be considered whenever there is significant soft-tissue compromise, diaphyseal extension, or open fractures (Fig. 3).

Fractures with large articular fragments that are minimally displaced or reduce after distraction (C1 and C2) are well suited to percutaneous screw fixation of the articular surface and hybrid frame application. C3 fractures in which adequate metaphyseal reconstruction can be achieved allows the application of an external fixator. This technique is less effec-

L. S. Weiner, M.D.: Department of Orthopaedic Trauma, Lenox Hill Hospital, and Department of Orthopaedics, Mt. Sinai Hospital, New York, New York 10021.

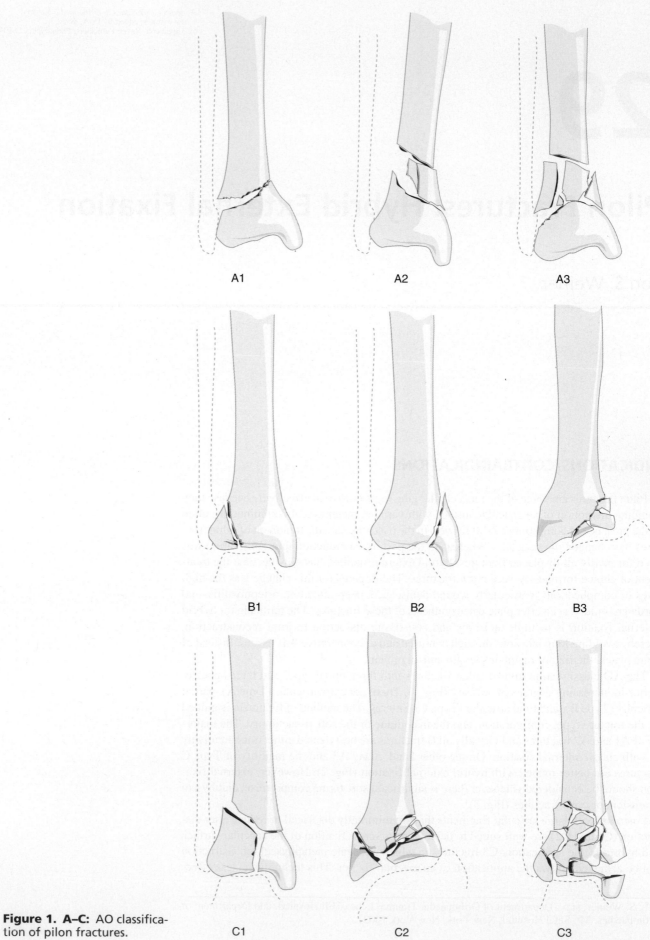

Figure 1. A–C: AO classification of pilon fractures.

A1

A2

A3

B1

B2

B3

C1

C2

C3

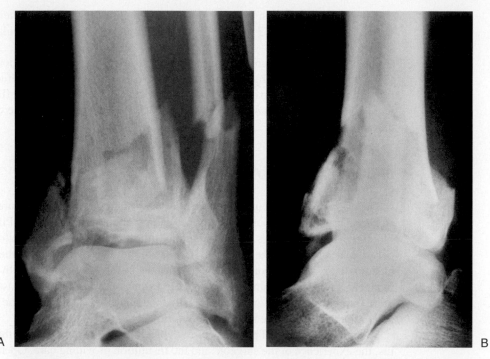

Figure 2. A, B: A comminuted pilon fracture within 3 cm of the joint. Fixation with distal wires can be difficult.

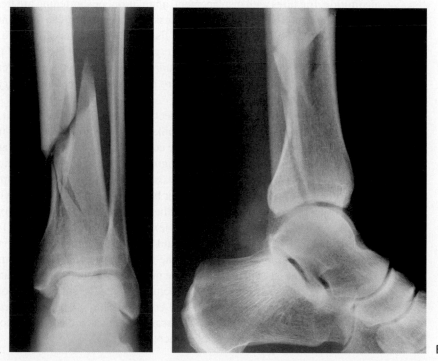

Figure 3. A, B: Fractures with metaphyseal–diaphyseal extension are an excellent indication for hybrid external fixation.

tive when there is extensive periarticular comminution (low C3) and often requires joint-spanning frames. Most C3 fractures require a formal arthrotomy for articular reduction and stabilization.

Open pilon fractures are a strong indication for hybrid external fixation. The location, size, and grade of open fractures are factors in decision making. Many Grade I and II open fractures are amenable to standard hybrid frames, whereas many Grade III open fractures require joint-bridging frames to allow serial debridement and soft-tissue coverage procedures.

PREOPERATIVE PLANNING

The evaluation in the emergency room of the patient with a pilon fracture should include a general trauma evaluation and a detailed examination of the extremity. Pilon fractures are often high-energy injuries, and concomitant injuries to the midfoot, hindfoot, knee, hip or pelvis, and spine should be ruled out. Because of the severe contusion to the soft tissue with bleeding and swelling, compartment syndromes of the leg or foot or both are not uncommon. Increasing pain, pain with passive toe extensions, or progressive loss of function require immediate evaluation. A careful and documented examination of the motor, sensory, and vascular status of the limb is mandatory.

The initial treatment of pilon fractures depends on the fracture pattern, the soft-tissue status, the experience of the surgeon, and the institution providing care. Open fractures, fractures with compartment syndromes, and patients with multiple injuries require immediate surgery. Provisional reduction with a joint-spanning fixator, with or without fibular plating, is required. In patients with isolated injuries, the timing of surgery is highly subjective. Some surgeons favor early external fixation, whereas others favor delayed fixation. In our institution, fractures with displacement, angulation, or shortening are treated with calcaneal pin traction on a Bohler Braun frame. Less severe fractures can be splinted. I prefer to wait 7 to 10 days to allow healing of the soft tissues before surgery. Fracture blisters are usually a sign of severe soft-tissue injury. Surgery is delayed until the base of the blister reepithelializes. After 3 days, the blisters are unroofed and treated with silver sulfadiazine (Silvadene) cream. I prefer to allow fracture blisters to heal before surgery, whether they are blood or fluid filled.

Preoperative planning is a critical aspect of the surgical procedure. Anteroposterior (AP), lateral, and oblique radiographs of the ankle and tibia are essential for initial fracture evaluation. Occasionally radiographs of the contralateral uninjured ankle are helpful for comparison. If the fracture is displaced, angulated, or comminuted, traction radiographs improve visualization of the metaphysis and joint surface. Preoperative computed tomography (CT) scans or tomograms or both may be useful in identifying the location and size of fracture fragments and whether they are amenable to internal fixation.

CT scans are most valuable for complex articular injuries (Type C; 14). To optimize the value of the CT scan, the fracture should be out to length or under distraction. Axial CT sections define the major fragment of the articular surface. The three main components of the fracture in the axial plane include the medial malleolus, the anterolateral corner, and the posterior malleolus. The size of the fracture fragments and presence of comminution can be assessed. Furthermore, metaphyseal comminution can be visualized, helping to determine whether a bone graft will be necessary. CT scans are useful in most C3 fractures and C2 fractures with significant displacement.

SURGERY

General or spinal anesthesia is administered. The patient is placed supine on a radiolucent table with a bolster beneath the buttock to maintain the leg in neutral rotation. A mobile C-arm image intensifier is positioned to allow visualization of the leg in both AP and lateral views with test images obtained before prepping and draping. The entire leg and ipsilateral iliac crest are prepped and draped. If needed, a sterile tourniquet can be applied to the thigh. A calcaneal traction pin, femoral distraction, or a simple tibial–calcaneal external fixator is used for initial indirect reduction (Fig. 4).

Intraoperative pin traction or a distractor are most useful for fractures with articular or metaphyseal comminution or both. Distraction achieves ligamentotaxis, which aids fracture reduction, decreasing the amount of dissection necessary for fracture exposure and fixation. Distraction by using a calcaneal pin alone is valuable in C2, C3, and B3 fractures with anterior subluxation of the talus.

If ligamentotaxis produces a near-anatomic joint surface, then percutaneous fixation is used. Fractures in which the articular surface is nondisplaced or reduces after distraction can be treated with percutaneous screw fixation and external fixation. If the joint cannot be closed reduced, then open reduction is mandatory to restore articular congruity. This also allows primary bone grafting of metaphyseal defects. Most operatively treated pilon fractures require two incisions. The fibula is approached through a posterolateral incision, which follows the posterior margin of the fibula. The tibial incision is anteromedial and remains medial to the tibialis anterior. The skin bridge between the two incisions should be

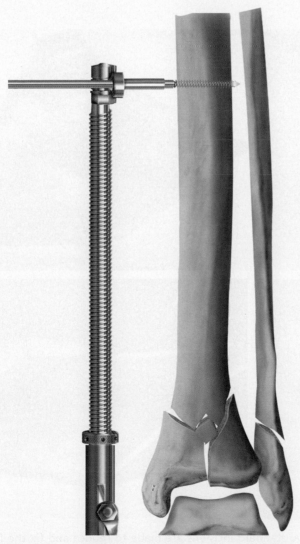

Figure 4. A femoral distractor or simple external fixator can be used to bring the fracture out to length by using indirect reduction.

at least 7 to 8 cm (Fig. 5A). The deep dissection should create full-thickness flaps from the skin to bone (Fig. 5B). The tendon sheath of the tibialis anterior should not be violated. Reduction can be facilitated with the use of calcaneal pins (Fig. 5C). During the deep dissection, care must be taken not to strip the soft tissues from comminuted fragments, which may devitalize the bone fragments. Capsular attachments to the articular fragment should not be detached. Dissection should be kept to the minimum necessary to allow fracture reduction and fixation (Fig. 5D).

Fixation of the fibula is performed through the posterolateral incision. Decisions regarding the need for fibular stabilization are often difficult. I favor fixation of fibular fractures, which aids in the reduction of the lateral or posterior portion of the tibial joint surface. Fibula fractures that are not fixed include low comminuted fractures or high fractures not associated with ankle pathology. In other words, if reducing and fixing the fibula will reduce part of the articular surface of the tibia through ligamentotaxis, it should be performed. Plating of the fibula with a one-third tubular plate is the method of choice. Transverse fractures, particularly in elderly or osteopenic bone, can be treated with an intramedullary device. Comminuted or segmental fibula fractures require longer incisions and larger implants (dynamic compression plate; DCP). In these cases, my preference is to bring the fibula out to length and fix it in place with one of the transfixing wires used in the external fixator.

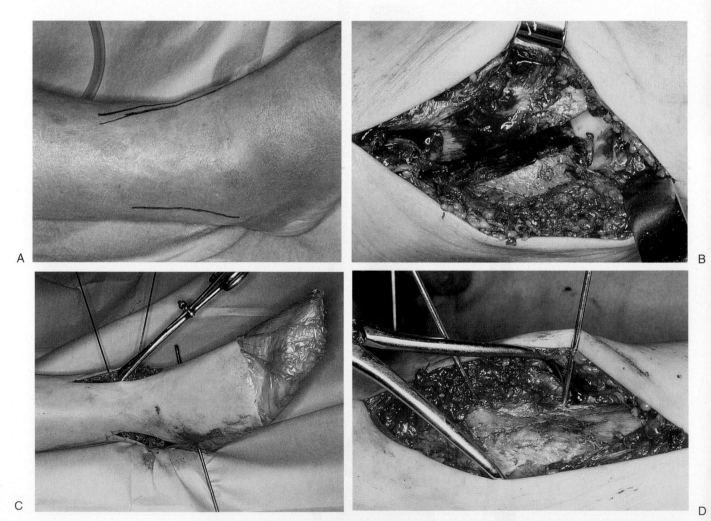

Figure 5. A: Two standard incisions are made to reduce and fix the fibula and tibia, respectively. **B:** Exposure of the fracture. **C:** Skin bridge shown; full-thickness flaps are created. A calcaneal pin is used for traction. **D:** Provisional reduction held with pins and bone-holding forceps.

Patients with open fractures or severely contused soft tissues are often treated with a staged approach. A spanning external fixator and primary plating of the fibula usually restores length and alignment of the tibia. When the soft tissues have recovered, formal fixation of the tibia and conversion to a hybrid external fixator can be done at 7 to 21 days.

Reconstruction of the metaphysis and articular surface is the next step. By using distraction and fracture manipulation, the major fragments of the metaphysis and the joint surface are reduced and stabilized with small bone-holding forceps or Kirschner wires (K-wires) or both. The metaphyseal fragments are usually fixed with screws for stability and to buttress the articular reconstruction. Fixation of the major metaphyseal fragments is performed with 3.5-, 4.0-, or 4.5-mm screws. The type and number of screws depend on the fracture configuration. Whenever possible, the anterolateral corner, the medial malleolus, and the posterior malleolus should be fixed. If there is metaphyseal bone loss, bone graft (iliac crest) should be used, although I have used bone-graft substitutes for small defects in the elderly. Iliac crest is important when the graft is used to recreate an anterior strut when the cortex of the tibia is severely comminuted.

Once the articular surface has been reconstructed, the metaphysis is reduced to the diaphysis with an external fixator. Application of the external fixator begins by inserting a thin (1.8-mm) wire from posterolateral to anteromedial (Fig. 6A). The wire may pass through the fibula or anterior to it. When the fibula is not plated, the posterolateral wire always passes through the fibula. If varus and shortening persists in the tibia after fibula fixation, then manipulation of the tibia is necessary. In this case, the posterolateral wire passes anterior to the fibula. My preference is to use a calcaneal pin to distract the tibia and restore length and alignment. A transfibular wire should not be inserted until the tibia is adequately reduced. The wire should not pass behind the fibula, where the peroneal tendons and sural

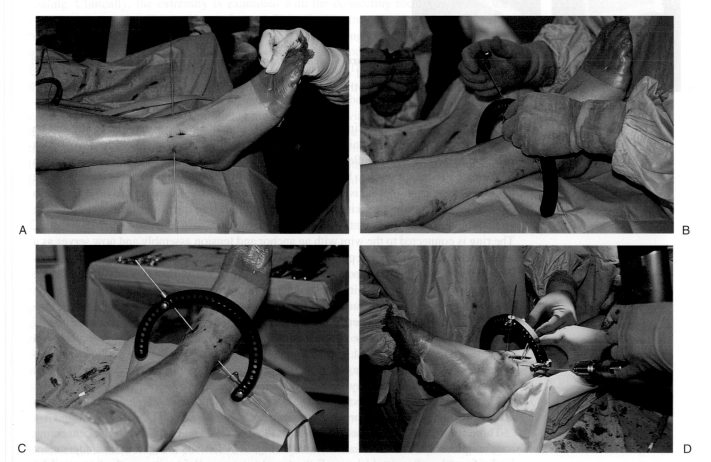

A   B   C   D

Figure 6. A: Wire one is inserted from posterolateral to anteromedial. **B–D:** Ring assembly. Wire two is inserted from posteromedial to anterolateral by using the ring as a template.

from the large-fragment set because they are stronger. Arrangements should be made for intraoperative radiography, and whenever possible, we use a mobile C-arm image intensifier. It is prudent, however, to obtain standard high-quality portable radiographs if the fluoroscopic images are not completely satisfactory. The OR staff should be informed of the surgeon's plans for postoperative immobilization such as casting or splinting. Specific arrangements may be required for anesthetic management, especially if surgery is done on an outpatient basis. In this situation, attention must be directed to giving adequate analgesia without excessive sedation or nausea. Local infiltration or regional nerve blocks with 0.5% Marcaine (bupivacaine) and Toradol (ketorolac), started intravenously and continued orally for only 48 hours, as well as adequate oral narcotics, limb elevation, and limited ambulation, help control pain postoperatively.

SURGERY

Positioning

After induction of general or spinal anesthesia, the patient is positioned supine, with a pad beneath the buttock on the injured side to aid access to the fibula (Fig. 1). All pressure points are padded. A pneumatic tourniquet is applied to the upper thigh for use during surgery, if required. A cephalosporin antibiotic (or an alternative if the patient is allergic) is given just after induction of anesthesia. The leg is prepared and draped free. A plastic adhesive drape covers the toes and seals an impermeable stockinette to the calf above the operative field.

Lateral Incision and Exposure

The incision(s) planned preoperatively are adjusted based on the examination of the soft tissues and the location of the fracture. Subcutaneous flaps should be avoided because they may compromise skin perfusion. We approach the fibula through a straight incision, between the lateral and anterior compartments, angling slightly anterior distally to allow access to the anterolateral corner of the ankle joint (Fig. 2). The superficial peroneal nerve, whose branches may cross the incision at a subcutaneous or fascial level, should be preserved (Fig. 3). Division or entrapment of the nerve in scar can lead to a symptomatic neuroma. The anterior inferior tibiofibular ligament (AITFL) is identified. It may be torn in substance or may be avulsed with a fragment of bone from the lateral malleolus or tibia. Its repair provides a helpful guide to anatomic reduction of the syndesmosis and hence the

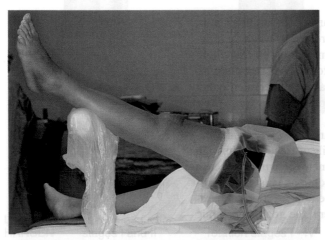

Figure 1. Before prepping and draping the extremity, a thigh tourniquet is applied, and a roll is placed beneath the ipsilateral buttock.

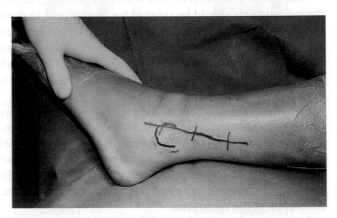

Figure 2. An oblique incision over the distal fibula affords access to the anterolateral joint space.

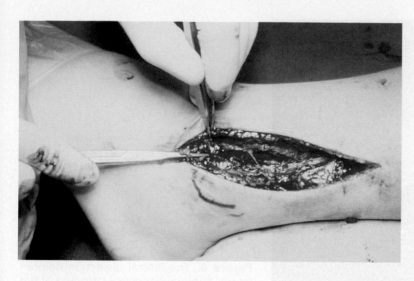

Figure 3. Care should be taken to avoid injury by protecting the superficial peroneal nerve during the lateral approach. Full-thickness flaps are carried down through the deep fascia without creating subcutaneous flaps.

proper relation of the fibula to the tibia. AITFL disruption also is present in higher fibula fractures (i.e., Lauge-Hansen pronation–external rotation or Danis–Weber C) as part of a compromised or torn syndesmosis. Its exposure, together with visualization of the anterolateral ankle joint, is important in this fracture pattern, especially when there is comminution of the fracture, because of difficulty gaining an anatomic mortise reduction if the surgeon focuses only on the extraarticular fracture and disregards the primary goal of articular-surface reduction.

Soft-tissue stripping, including the periosteum, is kept to a minimum, especially if there is significant comminution. Attempted anatomic reduction of the fibular-fracture fragments may be difficult. In this situation, an indirect reduction better preserves the soft-tissue attachments. Using a distracting device, such as a temporary external fixator or a properly contoured plate attached distally and advanced with a bone spreader against a pusher screw in the proximal fragment, helps restore length. If the fracture is noncomminuted, its ends are exposed by reflecting periosteum 2 mm, and clot is removed with irrigation and suction, avoiding curettes that might displace small fracture-surface fragments that can be valuable clues to an anatomic reduction.

Exposure must be sufficient to allow placement of reduction forceps and for insertion of fixation devices, and especially to evaluate visually the articular reduction of talus, anterolateral tibial plafond, and lateral malleolus. A narrow right-angled retractor placed into the anterior ankle capsule allows inspection of the ankle joint, after irrigation and removal of clot and any loose intraarticular fracture fragments (Fig. 4).

Lateral Reduction and Fixation

Fibular fractures with sufficient obliquity are first fixed with one (or rarely two) interfragmentary lag screw(s), supplemented with a one-third tubular plate (Figs. 5 and 6). With transverse fractures, a lag screw is impossible, and interfragmentary compression is achieved with a plate. If significant comminution is present, the plate is used in a bridging mode, bypassing the comminuted fragments and securing proper length, rotation, and angulation to the fibula by using the talofibular joint as a template for proper reduction (after anatomically reducing and temporarily transfixing this joint). Reference to radiographs of the intact opposite side may be helpful when comminution is extensive. Radiographic confirmation before plate application may be required to avoid malalignment. Bone grafting may be advisable, especially if fragments are small or devascularized by the injury. Fibular plates can be applied to the lateral aspect of the bone, or, in the case of supination–ex-

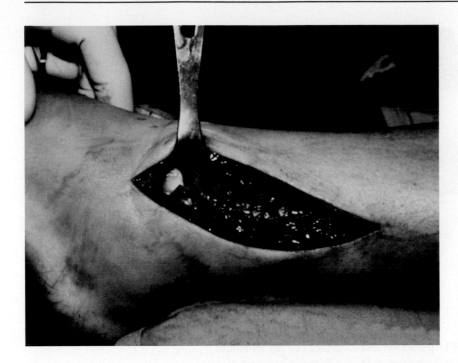

Figure 4. The lateral dissection demonstrates minimal periosteal stripping of the fibula and an excellent view of the talar dome. Vigorous irrigation and suction to evacuate the hematoma allows inspection for articular damage.

ternal rotation Type B fractures, to the posterior or posterolateral surface in the manner described by Weber as an antiglide plate (6).

For Danis–Weber Type A fractures, the anterior and lateral aspects of the fibula are exposed, along with the articular surface margin. The distal fracture fragment can usually be reduced anatomically. A dental pick or a bone hook is helpful to hold the fracture reduced while K-wires are inserted across the fracture for provisional, or more typically, definitive fixation. Reduction is confirmed visually and, if needed, radiographically. Usually Danis–Weber Type A fractures can be fixed with two small K-wires and a laterally applied tension-band wire placed distally around the K-wires and proximally around an anchoring

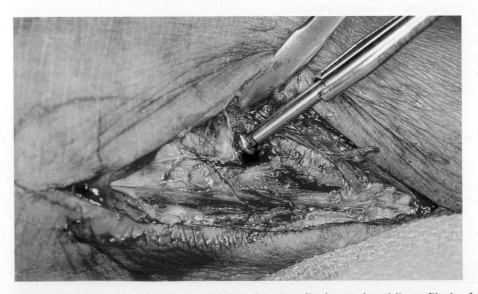

Figure 5. A 3.5-mm cortical screw is placed perpendicular to the oblique fibular fracture, after it is provisionally reduced with a pointed reduction forceps.

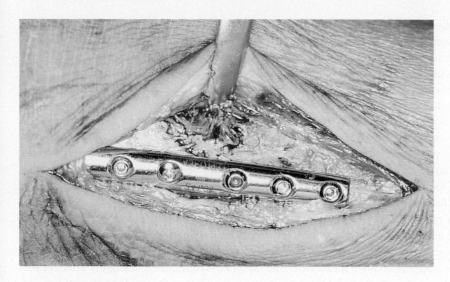

Figure 6. A 1/3-tubular plate is contoured and applied to the lateral or posterolateral surface of the fibula. Fully threaded 4.0-mm cancellous screws may improve purchase in distal metaphyseal bone. Care should be taken to avoid penetration of the talofibular joint.

screw or through a drill hole. Wire ends should be bent and impacted to minimize their prominence. Occasionally a lag screw is inserted slightly oblique to the fracture and through the proximal cortex. Alternatively, a one-third tubular plate can be contoured to fit a larger Type A fracture. Its distal end can be cut in the last hole and bent for impaction into the bone distally, producing a "hook–plate" configuration (Fig. 7).

Danis–Weber Type B fibular fractures are usually reduced by using traction on the distal fragment with a pointed reduction forceps with gentle internal rotation of the distal fragment. The reduction is "fine-tuned" by using a dental pick or reduction forceps on the fibula above the fracture, which typically permits some repositioning even with an intact in-

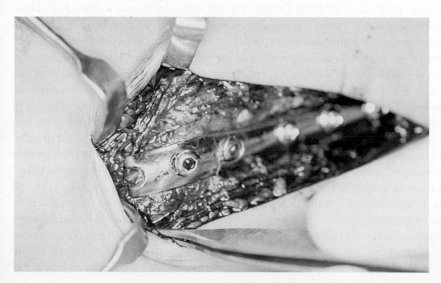

Figure 7. A "hook plate" is made by cutting through the last hole of a 1/3-tubular plate and bending the plate to create two small hooks. The plate is applied in such a way as to "hook" the tip of the fibula. This technique helps stabilize distal fractures.

terosseous membrane. Reduction is then achieved with a small reduction forceps inserted obliquely across the fibula, perpendicular to the fracture plane. Tightening the reduction forceps compresses the fracture without translating it, which can occur if the clamp is not perpendicular to the fracture plane. Danis–Weber Type B fibular fractures are usually supination–external rotation injuries with an oblique fracture plane extending from proximal posterior to distal anterior just above the joint. A single oblique 3.5-mm cortical lag screw is usually placed across the midportion of this fracture plane. Because an interfragmentary screw fixation does not provide adequate fixation alone, a one-third tubular neutralization plate is recommended. Care should be taken to ensure that distal screws do not enter the ankle joint. This neutralization plate can be applied extraperiosteally to the lateral aspect of the fibula, usually with three screws proximal and three screws distal to the fracture. It is necessary to contour the plate so it fits the shape of the lateral fibula, concave just above the plafond level, and gently convex over the larger lateral malleolus itself. Alternatively, an antiglide plate can be applied posterolaterally, on the flat fibular surface. Such a plate is placed beneath the peroneal tendons, with minimal contouring, so that a compressive force is applied to the fracture when the flat plate is tightened to a slightly concave surface (21,26). Although Weber described using such a plate without a lag screw anteriorly, we believe that a lag screw aids reduction and fixation. It can also be inserted from posterior to anterior through the plate, although this is more difficult.

Pronation–abduction lateral malleolus fractures also are typically classified as Danis–Weber Type B injuries. This pattern requires a lateral buttress plate, usually applied extraperiosteally to bridge the fracture zone after indirect fracture reduction of the lateral malleolus to the previously reduced talus. The reduction may be difficult because of lateral impaction. Occasionally the lateral tibial plafond is impacted and requires elevation and bone grafting similar to medial lesions or supination–adduction injuries (13). With significant fibular comminution after supination–external rotation, pronation–external injuries, we reverse the fixation sequence and approach the medial malleolus first. The fibula is easier to reduce if the usually simpler medial malleolar fracture is reduced and fixed first by stabilizing the talus in the mortise. The fibula can then be reduced to the lateral talar facet, by using direct or indirect reduction techniques, achieving the goal of a congruent ankle mortise. It is important to recognize such lateral tibial impaction injuries preoperatively. Last, it is important to assess syndesmosis stability intraoperatively, after fixation of any Type B lateral malleolar fractures, because soft-tissue disruption may render the ankle unstable despite fibular fixation.

Danis–Weber Type C lateral malleolar fractures are typically short oblique or nearly transverse pronation–external rotation injuries, although pronation–abduction and supination–external rotation patterns may be seen as well. Reduction is achieved by using indirect techniques, such as an external fixator, a small bone distractor, a plate with bone spreader and pusher screw, or manual traction with a pointed reduction forceps. This may be valuable in minimizing unnecessary exposure that might interfere with healing. Direct visualization of the anterolateral ankle corner of the ankle joint, the osseous syndesmotic relationship, restoration of the AITFL, and an intraoperative mortise radiograph all may be necessary to achieve fracture reduction (Fig. 8). The "high" lateral malleolus fracture is usually fixed with a 6- to 8-hole plate, which may be either a one-third tubular plate, or if higher stresses are anticipated, a small-fragment (3.5-mm) dynamic compression plate. Indirect reduction of the fracture may be performed with the plate. It can be attached distally in line with the proximal fibula and then pushed to length after ensuring that rotation and angulation are also correct. It is then fixed with screws to the proximal portion of the bone. Little, if any, plate contouring is required for most "high" fractures of the fibula. Occasionally the fibular fracture is sufficiently oblique that a lag screw can be inserted across the fracture. A properly applied plate can, however, be used to achieve interfragmentary compression, thus enhancing stability and promoting direct bone healing in noncomminuted fractures. Proximal fibular-shaft fractures rarely require plate osteosynthesis, which risks injury to the peroneal nerve. Syndesmosis reconstruction is achieved by reducing the fibula anatomically to tibia and talus in the mortise.

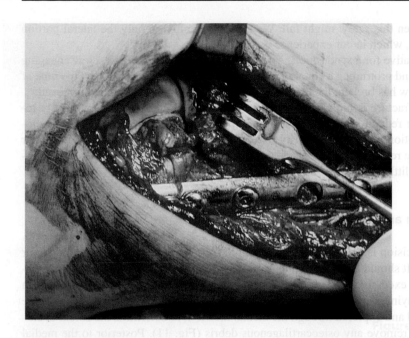

Figure 8. At the conclusion of the case, the joint should be reevaluated for reduction and articular damage. Note that the articular surfaces of the talus, lateral malleolus, and tibial plafond meet at the anterolateral corner of the ankle joint and should be inspected here for congruence.

Syndesmosis Fixation

After secure fibular-fracture fixation has been achieved, it is important to assess the stability of the mortise by directly observing the anterolateral corner of the joint. Syndesmotic instability can be assessed by pulling laterally with an instrument hooked around the distal fibula or manually displacing the talus laterally with external rotation. Displacement of more than a few millimeters, especially if there is failure of elastic recoil to the anatomic position, is an indication of soft-tissue disruption and need for transsyndesmotic screw fixation. Syndesmotic fixation is not necessary in all Danis–Weber Type C fibular fractures. Stable anatomic fracture fixation often restores adequate syndesmotic stability, especially after repair of a medial malleolus fracture, which restores the integrity of the deep deltoid ligament. It is important, however, to assess "high" fibula fractures for mortise stability and to insert a syndesmotic screw if instability is present. When mortise instability is noted, the fibula is reduced anatomically to the notch in the distal tibia, with the talus first reduced to the tibial plafond. After provisional fibulotibial K-wire fixation, radiographic confirmation of mortise alignment is obtained.

The size of the syndesmotic screw and the number of cortices of fixation remain controversial. However, we favor a 4.5-mm malleolar screw (from the AO/ASIF large-fragment set, not the 4.0-mm partially threaded small-fragment screws typically used for medial malleolar fixation). It is inserted parallel to the ankle joint, from the posterolateral fibula to the anteromedial tibia. If a plate was used for fibular fixation, it is often possible to place this screw through one of its holes. A 3.2-mm drill hole is made 2 or 3 cm above the joint from fibula to tibia. This is measured with a depth gauge, and a slightly shorter screw is chosen to prevent medial prominence. The fibula is tapped with a 4.5-mm cortical tap, which is advanced just into the tibia. The screw is then inserted with the ankle in maximum dorsiflexion, to avoid narrowing the mortise. Adjustment of the screw is done while inspecting the ankle joint, to provide sufficient but not excessive compression of the fibula into its proper relation with the tibia. Provisional K-wires, if used, are then removed, and a radiograph documenting reduction and implant location is taken before wound closure. The partially threaded 4.5-mm malleolar screw has several advantages: (a) it allows slight fibular motion, which minimizes stress on the screw; (b) it prevents mortise widening, but is durable enough to allow progression to full weight bearing within a few weeks; and (c) its larger head permits easier removal, 8 to 12 weeks after injury. Patients should be warned,

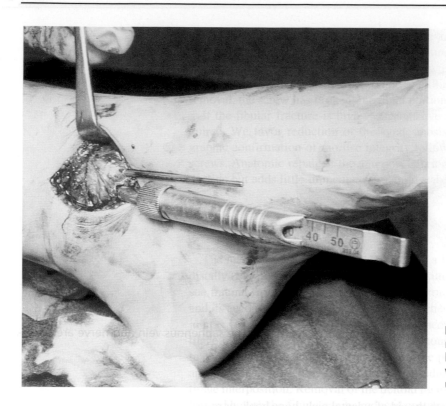

Figure 12. After reduction is achieved and maintained with the help of a dental pick or bone hook, the malleolus can be secured with one 2.5-mm drill bit, while another is used to make the second hole.

the fracture plane. For horizontal fractures, these are placed halfway between medial cortex and articular cartilage and angled proximally and laterally from the tip of the malleolus, so as to remain entirely within the malleolus and the distal tibial metaphysis. The bone can be very dense in this metaphyseal region and provides excellent anchorage for the cancellous screws. These should stop centrally in the cancellous bone. Fixation into the lateral cortex is unnecessary, and if attempted may cause the drill bit to walk along the far cortex, displacing the fracture. Generally, 40-mm screw lengths are sufficient, although this depends on patient size and fracture pattern. It is better to stay within the dense bone of the more distal tibial metaphysis, especially in osteoporotic patients, than to use longer screws. Small medial malleolar fractures may be fixed with one screw, typically in the larger anterior colliculus, with a parallel K-wire in the posterior colliculus to prevent rotation. Bending the K-wire so its tip lies on the screw head aids hardware removal and minimizes prominence. Comminuted fragments may be repaired with K-wires and a supplementary "tension-band" wire, which we prefer to anchor around a small screw above the malleolus (Fig. 13). Vertical medial malleolar fractures should not be fixed with oblique screws, but rather with horizontally placed ones that are perpendicular to the fracture. Washers may be required, or a one-third tubular plate, applied as a buttress in the case of osteoporosis or medial cortical comminution. Articular-surface impaction, which occurs in the medial tibial plafond during severe supination–adduction injuries, requires elevation and bone grafting of the resulting subjacent cancellous defect (23).

Because surgical repair of the deep deltoid ligament has not been shown to be effective, and anatomic reduction of the fibula with stable restoration of syndesmosis is successful in reestablishing the proper position of the talus in the mortise, we make no attempt to repair the deep deltoid ligament. Thus when treating an unstable lateral malleolar fracture associated with a deltoid ligament disruption, we do not expose the medial side of the ankle, unless required to reduce the talus.

Posterior Malleolus

Small posterior malleolar fragments (Volkmann's triangle) are often extraarticular. They are attached to the posterior inferior tibiofibular ligament and are usually reduced with anatomic reduction of the fibula. When large, such a fragment should be reduced and fixed to help stabilize the ankle mortise by reattaching the tibial anchorage of the posterior syndesmotic ligament. This frequently obviates the need for a transsyndesmotic screw. If the fragment is large and involves more than 25% of the articular surface of the distal tibia, we favor fixation, particularly if associated with posterior talar subluxation or dislocation.

The decision to fix a posterior malleolus fracture should be made preoperatively with a specific plan for medial or lateral exposure dependent on the fracture location and associated injuries. Restoration of fibular length and dorsiflexion of the foot frequently reduces the posterior fragment indirectly.

If open reduction is necessary, however, it can be done by a posterolateral or posteromedial approach. Most posteromedial articular fragments can be visualized satisfactorily through the bed of the medial malleolus before its reduction and fixation. We use anterior-to-posterior screws for the medial fragment and posterior-to-anterior screws for posterolateral fragments. Occasionally dissection behind the fibula is necessary to reduce a large displaced osteoarticular fragment.

Provisional fixation with K-wires is followed by confirmation of reduction by direct articular-surface inspection. It is wise to use intraoperative fluoroscopy or to obtain intraoperative radiographs before definitive lag-screw fixation. We usually use 3.5-mm cortical screws as lag screws, drilling gliding holes in the anterior distal tibia before reduction of the fracture, following which 2.5-mm threaded holes are drilled through the reduced and stabilized posterior fragment, by using an appropriate guide in the gliding hole.

Occasionally a significant posterior malleolar fracture can be reduced well with percutaneous manipulation under fluoroscopic control. In such cases, we perform percutaneous fixation with cannulated screws. Small posterior malleolar fractures, involving less than 25% of the articular surface, are typically lateral and extraarticular. These are not routinely fixed, as they typically reduce with reduction and fixation of the lateral malleolus because they are attached to the posterior–inferior tibiofibular ligament. They usually heal satisfactorily without fixation.

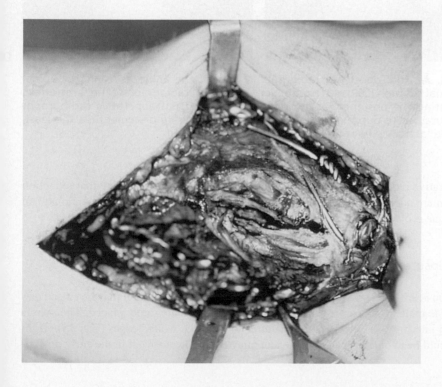

Figure 13. A tension band, fixed around two Kirschner wires in the medial malleolus, and a screw anchored in the tibial metaphysis is better than screws when the medial malleolus is comminuted or small.

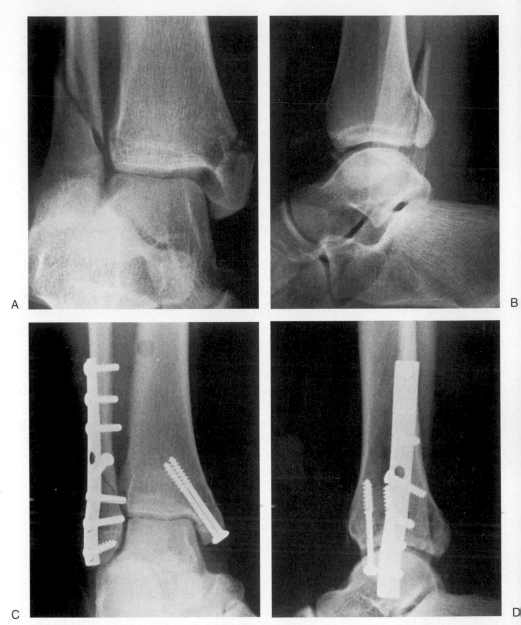

Figure 14. A: Anteroposterior radiographic view of the ankle, revealing a supination–external rotation (SER) pattern of injury. **B:** Lateral radiograph of the same ankle, demonstrating the posterior malleolar fragment. **C, D:** Intraoperative radiographs must be obtained to document the reduction and hardware placement. At the least, mortise and lateral views of the ankle are required.

Intraoperative radiographs must be taken before wound closure to ensure that reduction and fixation are adequate (Fig. 14A–D). We obtain a mortise and lateral view and add an AP or oblique projection if there is a specific need.

Wound Closure

The fascia is left open proximally over calf-muscle compartments but may be closed distally over the malleoli. Separate subcutaneous-layer sutures are rarely placed. The skin is closed with interrupted vertical mattress sutures to evert the wound edges (Fig. 15). Tight closure should be avoided because of the tendency for the leg to swell in the early postop-

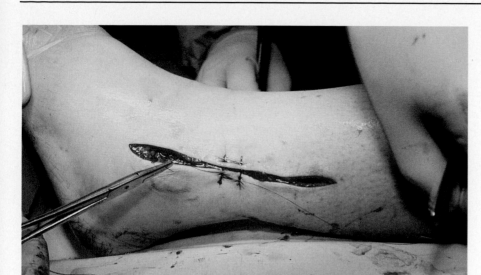

Figure 15. The fascia is closed with interrupted sutures. Subcutaneous sutures are not usually necessary. The surgical incision is closed with vertical mattress sutures to evert and oppose the wound edges. Forceps are not used to handle the skin.

erative period. Any skin at risk is either left open or closed with unilateral subcuticular sutures, as described by Allgöwer and Donati (17). If the wound is too swollen to close without excessive tension, the wound should be left open. We recommend delayed wound closure for all but the most minor open malleolar fracture wounds and use the tobramycin–polymethylmethacrylate bead-pouch technique of open wound care, as described by Ostermann et al. (18). Severely contaminated or worrisome ankle wounds are reassessed in the operating room (OR) within 24 to 48 hours. Our goal is to close all wounds within 5 to 7 days of injury. Rarely, plastic surgical flap-closure techniques are required. If free tissue transfer will be necessary, intraoperative plastic surgical consultation is advisable early in the patient's care. Long delays in wound closure increase the risk of wound complications.

Bupivacaine (Marcaine), 0.5%, is infiltrated liberally in the soft tissues to decrease postoperative pain. A nonadherent dressing and sterile gauze pads are held in place with a layer of loosely applied sterile cast padding. Ample additional padding is applied over this, with the ankle held in full dorsiflexion. Afterward, a short-leg posterior plaster splint is applied with the foot dorsiflexed (Fig. 16).

Open Fractures

Patients with open ankle fractures should be reduced, their wounds covered with a sterile dressing, splinted, and brought to the OR urgently for irrigation and debridement. Antibiotics and tetanus prophylaxis are administered promptly.

If there is any concern about the status of the soft-tissue envelope, additional surgical incisions, beyond what is required for adequate debridement, should be avoided until the soft tissues have recovered. It is important, however, to recognize that immediate surgical stabilization of open fractures is beneficial. Whenever possible, definitive internal fixation is recommended. Fixation that can be performed through the debrided wound should usually be done on completion of wound debridement. Definitive reduction and fixation of the opposite side of the ankle may be performed primarily as well, but only if the soft-tissue condition permits this to be done safely.

Comminution, bone loss, and severe soft-tissue injury that requires delayed internal fixation should be immobilized and stabilized with an external fixator until the surgery can be safely performed. An external fixator that eliminates ankle motion is applied, extending

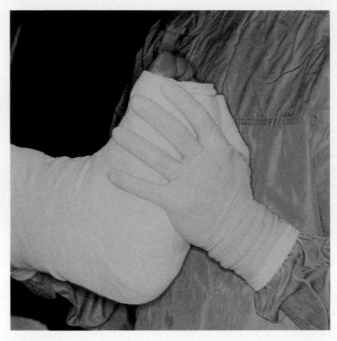

Figure 16. Generous padding should be applied after sterile dressings, followed by a posterior splint, which holds the ankle in neutral or slight dorsiflexion to prevent an equinus contracture.

from the tibia into both the calcaneus and forefoot. A tobramycin bead-pouch dressing is applied to open wounds, and the opposite side's fixation delayed (18). Primary wound closure is not performed during the initial visit to the OR. Open ankle fractures should rarely be stabilized with only a splint or cast, because skeletal stability is essential to protect the injured soft tissues. If internal fixation is inappropriate, a bridging external fixator is a good temporary alternative.

POSTOPERATIVE MANAGEMENT

In the recovery room, the leg is elevated, analgesia is administered, and treatment of nausea is provided. Patients may often be discharged directly home from the recovery room, with instructions to maintain limb elevation and avoid weight bearing. For outpatients, analgesics should be filled preoperatively to avoid delays on the way home.

At approximately 10 days, the patient is seen in the office to remove the splint and dressings. If satisfactory wound healing is noted, sutures are removed. If bone density is normal and fixation is secure, and there is no involvement of the tibial plafond, we usually allow protected weight bearing. An Aircast (Aircast, Inc., Summit, NJ) short-leg walker, or equivalent, is applied, and the patient is instructed to walk with crutches or a walker and place as much weight as is comfortable on the injured ankle. Generally, the Aircast is removed for sleeping as soon as comfort permits, as well as several times a day for active range-of-motion exercises. As the patient becomes more comfortable, gentle but progressive passive dorsiflexion stretching is added.

The postoperative radiographs are obtained at 2 and 6 weeks. At 6 weeks, the Aircast is replaced with an elastic support stocking and well-cushioned athletic training shoes with a mild rocker bottom.

The patient is advised to use crutches as needed while progressively resuming normal activities, either independently or with physical therapy if progress is delayed. Should non–weight bearing be advisable because of osteoporosis, comminution, or significant joint involvement, we recommend a fiberglass bivalved short-leg cast in neutral or, preferably, some dorsiflexion. This is worn night and day but removed at least 4 times daily for non–weight bearing range-of-motion exercises. Once stable fracture union is secure, usually by 3 months, progressive weight bearing is begun, often by using an Aircast short-leg walker for initial protection.

Whereas most malleolar fractures have fairly secure bone union 6 to 8 weeks after fixation, functional rehabilitation typically requires at least another 6 to 8 weeks before most patients can comfortably resume most low-demand activities or begin progressive athletic training of any significance. Lower impact activities such as cycling are better tolerated and walking in appropriate shoes (thicker, well-cushioned heels) before running. Return to running and competitive athletics typically requires 4 to 6 months. Most patients with anatomically reduced and fixed bi- or trimalleolar fractures have at least some functional deficit for months and benefit from sustained independent or supervised exercise programs (20).

Recovery rate and residual impairment typically closely correlate with the severity of the injury and accuracy of the reduction. Tibiotalar dislocation has a poorer outcome than malleolar fractures without complete dislocation. We suggest that patients begin with lower impact activities once comfort permits and build endurance gradually.

Local swelling lasts for months and may require elastic support. Some permanent thickening of the fractured ankle almost always occurs.

Syndesmosis screw removal is recommended, but it is deferred for at least 3 months after repair. Symptomatic fracture-fixation hardware is removed electively after mature healing but is not necessary in the absence of symptoms. After hardware removal, metaphyseal regions are generally protected with a splint and crutches for a week or 2 during soft-tissue wound healing. More proximal screw holes, however, should be protected from significant stresses until bone remodeling has occurred, which may require 6 to 12 weeks. Typically this can be achieved by avoiding contact sports and risk activities, but with full weight bearing out of protective devices.

Patients with diabetic or other peripheral neuropathy are particularly prone to complications after malleolar fractures, such as failure of fixation, loss of reduction, and development of a Charcot joint. Therefore they must be evaluated and managed with great care. It should be noted, however, that such patients often do very poorly with nonoperative care. In neuropathic patients with adequate arterial perfusion, we recommend stable internal fixation and strict non–weight bearing until their fractures are healed. This includes construction of a well-padded cast with the ankle in neutral for protective purposes, which occasionally can be bivalved to allow the cooperative patient to remove it intermittently for range-of-motion exercises.

Once the fractures have healed, weight bearing is begun in the cast or fracture brace; a padded ankle–foot orthosis (AFO) with a rocker-bottom shoe is used for the next 6 months, in an effort to provide protection against the possible development of Charcot osteoarthropathy.

COMPLICATIONS

Complications of malleolar surgery are increased in patients with malnutrition, osteoporosis, diabetes, peripheral vascular disease, and by local factors such as soft-tissue trauma and swelling. Wound slough, infection, and loss of fixation are best avoided by proper recognition and respect of soft-tissue injury. Posttraumatic arthritis of clinical significance is uncommon, except in high-energy fracture–dislocations with greater comminution, displacement, and overall cartilage injury. Malunion is also more likely under these circumstances, or after inadequate closed or open reduction. Perhaps the two most common complications of ankle surgery include loss of motion and hardware prominence. Ankle stiffness, particularly loss of dorsiflexion, can be minimized by appropriate early motion exercises and functional rehabilitation. Hardware prominence is an issue only if it is bothersome to the patient or threatening to the skin, and in either case, is addressed with removal of the screws or plate after fracture union.

Stiffness

Loss of dorsiflexion can be problematic. Aggressive independent stretching, if not rapidly successful, should be supplemented with formal physical therapy, as some patients do not stretch effectively. We have limited and unsuccessful experience with arthroscopic lysis of adhesions and with manipulation under anesthesia. Most patients can accommodate to this deformity, especially with the use of shoes with thicker heels. Rarely a posterior soft-tissue release, often including lengthening of the Achilles and occasionally other flexor tendons, is required. Some have suggested progressive stretching of the joint with an Ilizarov external fixator. Rarely a supramalleolar dorsiflexion osteotomy might be considered.

Infection

Infection usually is seen as wound breakdown or drainage. Pain or swelling that persists, or is worse than expected, should raise suspicion of infection, which is more common after open fractures and the use of percutaneous fixation wires. Whenever an infection is considered, diagnostic aspiration of the ankle is indicated. Open debridement is required for postoperatively infected joints, as well as for any operative wounds that develop an infection. Culture-specific antibiotics, stabilization of soft tissues, and delayed closure once all tissues are sufficiently healthy are important aspects of treatment for infected malleolar fractures.

Posttraumatic Arthritis

This may be due to initial cartilage injury, to postinfectious changes, or to malreduction leading to excessive focal joint contact pressure and resulting articular cartilage damage. Occasionally an anterior osteophyte develops, which is painful and limits dorsiflexion. Its resection may improve symptoms for long enough to be significantly beneficial. More typically, damage is more extensive, and the articular surface is unsalvageable. In such cases, if symptoms cannot be tolerated with appropriate shoes, activity reduction, occasional bracing, and analgesia or antiinflammatory medication, ankle arthrodesis should be considered. Much of the articular subchondral bone can be retained and fusion obtained by resection of the cartilage, bone feathering, and fixation in a neutral position with three large cannulated screws.

Malunion

Malunion is most common after cast immobilization of ankle fractures. The malunion should be corrected if the patient's general and local conditions permit surgery, the bone is of adequate quality to permit secure fixation, and the articular cartilage has not been significantly destroyed. Weight-bearing radiographs are very helpful for this assessment. The fracture must be taken down, the talus reduced satisfactorily under the tibial plafond, and the malleoli reduced so as to provide stable alignment in this position. Standard fixation is usually sufficient, although bone defects may require grafting, and buttress plates may be needed to ensure support of either malleolus.

Nonunion, although rare, usually responds to stable fixation, occasionally supplemented with bone graft, especially if a bone defect is present. Smokers have more difficulties with fracture healing, and should stop if at all possible.

ILLUSTRATIVE CASE FOR TECHNIQUE

A 38-year-old woman fell 5 feet from a ladder, sustaining an isolated injury to her ankle. Examination showed a swollen, ecchymotic ankle with painful fracture crepitus. There was posterior displacement of the foot and ankle on the leg. The patient could weakly flex and extend her toes. The dorsalis pedis and posterior tibial pulses were palpable, and sensation was intact on the dorsum and plantar aspect of the foot. There was no evidence of a compartment syndrome. Radiographs showed a trimalleolar fracture of the ankle with posterior subluxation of the talus (Fig. 17 A and B). The ankle was reduced and immobilized in a well-padded posterior splint. Because of significant swelling and ecchymosis, surgery was delayed. A CT scan was obtained to assess the posterior malleolar fracture (Fig. 17C). At surgery, a hook plate was used to fix the relatively distal lateral malleolus fracture. The pos-

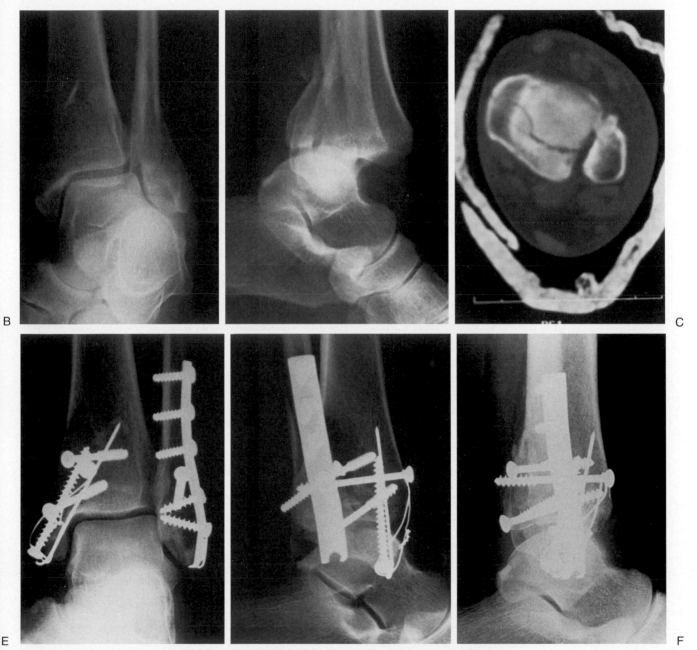

, B   C

E   F

Figure 17. A, B: Anteroposterior (AP) and lateral of the ankle shows a Danis–Weber B, Lauge-Hansen supination–external rotation (SER) IV trimalleolar fracture–dislocation. **C:** Axial view on the computed tomography scan shows a large posterior malleolar fragment involving 40% of the articular surface. **D–F:** Postoperative radiographs showing "hook–plate" fixation of the fibula, tension band wiring of the medial malleolus, and screw fixation of the posterior malleolus.

terior malleolar fragment was fixed through the medial incision with two screws placed from posteromedial to anterolateral. A tension band was used to stabilize the comminuted medial malleolus (Fig. 17D–F). An anterior-to-posterior screw was also used as the "cleat" for the tension band. Postoperative radiographs show an anatomic reduction of the fracture with restoration of the ankle mortise. Postoperatively, the patient was placed into a bivalved cast to allow active-assisted range-of-motion exercises. At 4 weeks, protected weight bearing was begun and gradually increased over the next month. At 3 months, the patient walked without external support but with a slight limp. There was minimal tenderness and residual swelling around the ankle. There was 5 degrees of dorsiflexion and 40 degrees of plantar flexion. Radiographs showed uneventful healing.

RECOMMENDED READING

1. Baird, R.A., Jackson, S.T.: Fractures of the distal part of the fibula with associated disruption of the deltoid ligament. Treatment without repair of the deltoid ligament. *J. Bone Joint Surg. [Am]*, ;69(9):1346–52, 1987.
2. Bauer, M., Jonsson, K., Nilsson, B.: Thirty-year follow-up of ankle fractures. *Acta. Orthop. Scand.*, 56(2):103–106, 1985.
3. Belcher, G.L., Radomisli, T.E., Abate, J.A., et al: Functional outcome analysis of operatively treated malleolar fractures. *J. Orthop. Trauma*, 11(2):106-9, 1997.
4. Bone, L., Stegemann, P., McNamara, K., Seibel, R.: The use of external fixation in severe fractures about the ankle. *Orthop. Trans.*, 14:265, 1990.
5. Bray, T.J., Endicott, M., Capra, S.E.: Treatment of open ankle fractures. Immediate internal fixation vs closed immobilization and delayed fixation. *Clin. Orthop.*, 240:47–52, 1989.
6. Brunner, C.F., Weber, B.G.: *Special Techniques in Internal Fixation*. Springer-Verlag, Berlin, 1982.
7. DeSouza, L.J., Gustillo, R. B., Meyer, T.J.; Results of operative treatment of displaced external rotation-abduction fractures of the ankle. *J. Bone Joint Surg.*, 67A:1066–1074, 1985.
8. Franklin, J.L., Johnson, K.D., Hansen, S.T.: Immediate internal fixation of open ankle fractures. *J. Bone Joint Surg.*, 66A:1349–1356, 1984.
9. Heim, U., Pfeiffer, K.M.: *Small fragment set manual*. Technique recommended by the ASIF Group, ed. 2., Springer-Verlag, New York, 1981.
10. Hughes, J.L., Weber, H., Willenegger, H., Kuner, E.H.: Evaluation of ankle fractures: Non-operative and operative treatment *Clin. Orthop.*, 138:111–119, 1979.
11. Konrath, G., Karges, D., Watson, J.T., et al: Early versus delayed treatment of severe ankle fractures: a comparison of results. *J. Orthop. Trauma*, 9(5):377–80, 1995.
12. Lauge-Hansen, N.: Fractures of the ankle. Analytic historic survey as basis of new experimental roentgenologic and clinical investigations. *Arch. Surg.*, 56:259–317, 1948.
13. Limbird, R.S., Aaron, R.K.: Laterally comminuted fracture dislocation of the ankle. *J. Bone Joint Surg.*, 69A:881 885, 1987.
14. Lindsjö, U.: Classification of ankle fractures: the Lauge-Hansen or AO system? *Clin. Orthop.*, 199:12–16, 1985.
15. Marti, R.K., Raaymakers, E.L.F.B., Nolte, P.A.: Malunited ankle fractures. The late results of reconstruction. *J. Bone Joint Surg.*, 72B-709–713, 1990.
16. Mast, J., Jakob, R., Ganz, R.: *Planning and reduction technique in fracture surgery*. Springer-Verlag, New York, 1989.
17. Müller, M.E., Algöwer, M., Schneider, R., Willenegger, H.: *Manual of internal fixation*, ed. 3., Springer-Verlag, New York, 1991.
18. Ostermann, P.A., Seligson, D., Henry, S.L.: Local antibiotic therapy for severe open fractures.A review of 1085 consecutive cases. *J. Bone Joint Surg. Br.*, 77B(1):93–7, 1995.
19. Ramsey, P., Hamilton, W.: Changes in tibiotalar area of contact caused by lateral talar shift. *J. Bone Joint Surg.*, 58A:356357, 1976.
20. Sammarco, G.J.: *Rehabilitation of the foot and ankle*. Mosby, St. Louis, 1995.
21. Schaffer, J.J., Manoli, A. II.: The antiglide plate for distal fibular fixation. A biomechanical comparison with a lateral plate. *J. Bone Joint Surg.*, 69A:596–604, 1987.
22. Tile, M.: Fractures of the ankle, pp. 523–561 In: Schatzker, J., Tile, M.(eds.): *The Rationale of Operative Fracture Care*. ed 2., Springer-Verlag, New York, 1996, pp. 371–405.
23. Trafton, P.G.: Medial ankle plafond impaction fractures due to supination-adduction: technique of surgical repair. *Techniques Orthop* 6:90–94, 1991.
24. Trafton, P.G., Bray, T.J., Simpson, L.A.: Fractures and soft tissue injuries of the ankle. 52 in *Skeletal Trauma*, ed 1. WB Saunders, Philadelphia, 1992.
25. Weber, B.G., Simpson, L.A.: Corrective lengthening osteotomy of the fibula. *Clin. Orthop.*, 199:61–67, 1985.
26. Wissing, J.C., van Laarhoven, C.J., van der Werken, C.: The posterior antiglide plate for fixation of fractures of the lateral malleolus. *Injury* 23(2):94–6, 1992.
27. Yablon, I.G., Leach, R.E.: Reconstruction of malunited fractures of the lateral malleolus. *J. Bone Joint Surg.*, 7 IA:521–527, 1989.

Master Techniques in Orthopaedic Surgery,
FRACTURES, edited by D. A. Wiss,
Lippincott–Raven Publishers, Philadelphia © 1998.

31

Talar-Neck Fractures: Open Reduction Internal Fixation

Timothy J. Bray

INDICATIONS/CONTRAINDICATIONS

Fractures of the talus account for approximately 1% of all fractures seen in major trauma centers; however, complications encountered after injury and treatment are some of the most challenging problems for the orthopaedic surgeon (6). The types of injuries that occur to the talus are variable, ranging from small chip fractures or articular surface avulsions to displaced, open fracture–dislocations of the neck or body of the talus.

Fractures of the talar neck are usually caused by high-energy motor vehicle or motorcycle trauma and are frequently associated with other skeletal or abdominal injuries. The most widely used classification is that proposed by Hawkins (Fig. 1). Most authors agree that nondisplaced fractures of the talar neck (Hawkins I) can be treated nonoperatively (6). Hawkins II fractures, with as little as 5 degrees of angulation or more than 2-mm offset should be treated with open reduction and anatomic, stable internal fixation. Virtually all Hawkins III and IV fractures with displacement are very strong indications for early open reduction, internal fixation (4).

Open talus fractures pose even greater urgency for treatment because of the tenuous blood supply to the bone after injury. Significant fracture displacement often dictates emergency reductions to prevent skin necrosis and infection and to enhance bone revascularization (Fig. 2). A high index of suspicion is necessary in the polytraumatized patient, as missed injuries in the foot can lead to difficult, delayed reconstructive problems.

T. J. Bray, M.D.: Department of Orthopaedic Surgery, University of California, Davis Medical Center, Sacramento, California; and Reno Orthopaedic Clinic, Reno, Nevada 89503.

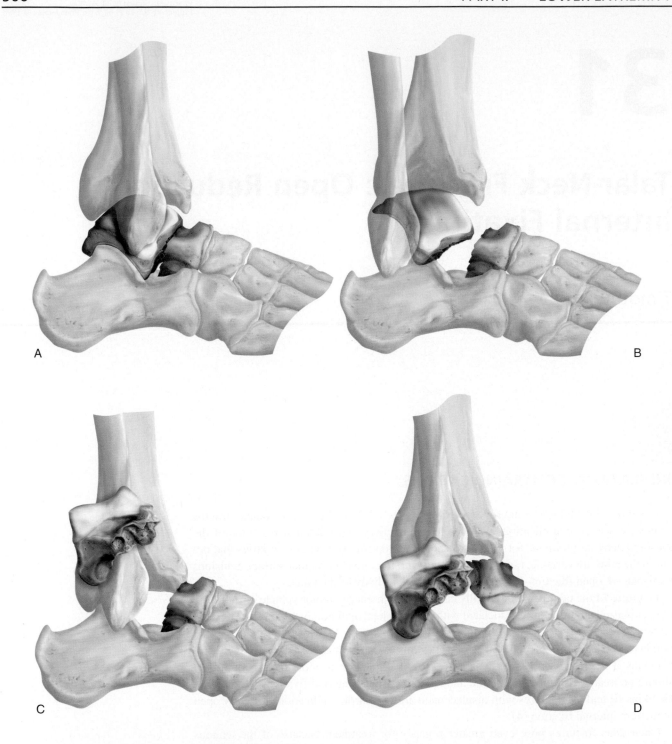

Figure 1. The Hawkins classification for talus fractures. **A:** Type I. **B:** Type II. **C:** Type III.
D: Type IV.

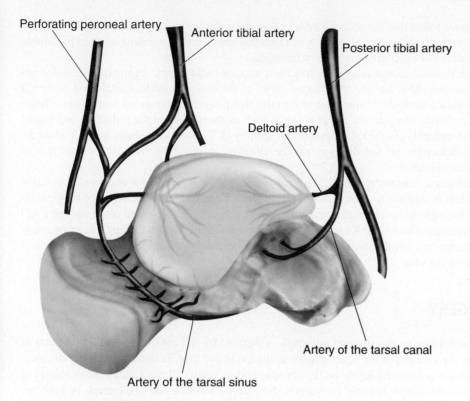

Perforating peroneal artery

Anterior tibial artery

Posterior tibial artery

Deltoid artery

Artery of the tarsal canal

Artery of the tarsal sinus

Figure 2. The vascular anatomy of the talus.

PREOPERATIVE PLANNING

Open or closed fracture–dislocations of the talar neck in multiply injured patients do not afford the clinician the luxury of a controlled preoperative plan. If the fracture is open, treatment consists of formal irrigation and debridement, anatomic reduction, and screw fixation from either an anterior or posterior approach. The joint capsule is closed whenever possible, and the traumatic skin and soft tissues are left open and closed in a delayed fash-

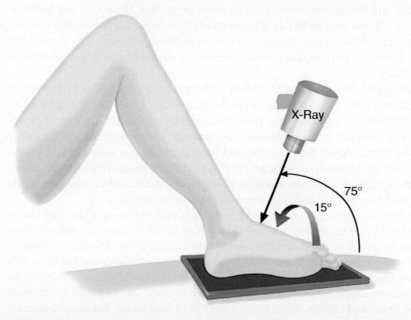

X-Ray

75°

15°

Figure 3. A pronated, oblique view of the foot helps to assess the fracture pattern and reduction.

ion. I have found that fluoroscopy tables allow the orthopaedic surgeon to scan the foot and ankle, permitting rapid confirmation of reduction and screw placement, and are preferable to multiple intraoperative portable radiographs.

With isolated closed talar-neck fractures, routine radiographic evaluation includes anteroposterior (AP), lateral, and oblique views of the foot and ankle. Canale and Kelly (2) described a pronated, oblique view of the talus that projects the bone on profile and is helpful in assessing the fracture morphology as well as the quality of the reduction and placement of implants (Fig. 3). Computed tomography (CT) scans have been helpful when articular defects occur but rarely assist the clinician in planning reduction maneuvers or selection of implants.

Mechanical, histomorphologic, and cadaveric studies have shown that posterior screw placement is superior to anterior screw fixation (6). Therefore, in the absence of multiple injuries, the patient is positioned laterally on a fluoroscopic table. Basic and small-fragment AO instrumentation including Kirschner wires (K-wires) and reduction clamps should be available. Large and small cannulated screws can be extremely helpful and should be available whenever possible.

SURGERY

In polytraumas, the surgical approach is dictated by the patient's overall condition as well as the location of the open wounds in the ankle and foot. In the vast majority of cases, patients are positioned supine on the operating table, which allows concurrent treatment of chest or abdominal injuries. Frequently the anterior medial, anterior lateral, or both approaches are required for fixation of the talus (5).

Anterior Screw Placement

The entire lower extremity is prepped and draped free. The forefoot is covered with a surgical glove to keep the toes out of the surgical field. The anteromedial approach is used most frequently (Fig. 4A and B). The skin incision begins just anterior to the medial malleolus, extending to the level of the talonavicular joint distally. The deep dissection is medial to the anterior tibial tendon and extends posterior if a malleolar osteotomy is necessary. The retinaculum over the tibialis posterior is incised, allowing posterior retraction of the tendon. If a medial malleolar osteotomy is performed (Fig. 4C), the intact malleolus is predrilled with a 2.5-mm drill bit before the osteotomy. The bone cut is completed with a small oscillating saw or osteotome, taking care not to cut through the articular surface. By using a small osteotome, the articular surface is carefully divided to facilitate subsequent reduction and fixation.

Anteromedial approaches can be used with or without a medial malleolar osteotomy. If the medial malleolus is fractured, then access to the talar neck or body is accomplished by a limited capsulectomy through the same incision described previously. Care must be exercised during this approach as the saphenous vein and nerve lie superficial and are easily damaged. Distal retraction of the osteotomized medial malleolus with a small lamina spreader or a small Hohmann-type retractor provides excellent visualization of the articular surface of the talar neck and body. Fixation of the medial malleolar fragment is usually accomplished with two 4.0-mm partially threaded cancellous screws.

The anterior lateral approach (Fig. 5A and B) allows access to the sinus tarsi and lateral talar body and neck (5). This approach is helpful for fractures that cannot be reduced from an anteromedial approach or if the subtalar joint requires exploration. The artery of the sinus tarsi may be jeopardized with this approach; however, in most displaced fractures, this vessel is usually damaged, and the surgical approach does not contribute to additional injury. The anterolateral approach uses a curvilinear skin incision that begins 2 cm anterior to the tip of the fibula and extends to the base of the fourth metatarsal. The deep dissection is carried through the extensor retinaculum and lateral to the extensor tendons. By retracting the tendons medially, the sinus tarsi and the talar neck are easily visualized.

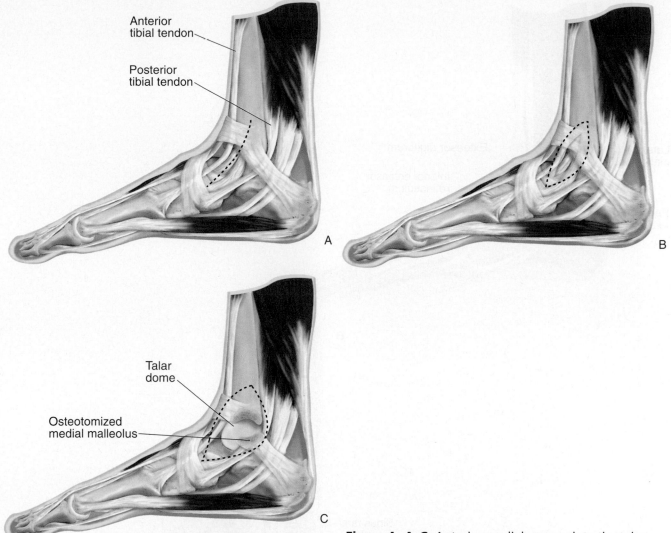

Anterior
tibial tendon

Posterior
tibial tendon

A

B

Talar
dome

Osteotomized
medial malleolus

C

Figure 4. A–C: Anterior medial approach to the talus.

Internal fixation by an anterior approach is best accomplished with either 4.0-mm cancellous or 3.5-mm cortical screws (3; Fig. 6A and B). Once the fracture site has been identified, the bone debris and clot should be copiously irrigated to allow anatomic reduction.
Dorsiflexion of the foot usually assists in fracture reduction while Weber reduction clamps
or large pointed pelvic reduction clamps hold the fracture while provisional fixation is undertaken. The tips of the large clamps can be placed percutaneously on the back of the ankle spanning the joint from front to back. Provision fixation with 1.6-mm or 2.0-mm K-
wires are helpful before definitive fixation.

Although titanium screws are magnetic resonance imaging (MRI) compatible and seem
attractive to use in a bone that is susceptible to avascular necrosis, their use is not mandatory. Stainless steel screws, physical examination, and good-quality plain radiographs will
usually allow the clinician accurately to follow up the bone to union. Avascular necrosis
can be diagnosed, treated, and followed up in the presence of stainless steel screws. Bone
scans are very effective in evaluating blood supply to the talus and provide sufficient information for therapeutic decision making.

Cortical lag screws (3.5 mm) are placed from either the anteromedial, anterolateral, or
occasionally both approaches and directed from anterior to posterior. Care must be exercised not to break the small bridge of bone that exists between the fracture and screw-in-

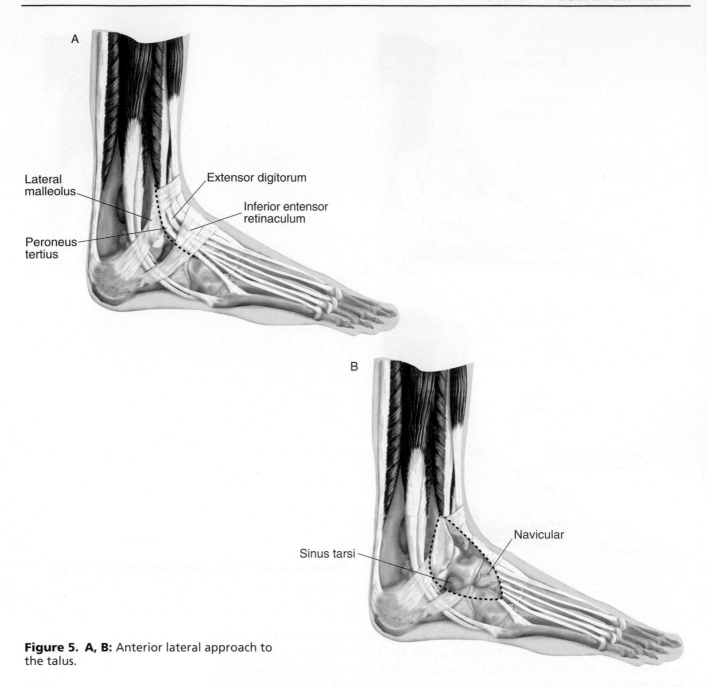

A

Lateral
malleolus

Extensor digitorum

Inferior entensor
retinaculum

Peroneus
tertius

B

Sinus tarsi

Navicular

Figure 5. A, B: Anterior lateral approach to the talus.

sertion site when stabilizing talar-neck fractures. Overdrill the near cortex with a 3.5-mm drill, and then place the 2.5-mm drill guide into the glide hole. Drill the far cortex with the 2.5-mm drill guide. Then depth gauge, tap, and place the screw in the standard fashion. Countersink the screwhead to avoid prominence or impingement of the talonavicular joint.

In complex fracture patterns in which screw placement is difficult, cannulated 4.5-mm screws can be placed in a retrograde fashion. This is performed by placing a guide wire from anterior to posterior. Posterior access is achieved through a limited approach and retrograde placement of a 4.5-mm cannulated screw. This technique provides the advantage of posterior screw placement while achieving anatomic reduction from an anterior portal.

Closure is routine by using subcutaneous suture and 3-0 nylon skin suture over a drain. A true "Robert Jones" dressing with roller gauze and a posterior splint with the ankle at 90 degrees is applied routinely.

In patients with severe comminution, it is worthwhile to reduce the fracture fragments by using miniscrews or multiple K-wires, if necessary. Multiple K-wires, with tibial or cal-

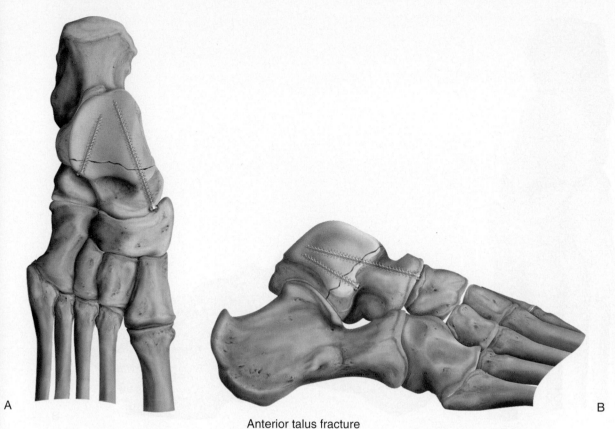

Anterior talus fracture

Figure 6. A, B: Optimal screw placement for fixation.

caneal external fixation to stabilize the hindfoot, can be an acceptable salvage alternative in these difficult, complex, comminuted cases. Only rarely is primary fusion or talectomy indicated as initial treatment.

Posterior Screw Placement

Posterior screw placement for talar neck and body fractures has multiple histologic, mechanical, and anatomic advantages (1). Whenever possible, screws are placed from a posterior to anterior direction, even if the reduction is obtained from an anterior portal (Fig. 7A–D). With this approach, the talonavicular joint is protected, the screws are more likely to be perpendicular to the fracture plane, and the anterior vascular structures are protected with this fixation technique.

The patient is placed in a true lateral position on a beanbag with the fluoroscopy table well padded with blankets to give adequate support for the foot and ankle (Fig. 8A and B). A tourniquet is placed on the thigh. After the leg is prepped and draped, a 3-cm vertical incision is made 1 cm lateral to the Achilles tendon. Identify and develop the interval between the peroneus brevis and flexor hallucis longis tendons (Fig. 9A and B) and open the posterior capsule exposing the talus posteriorly. Use the image intensifier to identify the posterior talus with the drill guide. With Hawkins I fractures in situ, fixation is accomplished

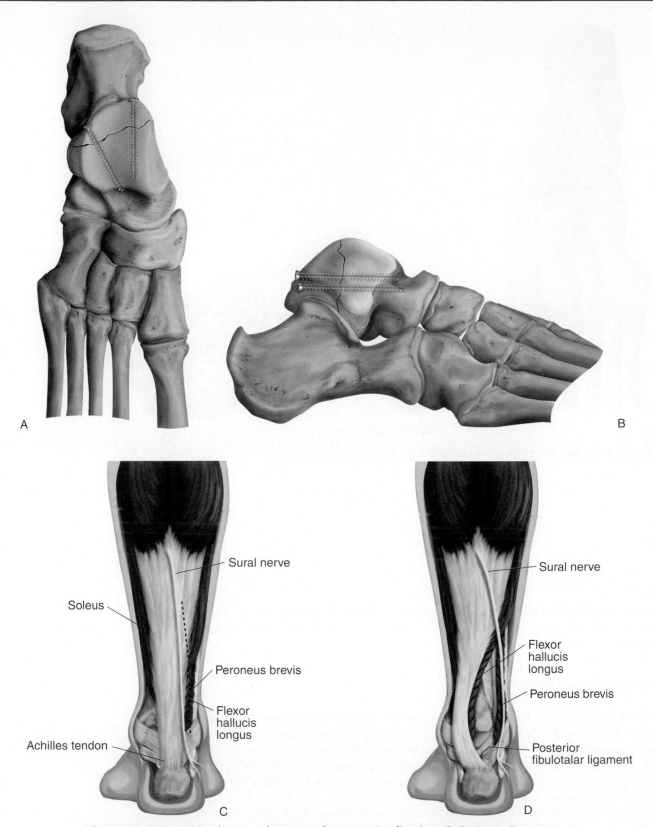

Figure 7. A, B: Optimal screw placement for posterior fixation. **C, D:** Posterior screw-placement landmarks.

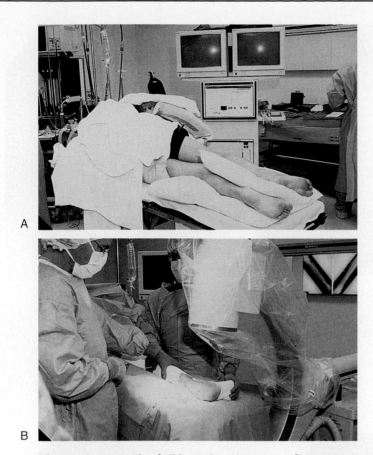

Figure 8. A, B: The full lateral position on a fluoroscopy table with a beanbag, using the fluoroscopy unit from the anterior side of the patient.

with 4.5-mm cannulated lag screws. Place the guide pin through the posterior portal and enter the body of the talus inferior lateral, if possible. The guide wire should enter the neck of the talus perpendicular to the fracture line, as documented on fluoroscopy (Fig. 10A and B). Use the oblique, pronated talar view to be certain the talonavicular joint is not violated. Then, depth gauge, tap, and place the 4.5-mm cannulated screws in a standard fashion. Cortical lag screws (3.5 mm) may be necessary to achieve compression for fractures anterior in the talar neck (3) or for surgeon's preference.

Hawkins II fractures require a reduction before fixation. By dorsiflexing the foot and using a 2.0-mm K-wire as a "joystick" in the talar neck, reduction can usually be obtained (Fig. 11). As previously noted, two 4.0-mm cancellous screws are preferred or one 6.5-mm cancellous screw, supplemented with 2.0-mm derotational guide wire placed from a posterior approach. If the reduction cannot be obtained, anterior reduction via an anterior lateral approach with posterior screw placement is our preferred method.

Hawkins Type III and IV fractures may have open wounds or require anterior reduction approaches and may be stabilized more time efficiently with anterior techniques. These fractures frequently occur in the multiply injured patient, where a supine position is preferred to manage associated injuries to the head, chest, or abdomen. If possible, the fracture is reduced from the front, whereas fixation is placed from the back.

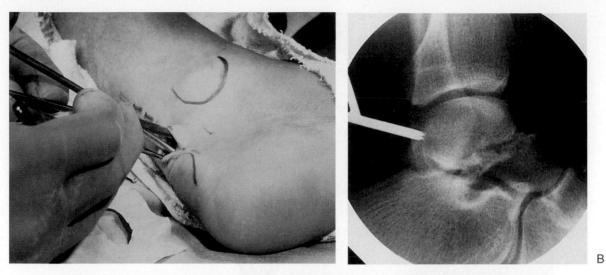

Figure 9. A: The incision is 2 cm in length, lateral to the Achilles tendon, inferior to the tip of the lateral malleolus. The interval between the peroneal brevis and the flexor hallucis longus is developed to the posterior joint capsule. **B:** The 2.0-mm AO drill guide is positioned through the soft tissues and fluoroscopically positioned for guide wire placement.

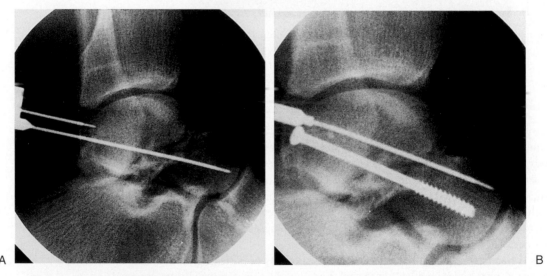

Figure 10. A: After the fracture is reduced, two guide wires are passed across the fracture site, and the reduction is checked fluoroscopically or radiographically as necessary. **B:** The depth is checked, taped, and two cannulated, 4.5-mm partially threaded screws are passed in lag mode.

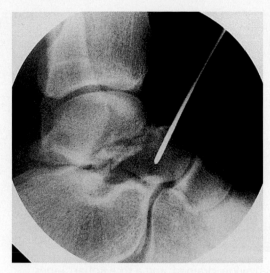

Figure 11. If a reduction maneuver is necessary, the foot can be dorsiflexed and a 2.0-mm guide wire used as a joystick to aid in the reduction maneuver.

POSTOPERATIVE MANAGEMENT

When stable fixation has been achieved, ankle and subtalar motion begins when the soft tissues appear benign, usually in 10 to 14 days. For the first 10 days, the foot should be supported in a Robert Jones–type bulky dressing with the foot splinted in neutral dorsiflexion (Fig. 12A and B). After the sutures are removed, the patient is started on a formal therapy program, consisting of active and passive range of motion of the foot, ankle, and hindfoot. A removable fracture brace facilitates therapy visits and patient involvement, if appropriate. Patients are usually seen at 2-week intervals initially to check motion and wound healing and to provide encouragement. Radiographs should include AP, lateral, and pronated oblique views obtained at 6-week intervals until the patient is fully functional at 4 months. Correlating the radiographs with the clinical course, the patient can usually begin partial weight bearing at 6 to 8 weeks. If union is slow, protected weight bearing is advised for an additional 6 weeks. When union occurs, full weight bearing is encouraged.

In 1970, Hawkins (4) described a subchondral lucency in the talar dome seen on radiographs 6 to 12 weeks after talar fractures. This finding indicated hyperemia and continued blood supply, suggesting avascular necrosis was unlikely to occur. If Hawkins' sign is present at 6 to 8 weeks, revascularization is occurring, and a united vascularized talus can be anticipated.

If Hawkins' sign is *not* present 6 to 8 weeks after fracture, either complete or incomplete avascular necrosis may occur. Several investigators have shown that bone union can occur in the presence of avascular necrosis with minimal resulting dysfunction. Prolonged immobilization or non–weight bearing has not been shown to enhance revascularization and may be detrimental to functional recovery. It may be more appropriate to allow maximal functional recovery of the extremity and then to perform an elective arthrodesis on a delayed basis.

In general, the outcomes of talar-neck fractures correlate well with the Hawkins' classification. If the early complications of sepsis and wound breakdown are avoided, the long-term results are favorable in Type I and II injuries and guarded in Type III and IV injuries. Hawkins I and II should have 70% to 90% good treatment results, whereas Hawkins III and IV have 40% to 60% good results. Patients may require hardware removal and should be advised of motion loss, prolonged therapy, and a prolonged time frame for full functional recovery. If avascular necrosis or nonunion occurs, recovery may be delayed or compromised.

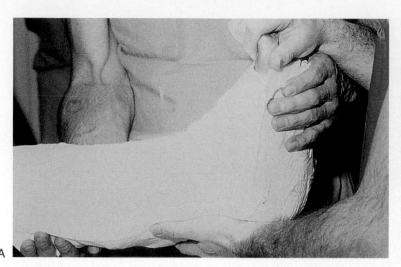
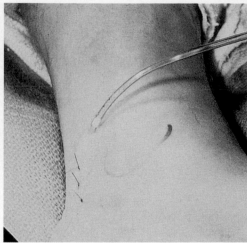

Figure 12. A, B: The wound is closed with 3-0 nylon, drained, and a true Robert Jones cotton-roll dressing is applied with a posterior splint holding the foot in the neutral position.

COMPLICATIONS

Avascular Necrosis

Avascular necrosis has been reported to occur in between zero and 50% of cases (6). These results are clearly dependent on the fracture classification, type, and timing of surgery. It would make empiric sense that Hawkins I and II injuries treated with early stable fixation should have a low rate of avascular necrosis (0 to 15%), whereas Types III and IV should be significantly higher.

The presence of a Hawkins' sign at 6 to 8 weeks seems to indicate that revascularization is occurring. However, small zonal areas of avascular necrosis may occur despite its presence. If the fracture unites, there is no indication for prolonged immobilization.

Bone grafts or electrical stimulators to enhance revascularization have little role in the management of avascular necrosis after talar-neck fractures. In general, arthrodesis is the treatment of choice to salvage most complications associated with avascular necrosis.

Infection

The principles of open fracture management apply to wound complications of the talus. Fever, pain, discharge, and wound slough all mandate early aggressive attempts to identify an organism. If the wound looks suggestive, aspiration, needle biopsy, and deep cultures are far more appropriate than a few days of outpatient oral antibiotics. If infection occurs, operative debridement, assessment of fracture-fixation stability, closure of the wound over tubes, and appropriate antibiotics are indicated. With the ever-changing field of antibiotic regimens, a close working relationship with an orthopaedic infectious disease colleague can be helpful. When appropriate, free tissue transfers, ring fixation, and even amputation may be indicated to control the complications associated with deep infection.

Delayed Union, Nonunion, and Malunion

A delay in union can occur after talus fractures. Attempts should be made to investigate concurrent variables, such as infection, metabolic and immunologic factors, nutrition, medications, and smoking. If repeated intervention is elected to treat a nonunion, revision fixation with supplemental bone graft is usually required (5). Avascular bone can be extremely difficult to negotiate when reoperating; therefore, it is critical to assess the vascularity before revision fixation. Malunions are more frequent and have been reported to occur in 25% of the cases. With care in open anatomic reduction, the incidence of malunion should decline. Dorsal beak resection for dorsal impingement and isolated hindfoot fusions usually result in acceptable outcomes for malunited hindfoot pathology.

Posttraumatic Arthritis

The talus plays a pivotal role in the weight-bearing mechanics of the hindfoot. Minor injury to any of the multiple articular surfaces can result in posttraumatic arthropathy with associated pain. Evaluation requires precise isolation of the offending joint, including CT, bone scans, and provocative lidocaine (Xylocaine) injections. Although not well defined, diagnostic/therapeutic arthroscopy may play a role in the evaluation and documentation process. Talotibial debridement and arthroscopic arthrodesis have been reported to be successful in certain cases. However, traditional open subtalar, talotibial, and talonavicular arthrodesis are usually successful in alleviating posttraumatic arthritic pain in these circumstances.

RECOMMENDED READING

1. Bray, T.J., et al.: Fracture fixation of the foot and hand. In (ed.): *Techniques in Fracture Fixation.* Gower, New York, 1992, pp. 14–20.
2. Canale, T.S. Fractures of the neck of the talus. *Orthopaedics,* 13(10):1105–1115, 1990.
3. Hanson, S.: Fractures of the talus: lower extremity; foot injuries. In Browner, B.D., Jupiter, J.B., Trafton, P.G., (eds.): *Skeletal Trauma.* Saunders, St. Louis, pp. 1960–1967.
4. Hawkins, M.D.: Fractures of the neck of the talus. *J. Bone Joint Surg. [Am],* 52:991–1002, 1970.
5. Mayo, K.: Fractures of the talus: principles of management and techniques of treatment. *Tech. Orthop.,* 2(3):42–54, 1987.
6. Swanson, T.V.: Fractures and dislocations of the talus. In Chapman, M. W. (ed.): *Operative Orthopaedics,* 2nd ed. Lippincott, Philadelphia, 1993.
7. Swanson, T.V., Bray, T.J., Holmes, G.B., Jr.: Fractures of the talar neck: a mechanical study of fixation. *J. Bone Joint Surg. [Am],* 74:544–551, 1992.

Master Techniques in Orthopaedic Surgery,
FRACTURES, edited by D. A. Wiss,
Lippincott–Raven Publishers, Philadelphia © 1998.

32

Calcaneal Fractures: Open Reduction Internal Fixation

Paul Tornetta III

INDICATIONS/CONTRAINDICATIONS

The indications for open reduction and internal fixation (ORIF) of the calcaneus are controversial. Results after surgery are superior to nonoperative management only if the posterior facet is anatomically reduced and if complications are avoided (3,12,15). The best indication for ORIF of the calcaneus is an intraarticular fracture of the calcaneus with displacement of the posterior facet in a young, active patient with no medical problems. Middle-aged patients should be considered operative candidates based on their lifestyles and fracture patterns. The more active a patient is, the more likely that he or she would benefit from properly performed ORIF. Even in less active patients, surgery may improve the functional result if the fracture displacement produces significant widening or shortening of the heel, because these problems increase the chances of a poor result when the fracture is treated nonoperatively.

Contraindications to surgery may be related to the overall health of the patient, the mental status, the fracture pattern, or the experience of the surgeon. Contraindications to internal fixation include neuropathy, insulin-dependent diabetes, peripheral vascular disease, venous stasis or congestion, lymphedema, immune compromise, heavy smoking, and other disorders that might impede healing. Older age is a relative contraindication. Finally, patient compliance is important in obtaining a good functional result after surgical intervention and must be considered preoperatively. Patients with a history of jumping from a height must be carefully scrutinized for signs of mental illness or depression. When appropriate, these patients should be evaluated by a mental health professional. Despite improved surgical techniques and implants, there is a subset of calcaneal fractures with severe comminution of the posterior facet that precludes reduction and internal fixation. In these injuries, primary fusion may be a good alternative to internal fixation. Less comminuted but

---

P. Tornetta III, M.D.: Department of Orthopaedic Surgery, Boston University Medical Center, Boston, Massachusetts 02118.

complex injuries with multiple fractures through the posterior facet offer a relative contraindication for surgeons without significant experience in the operative treatment of calcaneal fractures.

Open fractures present difficult management problems. A thorough irrigation and debridement of the traumatic wounds and the fracture is the first priority after resuscitation and trauma evaluation. If the wound is lateral and allows reduction of the posterior facet, then it is reduced and fixed with lag screws. This is performed only after reprepping and redraping after the debridement. If the wound is medial, I prefer to delay internal fixation until the soft-tissue environment has been addressed. Temporary triangular external fixation on the lateral side of the foot and ankle can be used to maintain the general alignment of the heel while awaiting definitive management. The external fixation pins (size 2.5 mm from the wrist external-fixation set) are placed in the tuberosity, the cuboid, and the talus. Definitive ORIF is performed 2 to 3 weeks after wound closure if the soft tissues are in good condition.

PREOPERATIVE PLANNING

Initial Survey

Physical examination of the patient with a calcaneus fracture must include a careful and complete survey of the axial as well as the appendicular skeleton. Spine fractures are common in patients with calcaneal fractures because the mechanism of injury is often axial loading caused by a fall from a height. Radiographs of the affected extremity and spine should be routine.

Physical examination of the foot and ankle begins with evaluation of the soft tissues to rule out open fracture or compartment syndrome. Compartment syndrome of the foot is difficult to diagnose clinically. Calcaneal fractures are painful but usually respond to splinting, elevation, ice, and analgesics. Severe and unrelenting pain should be considered a compartment syndrome until proven otherwise. Significant swelling in the foot is common after calcaneal fracture, and the region may not feel tense even in the face of compartment syndrome. Sensation is rarely affected, and its absence does not rule out compartment syndrome. Pain on passive extension of the metatarsophalangeal joints is the best method of clinical examination but is not sensitive enough safely to rule out compartment syndrome. Direct intracompartmental pressure measurement is the most accurate method of diagnosis. Pressures should be taken in the central (interosseous) and medial compartments. Hand-held devices, monometers, or arterial line monitors are equally effective in measuring compartment pressures. I perform a fasciotomy if the compartment pressure is within 30 mm Hg of the diastolic pressure. If the pressure measurements are borderline, then in the absence of significant clinical symptoms, the foot may be observed and pressures rechecked in 30- to 60-minute intervals. If a fasciotomy is required, the calcaneal fracture is not usually fixed at this time because the incisions necessary for the fasciotomy are not useful for reduction and fixation of the calcaneus.

The remainder of the physical examination of the foot and ankle is directed at diagnosing concomitant injuries. Palpation of the entire lower leg, ankle, and foot may help in identifying such injuries. Commonly associated regional injuries include ankle fractures (especially the lateral malleolus), ankle-ligament injury, peroneal dislocation, midfoot fractures, talar fractures, and metatarsal fractures. Radiographic evaluation of symptomatic areas is essential.

Specific Radiographs

The specific radiographs that are necessary to evaluate an injury to the hindfoot include anteroposterior (AP), lateral, and mortise views of the ankle; AP, lateral, and oblique views of the foot; and an axial view of the calcaneus (Harris view). Contralateral axial and lateral

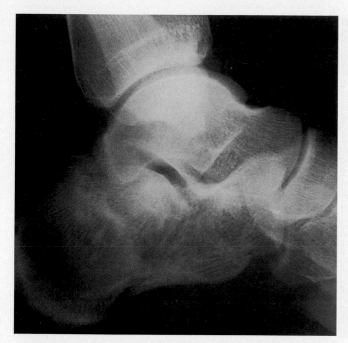

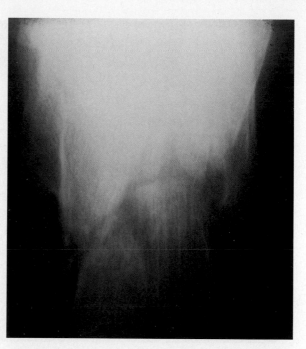

Figure 1. The lateral view of the calcaneus demonstrates a joint-depression fracture with a portion of the posterior facet impacted into the cancellous bone of the tuberosity. The sagittal-plane rotation of the displaced posterior facet is best seen on this view.

Figure 2. The axial or "Harris" view demonstrates the primary fracture line, medial comminution, the fractures into the facet, and the varus angulation of the tuberosity.

views of the calcaneus and an oblique view of the contralateral foot may be useful in delineating the patient's normal anatomy. The ankle radiographs are necessary to rule out concomitant ankle or talar fractures, as well as to evaluate the calcaneus, subtalar joint, and calcaneocuboid joint. The lateral view of the calcaneus allows preliminary classification of the fracture and information about the integrity of the posterior facet (Fig. 1). Even in comminuted and displaced fractures, a portion of the facet is usually intact, and the relationship of the subtalar joint can be evaluated. With impaction or depression of part of the posterior facet, the lateral radiograph may demonstrate a double density in this region, which may be confused with an oblique view of the joint. This can be clarified easily because in a true oblique view, the posterior facet of the talus will also appear as a double density, and in a calcaneal fracture, it will be only one line. The calcaneocuboid joint and anterior calcaneus are best visualized on the foot films. The axial view demonstrates the position of the tuberosity, the status of the medial wall, and the location of the fracture(s) through the facet (Fig. 2).

Computed Tomography Scans

To gain a better understanding of the fracture morphology, biplanar CT scans with 2- or 3-mm cuts are obtained. The scan should include images in the plane of the foot as well as in a plane perpendicular to the posterior facet of the talus. The most important of these are the axial images of the hindfoot perpendicular to the posterior facet of the talus. It is described in reference to the talus because the posterior facet of the calcaneus is displaced. This view is obtained with the foot flat on the table, the knee flexed, and the gantry angled 30 degrees forward. The axial images are used to classify the fracture and to evaluate the fracture anatomy. Pertinent anatomic points to make note of are the position and integrity of the tuberosity, the location and number of fractures in the posterior facet, displacement of the lateral wall, the location of medial-wall comminution or fracture lines, the size of the sustentacular fragment, fractures in the anterior calcaneus, the presence or absence of an

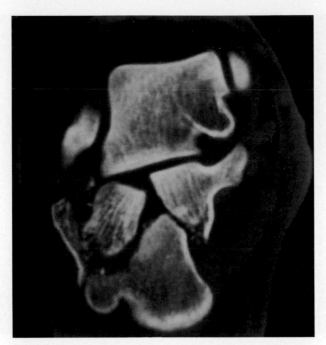

Figure 3. The 30-degree semicoronal computed tomography (CT) image demonstrates the comminution and degree of depression of the posterior facet. The separation and step-off are easily seen, but the sagittal-plane rotation of the fragments is not well visualized. The wedging effect of the tuberosity fragment separating the facet fragments and the lateral wall blowout is well visualized.

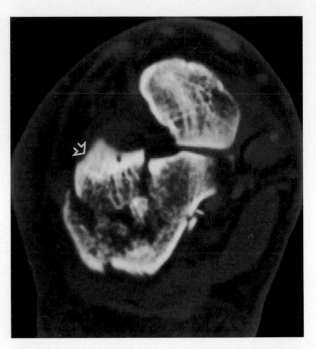

Figure 4. A computed tomography (CT) image farther anterior demonstrates a separate anterolateral fragment (open arrow).

anterolateral fragment, and the position of the peroneal tendons (dislocated or not; Figs. 3 and 4). The CT images in the plane of the foot are used to evaluate the anterior calcaneus and sustentaculum tali. Fractures of the sustentacular fragment in the coronal plane may decrease the bone available for fixation of the facet. These fractures may not be seen in the other radiographs or axial CT but are visible on the CT images in plane of the foot (Fig. 5).

Classification

The fracture is classified by the system of Essex Lopresti (5) by using the plain films and by that of Sanders (11) from the 30-degree semicoronal CT scan (Fig. 6). The initial division into joint depression versus tongue-type fracture will help in the reduction tactic. The Sanders classification was devised based on the ease of reduction and fixation via the lateral approach and has been predictive of outcome (11,12). The greater the number of fractures in the facet and the more medial their location, the harder will be the reduction. In the Sanders classification, the fracture lines are designated A through C by their location from lateral to medial, respectively. In a Type 2C fracture, the entire facet is displaced from the intact medial calcaneus.

Planning the Reduction and Fixation

The anatomy of the fracture must be well understood before surgery, not only as it relates to displacement, but also as it relates to the tactic for surgical reduction. There are two critical steps in planning the reduction and fixation of a calcaneal fracture. First are references for reduction, which include the anteroinferior margin of the facet (the angle of Gissane), the posterior facet of the talus, the intact posterior facet of the calcaneus, the calca

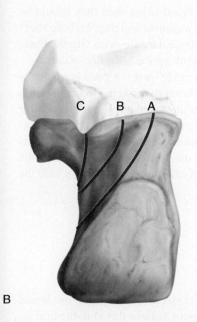

Figure 5. The computed tomography (CT) scan in the plane of the foot is the best view to evaluate the sustentaculum region. On this CT image, a vertical fracture through the sustentaculum is visible that is not seen on any other projection (solid arrow). The displaced lateral portion of the posterior facet is seen to be impacted into the tuberosity adjacent to the sustentacular region. Finally, the separate anterolateral fragment is seen on this view as well (open arrow).

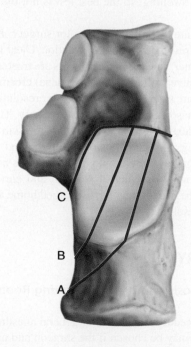

Figure 6.   A, B: The computed tomography (CT) classification of Sanders. The fracture is described by the number and location of fracture lines in the posterior facet. Each fracture is given a number and a letter corresponding to the number of fragments of the posterior facet and their location. For example, a 2B fracture has one fracture line in the "B" location (see Fig. 3), and a 3BC has two fracture lines, one in the B position and one in the C position.

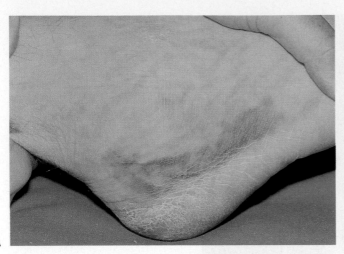
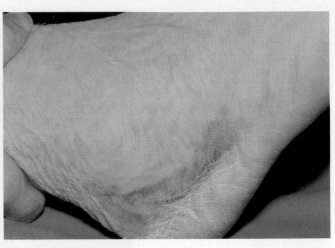

A   B

Figure 7. The "wrinkle test" is done by bringing the foot from the plantarflexed position **(A)** into dorsiflexion **(B)** and observing the wrinkles that form on the lateral side of the ankle and foot.

neocuboid joint, the tuberosity, and the lateral wall. Second are the standard fixation points used, which include the sustentaculum tali, medial wall, tuberosity, and anterior calcaneus. The status of these anatomic regions must be clearly understood before proceeding with surgery.

Evaluation of the Soft Tissues

To avoid wound complications after surgery, the initial postinjury swelling must be resolved. This commonly takes 10 to 21 days to occur but dramatically improves the condition of the soft tissues. The lateral bulge caused by lateral wall displacement can be confused with swelling, so the best test is not the apparent swelling, but the pliability of the skin.

Blisters are a contraindication for surgery. If they are blood filled, then they should be allowed to resolve without intervention. Clear blisters are aspirated and then unroofed several days later. In either case, blisters are treated as burns once they are open. Sterile dressings with silver sulfadiazine (Silvadene) cream are used until epithelialization occurs.

If there are no blisters or after blister resolution, the "wrinkle" test is a good predictor of whether the soft tissue will tolerate surgery. This is performed by bringing the ankle from a plantar-flexed position to neutral. If the skin wrinkles with this maneuver it is ready for surgery (Fig. 7). Ecchymosis is common and is often distributed along the peroneal tendons. As long as there are no blisters, this is not a contraindication to surgery. The foot is kept in a bulky dressing of soft roll and elevated until the soft tissues will tolerate the surgery. The patient may be discharged home and the foot examined every 5 days until the swelling resolves.

SURGERY

Patient Positioning and Operating Room Setup

The procedure is done under general anesthesia with complete muscle paralysis. Spinal anesthesia may be chosen if the surgeon and anesthesiologist believe this is in the best interests of the patient. Before positioning the patient, a first-generation cephalosporin is given intravenously and a Foley catheter inserted in the bladder. The patient is moved into the lateral decubitus position with the operative side up. Care is taken to pad the chest, ax

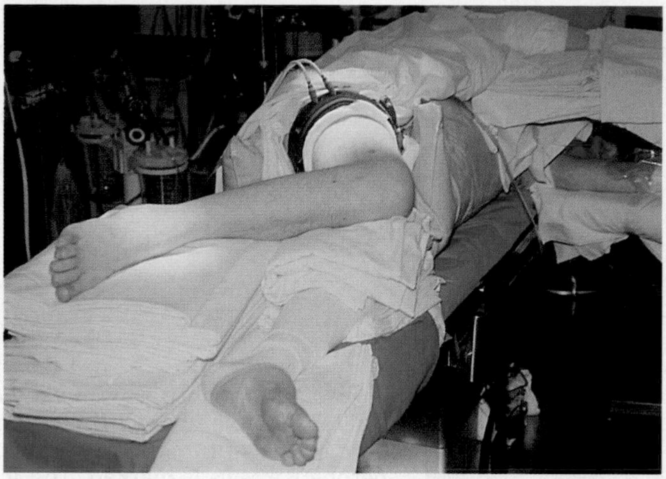

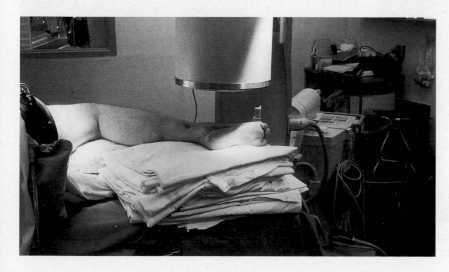

Figure 8. The patient is placed in the lateral decubitus position. Sheets are placed under the affected leg to keep it level during the surgery.

illa, and nonoperative leg, which is flexed at the hip and knee so that the tibia is just up to and parallel with the edge of the table anterior to the patient. A tourniquet is placed on the operative thigh. Folded sheets are placed behind the down leg so that the affected leg lies parallel to the floor. Padding is placed between the legs, and the affected leg rests on the sheets (Fig. 8). The image intensifier is brought in at an approximately 45-degree angle to the bottom of the table in front of the patient (Fig. 9). This will allow good-quality lateral, axial, and Broden's images intraoperatively. The radiographs and computed tomography (CT) scans are displayed for reference during surgery.

Operative Approach

Under pneumatic tourniquet control, the lateral aspect of the calcaneus is exposed through a full-thickness L-shaped incision (6,17). It begins 2 to 3 cm superior to the tip of the fibula just anterior to the Achilles tendon and parallels the tendon over the calcaneus, taking a 90-degree turn at the inferior aspect of the calcaneus. This is generally at the border of the thick plantar skin with the normal lateral skin. The incision is extended distally for approximately 3 cm and then angles slightly dorsal to the base of the fifth metatarsal (Fig. 10).

Figure 9. The fluoroscope is brought in at a 45-degree angle from the anterior and distal corner of the table.

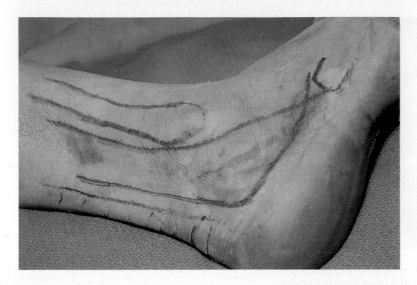

Figure 10. The incision is marked on the skin in reference to the fibula, Achilles tendon, and the base of the fifth metatarsal. The course of the peroneus brevis is marked. The incision angles anteriorly at its distal end.

The deep dissection begins over the tuberosity of the calcaneus and proceeds down to bone in one cut. Care is taken not to bevel the deep cut. Proximally, dissection is performed in line with the incision by using scissors to avoid damage to the sural nerve. This is normally located in the flap, but its location can vary. Distally the incision is deepened until the fascia of the abductor digiti minimi muscle is identified (Fig. 11). Sharp retractors are used to apply traction on the flap during the dissection. The flap should be full thickness and take the periosteum, ankle ligaments, and peroneal tendons with it. To accomplish this, a no. 15 blade is held almost parallel with the lateral surface of the calcaneus, and counterpressure is provided by the surgeon pushing medially on the corner of the heel or by using a pickup (Fig. 12). Placing several folded sterile towels under the distal tibia allows the foot to be adducted, which increases the exposure. The knife blades must be replaced often, as they dull quickly. The surgeon must pay particular attention to stay on the lateral wall and not fall into the lateral wall fractures. Proximally the incision is deepened over the top of the tuberosity. Distally the dissection proceeds over the short abductor fascia to the inferior surface of the calcaneus without damaging the fascia. The dissection is completely subperiosteal from this point on. The peroneal tendons are at risk distally in the wound, and dissection in this region should be done only after the tendons have been identified and are protected with a retractor. The dissection proceeds until the subtalar joint is reached. It is

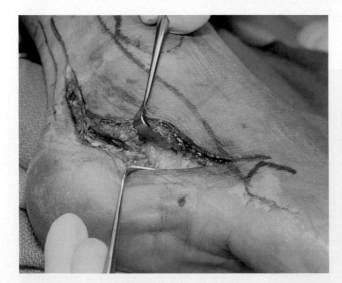

Figure 11. The abductor digiti minimi fascia is visible in the distal part of the incision and should not be divided.

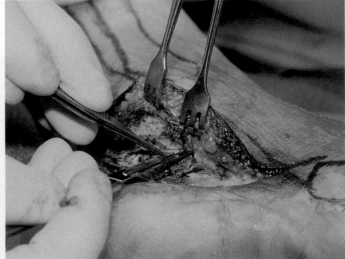

Figure 12. The scalpel is held almost parallel with the lateral wall during the elevation of the full-thickness flap.

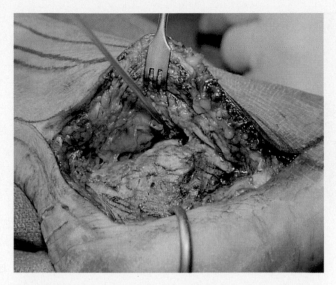 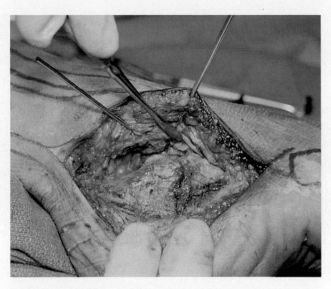

Figure 13. The first K-wire is placed just above the corner of the lateral process of the talus and directed into the talar body.

Figure 14. With the flap held by the K-wires, there is excellent exposure of the lateral calcaneus. The Freer elevator is pointing to the peroneal tendons within the flap.

common for a significant amount of tissue to be interposed in the joint laterally; this must be removed. The posterior facet of the talus is identified. Two Kirschner wires (K-wires) are placed as retractors for the flap. One is placed in the lateral process of the talus and aimed toward the body of the talus (Fig. 13). The second is placed in the fibula. These are then bent away from the field to retract the flap without tension during the procedure. The impacted lateral portion of posterior facet and the entire lateral wall are visible at this point (Fig. 14).

Reduction and Fixation

Full exposure of the fractured fragments necessitates removal of the fractured lateral wall. This is performed by using a curved osteotome to reflect the wall (Fig. 15). The displaced and impacted lateral portion of the posterior facet is freed from the body of the cal-

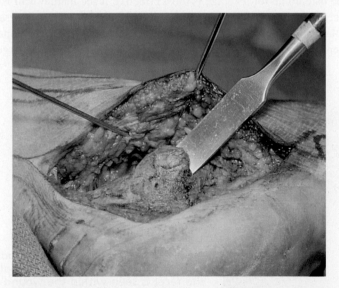

Figure 15. The fractured lateral wall is removed with an osteotome.

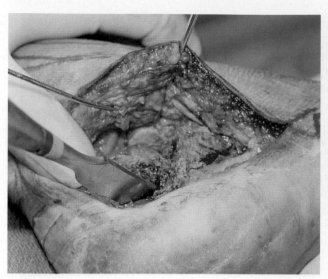

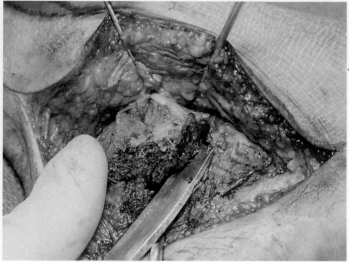

A

B

Figure 16. A curved osteotome is introduced below the displaced posterior facet **(A)** and used to disimpact it from the cancellous bone **(B)**.

caneus by using an osteotome (Fig. 16). The exact location of the anterior and inferior extent of this portion of the facet is predetermined on the semicoronal CT scan. Once the posterior facet is dislodged from the calcaneus, there is no soft tissue attached to it, and it is easily mobilized. Because of the lack of soft-tissue attachments in joint-depression fractures, the surgeon must be careful not to allow the facet fragment to fall off the field. In tongue-type fractures, the tuberosity fragment attached to the facet allows it to be rotated externally without stripping all attachments. Once the posterior-facet fragment has been mobilized, the fracture site should be cleaned of all callus and debris. The intact medial portion of the facet is probed and inspected. Adduction of the foot allows better examination of the talar side of the joint for injury (Fig. 17).

Reduction of the facet cannot be successfully accomplished until the tuberosity is reduced. A common mistake is attempting to reduce the posterior facet first. Reduction of the tuberosity corrects the calcaneal height and tuberosity varus and may be accomplished by levering with an osteotome, pulling with a large-radius bone hook, placement of a femoral distractor, use of a traction pin, or use of a Gissane spike (Fig. 18). Each has its advantages. The use of the osteotome for leverage is most effective if the medial wall is not comminuted. It is placed into the primary fracture line, as determined on the preoperative CT scan, and levered plantarward to reduce the tuberosity (Figs. 18 and 19). The bone hook is useful in joint-depression fractures if the tuberosity is not comminuted. A large-radius bone

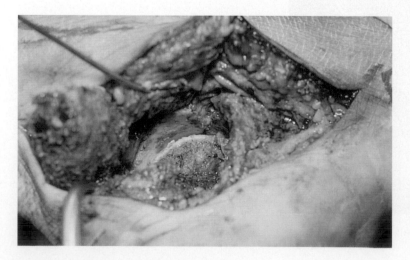

Figure 17. With the displaced portion of the facet removed, the intact medial portion of the facet is seen within the wound. In this case, there is significant injury to the cartilage of the posterior facet of the talus.

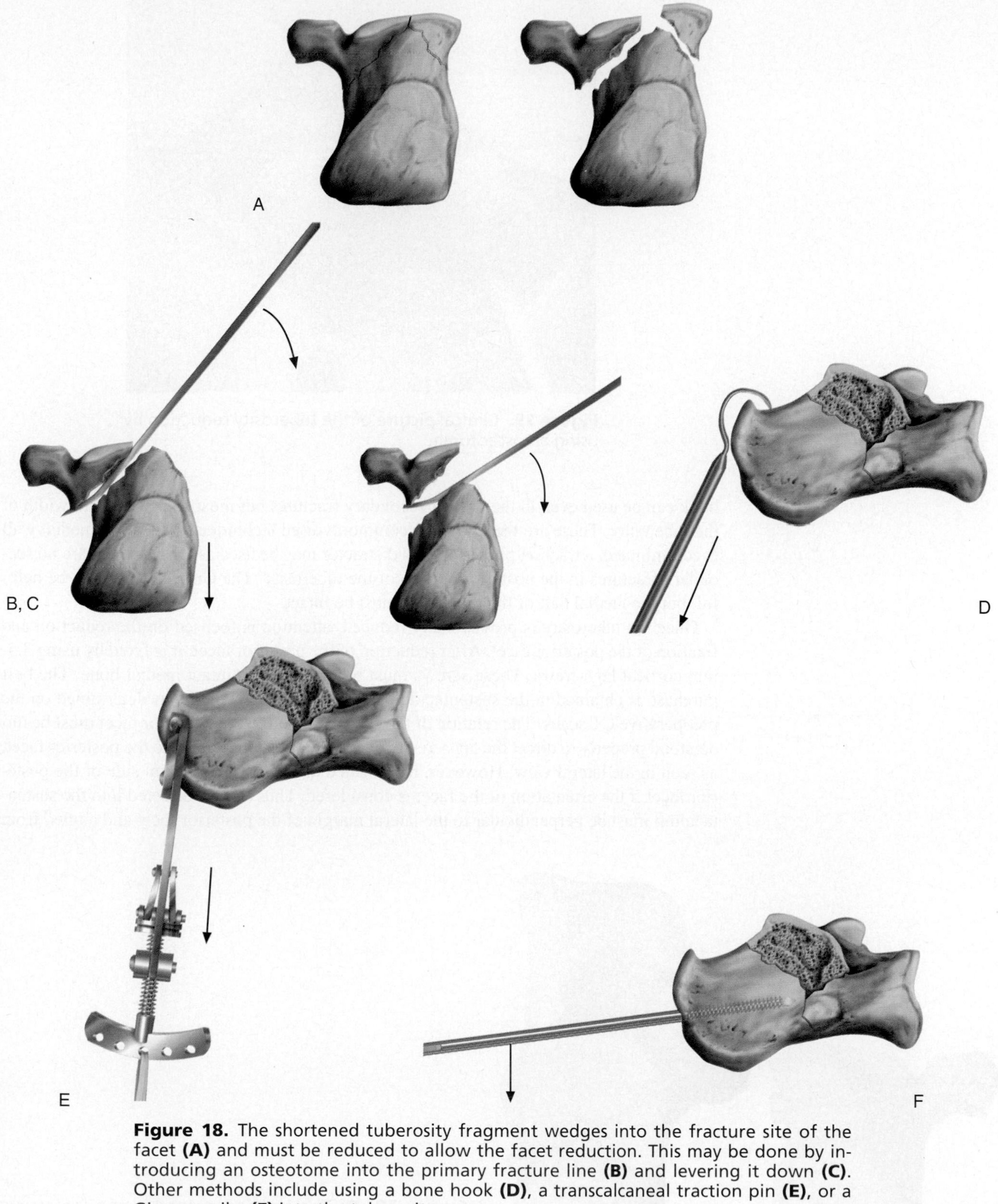

Figure 18. The shortened tuberosity fragment wedges into the fracture site of the facet **(A)** and must be reduced to allow the facet reduction. This may be done by introducing an osteotome into the primary fracture line **(B)** and levering it down **(C)**. Other methods include using a bone hook **(D)**, a transcalcaneal traction pin **(E)**, or a Gissane spike **(F)** into the tuberosity.

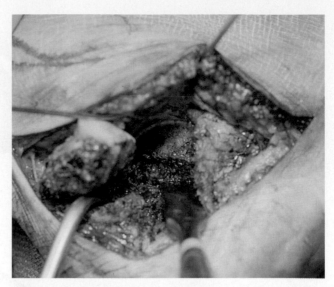

Figure 19. Clinical picture of the tuberosity reduction by using an osteotome.

hook can be used even in the face of secondary fractures but must span the entire width of the tuberosity. These are the two most commonly used techniques. When the medial wall is comminuted, a traction pin or femoral distractor may be used as long as there are no secondary fractures in the posterior portion of the tuberosity. The Gissane spike can be helpful, but the medial half of the tuberosity must be intact.

Once the tuberosity is provisionally reduced, attention is focused on the reduction and fixation of the posterior facet. After reduction of the posterior facet, it is fixed by using 3.5-mm cortical lag screws. These screws must be directed into intact medial bone. The best purchase is obtained in the sustentaculum tali if it is intact, which was determined on the preoperative CT scans. The relation of the sustentaculum to the posterior facet must be understood properly to direct the lag screws. The sustentaculum is distal to the posterior facet, as seen in the lateral view. However, it is located directly on the medial side of the posterior facet if the orientation of the facet is considered. Thus screws directed into the sustentaculum must be perpendicular to the lateral margin of the posterior facet and angled from

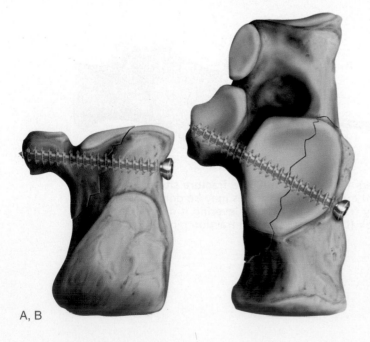

A, B

Figure 20. A: The starting point for the lag screws should be slightly inferior to the joint to ensure placement into the intact medial facet or tuberosity without penetrating the joint. **B:** The lag screws should be positioned perpendicular to the posterior-facet fracture. This necessitates directing the screws from posterolateral to anteromedial, as seen from the superior surface.

proximal and lateral to distal and medial with respect to the lateral border of the foot (Fig. 20B). Additionally, starting slightly inferior to the lateral margin of the posterior facet will help avoid penetration of the joint (Fig. 20A). Lag screws are easiest to place with fractures that are lateral in the facet (Sanders A location), because more medial bone stock is available. If the fracture is more medial, at the junction of the facet and the sustentaculum (Sanders C location), only a small area of bone is available for fixation. Although not commonly performed, the gliding hole for the lag screw can be drilled in the reverse direction to assure placement into the sustentaculum. This technique is useful for Type C fractures in particular. If the lag holes are reverse drilled, this can be done on a side table by holding the facet fragment with two sets of bone tenaculums. After placement of the lag holes, the reduction of the facet is obtained.

To accurately reposition the posterior facet, the tuberosity must be reduced so that it does not block the reduction. If the facet is comminuted, the most lateral fragments are reduced to each other first and held with K-wires while the now intact unit is reduced to the medial fragment. The displaced portion of the facet is rotated to match the intact fragment and then placed in the fracture bed against the posterior facet of the talus. If cortical bone of the lateral wall interferes with the reduction, it may be trimmed with a rongeur without concern.

Evaluating fracture reduction is the most important part of the procedure. Starting at the posterior aspect of the facet, the reduction is visualized directly by applying a varus moment to the heel and directing the light (a headlight is helpful) into the subtalar joint (Fig. 21). Light directed against the posterior facet of the talus will be reflected onto the posterior facet of the calcaneus. If the fracture is medial, it may not be directly visible. A Freer elevator is an excellent tool for "feeling" the reduction and is used in most cases (Fig. 22). Anteriorly, the inferior margin of the facet at the angle of Gissane should line up with the intact calcaneus. This area is useful to judge rotational alignment of the facet but is accurate only if the anterolateral calcaneus is nondisplaced or reduced. A displaced anterolateral fragment (6) takes with it the bone adjacent to the inferior margin of the posterior facet, and this area cannot be used as a reference for the reduction of the facet (Fig. 23). Ideally, the posterior facet of the calcaneus should be perfectly congruent with the posterior facet of the talus anteriorly, laterally, and posteriorly. Finally, the reduction is confirmed fluoroscopically. The lateral view will demonstrate a double density if the facet if displaced. The best guide, however, is to obtain fluoroscopic Broden's views (Fig. 24). Any step-off or gap at the fracture site can be appreciated by using these views. Only rotational deformity in the

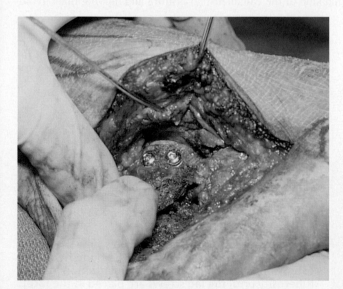

Figure 21. A varus force on the calcaneus helps assess the reduction. Light directed against the posterior facet of the talus reflects onto the calcaneus and helps with direct visualization of the reduction.

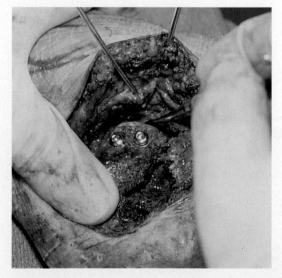

Figure 22. A Freer elevator is an excellent tool to feel the reduction for step-off and gap.

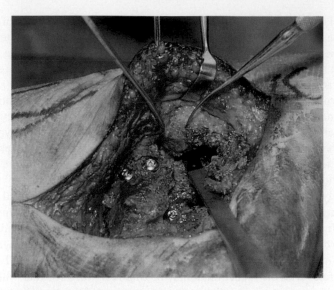

Figure 23. When a displaced anterolateral fragment exists, then the reduction of the anterior portion of the facet is more difficult to judge. The osteotome demonstrates the anterolateral fragment. Note the displacement from the anterior portion of the facet, which is reduced to the sustentaculum.

sagittal plane is not visible on the Broden's view. Although the lateral fluoroscopic view will demonstrate large rotational displacements, this is the one plane of reduction that must be determined clinically. Careful evaluation of the posterior and anterior margins of the facet will reveal malrotation with respect to the medial fragment.

The reduction is generally stable, but it is prudent to insert a temporary K-wire(s) before lag-screw placement. If the gliding holes are predrilled, then the inner drill sleeve is used to ensure central placement of the screws in the gliding hole. If the sustentaculum is intact, it is used for fixation. If the sustentaculum is fractured, then the lag screws must be directed more posteriorly into the medial portion of the facet, as determined on the preoperative CT scan (Fig. 5). The posterior tibial neurovascular bundle lies close to the medial side of the calcaneus, so drilling and tapping must avoid

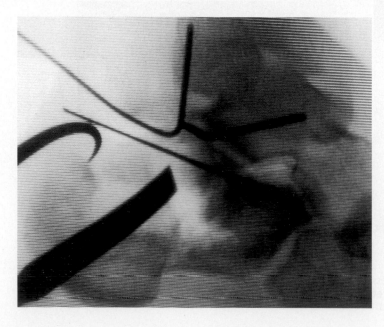

Figure 24. The fluoroscopic Broden's view shows the reduction of the posterior facet. The bone hook and osteotome are maintaining the reduction of the tuberosity until the lag screws are placed in the facet. A K-wire is holding the reduction of the facet. Note the parallelism of the posterior facet of the talus and the calcaneus.

unnecessary penetration beyond the medial cortex (1). As the bone in this region is quite dense, the use of a new drill bit helps to avoid thermal injury to the bone. The 3.5-mm cortical lag screws are then placed with washers and tightened.

Once the facet is reduced and fixed, attention is turned to the reduction and fixation of the tuberosity and the anterior calcaneus, usually with a plate. Several plates are available for this purpose, including some specifically designed for the calcaneus. I prefer a 2.7-mm minifragment metacarpal plate (Synthes, Paoli, PA, U.S.A.) because they are easily contoured, positioned, and can accommodate either 2.7- or 3.5-mm screws. The reduction of the anterior calcaneus is performed first. This is especially important if there is a separate anterolateral fragment or the fracture enters the calcaneocuboid joint. Additional dissection for exposure of the anterior calcaneus and the calcaneocuboid joint may be necessary (Fig. 25). If there is a displaced anterolateral fragment, it is reduced by direct pressure by using an osteotome or bone tamp. Fixation varies depending on the size and location of the fragment. Either a plate to the tuberosity or a lag screw placed percutaneously through the flap is necessary (15). Care must be taken when placing a percutaneous screw to avoid injury to the sensory branches of the peroneal nerve.

In tongue-type fractures, the tuberosity is reduced with the posterior facet. For joint-depression fractures, the tuberosity reduction must be maintained during plate placement. This can be done with a bone hook or by temporary K-wire placement into the posterior-facet fragment. The lateral wall fragment(s) are replaced or used as graft, and the plate is contoured to the lateral calcaneus (Fig. 26). Bone grafting is rarely required as the tension trabeculae of the bone are restored. In most instances, one plate from the tuberosity to the anterior calcaneus will suffice. However, if there is a bone defect, several small plates may be used. A three-hole plate running from the posterior tuberosity to the posterior part of the facet acts in tension and can maintain calcaneal height.

After the plate is contoured and secured with one screw proximally and distally, a lateral and an axial image are obtained (Fig. 27). If these show adequate restoration of the height and width of the calcaneus, as well as the angle of the tuberosity, the remaining screws are placed. Two screws into the tuberosity, two into the anterior calcaneus, and one into the medial part of the facet are sufficient to ensure fracture stability.

The wound is irrigated and closed over a drain (medium hemovac). Closure is done by using interrupted figure-of-eight sutures from the periosteum of the flap to the deep tissues. In the distal part of the flap, the repair includes the fascia of the abductor digiti minimi. The sutures are all placed and clamped before any one is tied. They are then tied from proximal

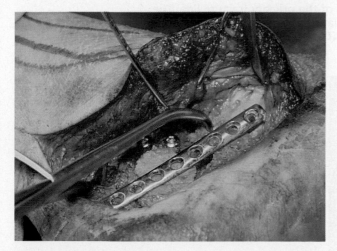

Figure 25. The small Hohmann retractor is in the calcaneocuboid joint. Complete exposure of the lateral calcaneus is obtained for plate placement. The anterolateral fragment is now reduced.

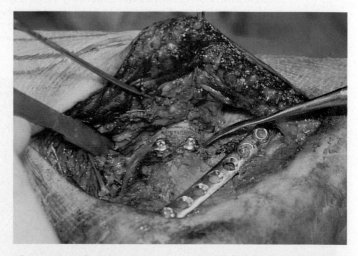

Figure 26. The plate is contoured and fixed with two screws at each end. Note the reduction of the posterior facet of the calcaneus to that of the talus and of the anterolateral fragment (Freer elevator).

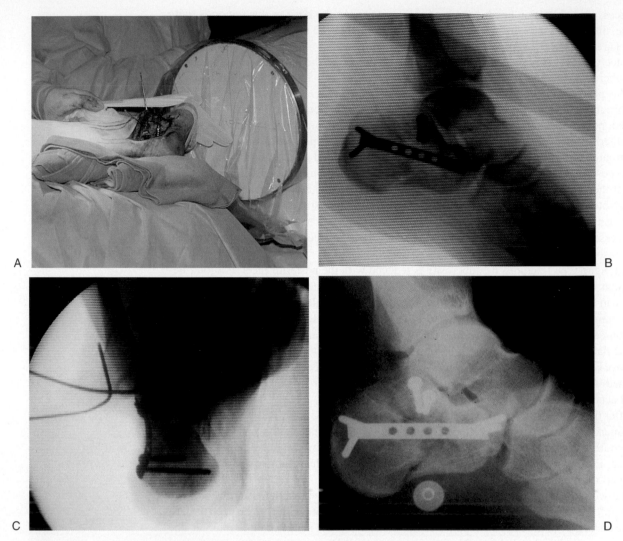

Figure 27. An axial image is easily obtained with the C-arm by dorsiflexing the foot with a lap pad **(A)**. The lateral **(B)** and axial **(C)** views must confirm the reduction before closure. Correction of the tuberosity varus is demonstrated by the axial view. There is a free fragment of medial bone visible at the level of the primary fracture line. The reconstitution of the height of the calcaneus, the relation of the posterior facet, and the angle of Gissane is seen on the final lateral view **(D)**.

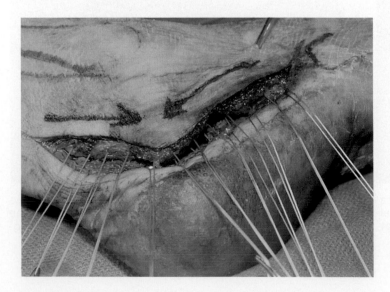

Figure 28. The deep sutures are all placed and tagged before any is tied. They are then tied from the edges of the incision toward the apex (arrows on foot). This allows closure with minimal tension.

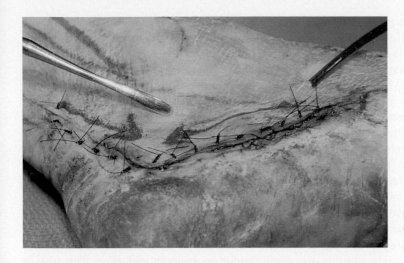

Figure 29. After the skin sutures are placed, the foot has a normal contour. The lateral bulge seen preoperatively (Fig. 11) is gone.

and distal toward the apex of the flap (Fig. 28). The skin is closed with vertical mattress sutures or a running baseball stitch (Fig. 29). The tourniquet is released after the dressing is applied. If the ankle comes easily into neutral, then only a bulky dressing is applied. If the Achilles tendon feels tight with dorsiflexion of the ankle, then a well-padded short-leg cast or splint is applied with the ankle in neutral dorsiflexion.

Final radiographs are taken in the operating room, and the patient moved to the recovery room if the films are acceptable.

POSTOPERATIVE MANAGEMENT

Postoperatively the foot and leg are elevated. A first-generation cephalosporin is administered until 24 hours after the drain is removed. The patient is mobilized on crutches, non–weight bearing. The drain is removed when it drains less than 30 ml over a 24-hour period. Once the drain is out, the patient is discharged with instructions to elevate the leg and wiggle the toes frequently. Depending on the degree of postoperative swelling in the flap, ankle and subtalar motion can begin as early as 2 days after surgery. If the flap is swollen, then motion should be delayed and the patient splinted in neutral for 2 to 3 weeks.

The need for physical therapy varies from patient to patient. Early therapy consists of isometric quadriceps and hamstring exercises and active range of motion to the ankle, subtalar, and midfoot regions. Having the patient attempt to "write" the letters of the alphabet with his foot is a good method of encouraging motion of the ankle, hindfoot, and midfoot joints. The sutures are removed at 3 weeks, as long as the wound looks well healed. A lateral radiograph should be taken at this time to confirm maintenance of the reduction.

By 6 weeks, the patient should have recovered full ankle motion and have more than 50% of the normal subtalar motion. If this is not the case, then passive mobilization with a therapist should be started. By 8 to 10 weeks, the patient should have functional motion and minimal pain in the ankle and hindfoot. If radiographs at this time show healing with maintenance of the reduction, then partial weight bearing (30 lb) is begun. Full weight bearing is allowed at 12 weeks. Coincident with full weight bearing, the patient is started on a program of ankle strengthening (especially the peroneal muscles) and proprioceptive training. An aircast may make the patient feel more comfortable until his coordination returns.

COMPLICATIONS

Early after the surgery, a hematoma may form under the flap, especially if the drain comes out too early. If this occurs, then the hematoma should be aspirated to avoid healing problems. If it is large or tense and cannot be aspirated, then it should be evacuated surgically by opening of the inferior edge of the incision. If it is not removed, the risks of flap failure and infection increase.

The most common complication after open calcaneal surgery is related to wound healing. The apex of the flap may not heal and leave a partial or even full-thickness wound. As long as the rest of the incision is healing and there is no fluid under the flap, this complication responds well to conservative measures. Wet to dry dressing changes or the use of petroleum gels in conjunction with elevation and delaying therapy usually allow the wound to heal.

Wound infection is fortunately not common but can be devastating. Emergency surgical debridement of the infection is necessary. The incision should be opened completely and all necrotic tissue removed. If infection occurs within the first 6 weeks and is acute in its presentation, then hardware is maintained. If the infection occurs more than 6 weeks after surgery, then the plate(s) should be removed. The posterior facet lag screws may be maintained. Not infrequently, multiple debridements are needed. Occasionally, exposed hardware or bone require plastic surgical consultation and free tissue transfer.

Posttraumatic subtalar arthritis may occur despite an anatomic reduction. This may be due to the initial cartilage injury. If modification of activity and medication do not provide relief, then a subtalar fusion may be indicated. The surgical restoration of the calcaneal height and width from the internal fixation makes late fusion less difficult.

Other late complications include peroneal irritation and cold intolerance. If peroneal irritation occurs over the plate, or more commonly, a screw head, then the hardware should be removed. Single screws can be removed through a small stab wound rather than elevating the entire flap. If the patient complains of discomfort while working in a refrigerated or cold environment, then plate removal may help to decrease discomfort.

ILLUSTRATIVE CASE FOR TECHNIQUE

A 23-year-old man jumped down a flight of nine stairs. He sustained a Sanders Type 2B, Essex Lopresti joint-depression type fracture of his calcaneus (Fig. 30). The leg was elevated until the swelling resolved, and he underwent surgery on postinjury day 17. The fracture was reduced anatomically and fixed with lag screws and a minifragment plate (Fig. 31).

His postoperative course was uneventful. At 12 weeks, he began full weight bearing. By 16 weeks, he was walking without any assistive device, had 10 degrees of dorsiflexion and 30 degrees of plantarflexion at the ankle, and had 80% of the subtalar motion of the contralateral foot. He returned to work as a laborer with minimal complaints of pain. At 2 years, he has minimal pain after long work days and is fully functional (Fig. 32).

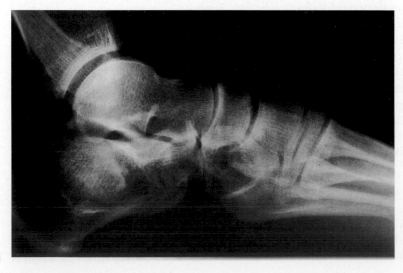

Figure 30. The lateral radiograph **(A)** demonstrates a joint-depression fracture with significant impaction of the posterior facet. *(figure continues)*

A

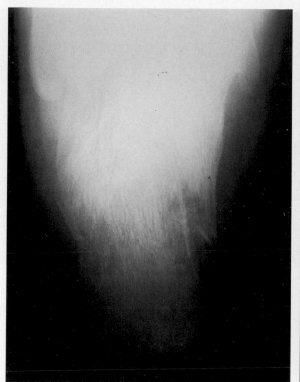

B

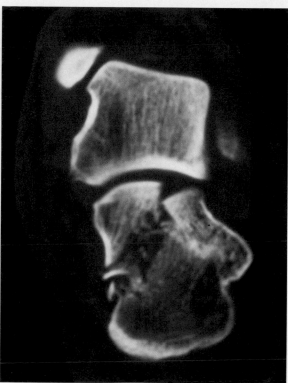

C

Figure 30. *(continued)* The primary fracture line exiting the medial cortex and the tuberosity is in varus on the axial view **(B)**. The 30-degree semicoronal computed tomography (CT) scan reveals a Type 2B fracture of the facet with comminution of the medial cortex **(C)**.

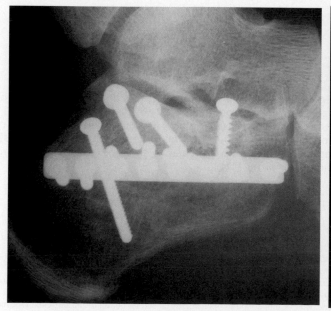

A

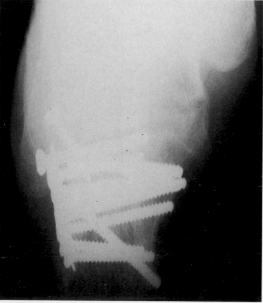

B

Figure 31. The postoperative lateral **(A)** view demonstrates an anatomic reduction of the calcaneus with two lag screws in the facet, a minifragment plate, and lag-screw fixation of the anterolateral fragment, which was placed percutaneously. The reduction of the tuberosity and medial cortex is seen on the axial view **(B)**.

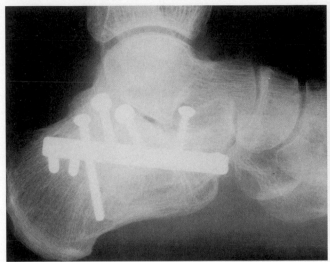

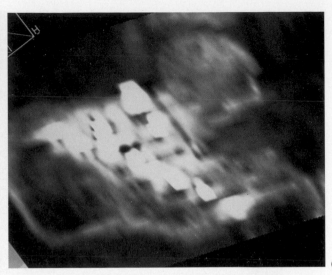

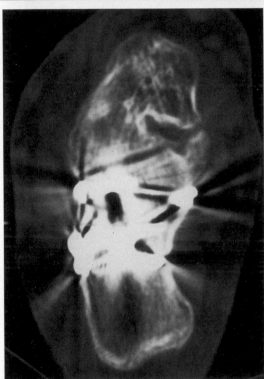

Figure 32. At 2 years, the patient had only minimal pain. The trabeculae have remodeled **(A)**. The 30-degree semicoronal computed tomography (CT) image demonstrates an anatomic reduction of the facet and good alignment of the tuberosity **(B)**. The sagittal-plane CT reconstruction shows excellent congruence of the posterior facet **(C)**.

RECOMMENDED READING

1. Albert, M.J., Waggoner, S.M., Smith, J.W.: Internal fixation of calcaneus fractures: an anatomical study of structures at risk. *J. Orthop. Trauma,* 9(2):107–112, 1995.
2. Bordeaux, B.D.: Reduction of calcaneal fractures by the McReynolds medial approach technique and its experimental basis. *Clin. Orthop.,* 177:87, 1983.
3. Buckley, R.E., and Meek, R.N.: Comparison of open versus closed reduction of intraarticular calcaneal fractures: a matched cohort in workmen. *J. Orthop. Trauma,* 6(1):216, 1992.
4. Carr, J.B., Hamilton, J.J., Bear, L.S.: Experimental intraarticular calcaneus fractures: anatomic basis for a new classification. *Foot Ankle,* 9:81, 1988.
5. Essex Lopresti, P.: The mechanism, reduction technique and results in fractures of the os calcis. *Br. J. Surg.,* 39:395, 1952.
6. Langdon, I.J., Kerr, P.S., Atkins, R.M.: Fractures of the calcaneum: the anterolateral fragment. *J. Bone Joint Surg. [Br],* 76(2):303, 1994.
7. Letournel, E.: Open treatment of acute calcaneal fractures. *Clin. Orthop.,* 290:60, 1993.
8. McLaughlin, H.L.: Treatment of late complications of os calcis fractures. *Clin. Orthop.* 30:111, 1963.

9. Palmer, I.: The mechanism and treatment of fractures of the calcaneus: open reduction with the use of cancellous grafts. *J. Bone Joint Surg. [Am],* 30:2, 1948.

10. Ross, S.D., Sowerby, M.R.: The operative treatment of fractures of the os calcis. *Clin. Orthop.,* 199:132, 1985.

11. Sanders, R.: Review article: intra-articular fractures of the calcaneus: present state of the art. *J. Orthop. Trauma,* 6(1):252, 1992.

12. Sanders, R., Fortin, P., DiPasquale, T., et al.: Operative treatment in 120 displaced intraarticular calcaneal fractures: results using a prognostic computed tomography scan classification. *Clin. Orthop.,* 290:87, 1993.

13. Stephenson, J.R.: Treatment of displaced intra-articular fractures of the calcaneus using medial and lateral approaches, internal fixation, and early motion. *J. Bone Joint Surg. [Am],* 69:115, 1987.

14. Thoren, O.: Os calcis fractures. *Acta. Orthop. Scand.,* (suppl)70:1 1964.

15. Tornetta, P., III.: Open reduction and internal fixation of the calcaneus using minifragment plates. *J. Orthop. Trauma,* 10(1):63–67, 1996.

16. Tornetta, P., III., and Sheskier, S.: Fractures of the os calcis: a method of choosing the surgical approach. *J. Orthop. Tech.,* 2(2):46, 1994.

17. Zwipp, H., Tscherne, H., Wulker, N.: Osteosynthese dislozierter intraartikulaar calcaneusfrakturen. *Unfallchirurgie* 91:507, 1988.

Master Techniques in Orthopaedic Surgery,
FRACTURES, edited by D. A. Wiss,
Lippincott–Raven Publishers, Philadelphia © 1998.

33

Tarsometatarsal "Lisfranc" Injuries: Evaluation and Management

Bruce J. Sangeorzan and Stephen K. Benirschke

INDICATIONS/CONTRAINDICATIONS

The primary indication for treating an injury is the knowledge that the injury that does poorly without treatment. Conceptually, those tarsometatarsal injuries that will, if untreated, lead to a loss of the arch or significant deformity should be treated surgically. This includes both displaced injuries and subtle injuries that have instability in two planes. The decision to treat a tarsometatarsal injury surgically is based on both physical examination and radiographic studies.

The transverse and longitudinal arches of the foot depend on the tarsometatarsal joints to make the foot sufficiently rigid to support the body, much as the apical blocks of ice support an igloo. Unstable tarsometatarsal injuries constitute a loss of this structural integrity and may result in deformity of the foot. In the majority of displaced injuries, the metatarsals displace dorsally and laterally on the tarsal bones, which produces pes planus with forefoot abduction. As a result, when weight is borne on the foot, it collapses. During heel lift, further deforming forces that act on the midfoot tend to exacerbate the deformity. For the metatarsals to displace in this direction, the plantar tarsometatarsal (Lisfranc) ligaments must be disrupted. Operative treatment is indicated when an ambulatory patient has an injury that renders the foot mechanically unsound, deformed, or both.

Ambulatory patients with displaced Lisfranc joints apparent on the plane radiographs and all the stabilizing ligaments disrupted are candidates for surgery. When the injuries are subtle or apparently undisplaced, operative treatment is indicated only when two-plane instability is detected on clinical examination or stress radiographs. Because the foot functions in weight bearing, the integrity of the plantar ligaments is of greater importance than that of the dorsal ligaments. Lisfranc injury is so often missed as to warrant discussion of diagnosis in the Indications section. There are few injuries in orthopaedics in which the

B. J. Sangeorzan, M.D.: Department of Orthopaedics, University of Washington, Harborview Medical Center, Seattle, Washington 98104.

S. K. Benirschke, M.D.: Department of Orthopaedics, Harborview Medical Center, Seattle, Washington 98104.

maxim "the eye doesn't see what the mind doesn't search for" is more appropriate. Swelling and tenderness in the midfoot with no obvious fracture should trigger a high index of suspicion.

Physical Examination Criteria

Instability should be determined by physical examination. The physician grasps the metatarsal heads and applies a dorsal force to the forefoot while the other hand palpates the tarsometatarsal joint. Dorsal subluxation or dislocation of the bases of the metatarsals suggests instability. If the first and second metatarsal can be displaced medially or laterally as well, global instability is present, and surgical treatment is needed. Low-energy injuries interrupt the medial capsule but do not disrupt the plantar ligaments. When the plantar ligaments are intact, no dorsal subluxation will occur with stress examination. These injuries may be treated nonoperatively or with less rigid fixation at the discretion of the examining surgeon.

Radiographic Criteria

With ligamentous disruption of the midfoot without fracture, non–weight bearing radiographs may be deceptively benign. The ligaments are torn with initial displacement however, when the deforming force is removed, the foot may spring back into a neutral position, concealing gross instability. The physician should be suspicious whenever there is gross midfoot swelling and pain. Three radiographic findings on plane films, when disrupted, suggest subtle tarsometatarsal injury. The first and most reliable is disruption in the continuity of a line drawn from the medial base of the second metatarsal to the medial side

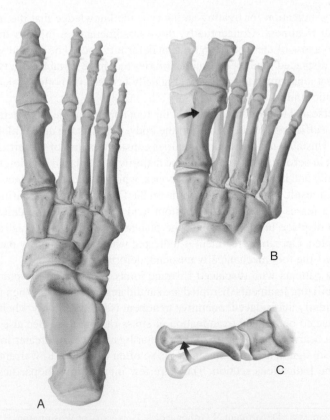

Figure 1. A–C: Diagrammatic representation of a dorsal view of the foot. The metatarsal bases are forced laterally and dorsally.

of intermediate cuneiform on the anteroposterior (AP) and oblique views (Fig. 1). Second, widening of the interval between first and second ray should be viewed with suspicion. If there is tenderness to palpation, stress views should be obtained. Third, the medial side of the base of the fourth metatarsal should line up with the medial side of the cuboid on the oblique view. This is a soft sign because the cross section of the base of the metatarsal is not equal to the cross section of the cuboid. As a result, it is possible for a step-off to be present if the angle of the beam is slightly misdirected. On the lateral view, the metatarsals are aligned with the cuneiforms at the dorsal cortex. When there is ligament injury, the metatarsals are typically dorsally displaced in relation to the cuneiforms.

Contraindications to surgical intervention include nonambulatory individuals, patients with serious vascular disease unlikely to heal a surgical incision but who have no significant deformity, or an injury that is unstable in only the transverse plane. Lisfranc injuries with only bone injuries can be treated by closed means or by closed reduction with percutaneous pinning. When there is deformity and compromised circulation, the surgeon faces a dilemma. Leaving a deformity puts the patient at risk for ulceration, while treating it surgically puts the patient at risk for wound-healing problems. In this circumstance, it is worth considering a vascular surgical consultation to evaluate whether an inflow procedure would be beneficial prior to orthopaedic intervention.

Neurologic impairment is also a cause for concern. The physician must decide whether sufficient energy produced the injury or whether an underlying neuropathic condition exists. Trivial injuries that cause significant displacement should stimulate an investigation into a possible neuropathic condition. Treatment of a Charcot neuropathic foot has different indications for treatment as well as different technique. When treating a Lisfranc injury in the presence of peripheral neuropathy, more fixation will be required, and a longer period of postoperative protection is indicated.

PREOPERATIVE PLANNING

Physical examination should document the status of the dorsalis pedis and posterior tibial pulses, the integrity of the skin, and the habitus of the foot. Tendon entrapment may be demonstrated by altered, uncorrectable position of the toes or midfoot. Intact or altered sensation should be documented.

Preoperative imaging should include a simulated weight-bearing AP and lateral of the foot, as well as an oblique view. Oblique views are essential to evaluating a midfoot injury and should be included in the foot-trauma series. If there is uncertainty as to the presence, location, or degree of injury, stress radiographs should be performed in two planes. Typically they are done by using fluoroscopy to make certain that the correct plane is achieved for the image. When the index of suspicion is high, the stress roentgenogram is performed in an operating room (OR) so that if the injury is confirmed, surgery can be done under the same anesthetic. An appropriate anesthetic is given, and the fluoroscopy unit is brought into the OR suite. The table is bent at the knees so the foot is relatively parallel to the floor.

While wearing lead gloves, the first and second metatarsal heads are grasped with one hand and the hindfoot with the other. With the thumb placed over the cuboid to act as a fulcrum, the forefoot is abducted and an AP radiograph is obtained. Instability is present if a gap occurs on the medial side of the first or second tarsometatarsal joint (Fig. 2D). Stress views in the lateral plane are performed if uncertainty exists. This is done by grasping the midfoot with one hand and the forefoot with the other, and acutely plantarflexing through the tarsometatarsal joint. Orient the fluoroscopy unit across the table and obtain an image. Although the tarsometatarsal joints may angulate, they should not open asymmetrically. Subluxation indicates that the joints are unstable.

Look also for instability at the intercuneiform level (Fig. 3A and B). These injuries are not rare, but because they are subtle, out of the plane of standard radiographs, and not well described, they are easily missed. Treatment follows the same principles as those at the

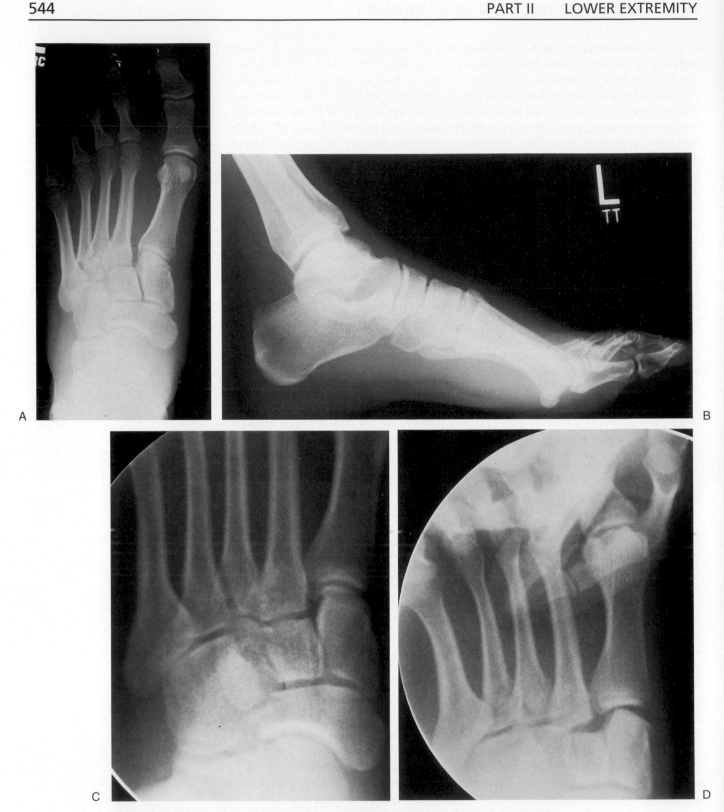

Figure 2. A: An anteroposterior (AP) radiograph demonstrating a subtle Lisfranc injury. The base of the second metatarsal is displaced laterally. **B:** This non–weight bearing lateral radiograph shows that the dorsal cortex of the second metatarsal is subluxed dorsally relative to its cuneiform. **C:** A scout view is used to confirm that the foot is in the correct position for assessing the tarsometatarsal joints. **D:** The stress radiograph reveals instability in the first, second, and probably third tarsometatarsal joints.

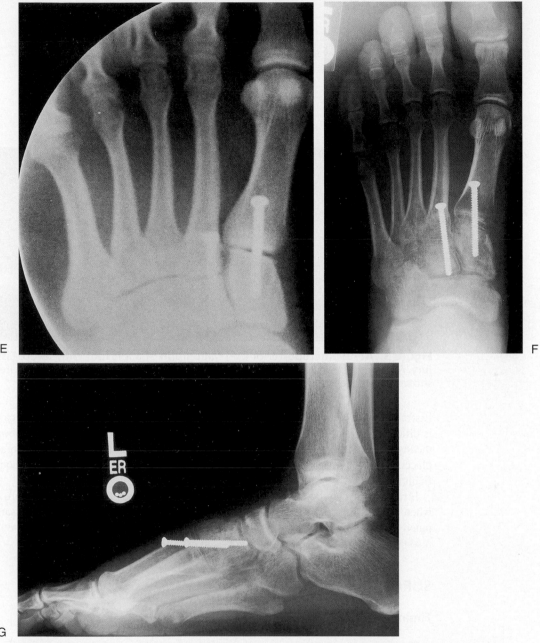

Figure 2. *(continued)* **E:** An intraoperative fluoroscopic taken after fixation reveals that the third metatarsal is stable. **F:** Six weeks following surgery, the reduction appears anatomic, and the clinical position of the foot is good. **G:** Alignment of the metatarsal bases is restored in both planes.

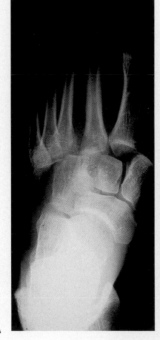

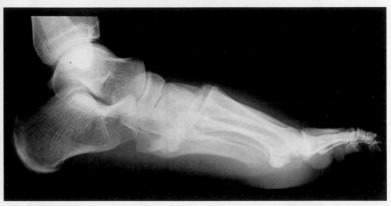

A   B

Figure 3. A: An anteroposterior (AP) radiograph of a left foot with severe Lisfranc injury. All five metatarsals are displaced laterally. **B:** The non–weight bearing lateral view shows that there is a dorsal dislocation.

Lisfranc level. Stress views in the AP plane are used to confirm the injury. Because there is little motion in most of the intercuneiform joints, any significant motion is abnormal. If the instability is great enough to allow subluxation of the midfoot, it should be treated. Displacement of the intercuneiform joints leads to deformity that is poorly understood and difficult to treat.

If radiographs are done in AP, lateral, and oblique planes, and stress views are obtained when there is uncertainty, additional imaging modalities should not be necessary. Computed tomographic scans of the midfoot are difficult to interpret. The role of the magnetic resonance imaging (MRI) scan has not been established.

SURGERY

Timing

There are several factors that must be considered when surgical intervention is necessary. These include the amount of soft-tissue swelling, the availability of imaging studies, and the degree of displacement. Surgery should be done emergently only in the presence of a compartmental syndrome, an open injury, or a deformity that threatens the integrity of the skin. Open injuries should be stabilized as soon as possible. If emergency stabilization threatens the survival of the limb, the soft tissue may be treated, and the bony stabilization performed when the safety of the soft-tissue envelope is restored. If there is gross instability, stabilizing the bone may help the soft tissue to heal, as it does in a long-bone fracture.

Technique

The patient is positioned supine with a roll beneath the greater trochanter to rotate the limb internally to a neutral position. A second roll is placed beneath the popliteal fossa. Knee flexion allows plantarflexion of the foot for easier exposure and imaging.

A longitudinal incision is made in the web space between the first and second rays (Fig. 4B), taking care to avoid damage to the dorsal cutaneous nerves. Expose the first tarsometatarsal joint between the long and short hallux extensor tendons (Fig. 4C). There is typically significant hemorrhage in this area, making identification of the structures somewhat difficult. The capsule may be enfolded into the joint and should be removed and preserved for later reapproximation. A small periosteal elevator is placed along the medial side of the first tarsometatarsal joint to confirm its reduced position. Remove the enfolded joint capsule medially so that the medial edge of the joint can be seen. Because the displacement is most often dorsal and lateral, the first metatarsal usually reduces with a plantar and medial force. When the first metatarsal is reduced relative to the medial cuneiform, place a Kirschner wire (K-wire) across the joint at its periphery, preventing loss of reduction before definitive fixation (Fig. 4D). Place the K-wire in the area of the joint that will be used for definitive fixation.

Before reducing the second metatarsal, check for injury between the medial and middle cuneiforms. Although not as common as Lisfranc-level injuries, disruption of the medial/middle cuneiform junction is the most common of the intertarsal disruptions. If there is first–second intertarsal instability, it should be addressed before the tarsometatarsal repair because it is difficult to secure the metatarsals to mobile tarsals. Under direct vision, the cuneiforms are reduced and held together with a pointed reduction clamp. Through a small stab wound, drill from medial to lateral, beginning in the middle of the dorsal one third of the medial cuneiform. This starting position is necessary because the middle cuneiform is smaller in its dorsoplantar and proximal-to-distal direction than is the medial. It also keeps the screw out of the way of the screws that will traverse the tarsometatarsal joints. Measure the drill hole and place a 3.5-mm screw from medial to lateral. Do not place the screw into the lateral cuneiform.

Next reduce the second metatarsal base into its mortise, between the three cuneiforms. This is accomplished by directly reducing the base of the second metatarsal against the intermediate cuneiform. If it is difficult to reduce, look plantarly for interposition of bone. Occasionally, part of the base of the second metatarsal is avulsed by Lisfranc plantar ligament and blocks reduction of the second metatarsal. Use a small elevator to push the fragment plantarly and medially. When it is reduced, place a large pointed reduction clamp from the base of the second metatarsal to the middle of the medial cuneiform and compress. Place a K-wire at the periphery of the joint to maintain the position. Notch the dorsal cortex of the second metatarsal 12 to 15 mm from the joint and prepare a hole for the 3.5-mm screw with a 2.5-mm drill. Before advancing the drill, center it over the second toe, and advance it in a position almost parallel to the plantar surface of the foot. This is necessary because the intermediate cuneiform is quite small in cross section, and if the screw is directed too plantarly, it is easy to miss the cuneiform altogether. The drill hole should be tapped before inserting a 3.5-mm cortical screw to prevent subluxation as the screw is advanced across the joint. When the screw has been seated, remove the K-wire.

Next, reassess the position of the first metatarsal relative to the medial cuneiform. If it has moved or is overreduced, reposition it and place a K-wire at the edge of the joint. Again, drill, tap, and place a 3.5-mm cortical screw. This screw should start 15 to 20 mm from the joint, although it need not be quite as parallel to the plantar surface of the foot, because the shape of the medial cuneiform is greater in the dorsoplantar direction. This screw should be approximately 40 mm in length. If the measured length is less than 30 mm, the starting hole was placed too close to the joint or the drill was directed obliquely out of the cuneiform. A screw this short may not provide adequate purchase in the cuneiform.

The third tarsometatarsal joint should be directly evaluated. If it requires fixation but the fourth does not, no further incision is required. Develop a full-thickness flap through the original incision until the third tarsometatarsal joint can be visualized. It will usually follow the second into a reduced position. Hold it in place with a reduction clamp, and place the screw through a small stab wound. However, if the third and fourth metatarsal bases both require reduction and fixation, it is helpful to make a second incision. A longitudinal incision is made over the base of the fourth ray parallel to the first incision (Fig. 4B). Depending on the size of the extensor brevis muscle, it may be possible to elevate the lateral border of the muscle. If it is too large, split the muscle belly bluntly in line with its fibers to visualize the tarsometatarsal joints. Reduce the third first. Again, use a K-wire as provisional fixation. Definitive fixation is provided by a 3.5-mm cortical screw.

Because the fourth and fifth tarsometatarsal joints are mobile, the goals of treatment are slightly different. These joints must be held in place only long enough to develop a scar capsule. Screws may break because of the motion in this joint. The fourth and fifth are held in place and pinned with 0.062-inch K-wires (Fig. 4E–G). The preferred fixation is a 3.5-mm screw across the injured tarsometatarsal joint. Screws may be used obliquely when reduction is difficult or intertarsal injuries require fixation (see Fig. 4A).

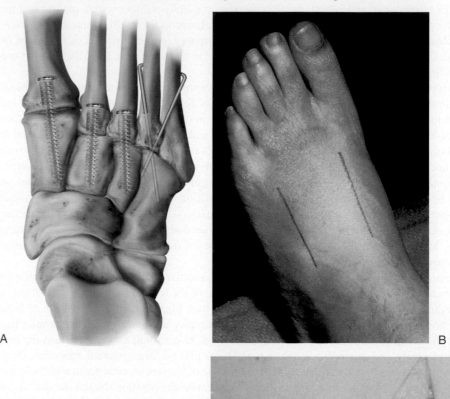

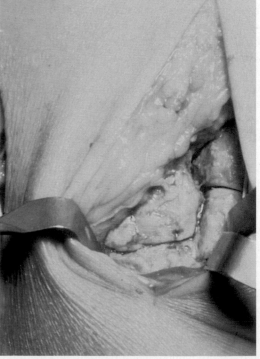

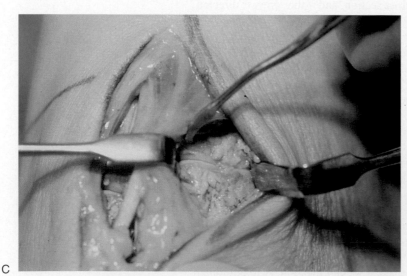

Figure 4. A: Idealized fixation. A small screw, usually 3.5 mm, transfixes the base of the metatarsal and cuneiform. The screw should be directed from distal to proximal and begin approximately 15 mm from the joint, or a little farther in the first ray. If there is intercuneiform injury, an additional screw is directed from medial to lateral. **B:** The preferred position of the two dorsal incisions. **C:** This figure shows the intraoperative exposure through the more medial of the two dorsal incisions. **D:** Intraoperative photograph showing the base of the second metatarsal reduced into its mortise.

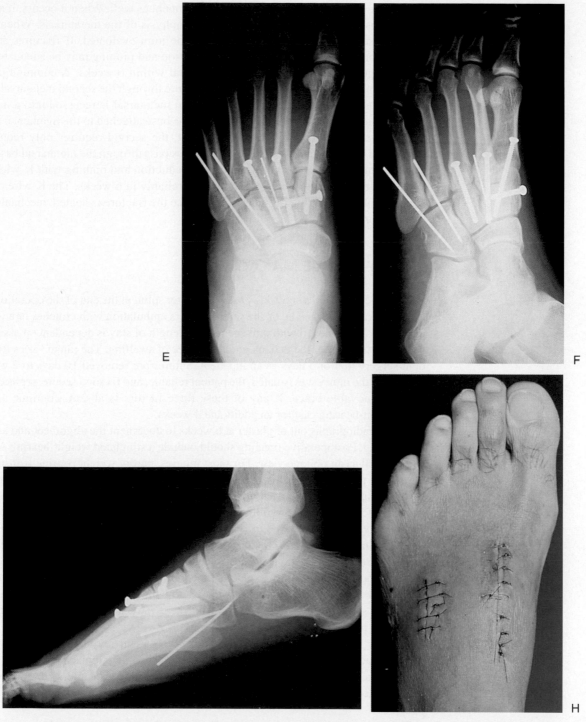

Figure 4. *(continued)* **E:** The 3.5-mm screws bridge the first, second, and third tarso-metatarsal joints and the joint between the medial and intermediate cuneiform. The fourth and fifth tarsometatarsal joints are transfixed by 0.062-inch Kirschner wires. **F:** This oblique view shows that the base of the fourth metatarsal, on its medial side, lines up with the medial side of the cuboid. **G:** A lateral radiograph of the same foot shows that the dorsal cortex of the metatarsal and tarsal bones are sligned. **H:** A post-operative photograph of the operated foot at 2 weeks.

Lisfranc injuries may have a fracture component as well. When it occurs, it most commonly presents as a fracture through the metaphysis of the metatarsals. When unstable, the fracture should be stabilized, and then the joint evaluated. If fractures are present without concomitant ligament injuries, reduction and pinning may be adequate, because fractures get "sticky" within 3 weeks and heal within 6 weeks. A common pattern includes a joint disruption at the first ray, a fracture through the second metatarsal base, and a joint injury at the third. Because the second metatarsal is recessed into a mortise between the cuneiform, it fractures and leaves the base attached to the ligaments. If the first and third rays are stabilized across the joint, the second requires only reduction and sometimes pinning for 4 weeks. When fractures pass through the metatarsal bases and the joint is intact, treatment is not so involved. Reduction and pinning with K-wires may be enough. Unlike the ligaments, fractures heal reliably in 6 weeks. The K-wire can be left in place until the fracture becomes stable. Once the fracture is healed, mechanical stability is restored.

POSTOPERATIVE MANAGEMENT

Place the patient in a short-leg posterior plaster splint at the end of the operation. The patient is discharged when he or she safely masters ambulation with crutches or a walker and pain control is achieved with oral agents. The length of stay is dependent on associated injuries, the fragility of the patient, and the degree of swelling. The range varies from outpatient surgery to 4 or 5 days as an inpatient. Sutures are removed 10 days to 2 weeks after surgery. If the injury was isolated, the patient reliable, and fixation secure, replace the splint with a removable brace. If any of these three factors is absent, continue a short-leg non–weight-bearing cast for an additional 4 weeks.

Obtain radiographs out of plaster at 6 weeks to document the alignment and assess fracture healing. Postoperative imaging should include a simulated weight-bearing AP and lateral, as well as an oblique view. For most injuries, partial weight bearing is instituted in a removable protective boot at 6 weeks. Self-directed physical therapy (PT) is begun at this time. Swimming is encouraged, and riding an exercise bike is allowed. Encourage the patient to gradually advance to full weight bearing over the next 2 to 4 weeks, depending on the stability and fixation. At 8 to 10 weeks, the patient can begin wearing a regular shoe if the foot is not too swollen. The screws are left in place for a minimum of 16 weeks. If the implants are asymptomatic and transfix only the first through third tarsometatarsal joints, they may be left permanently in place. If the joint has become sufficiently stiff, the screws will not be symptomatic. However, a small amount of motion frequently occurs, which causes the screws to loosen. If this happens, the screws can often be removed under local anesthesia in the office or outpatient center.

Because swelling may persist for months, the patient may begin by wearing athletic shoes. As activity level increases, a standard work shoe may replace the athletic shoe for a few hours a day in increasing amounts until normal shoes can be tolerated. The process may be facilitated by a custom-molded full-length insole of a nonrigid material such as cork or pelite.

The patients may return to work at 10 days to 2 weeks if they work in an office. They should return to work in 3 to 4 months if involved in heavy labor activities. Patients should avoid jumping-type recreational activities, such as basketball and volleyball, and running for 9 to 12 months. The degree of return to work and recreational activities depends on the amount of trauma, the degree of articular surface injury, and the quality of the bone. Most patients will continue to have some symptoms in the foot for up to 2 years. Many will have life-long symptoms. Only a small percentage will go on to midfoot arthrodesis if reduced and held rigidly. If symptoms are mechanical (i.e., midfoot pain during heel rise), a custom, full-length, semirigid insole may be beneficial. Generally, this should be fabricated when the patient has returned to full weight bearing and the swelling has resolved.

COMPLICATIONS

Associated injuries following midfoot fractures and dislocations include intercuneiform injuries, tendon entrapment, and vascular injury. The interval between the medial and intermediate cuneiform is the most common associated intercuneiform joint injury. The tibialis anterior is the most commonly entrapped tendon. The tibialis anterior tendon inserts in part on the base of the first metatarsal. As the first metatarsal is displaced laterally, it takes the tendon with it. As the deforming force is removed, the metatarsal moves medially, and the tendon is trapped by the medial cuneiform. This complication is treated during open reduction. At the time of surgery, the anterior tibia tendon will be in the way of reduction and can be reduced to its normal position. The most common vascular injury is to the plantar branch of the dorsalis pedis, where it is tethered between the first and second metatarsal. Damage to this vessel, however, is of little clinical significance, but there are historic references documenting the potential for more severe injuries, resulting in forefoot ischemia.

Injury to the dorsal cutaneous branches of the superficial peroneal nerve also may occur. Because the tissues are edematous and displaced and there is significant hemorrhage in the subcutaneous tissue, identification of these small nerves is challenging. Care should be taken to preserve the nerves, and patients should be warned preoperatively that nerve injury is possible. If one of these nerves is divided during surgery, the proximal end can be tucked into the extensor brevis muscle belly, or the two ends can be reapproximated.

Soft-tissue problems are not uncommon, particularly after direct trauma. There is little muscle to absorb the load or augment the blood flow. Patients should be warned that eschar may develop in areas that were injured and may include the surgical incision. It is uncommon for these soft-tissue problems to require free tissue transfer, but skin grafts are common in direct injuries. Full-thickness wounds are managed with dressing changes until there is an adequate bed of granulation tissue to support a split-thickness graft.

Nonunion is uncommon in metatarsal fractures but occasionally occurs and will require treatment if it is painful or leads to instability. There are times when, in spite of nonunion, there is sufficient "splinting" by the surrounding structures that symptoms are minimal and surgical treatment is unnecessary.

Incomplete reduction is a common problem that may lead to loss of the arch and abduction of the forefoot. Great care should be taken to adequately plantar flex and adduct the metatarsals. It is essential to be certain that the first metatarsal is brought medially and plantarly before trying to reduce the second. This will lessen the likelihood of incomplete reduction. A prominent cuneiform may be observed on the dorsomedial aspect of the foot when the first metatarsal is incompletely plantarflexed and adducted. At times this deformity may also be due to unrecognized intercuneiform injury.

RECOMMENDED READING

1. Arntz, C.T., Veith, R.G., Hansen, S.T.: Fractures and fracture-dislocations of the tarsometatarsal joint. *J. Bone Joint Surg.*, 70(2):173–181, 1987.
2. Blair, W.F.: Irreducible tarsal metatarsal fracture dislocation. *J. Trauma,* 21:988–990, 1981.
3. DeBenedetti, M.J., Evanski, P.M., Waugh, T.R.: The unreducible Lisfranc fracture. *Clin. Orthop.*, 136:238–240, 1978.
4. Foster, S.C., and Foster, R.R.: Lisfranc tarsal metatarsal fracture dislocation. *Radiology,* 120:79–83, 1976.
5. Sangeorzan, B.J., Veith. R.G., Hansen, S.T., Jr.: Fusion of Lisfranc's joint for the salvage of tarsometatarsal injuries. *Foot Ankle* 10(4):193–200, 1989.

Master Techniques in Orthopaedic Surgery,
FRACTURES, edited by D. A. Wiss,
Lippincott–Raven Publishers, Philadelphia © 1998.

34

Gastrocnemius and Soleus Rotational Muscle Flaps: Soft-Tissue Coverage

Randy Sherman

INDICATIONS/CONTRAINDICATIONS

A muscle flap is indicated when vital structures such as bones, joints, tendons, or hardware are exposed and require coverage. In the lower leg and particularly the tibia, a muscle flap must be well vascularized and durable. Of all the local rotational flaps, the gastrocnemius is one of the most reliable. It is a broad muscle with a single proximal vascular pedicle, which is well protected in the popliteal fossa. The gastrocnemius muscle or myocutaneous rotational flap is the procedure of choice for soft-tissue coverage of complex open wounds about the knee and proximal third of the tibia and fibula. The use of this flap is indicated in the following circumstances: (a) coverage of acute, Grade IIIB open tibial fractures with or without hardware, involving exposure of the knee joint, capsule, fracture site, or exposed cortex (Fig. 1); (b) obliteration of dead space and wound closure after radical debridement of osteomyelitic wounds in this region, as well as infected nonunions (Fig. 2); (c) coverage of exposed total knee arthroplasties or prearthroplasty tissue augmentation in densely scarred wound beds (Fig. 3); and (d) limb salvage and coverage of endoprostheses or allograft material after resection of musculoskeletal neoplasms (Fig. 4).

The soleus muscle, without a myocutaneous correlate, has a much more limited area of rotation and is used primarily for small, medially based, open wounds in the middle third of the leg. Indications include coverage of acute open fractures and chronic osteomyelitic wounds (Fig. 5).

Contraindications to the use of a gastrocnemius flap include vascular compromise of the muscle itself by disruption of the sural artery pedicle, compromise of the popliteal artery from which it emanates, or occlusion of the proximal arterial tree. Significant local trauma to the muscle itself, although rare, prevents its successful rotation. Recipient-site contraindications include a wound in the proximal third region whose size and dimension is too

R. Sherman, M.D.: Division of Plastic and Reconstructive Surgery, University of Southern California–University Plastic Surgeons, Los Angeles, California 90033-4680.

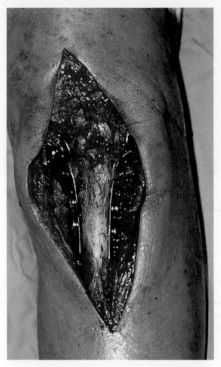

Figure 1. Grade III B open tibial-plateau fracture with exposed knee joint after internal fixation and unsuccessful attempt at primary wound closure.

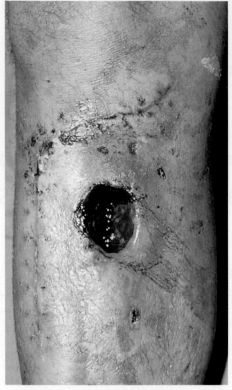

Figure 2. Dead space involving skin, subcutaneous tissue, muscle, and bone in a proximal-third infected nonunion.

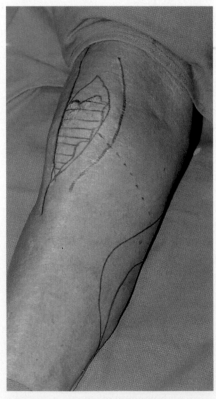

Figure 3. Scarred, atrophic prepatella skin in an elderly patient after removal of an infected total knee arthroplasty.

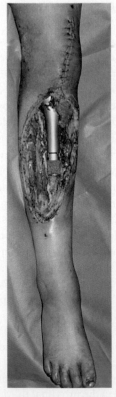

Figure 4. A 10-year-old girl immediately after tumor extirpation of a proximal tibial osteosarcoma and placement of endoprosthesis after loss of anterior skin.

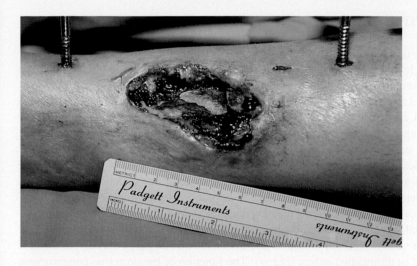

Figure 5. Middle-third Grade III B open tibial fracture with a bony sequestrum and loss of overlying soft tissue.

large for coverage by the gastrocnemius muscle. Similarly, injury to the substance of the soleus muscle will hinder its ability to be transposed. Vascular compromise to the soleus muscle is extremely rare because of its segmental inflow. Because of minor perforators that exit from the posterior tibial artery distally, the surgeon must take great care to assure adequate vascularity to the most distal aspect of the soleus muscle when a large transposition is undertaken. As with the gastrocnemius, a large anterior or laterally located wound in the middle third of the leg may not be completely covered by the soleus muscle (Fig. 6), and free tissue transfer may be a better option. As with any muscle-coverage procedure, infection or tumor recurrence is best avoided by thorough debridement or excision before wound closure. No muscle flap will successfully combat retained sequestrum or loose infected hardware as a nidus for continued infection.

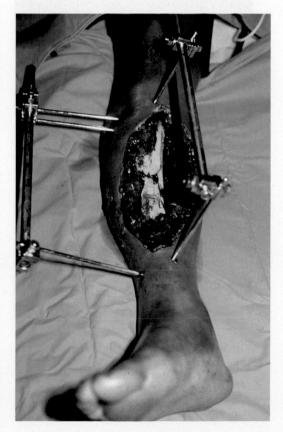

Figure 6. Large, middle-third Grade III B open tibial fracture cannot be closed by a local soleus flap and requires free tissue transfer.

PREOPERATIVE PLANNING

A thorough examination of the patient is crucial when planning either a gastrocnemius or soleus muscle flap for coverage of a complex open wound. Radiographs should be viewed with particular attention as to the location of the fracture and the presence or absence of internal fixation devices. For acute fractures, if an external fixator is indicated, the surgeon should anticipate the need for subsequent soft-tissue closure and construct the frame to allow unrestricted transposition of the muscles from posterior to a medial or anterior plane. The zone of injury around the fracture site should be recognized because aggressive or radical debridement may significantly alter the dimensions of the wound (Fig. 7). Clinical examination of the leg should be made, with particular attention to the wound size including length, width, and depth. Other factors such as induration, discoloration, ecchymosis, and cellulitis must be considered. A detailed vascular examination with palpation of the dorsalis pedis and posterior tibial pulses for arterial inflow, as well as Doppler examination for venous outflow, should be documented. Arteriography may be indicated if there are absent or diminished pulses (Fig. 8). The function of the posterior-compartment muscles should be assessed whenever possible. Sensory examination of the foot must be documented, with particular attention to the posterior tibial nerve, sural nerve, and saphenous nerve. The surgical incisions can be planned in conjunction with the need for additional debridement and internal or external fixation of the fracture.

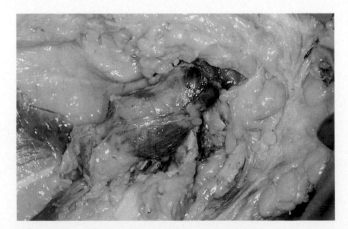

Figure 7. Large amount of retained titanium from a previously removed infected total knee arthroplasty.

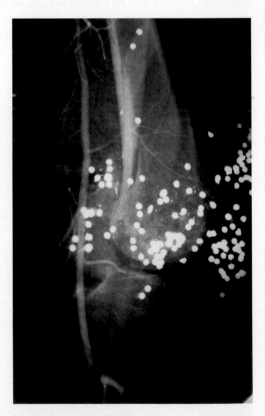

Figure 8. Angiogram demonstrating patency of the popliteal artery and continuity of the sural arteries despite the fracture comminution and retained gunshot pellets.

SURGERY

Gastrocnemius

A muscle flap is undertaken only after complete and definitive debridement of a traumatic or infected wound has been completed or a tumor has been extirpated (Fig. 9). A tourniquet is placed on the thigh, and the entire leg is prepped and draped. The approach to the gastrocnemius muscle can be made through perpendicular, oblique, or parallel incisions. If a parallel incision is used, the gastrocnemius muscle must be tunneled beneath the resulting bipedicled fasciocutaneous flap. The gastrocnemius muscle is identified by incising the deep investing fascia of the leg longitudinally along the anterior border of the muscle (Fig. 10). The fascia can be opened proximally toward the origin of the muscle and distally to its insertion on the Achilles tendon if necessary. The fatty plane between the gastrocnemius and soleus is developed by either sharp or digital dissection. This areolar plane is confirmed by visualization of the plantaris longus tendon, which lies adjacent to the soleus at or near its medial border (Fig. 11). The white investing fascia on the posterior border of the soleus and the deep border of the gastrocnemius make this plane unmistak-

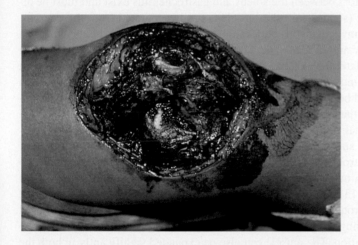

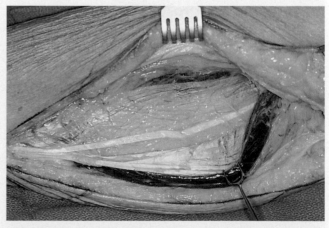

Figure 9. Completed debridement of infected fracture of the knee with removal of all nonviable soft tissue and bony sequestrum.

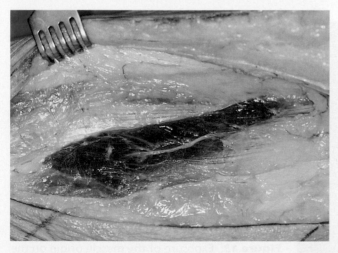

Figure 10. The gastrocnemius muscle is visible once the deep investing fascia is incised longitudinally.

Figure 11. The plantaris longus tendon confirms the plane between the gastrocnemius and soleus muscles.

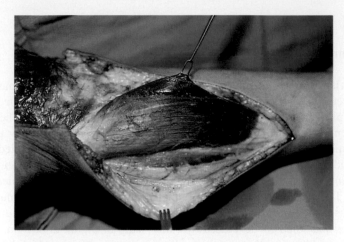

Figure 12. The median raphe separates the medial and lateral heads of the gastrocnemius and carries the neurovascular structures that must be protected.

able. Occasionally perforators between the soleus and gastrocnemius exist and must be divided. Moving posteriorly (superficial), the muscle is easily separated from the deep investing fascia. One or two myocutaneous perforators must be saved if a myocutaneous flap is planned; otherwise, they are divided. The gastrocnemius is separated along its median raphe into a medial and a lateral head. The raphe is easier to identify and more prominent in the distal portion of the muscle (Fig. 12). The sural nerve and lesser saphenous vein run along the raphe and should be preserved. These are constant landmarks and facilitate separation of the medial from the lateral head. Once the median raphe has been identified, dissection proceeds from distal to proximal, staying along the posterior midline while protecting the neurovascular structures at all times. When both the posterior and anterior surfaces are freed, the gastrocnemius can be released from its attachment to the Achilles tendon. The dissection continues proximally to the origin of the gastrocnemius muscle from the femoral condyle (Fig. 13). With proximal dissection in the popliteal space, care must be taken to visualize and protect the vascular pedicle (Fig. 14). The muscle can be released from the condyle by resecting its tendinous attachments, resulting in a 2- to 3-cm increase in the length for arc of rotation. The muscle can also be expanded significantly in both the

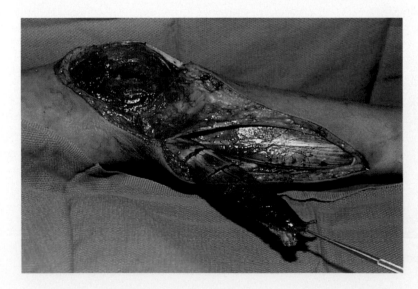

Figure 13. Exposure of the muscle origin on the femoral condyle requires adequate muscle retraction and sufficient proximal exposure.

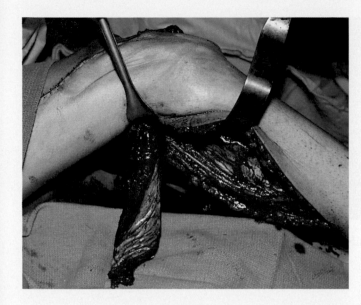

Figure 14. When needed, the sural artery pedicle can be visualized on the deep surface of the gastrocnemius in the popliteal fossa.

transverse and longitudinal planes by crisscross incisions through its heavily fused bilaminar myofascia both anteriorly and posteriorly (Fig. 15). Furthermore, the gastrocnemius muscle can be split longitudinally in the distal portion so that part of the muscle can be used to obliterate deep dead space, while using the remainder of the muscle for superficial coverage.

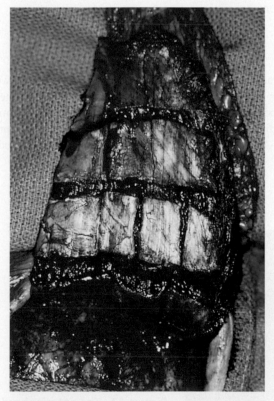

Figure 15. Transverse and longitudinal myofascial release on both deep and superficial surfaces allows significant expansion of muscle area to be used for coverage.

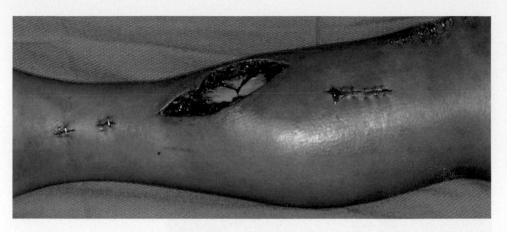

Figure 16. Ideal wounds for soleus coverage are small, medial wounds located in the middle third of the leg.

The lateral gastrocnemius flap is raised in a similar fashion from a lateral cutaneous approach by using one of the three incisions described. Of paramount importance is the identification and protection of the peroneal nerve just below the head of the fibula as it penetrates from superficial to deep into the lateral compartment. Once the safety of this nerve is assured, raising the lateral gastrocnemius muscle is done in a fashion similar to that described for the medial head. It should be noted, however, that the lateral gastrocnemius muscle is smaller than the medial head and will not provide the same quantity of muscle for laterally based lesions.

Soleus

The soleus is almost always raised from a medial approach and is used to cover small medial and anterior-based middle-third wounds (Fig. 16). A curvilinear incision is made over the medial aspect of the calf. The plane between the gastrocnemius and soleus muscles is easily identified and serves as an excellent starting point. When raising the soleus, the gastrocnemius–Achilles musculotendinous unit must be preserved at all times. Alice

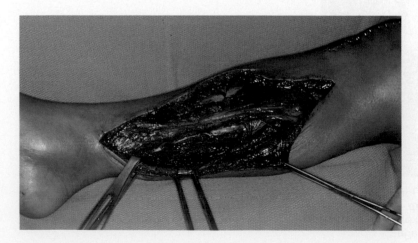

Figure 17. The anterior border of the Achilles is identified and retracted with Alice clamps to aid dissection of the posterior surface of the soleus from the tendon.

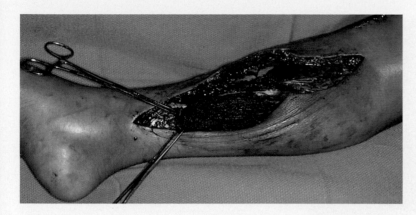

Figure 18. Once freed from its anterior and posterior attachments, the soleus muscle is transected distally.

clamps are placed on the edge of the Achilles tendon the better to demonstrate the area where the two merge. The fascia that fuses the posterior soleus to the Achilles is divided (Fig. 17). Proceeding from proximal to distal, the muscle is dissected off the Achilles tendon with either a knife or Metzenbaum scissors from medial to lateral. A pseudoraphe is encountered approximately three fourths of the way through the dissection. It is important to separate this and continue the dissection both posteriorly and then laterally to include the entire soleus muscle. The muscle is released distally to include as much length as possible (Fig. 18). The plane between the deep side of the soleus and the deep flexor compartment is identified and can be digitally dissected. Care must be taken to identify the distal perforators arising from the posterior tibial artery and vein. These can be very short and, if inadvertently injured or cut, may retract beneath the deep fascia, making them difficult to ligate. Once these distal perforators have been identified, ligated, and divided, the soleus attachments on the lateral side are dissected free under direct visualization. The muscle must be freed quite proximally, especially on its lateral side, to achieve any significant rotation of the muscle into the wound (Fig. 19). Crisscross release of the myofascia of the soleus can be done on the deep or anterior surface of the muscle to expand the size and the dimensions of the flap (Fig. 20).

Each muscle, once transferred, is secured into place with absorbable sutures. It is worth emphasizing that the muscle, particularly the gastrocnemius, can be split longitudinally,

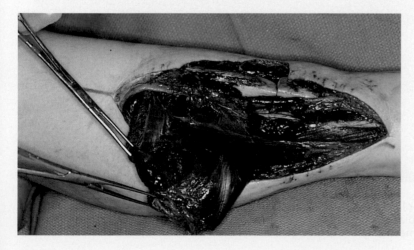

Figure 19. Because of the broad attachments on both the tibial and fibular sides, dissection must continue quite proximally to achieve any significant transposition.

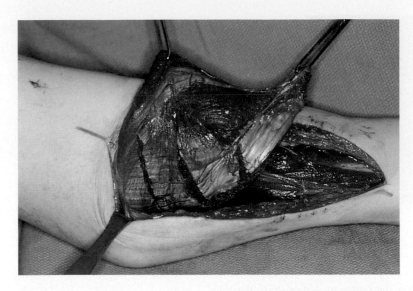

Figure 20. Scoring of the myofascia on the anterior surface of the soleus allows great dimensions for coverage.

with one slip obliterating dead space and the remainder addressing the requirements of the open wound. Finally, a skin graft over the flap is necessary and can be harvested from either the ipsilateral calf, thigh, or buttock after application of aerosolized thrombin. The thickness of the graft is usually 15 to 18 thousandths of an inch (Fig. 21). Alternatively, a myocutaneous flap can be designed to include skin and subjacent subcutaneous tissue, based on perforators from the gastrocnemius (Fig. 22). The skin overlying the muscle is used and can extend 5 cm proximal to the medial malleolus. The ability to close the donor site must be considered before executing this myocutaneous flap. This possibility does not exist with the soleus. Before wound closure, a Jackson–Pratt drain is placed in the wound.

A well-padded short-leg posterior splint is applied with the foot and ankle in neutral dorsiflexion (Fig. 23).

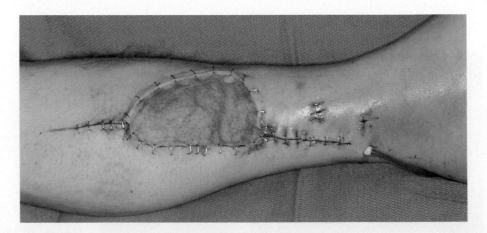

Figure 21. A split-thickness skin graft measuring between 15 and 18 thousandths of an inch can be placed immediately after successful flap transposition. I use sheet grafts as opposed to meshed grafts with equal success to improve recipient-site aesthetics.

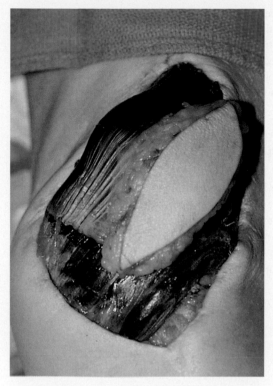

Figure 22. A cutaneous paddle can be reliably transferred with the gastrocnemius muscle if it contains at least one myocutaneous perforator.

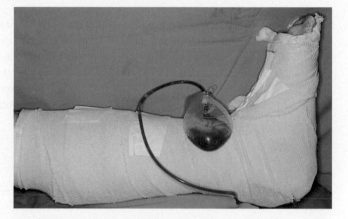

Figure 23. At the completion of the procedure, Jackson–Pratt drains are placed on suction, and the extremity is secured in a well-padded posterior splint, making sure the foot is plantigrade.

POSTOPERATIVE MANAGEMENT

The Jackson–Pratt drain is removed once drainage is less than 30 ml per day. The dressings are changed between 3 and 5 days, and the skin grafts are inspected. The patient is allowed to place the leg in a dependent position for a short period at 1 week and is trained to increase the tolerance over the course of the subsequent 3 to 5 weeks. Prolonged dependency is avoided for 6 to 8 weeks to avoid venous congestion. The timing of weight-bearing ambulation depends primarily on the orthopaedic injury, rather than on the muscle flap. The patient is seen weekly in the office until the wound is completely closed and dry. Patients must be counseled preoperatively as to the deformity caused by muscle rotation, with loss of natural convexity in the proximal and middle third of the leg caused by rotation of the gastrocnemius muscle. It is well documented that both the gastrocnemius and soleus muscles will atrophy over time after transposition. After a gastrocnemius or soleus muscle flap, range of motion of the knee and ankle are usually started during the first week.

COMPLICATIONS

Because of the rich blood supply and durability of both the gastrocnemius and soleus muscles, flap death is rare. More common, however, is the development of a postoperative hematoma, which requires surgical evacuation, irrigation, and control of the bleeding site. Loss of power with plantar flexion is rarely a problem if the gastrocnemius or the soleus muscle is used alone. A combined gastrocnemius and soleus flap can lead to a greater incidence of muscle weakness and gait abnormalities. Pain and dysesthesias at the donor site resulting from flap transposition should be expected during the first 6 to 8 weeks and should not be considered a complication. Occasionally, with dissection of the soleus muscle and loss of its middle and distal perforators, the distal end of the soleus may become devascularized and, if recognized, should be resected. If unrecognized, this can lead to partial flap necrosis and subsequent wound infection with bone or hardware exposure or both. Reversed or distally based soleus flaps, although described, should not be considered reliable alternatives for muscle transposition.

ILLUSTRATIVE CASE FOR TECHNIQUE

A 36-year-old man sustained a Grade IIIB open, comminuted tibial-plateau and proximal-third fracture (Fig. 24). After open reduction and internal fixation, the wound broke down. The gastrocnemius muscle was harvested from the medial side through a transverse skin incision (Fig. 25). The muscle was rotated into place (Fig. 26) with release of its investing fascia, allowing the hardware to be entirely covered. A split-thickness skin graft was placed. The wound healed without incident (Fig. 27).

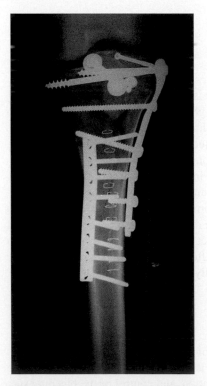

Figure 24. Grade IIIB open tibial-plateau and proximal-third fracture after open reduction and internal fixation.

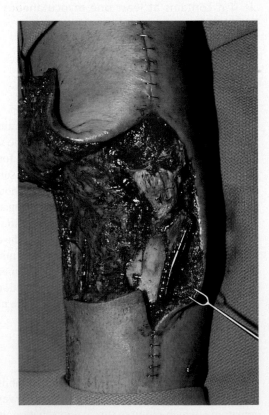

Figure 25. Exposure of the gastrocnemius is made through a transverse posterior incision from the wound.

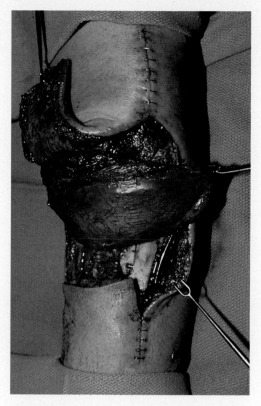

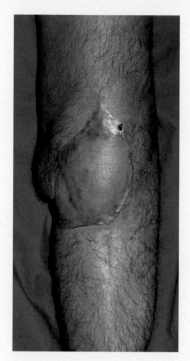

Figure 26. Once the muscle is freed, it is transposed into place for complete wound coverage.

Figure 27. A well-healed skin graft over the muscle completes the healing process, allowing the fracture to unite.

RECOMMENDED READING

1. Arnold, P.G., Mixter, R.C.: Making the most of the gastrocnemius muscle. *Plast. Reconstr. Surg.,* 72:38, 1983.
2. Chandrasekhar, B., Brien, W.: Coverage strategies in total joint replacement. *Orthop. Clin. North Am.,* 24:3, 1993.
3. Feldman, S.J., Cohen, B.E., Mayo, S.W., Jr.: The medial gastrocnemius myocutaneous flap. *Plast. Reconstr. Surg.* 61:531, 1978.
4. Guzman-Stein, G., Fix, R.J., Vasconez, L.O.: Muscle flap coverage for the lower extremity. *Clin. Plast. Surg.,* 18:545, 1991.
5. Lesavoy, M.A., Dubrow, T.J., Wackym, P.A., et al.: Muscle flap coverage of exposed endoprostheses. *Plast. Reconstr. Surg.* 83:90, 1989.
6. Malawar, M.M., Price, W.M.: Gastrocnemius transposition flap in conjunction with limb sparing surgery for primary bone sarcomas around the knee. *Plast. Reconstr. Surg.* 73:741, 1984.
7. Mathes, S.J., McCraw, J.B., Vasconez, L.O.: Muscle transposition flaps for coverage of lower extremity defects: anatomic considerations. *Surg. Clin. North Am.* 54:1337, 1974.
8. Mathes, S.J., Nahai, F.: *Clinical Application for Muscle and Musculocutaneous Flaps.* Mosby, St. Louis, 1982.
9. McCraw, J.B., Fishman, J.H., Sharzer, L.A.: The versatile gastrocnemius myocutaneous flap. *Plast. Reconstr. Surg.,* 62:15, 1978.
10. Stark, W.: The use of pedicled muscle flaps in the treatment of chronic osteomyelitis resulting from compound fractures. *J. Bone Joint Surg.,* 28:343, 1946.
11. Tobin, G.F.: Hemisoleus and reversed hemisoleus flaps. *Plast. Reconstr. Surg.,* 76:87, 1985.
12. Yaremchuck, M.V.: Acute management of severe soft tissue damage accompanying open fractures of the lower extremity. *Clin. Plast. Surg.,* 13:621, 1986.

PART III

Pelvis and Acetabulum

Master Techniques in Orthopaedic Surgery,
FRACTURES, edited by D. A. Wiss,
Lippincott–Raven Publishers, New York © 1998.

35

Pelvic Fractures: External Fixation

Mark S. Vrahas

INDICATIONS/CONTRAINDICATIONS

Pelvic external fixation is indicated for the immediate management of patients with hemodynamic instability after pelvic fractures. Depending on the location and type of pelvic fracture, external fixation can be used alone or in combination with internal fixation definitively to stabilize pelvic fractures. External fixation is widely recognized as a useful technique for controlling bleeding associated with displaced pelvic fractures. This type of hemorrhage usually results from disruption of the extensive pelvic venous plexuses and, to a lesser extent, from bleeding at the fracture surfaces (8). Achieving direct surgical control of these bleeding sites is difficult, and indirect methods are generally preferred. Because the disrupted pelvic ring can expand radially, the space for blood loss greatly increases after fracture. External fixation, by stabilizing the pelvis, reduces pelvic volume, facilitating tamponade (9).

Not all displaced pelvic fractures cause substantial blood loss, but certain fracture patterns are more likely to result in major bleeding. Fractures with disruption of the posterior sacroiliac ligaments are more prone to cause severe blood loss than are those with intact posterior ligaments. Similarly, fractures in which the pelvis opens like a book are more likely to cause significant bleeding than are fractures in which the pelvis collapses. The most ominous situation is when the pelvis opens like a book and the posterior ligaments are disrupted (2).

The indications for immediate pelvic external fixation are based on hemodynamic instability or expected continued bleeding. A careful assessment of the patient's vital signs, as well as serial blood counts, are useful in determining ongoing blood loss. If the initial blood loss has slowed or stopped, crystalloid replacement may be all that is necessary. However, it is often difficult to know whether or not the bleeding has completely stopped. If crystalloid and blood replacement do not correct the patient's hemodynamics, there is a good chance that the patient is still bleeding (1).

M. S. Vrahas, M.D.: Department of Orthopaedic Surgery, Louisiana State University, New Orleans, Louisiana 70112.

In a patient with clinical signs of shock, pelvic external fixation may be indicated after other sources of bleeding have been ruled out. Although pelvic fractures often result in severe blood loss, hemorrhage from intraabdominal sources should not be overlooked.

If an intraabdominal source of blood loss has not been identified, an exploratory laparotomy is contraindicated because it may decompress the pelvic hematoma and increase rather than decrease the blood loss (4). This is especially true if the retroperitoneal hematoma is opened. If intraabdominal bleeding has been ruled out, pelvic external fixation is an effective method to control bleeding. If blood loss continues after external fixation, angiography with embolization of the bleeding pelvic vessels may be helpful.

If the patient does require a laparotomy to control intraabdominal bleeding, the orthopaedic surgeon should be prepared to stabilize the pelvis with internal or external fixation at the same time.

Definitive Fixation

The pelvis comprises three bones, two innominate bones and the sacrum, held firmly together by several strong ligaments. In the front are the pubic symphyseal ligaments, and in the back are the anterior sacroiliac ligaments, the posterior sacroiliac ligaments, the sacrotuberous ligaments, and the sacrospinous ligaments. Fractures or disruption of the supporting ligaments can destabilize the pelvis. The degree of instability depends on the overall pattern of injury and is generally divided into three categories (10). In Type A injuries, the pelvis is disrupted without affecting stability. Isolated fractures to the iliac wings or avulsions of the ischial spine are in this category. In Type B injuries, the anterior pelvis is disrupted, but the supporting structures of the posterior pelvis remain intact. For example, the pubic symphyseal ligaments can tear, or the pubic rami can fracture, while the posterior sacroiliac ligaments and the bone surrounding the posterior sacroiliac joints remains intact. The pelvis can open and close like a book, but because the posterior pelvis remains intact in Type B fractures, there is no posterior or superior displacement. In Type C injuries, the posterior pelvis is disrupted either through the bone or through the sacroiliac ligaments in conjunction with an anterior injury. This leaves the pelvis unstable in all directions (10). Put more concisely, with Type A disruptions, the pelvis is completely stable; with Type B disruptions, the pelvis is rotationally unstable and vertically stable; and with Type C disruptions, the pelvis is rotationally and vertically unstable.

External fixation provides good control of the anterior pelvis. When the posterior pelvis has not been disrupted, as in a Type B fracture, an external fixator can serve as definitive stabilization. In contrast, external fixation alone does not produce adequate stabilization for Type C fractures. External fixation can be used in Type C fractures to stabilize the anterior pelvis, but internal fixation must be added adequately to stabilize the posterior pelvis. External fixation is particularly useful for Type C fractures in which there are extensive rami fractures anteriorly. Bridging the rami with an external fixator eliminates the need for an extensile, and potentially dangerous, anterior surgical approach.

If the patient is hemodynamically stable, external fixation should be avoided. In this circumstance, internal fixation gives better results. However, internal fixation can be delayed until the patient has been carefully evaluated, and the surgery scheduled semielectively. An external fixator placed immediately can limit the options for internal fixation. Infected or contaminated pin sites can make risky the approaches to the anterior sacroiliac joint and the iliac wing.

PREOPERATIVE PLANNING

Bleeding After Pelvic Fractures

Pelvic external fixation for patients who are hemodynamically unstable should be considered an urgent procedure. Many different frames are available, and almost any fixator properly applied provides adequate initial stabilization (11). More important than the actual frame type or configuration is the rapidity with which it is applied. Therefore to facilitate application, the surgeon should become familiar with an external fixator in advance. At our institution, a pelvic external fixator tray is wrapped and sterilized separately. This allows quick access in the event of an emergency.

In critically ill patients, an anteroposterior (AP) radiograph is all that is generally available for preoperative planning. However, in hemodynamically stable patients, 40-degree inlet and outlet views as well as computed tomography (CT) scans can be very helpful. The radiographs should be carefully evaluated to determine whether both the anterior and posterior pelvis are disrupted. This determination is important for the reduction maneuver necessary at the time of frame application. Posterior displacement greater than 1 cm suggests posterior pelvis disruption. Displacements greater than 2.5 cm at the pubic symphysis suggest anterior ligament disruption (3).

A full radiographic and clinical analysis should be made before proceeding with definitive fixation. The essential plain radiographs are the AP pelvis, the inlet view, and the outlet view. A CT scan is often necessary to evaluate the posterior pelvis. These multiple views help the surgeon to determine which components of the pelvis have been disrupted and which remain intact. In addition, they allow the surgeon to examine fracture displacement in multiple planes, thereby facilitating reduction. Ultimately, the overall fixation necessary will depend on pelvic stability.

SURGERY

Anatomic Considerations

The primary requirement for restoring pelvic stability with an external fixator is good pin placement and fixation. To achieve this, pins can be placed either along the iliac crest or in the supraacetabular region. It is easiest and safest to insert pins into the iliac crest. Occasionally, however, the iliac wing is fractured in the area where pins would be placed. In these cases, it may be necessary to place pins in the supraacetabular region.

When pins are inserted along the iliac crest, they should be placed in the anterior pillar of the crest. This is the thickest portion of the crest and offers the best fixation. If a patient with a nondisrupted pelvis is placed supine on an operating table, his pelvis is situated so that the pubic symphysis and the anterior superior iliac spines lie in a plane nearly parallel to the floor (Fig. 1). This means that the anterior pillar of bone is nearly parallel to the floor as well. With the disrupted pelvis, it is necessary to visualize how the displacements have affected the position of the anterior pillars. Pressure against the iliac crests will help to bring the pelvis into a more anatomic position. The crest of the ilium is asymmetric due to an

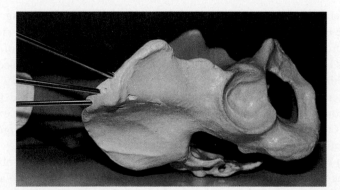

Figure 1. The thickest bone for pin insertion is in the anterior pillar of the iliac wing. This pillar of bone lies nearly parallel to the floor when the patient is supine on the operating table.

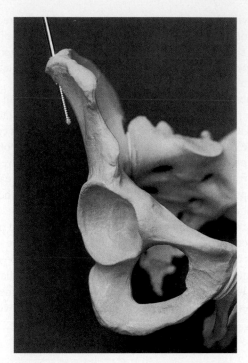

Figure 2. The iliac crest overhangs slightly laterally. Pins inserted in the center of the crest or toward the lateral edge will miss the bulk of the bone.

overhang of bone laterally. Pins inserted in the center of the crest or toward the lateral portion are likely to miss the bulk of the ilium. Because of this, the best starting position is along the medial one third of the crest (Fig. 2).

Pins positioned in the supraacetabular region should be inserted in a direction perpendicular to the floor. The bone in the supraacetabular region is very good, but its proximity to the hip joint makes placing pins in this area more risky. Pins inserted in this area can easily enter the hip joint, causing major complications. For this reason, they should always be inserted with C-arm guidance.

Approaches for Pin Placement Along the Crest

Three different methods can be used to insert half pins into the iliac wing. One option is to expose the entire iliac wing. This requires a larger dissection, but best ensures that the pins will be properly positioned. A second option is to expose only the top of the iliac crest. This requires less dissection, however, it is somewhat more difficult to place the pins correctly. The third option is to insert the pins through small stab wounds. This requires the least dissection, but is technically difficult and probably best left to very experienced surgeons. Moreover, the choice of approach is based primarily on surgeon experience and preference. If the surgeon only rarely places a pelvic external fixator it is probably best to expose the entire iliac wing.

Exposing the Entire Iliac Wing. To expose the entire iliac wing, an oblique incision is made in the region of the iliac crest. The incision should be made in the area where the iliac wing will be after the pelvis has been reduced. Incisions made directly over the crests of the unreduced pelvis will be in the wrong position after reduction has been achieved. We have found it helpful to perform a trial reduction and mark the skin before making an incision.

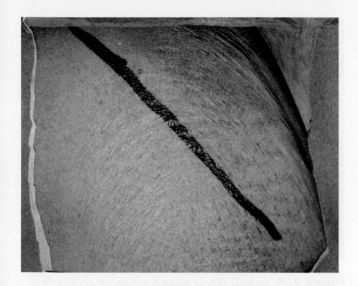

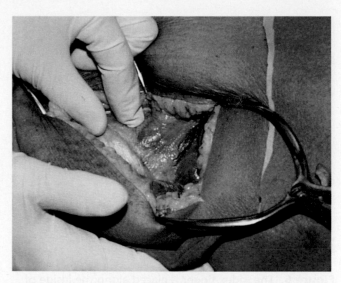

Figure 3. An 8-cm incision is made in the area where the iliac crest will be once the pelvis is reduced.

Figure 4. If the iliac wing is displaced laterally, push on the patient's side to bring the crest into the wound.

Make an 8-cm incision, but extend it as far as necessary to achieve adequate exposure (Fig. 3). This is often necessary in obese patients. Once through the skin and subcutaneous tissue, palpate for the iliac crest. If the pelvis is displaced, push on the patient's side to bring the crest into the wound (Fig. 4).

The remainder of the approach is similar to that used for harvesting an iliac-crest bone graft. Detach the insertion of the external oblique, and dissect subperiosteal along the iliac fossa deep enough to allow the entire index finger to be placed along the bone. Detach the origins of the hip abductors on the outside of the pelvis and again dissect subperiosteally to a similar depth (Fig. 5).

Identify the thick anterior pillar of bone by palpating along the crest. Place your index finger along the inner table of the pelvis and your thumb along the outer table to identify the proper direction for pin insertion. The first pin should be placed in the anterior portion

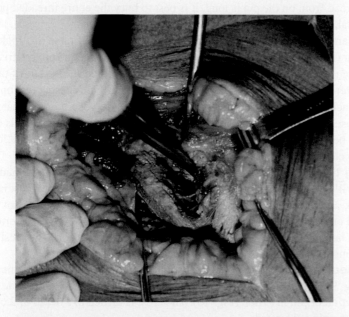

Figure 5. Dissect subperiosteal areas on the inside and outside of the pelvis.

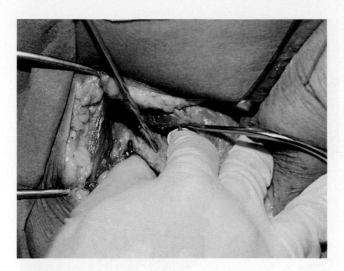

Figure 6. The index finger is placed along the inside of the pelvis, and the thumb is placed along the outside of the pelvis to guide pin insertion. The first pin is placed at the anterior edge of the anterior pillar.

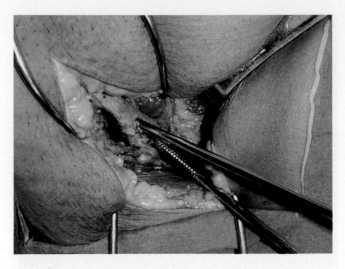

Figure 7. A second pin is placed posterior to the first, also in the anterior pillar.

of the anterior pillar. In this area, drill a hole 2 cm deep. The proper drill size will be determined by the type of external fixator being used. After drilling, insert a 4.5-, 5-, or 6-mm half pin. By grasping the crest between your thumb and index finger, it is possible to judge the proper direction for pin placement (Fig. 6). The pin should be inserted at least 4 cm. When the thread from on the pin is long, it is best to bury the entire threaded portion of the pin. In general, the deeper the pin is inserted the better.

With the same technique, insert a second pin posterior to the first in the thick bone of the anterior pillar (Fig. 7). Do not worry about the position of the second pin relative to the first. The objective is to get the pin into good bone. The pins can be stressed to fit the necessary pin clamp after insertion. It is possible to insert a third pin if you suspect that one of the first pins has not achieved good fixation. However, two pins are generally adequate.

Pins are inserted in the contralateral crest by using the same technique. It is best to close the incisions before constructing the frame because the frame obstructs the field and makes it difficult to close the wounds.

Exposing the Top of the Iliac Crest. An 8-cm oblique incision is made where the iliac crests will be after the pelvis has been reduced. The top of the iliac crest is exposed so that the thick anterior pillar of bone can be palpated, but the muscles are not stripped off the inner and outer walls of the crest. A small Kirschner wire (K-wire) is inserted along the iliac fossa to help the surgeon identify the direction for pin insertion. The crest is drilled to a depth of approximately 2 cm, and a half pin is inserted (Fig. 8).

Percutaneous Technique. A small incision is made perpendicular to the direction of the crest (Fig. 9). The crest is palpated, and a K-wire is placed along the iliac fossa to define the direction of pin insertion (Fig. 10). The crest is drilled to a depth of 2 cm in this direction, and the pin is inserted.

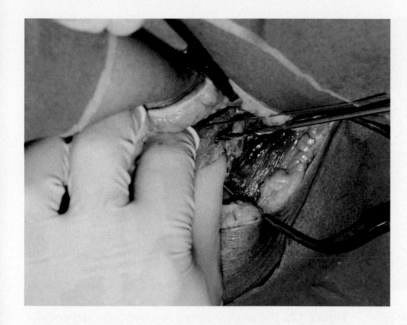

Figure 8. A K-wire is placed along the inside of the iliac wing to guide pin insertion when only the top of the crest has been exposed.

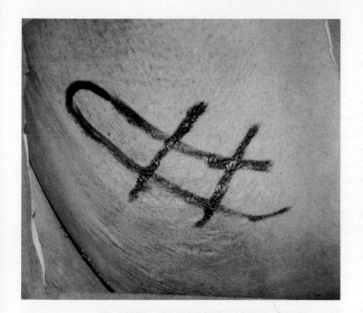

Figure 9. Skin incisions for percutaneous insertion are made perpendicular to the crest.

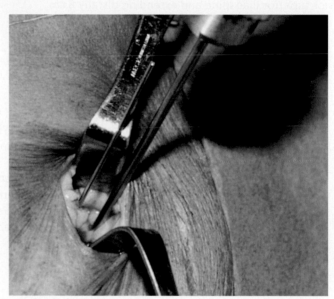

Figure 10. A K-wire is inserted along the inner iliac crest to guide pin insertion.

Approach for Pin Placement in the Supraacetabular Region

The patient is positioned supine on a radiolucent table. An 8-cm vertical incision is made beginning 2 cm proximal to the anterior superior iliac spine and extended distally (Fig. 11). The interval between the sartorius and the tensor fascia lata is identified and developed. The tissues are bluntly dissected, and the anterior inferior spine is palpated. The drill bit is positioned just below the anterior inferior spine, and its position is checked by using the image intensifier. The pin site is drilled to its full depth in a direction perpendicular to the floor. The pin is inserted and its position checked by using the image intensifier (Fig. 12). A second pin is inserted just above the first pin.

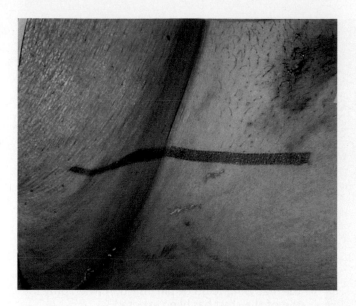

Figure 11. For pin placement in the supraacetabular region, an incision is made beginning just above the anterior superior iliac spine and extending distally 8 cm.

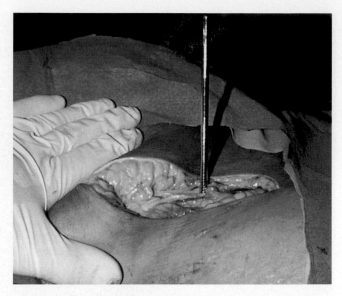

Figure 12. The pin is inserted in a direction perpendicular to the floor.

Frame Construction

A properly constructed frame allows access to the abdomen for surgical procedures and allows the patient to sit. The frame should be constructed on the half pins with the pin bar and bar connectors left loose. The pelvis should then be reduced and the connections tightened (Fig. 13).

Several frame constructions are acceptable. I prefer a Slatis-type frame. Two long bars are extended from the pins toward the lower extremities. These bars are connected by two cross bars. This frame construction leaves the abdomen free for surgical approaches and does not impinge on the abdomen when the patient is upright (Fig. 14).

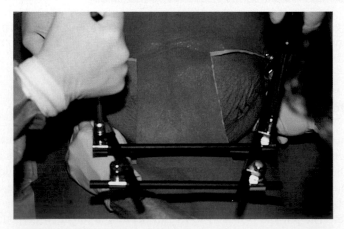

Figure 13. All pin–bar and bar–bar connectors are left loose. The pelvis is reduced, and the connectors are tightened.

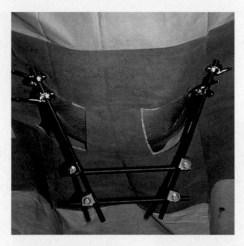

Figure 14. A long bar is attached to the half pins and directed distally. These bars are connected by two cross bars. This leaves the abdomen free for surgical procedures. The bars do not impinge on the abdomen when the patient sits.

Reduction Techniques

The proper reduction technique depends on the fracture pattern. For Type B fractures (posterior pelvis intact), the pelvis can be reduced by simply pulling the half pins toward the midline. If the posterior pelvis is disrupted (Type C fracture), this maneuver can cause the back of the pelvis to open. For fractures in which the posterior ligaments are disrupted, the half pins should be used as reduction aids. Attempt to use the pins like pincers to pull the front and the back of the pelvis together at the same time (Fig. 15). Additional force can be generated by pushing on the patient's sides or with longitudinal traction on the leg.

An alternative method for achieving reduction is to roll the patient into the lateral decubitus position. The patient's body weight helps reduce the pelvis. This technique is useful in patients who are hemodynamically stable and have no other injuries.

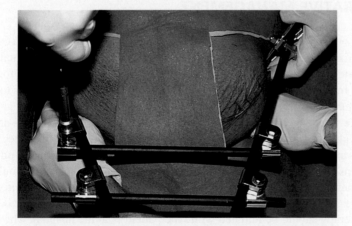

Figure 15. For Type C fractures, the pins are used as reduction aids. The pins are manipulated like pincers to bring the back and the front of the pelvis together at the same time. Additional reduction force can be generated by pushing on the patient's sides.

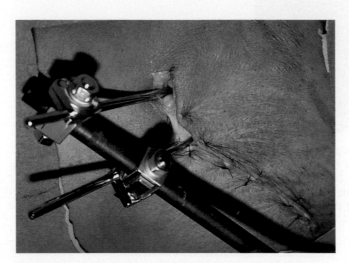

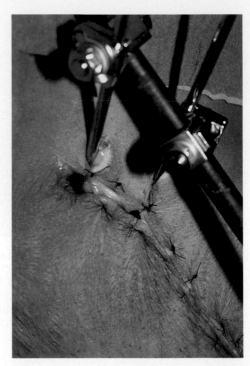

Figure 16. Pin causing tension on the skin. A relaxing incision should be made.

Figure 17. Pin sites after relaxing incisions.

Finishing Touches

Once the fixator connections have been tightened, the pelvic reduction and pin placement are checked with intraoperative radiographs. A repeated reduction should be performed if necessary. Once a satisfactory reduction has been achieved, check the pin sites to ensure that none of the pins is causing skin tension (Fig. 16). If this is the case, a relaxing incision should be made (Fig. 17).

POSTOPERATIVE MANAGEMENT

Depending on the fracture pattern, external fixation may be used alone or in combination with internal fixation for definitive management. More often, however, external fixation is used immediately to control blood loss and is converted to internal fixation for definitive management. In these cases, the first step in the postoperative management is to determine what, if any, further fixation is necessary.

Pin-site care should be initiated on the first postoperative day. The pin sites are left open to air and are cleansed twice daily with half-strength peroxide solution. Salves and occlusive dressings are not used. Before discharge, the patient should be instructed on proper pin care. If the pins are causing tension on the skin, a small relaxing incision should be made under local anesthesia to prevent skin necrosis. If the fixator is used as definitive fixation, it may be necessary to perform this procedure several times while the fixator is in place.

Physical therapy should be initiated while the patient is in the hospital. The exact regimen depends on the fracture pattern. Weight-bearing status is determined by the stability of the posterior pelvis. If the posterior pelvis is intact, the patient can bear full weight. If it has been disrupted on one side, the patient can bear touch-down weight only on the injured side and full weight on the uninjured side. For example, if the patient's right sacroiliac joint has been disrupted, but the left is intact, the patient can bear full weight on his left side, but only touch-down weight on his right. If the pelvis has been disrupted on both sides posteriorly, weight-bearing is not permitted. The patient should remain at touch-down weight bearing on the side of the posterior disruption for 8 weeks. At that point, weight bearing can be increased to 50%. At 12 weeks, the patient is allowed to bear full weight. Throughout the recovery period, the patient is allowed active hip range of motion and muscle-strengthening activities.

The patient should be evaluated at weekly intervals for the first 2 or 3 weeks with radiographs of the pelvis to ensure maintenance of reduction. If displacement occurs and is recognized early, it can be addressed more easily than if the pelvis heals with a malunion. A standard AP view and 40-degree inlet and outlet views provide the necessary information.

Once the patient is discharged from the hospital, he or she is seen in the outpatient clinic weekly for the first 2 or 3 weeks for clinical and radiographic evaluation. The next visit is 6 weeks later (8 weeks after surgery) when the patient is increased to partial weight bearing. One month later (12 weeks after surgery), the patient returns to have the fixator removed. This is usually done under local anesthesia in the clinic. However, on occasion it is removed in the operating room under light sedation. The patient is allowed to begin full weight bearing at that time. This schedule may vary depending on the condition of the pin sites. Patients require more frequent follow-up visits for pin-site problems.

Although it is safest to restrict the patient's weight bearing for 3 months, it is possible to accelerate this time frame based on the radiographic healing. Occasionally, pins become loose or infected and must be removed. If this should occur during the first 8 weeks after surgery, it is best to replace the pin and continue the external fixator. After 8 weeks, if the radiographs show sufficient healing, it may be possible to remove the external fixator. However, restricted weight bearing should continue for 12 weeks or until the surgeon is sure the pelvis has healed.

The patient's recovery depends not only on the pelvic fracture but also on associated injuries and other comorbidities (7). More than half of patients with unstable pelvic fractures will have concomitant injuries to the head, abdomen, or thorax, and nearly two thirds will have injuries to the lower extremities. These diverse patterns of injury make it difficult to predict functional outcomes. Nevertheless, by using the Sickness Impact Profile, Gruen et al. (6) found that patients with unstable pelvic fractures in which acceptable reduction and stable internal fixation were achieved had only mild disabilities at 1 year after injury. Seventy-six percent of the patients who had been working before injury returned to work; 62% returned full time, and 14% returned with job modifications. Lower-extremity injuries were a better predictor of work disabilities than were the pelvic disruptions (6). Sexual function also appears to be affected by pelvic fractures, although it is not clear whether this is a sequela of pelvic fractures in particular or of major trauma in general (7).

COMPLICATIONS

Pin-Site Infection

A pin-site infection is the most common complication after pelvic external fixation and frequently indicates pin loosening. Pin stability should be evaluated by manually attempting to move the pin in the bone. If the pin is loose, it should be removed or replaced. Another frequent cause of pin-site infection is skin necrosis that results from skin tethering by the pin. During the patient's stay in the hospital and at each postoperative visit, the pin sites should be checked. If the skin around a pin is causing tension, a small relaxing incision should be made while the patient is under local anesthesia. Occasionally, cellulitis develops around the pins in the absence of skin necrosis or pin loosening. If this occurs, the patient should be started on oral antibiotics. If the cellulitis does not clear, intravenous antibiotics may be indicated, or the pin should be changed.

Pin Penetration of the Hip Joint

Pin penetration of the hip joint is most often associated with pins placed in the supraacetabular region. A pin that inadvertently enters the hip joint and is recognized and removed at the time of the initial surgery is usually not a problem. However, a pin that is left in the hip joint can lead to septic arthritis or joint destruction.

Complications caused by an intraarticular pin are not easily treated. Therefore the surgeon should take great care to avoid placing a pin into the hip joint. Image intensification should be used any time pins are placed in the supraacetabular region. In addition, pin placement should be checked radiographically before the patient leaves the operating room regardless of how the pins are inserted.

Lateral Femoral Cutaneous Nerve Palsy

In 10% of patients, the lateral femoral cutaneous nerve courses over the iliac wing on its way to the thigh (5). This makes it vulnerable to injury during pin insertion. This complication can be avoided by looking for the nerve on the crest during the approach, but it is sometimes difficult to see. An injury to this nerve cannot be treated. However, the area of decreased sensation on the anterior thigh does not usually lead to functional impairment. Patients should be informed of this risk preoperatively whenever possible.

Pelvic Fracture Displacement

The patient should be evaluated radiographically weekly for the first 2 or 3 weeks to make sure that loss of reduction has not occurred. Poststabilization displacements are not uncommon. The patient should be informed of this risk preoperatively. Once a loss of reduction has been recognized, the next step depends on the fracture type and the amount of displacement. Frequently, conversion to internal fixation is appropriate.

ILLUSTRATIVE CASE FOR TECHNIQUE

A 36-year-old unrestrained driver was involved in a head-on motor-vehicle collision. The patient was conscious at the scene, but his car was destroyed, and a 1-hour extraction time was necessary. On evaluation in the emergency room, the patient was awake, alert, and complaining of pain in his pelvic region. His airway was patent, and he was having no dif-

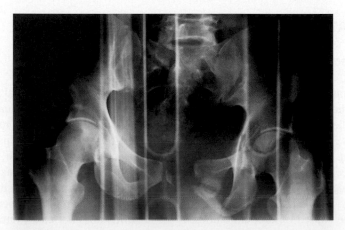

Figure 18. Initial anteroposterior pelvic radiograph showing Type C pelvis fracture.

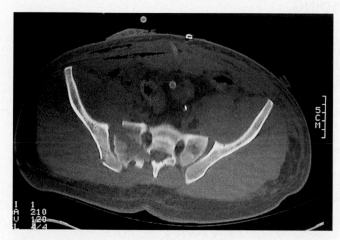

Figure 19. Initial computed tomography scan showing disruption of the sacrum and iliac wing.

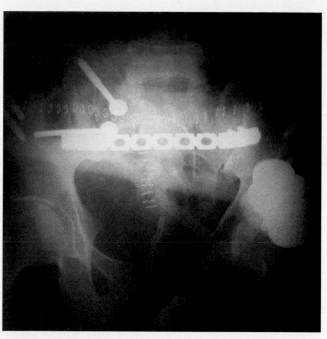

Figure 20. Anteroposterior pelvic radiograph after definitive stabilization.

ficulty breathing, although his respiration rate was increased at 30 breaths per minute. His pulse was 150 beats per minute, and his blood pressure was 120/70 mm Hg. Based on his rapid pulse, a diagnosis of class II shock was made, and 2 L of Ringer's lactate solution was infused.

The patient's abdomen was soft and nontender except when palpated in the pelvic region. Palpation of the pelvis caused pain. There was a right flank hematoma. There was no disruption of the skin in the pelvic region, and the rectal examination showed no occult blood or high-riding prostate. There was no blood at the urethral meatus. The patient was unable to dorsiflex or plantarflex his right foot, although the peripheral pulses were intact.

Cervical spine and chest radiographs were normal. An AP pelvis radiograph revealed widening of the pubic symphysis with displacement of the right hemipelvis superiorly. A sacral fracture with displacement greater than 1 cm also was noted (Fig. 18).

After infusion of 2 L of Ringer's lactate solution, the patient's pulse decreased to 110 beats per minute, but quickly drifted back up to 150 beats per minute. Blood transfusions were started as patient evaluation continued. A CT scan of the abdomen and pelvis revealed no intraabdominal source of blood loss. It also revealed a sacral fracture with vertical displacement as well as a fracture of the posterior iliac wing (Fig. 19).

Although the patient's blood pressure remained stable throughout the evaluation, his pulse continued at 150 beats per minute despite 4 units of blood and continued crystalloid transfusion. The hemodynamic instability was attributed to the pelvic fracture, and the patient was brought to the operating room for pelvic external fixation.

The fixator was applied by exposing the tops of the iliac crests. Two pins were inserted in each crest, and a Slatis-type frame was applied. After application of the external fixator and a total of 7 units of blood, the patient's pulse stabilized at 95 beats per minute. The patient required transfusion of another 2 units of blood over the next 24 hours. At day 4, the patient was returned to the operating room for internal fixation of the pelvis. The external fixator was left in place to stabilize the anterior pelvis. A transverse incision was made posteriorly, and the patient's sacral fracture was reduced and stabilized with a bridging 4.5-mm reconstruction plate (Fig. 20).

Postoperatively, the patient was maintained non–weight bearing on his right lower extremity for 2 months, and partial weight bearing for 1 month. The fixator was removed at 3 months, and the patient was allowed to bear full weight. His sciatic nerve injury did not resolve.

RECOMMENDED READING

1. American College of Surgeons Committee on Trauma: *Advanced Trauma Life Support.* American College of Surgeons, Chicago, 1993, pp. 86–87.
2. Dalal, S.A., Burges, A.R., Siegel, J.H., Young, J.W.: Pelvic fractures in multiple trauma: classification by mechanism is the key to pattern of organ injury, resuscitative requirements and outcome. *J. Trauma,* 29:981, 1989.
3. Edeiken-Monroe, B.S., Browner, B.D., Jackson, H.: The role of standard roentgenograms in the evaluation of instability of pelvic disruptions. *Clin. Orthop.,* 240:63–76, 1989.
4. Ghanayem, A.J., Wilber, J.H., Lieberman J.M., Motta, A.O.: The effect of laparotomy and external fixator stabilization on pelvic volume in an unstable pelvic injury. *J. Trauma,* 38(3):396–400, 1995.
5. Ghent, W.R.: Further studies on meralgia paresthetica. *Can. Med. Assoc. J.,* 6:871–875, 1961.
6. Gruen, G.S., Leit, M.E., Gruen R.J., et al.: Functional outcome of patients with unstable pelvic ring fractures stabilized with open reduction and internal fixation. *J. Trauma,* 39(5):838–844, 1995.
7. McCarthy, M.L., MacKenzie, E.J., Bosse, M.J., Copeland, C.E., Hash, C.S., Burgess, A.R.: Functional status following orthopaedic trauma in young women. *J. Trauma,* 39(5):828–836, 1995.
8. Mears, D.C., and Rubash, H.E.: *Pelvic and Acetabular Fractures.* Williams & Wilkins, Baltimore, 1984.
9. Tile, M.: *Fractures of the Pelvis and Acetabulum.* 2nd ed. Williams & Wilkins, Baltimore, 1995.
10. Tile, M.: Pelvic ring fractures: should they be fixed? *J. Bone Joint Surg. [Br],* 70:1–12, 1988.
11. Vrahas, M.S., Wilson, S., Paul, E.: Comparison of fixation methods for preventing pelvic ring expansion. 8th Annual Meeting of the Orthopaedic Trauma Association, Minneapolis, Minnesota, 1992.

Master Techniques in Orthopaedic Surgery,
FRACTURES, edited by D. A. Wiss,
Lippincott–Raven Publishers, Philadelphia © 1998.

36

Diastasis of the Symphysis Pubis: Open Reduction Internal Fixation

David C. Templeman and Andrew H. Schmidt

INDICATIONS/CONTRAINDICATIONS

The pubic symphysis is a cartilaginous joint where the pubic bones meet. The fibrocartilaginous disc is reinforced by a superior and inferior pubic ligament. The arcuate ligament forms an arch between the two inferior pubic rami and is thought to be the major soft-tissue stabilizer of the symphysis pubis (7).

Injuries to the pubic symphysis include (a) diastasis, (b) fractures into the symphysis, and (c) fracture–dislocations. When the pubic symphysis is not disrupted, the anterior-ring injury usually consists of pubic rami fractures. These fractures are usually vertically oriented but may be comminuted or horizontal (11). It is rare for diastasis of the symphysis pubis and fractures of the pubic rami to coexist (4,10).

Open reduction and internal fixation (ORIF) is indicated when diastasis of the pubic symphysis exceeds 2.5 cm. Fixation is performed to improve the stability of the anterior pelvic ring. The indications for surgery are based on the magnitude of displacement and the stability of the pelvic ring.

There are several classification schemes for pelvic fractures. Early classifications were based on either the location of the fracture or the mechanism of injury. Most modern classifications, however, are based on the degree of pelvic stability (1,19). The Tile classification of pelvic ring injuries attempts to predict the mechanical instability of the injured pelvic ring. Injuries are A, stable; B, rotationally unstable, but vertically stable, and C, rotationally and vertically unstable. Tile Type B and C injuries may have associated disruption of the symphysis pubis (19).

Diastasis of the symphysis pubis and external rotation of one innominate bone results in

D. C. Templeman, M.D.: Wayzata Orthopaedics, Plymouth, Minnesota 55441.

A. H. Schmidt, M.D.: Department of Orthopaedic Surgery, University of Minnesota, Hennepin County Medical Center, Minneapolis, Minnesota 55415.

the so-called "open-book" injury. This is a Tile-B injury, in which the posterior pelvic ligaments are intact and prevent cephalad displacement of the involved innominate bone.

When disruption of the symphysis pubis is greater than 2.5 cm, most traumatologists recommend ORIF. Displacement of this magnitude is thought to be accompanied by sprains of the sacrospinous ligament and the anterior sacroiliac ligaments. Injuries to these ligaments are thought to allow the involved innominate bone to rotate externally. Fixation of the symphysis is sufficient to correct this instability (11).

In contrast to Tile-B injuries, Tile-C injuries with disruption of the symphysis pubis and associated disruption of the posterior pelvic ring result in complete instability of the pelvis. Fixation of the anterior ring alone is insufficient and must be accompanied by reduction and fixation of the posterior pelvis (15,19).

Contraindications to internal fixation of the symphysis pubis include unstable, critically ill patients; severe open fractures with inadequate wound debridement; and crushing injuries in which compromised skin may not tolerate a surgical incision. The placement of a suprapubic catheter to treat an extraperitoneal bladder rupture may result in contamination of the retropubic space. We believe this constitutes a contraindication to ORIF of the adjacent symphysis pubis. Associated problems that may preclude secure fixation are osteoporosis and severe comminution of the pubis.

When diastasis of the symphysis pubis is less than 2.5 cm, internal fixation is seldom necessary. Patients may be safely mobilized, allowing toe-touch weight bearing on the side of the externally rotated hemipelvis. Radiographs are repeated within the first few weeks to ensure there is no further displacement. There is usually enough healing within 8 weeks to allow full weight bearing. Any increase in pain associated with activity must be evaluated with radiographs to detect the development of late instability.

PREOPERATIVE PLANNING

Anteroposterior, caudal, and cephalad views are required to determine the direction and magnitude of the symphysis pubis disruption and the relative position of the pubic bones. Differences in the height of the pubic rami usually indicate that the hemipelvis is displaced in more than one plane. The most common deformity associated with disruption of the symphysis pubis is cephalad migration, posterior displacement, and external rotation of one hemipelvis (1). This pattern indicates a posterior pelvic injury that requires posterior reduction and internal fixation to achieve a stable pelvis (Tile C; 14,15,19).

The severity of pelvic and visceral injuries requires immediate evaluation and resuscitation. A multidisciplinary team consisting of general surgeons, orthopaedists, and urologists is frequently required (2,8,20).

Urologic injuries are present in many patients with anterior pelvic trauma. In male patients, a retrograde urethrogram should be done to ensure that the urethra is intact before passing a Foley catheter. The presence of blood at the tip of the penile meatus is frequently cited as a sign of urethral trauma; however, it is not present in the majority of cases. When the urethra is intact, a Foley catheter is passed and a cystogram is obtained. Extravasation of dye during the urethrogram is a contraindication to blind passage of a Foley catheter and requires urologic consultation. Because the female urethra is only several centimeters in length, a retrograde urethrogram is not required before inserting a Foley catheter (8).

The bladder should be studied by cystography with an intravenous pyelogram or retrograde cystogram. External compression of the bladder is frequently caused by a pelvic hematoma.

The management of extraperitoneal bladder ruptures in patients with pelvic fractures is controversial. Traditional Foley catheter drainage of extraperitoneal ruptures avoids the need for a laparotomy and direct repair. Kotkin and Koch (5) found that patients with extraperitoneal bladder ruptures and pelvic fractures have higher rates of complications and stressed the need for adequate bladder drainage.

When an extraperitoneal bladder rupture exists, the patient is at an increased risk for infection due to seeding of the pelvic hematoma. When internal fixation of the symphysis is planned, the risk of infection from the ruptured bladder must be considered. We favor primary bladder repair, irrigation of the anterior pelvic ring injury, and the use of antibiotics. The timing of the bladder repair is determined for each individual injury (8).

After the initial evaluation and resuscitation of the patient, radiographic studies are obtained. In addition to the anteroposterior roentgenogram, 40-degree cephalad and 40-degree caudal views are used to determine the displacement of the pelvic ring (20). All three views are used to determine the three-dimensional anatomy of the pelvis (Fig. 1A–C). Computed tomographic scans are recommended to assess the posterior pelvic anatomy. The anterior structures are best studied with plain films (19,20).

Disruption of the symphysis with isolated external rotation of the innominate bone results in the so-called open-book injury. With this injury, the intact posterior structures of the pelvis prevent cephalad displacement. The injury is considered to be rotationally unstable but vertically stable (Tile B). The magnitude of the symphysis diastasis determines the method of treatment. When the diastasis is greater than 2.5 cm, internal fixation is usually performed (13,19).

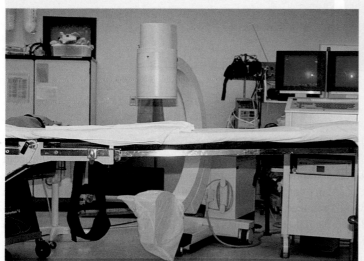

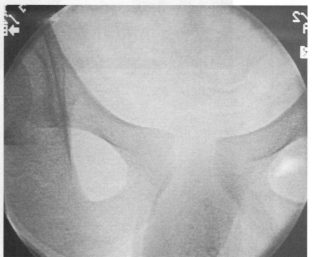

A   B

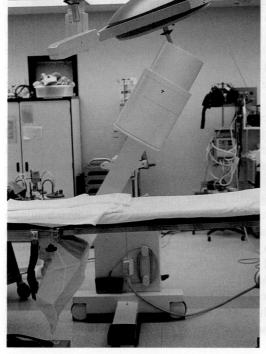

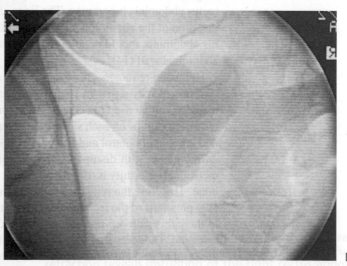

C   D

Figure 1. A, B: An operating room table with a radiolucent extension. This table allows tilting of the fluoroscopic unit to obtain cephalad **(C, D)** and caudad **(E, F)** images of the pelvis **(B, C)**. (*figure continues*)

receive some form of treatment, either to prevent thrombosis or to treat thrombi that have already formed.

Routine screening is not helpful because of the high percentage of patients who develop DVT. Screening is considered when surgery is planned after a delay of 2 to 5 days from the time of the injury. The diagnosis and treatment of thrombi that are identified preoperatively may help prevent an intraoperative pulmonary embolism (17).

The perfect form of prophylaxis and treatment for venous thrombosis remains elusive. Pharmacologic agents should be safe and easy to administer, monitor, and reverse. The use of pharmacologic anticoagulation in trauma patients is further complicated when there are associated head injuries, retroperitoneal bleeding, and thoracoabdominal injuries. Treatment cannot be started until bleeding is controlled (17). Mechanical devices that increase venous blood flow by intermittent mechanical compression offer an alternative to pharmacologic agents. However, when used as a sole form of therapy, they are ineffective. One study found that combined use of mechanical compression and low-dose heparin was effective in reducing the incidence of DVT (18).

Heparin, warfarin (Coumadin), and low-molecular weight heparins are all used as forms of pharmacologic prophylaxis. Low-dose heparin is ineffective as a single form of treatment in trauma patients. However, low-dose heparin used in conjunction with intermittent mechanical compression may be effective in reducing the incidence of DVT (18). Currently, low-molecular-weight heparins appear to offer an excellent form of prophylaxis for trauma patients. Monitoring is not required; the onset of action is rapid, and there are few bleeding complications. Geerts et al. (5) found in a double-blind study that low-molecular-weight heparin (Lovenox) administered in a dose of 30 mg subcutaneously every 12 hours, in comparison with low-dose heparin, resulted in 21% risk reduction for all DVT. A 73% reduction for proximal DVT was found in a subgroup of patients with lower-extremity and pelvic trauma.

The use of pharmacologic anticoagulation in multiply injured patients, some of whom may have intercranial or thoracoabdominal bleeding, is a complex issue. Although these variables prevent the use of rigid protocols, a few general guidelines are available: (a) In most patients, bleeding has stopped and resuscitation is complete within 24 to 48 hours after the injury; (b) once bleeding has stopped, pharmacologic anticoagulation can be started (17), and (c) patients who cannot receive pharmacologic anticoagulation may undergo repetitive screening or receive a vena cava filter. Vena cava filters are usually required when a significant thrombus is detected before surgery (17). Treatment should be continued for several weeks. The exact length of treatment has not been established. One group has used postoperative warfarin for 3 weeks after discharge (3).

With stable fixation, patients can be mobilized from bed to chair on the first or second day after surgery. Ambulation depends on the specific injury. For the isolated "open-book" injuries (Tile B), we recommend partial weight bearing on the injured side for 8 weeks. Follow-up radiographs at this time usually indicate some new bone formation in the region of the symphysis. This is interpreted as sufficient healing and stability. In patients with combined internal fixation of the anterior and posterior pelvic ring (Tile C), weight bearing should be delayed for 8 to 12 weeks.

When full weight bearing is permitted, physical therapy may be helpful. Most patients have muscle atrophy as a result of injury and convalescence. Physical therapy, directed at increasing hip abductor strength and aerobic conditioning, helps restore a normal gait. Lower back–strengthening exercises and work-increasing programs may be beneficial in patients who need to return to heavy labor.

Discharge from the hospital is dependent on the presence of associated injuries. Many patients can use crutches or are able to perform bed-to-chair transfers within a week after surgery.

Matta (15) reported the results of open reduction for anterior fixation of pelvic-ring injuries. In a series of 127 patients with pelvic-ring injuries, this author noted that 88 of 105 fractures of the obturator ring were not internally fixed, and none required subsequent treatment for nonunion or loss of reduction.

Based on this study, the author recommended that internal fixation of the anterior pelvic ring should be reserved for symphysis pubis dislocations and only a minority of pubis rami fractures that remain widely displace after ORIF of the posterior pelvic ring (13).

COMPLICATIONS

Complications related to internal fixation of the symphysis pubis are uncommon. Loss of fixation is usually associated with inadequate reduction and fixation of the posterior pelvic ring. If this occurs, the entire fixation construct, in both the anterior and posterior pelvic ring, requires revision, reduction, and fixation.

Because of physiologic motion at the symphysis pubis, screw backout or plate failure are occasionally seen. It is unusual for these to become symptomatic, and late hardware removal is infrequent.

Fortunately, wound dehiscence or infection are rare. Irrigation and debridement should include exposure of the plate and retropubic space. When there has been a prior urologic injury, reevaluation of the urinary system is necessary. This should include urinalysis, urine cultures, and may even require imaging studies. A consultation with a urologist is recommended.

Impotence may result from the initial injury. Because patients may be reluctant to discuss this issue, "polite questioning" in the private setting of an examination room may identify those patients with sexual dysfunction.

ILLUSTRATIVE CASE FOR TECHNIQUE

A 29-year-old man was injured in a high-speed snowmobile accident (Fig. 6A–C). ORIF was performed in two stages (Fig. 7).

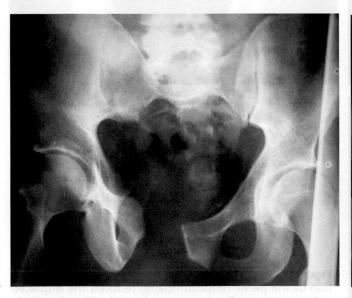
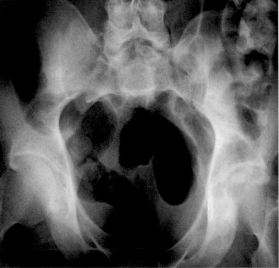

A   B

Figure 6. Anteroposterior **(A)**, caudal **(B)**, and cephalic **(C)** radiographs of the pelvis show a diastasis of the pubic symphysis and a fracture of the right sacral ala. The right hemipelvis is displaced posteriorly, cephalad, and is externally rotated. *(figure continues)*

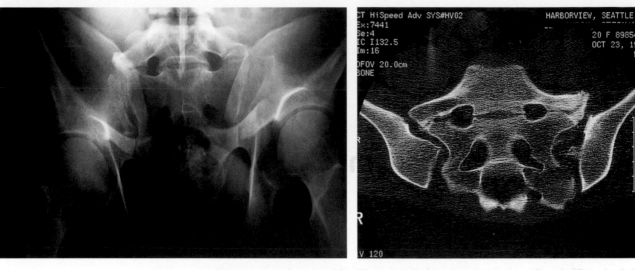

A

B

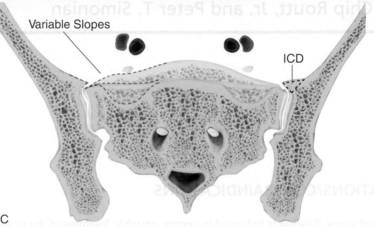

C

Figure 1. A: The pelvic-outlet radiograph alerts the surgeon to a potential sacral dysmorphism. The upper sacrum is located at the level of the iliac crests. The upper sacral foramina are oddly shaped. The ala are acutely angulated and often asymmetric. Mammillary processes are noted along the ala. A residual "disc space" may be present also between the upper two sacral segments. A true lateral sacral image confirms the upper sacral vertebral prominence with acutely angulated alar slopes. The alar slope is estimated based on the iliac cortical density (ICD), which is usually coplanar relative to the anterior alar surface. **B:** Computed tomography (CT) scan demonstrates "tongue-in-groove" articulations of the sacroiliac joint in sacral dysplasia. The CT scan also confirms the relation between the iliac cortical density and the anterior sacral ala. The small "danger zone" of the dysplastic upper sacral segment is recognized. Fluoroscopically guided iliosacral screw insertions are dangerous in these patients and are not recommended. **C:** The variable structure of the upper sacrum. The relation between the iliac cortical density and the alar slope must be understood to insert iliosacral screws safely by using fluoroscopic guidance.

Obesity is also a relative contraindication to iliosacral screw fixation for several reasons. Intraoperative fluoroscopic imaging in obese patients is compromised by the large abdominal panniculus. Fluoroscopic detail in these patients may be inadequate to safely guide screw placement. Additionally, extra-long instrumentation such as drills, taps, and screwdrivers are necessary for the obese patient. Fluoroscopic pelvic imaging is also complicated in some polytraumatized patients because of contrast agents that were used during the initial abdominal evaluations and should be avoided when possible. Finally, in patients with open fractures or compromised posterior skin and soft tissues, iliosacral screw placement should be done percutaneously rather than through an open approach.

PREOPERATIVE PLANNING

In the hemodynamically unstable patient with a pelvic-ring disruption, resuscitation efforts proceed simultaneous with the primary evaluation. Large-bore intravenous access allows rapid volume infusion, and the patient is kept warm. The potentially injured pelvis can be immobilized at the accident scene before patient transport by using a variety of simple techniques. A vacuum beanbag, a large circumferential sheet, or military antishock trousers (MAST) are recommended temporarily to stabilize the pelvis. Regardless of the chosen technique, pelvic overcompression is avoided.

The physical examination is a single evaluation performed by the most experienced physician. A detailed neurologic examination is documented in alert patients. Examination of the pelvic area notes abrasions, contusions, degloving injuries, or open wounds. Sterile pressure dressings are applied to open pelvic wounds to diminish ongoing bleeding. The lumbosacral cutaneous examination is performed along with the posterior spine assessment when the patient is log-rolled by a team of assistants. The mechanical evaluation of the pelvis is ideally performed under fluoroscopic imaging. Pelvic-ring instability is noted as gentle manual pressure is applied to each iliac crest. This maneuver produces significant pain in alert patients. To prevent clot disruptions, vigorous and repetitive manual pelvic examinations are not advocated. Digital rectal, prostatic, and vaginal examinations are performed, testing for both gross and occult blood.

The radiographic assessment begins with a screening anteroposterior pelvic radiograph. In certain hemodynamically unstable patients, pelvic angiographic embolization is helpful. A complete pelvic radiographic series includes orthogonal views (inlet/outlet), and a lateral sacral image should be obtained. A pelvic CT scan is essential to further delineate the pathologic conditions.

The timing of pelvic reduction and fixation is primarily dependent on the clinical condition of the patient. Hemodynamically unstable patients with unstable pelvic-ring injuries require some form of rapid pelvic stabilization. Anterior pelvic external-fixation frames and posterior pelvic antishock clamps have been advocated to rapidly stabilize the pelvic ring. We recommend application of such devices using fluoroscopy in the angiographic suite when possible. Emergency pelvic open reduction and internal fixation risks bleeding and has a higher complication rate. Percutaneous posterior pelvic internal fixation using iliosacral screws minimizes the bleeding risk and is useful when an accurate closed manipulative reduction is possible. Percutaneous iliosacral screws may be used in an emergency in combination with anterior pelvic external fixation. For hemodynamically stable patients, operative pelvic stabilization should be expeditious. Before surgery, distal femoral traction is useful to improve the reduction and to provide patient comfort.

Preoperative planning should consider the mechanism of injury, associated major system injuries, and the local soft-tissue conditions before surgery. Special attention is given to the radiographic studies. If the screening anteroposterior pelvic radiograph identifies the pelvic-ring disruption, then pelvic inlet and outlet views along with a lateral sacral plane radiographs should be obtained. These additional views demonstrate the specific sites of injury and the direction of displacement. Iliac and obturator oblique pelvic radiographs are obtained in patients with concomitant acetabular fractures. A two-dimensional CT scan further delineates the pelvic injury.

Based on the mechanism of injury, the physical examination, and the radiographic studies, the surgeon formulates a plan. The preoperative plan includes all of the surgical details including timing, patient positioning, exposures, reduction strategies, fixation techniques, and treatment alternatives. Even the anticipated rehabilitation goals are planned preoperatively, especially in polytraumatized patients.

Not all posterior pelvic fractures are amenable to iliosacral screw fixation, and the surgeon should be familiar with various anterior and posterior pelvic operative exposures, as well as percutaneous techniques. The treatment plan must be tailored to the individual patient. Insertion of iliosacral screws can be performed with the patient in the supine, lateral, or prone position, each with its own advantages and disadvantages. The lateral position complicates both anterior and posterior pelvic surgical exposures and is not recommended for patients with potential spinal injuries. Prone positioning facilitates posterior surgical exposures but denies the surgeon simultaneous anterior pelvic surgical access. Anterior pelvic external-fixation frames further complicate prone and lateral patient positioning for surgery.

If the supine position is selected, strict attention to detail during patient positioning, as well as skin preparation and draping, is mandatory. In polytraumatized patients, the supine position is familiar, allows several teams to work simultaneously on injured extremities, and also provides anterior pelvic access. Patient position changes and repeated drapings are avoided and save valuable time.

SURGERY

Positioning

A general anesthetic and a first-generation cephalosporin are administered before the patient is moved onto the operating room table. Spinal precautions protect the patient during transfer from the bed and positioning on a fluoroscopically compatible operating table. Several strong assistants are needed to elevate the patient from the operating table so the surgeon can position a soft lumbosacral support. This support consists typically of two stacked and folded operating room blankets. The support is necessary to allow posterior pelvic access. If needed, distal femoral pin traction is continued by using a pulley system attached to the operating table (Fig. 2).

Neurodiagnostic monitoring may be helpful, especially in patients with transforaminal sacral fractures undergoing closed manipulative reductions and percutaneous iliosacral screw fixations. Neurodiagnostic monitoring is not used as a substitute for either a detailed preoperative plan or inadequate intraoperative fluoroscopic imaging. Neurodiagnostic information also may be confusing, especially in patients with preoperative neurologic abnormalities.

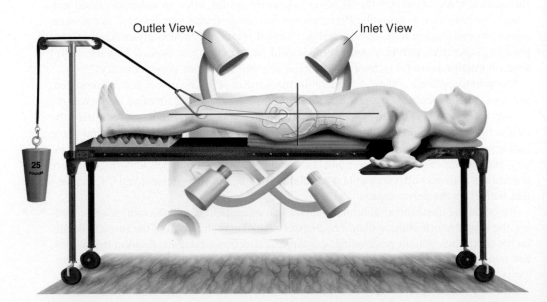

Figure 2. The patient is positioned supine and elevated on two folded and stacked blankets, a lumbosacral support. This operating table has no central support and allows extremes of fluoroscope rotation and therefore pelvic imaging. Distal femoral traction is possible by using a pulley system anchored to the foot of the table.

Imaging

The radiology technician and fluoroscope are positioned on the side opposite from the injured posterior hemipelvis. The initial anteroposterior pelvic fluoroscopic image is used simply to assess proper patient positioning. Minor positional corrections are made and confirmed.

The fluoroscope tilt is then adjusted until "perfect" inlet and outlet posterior pelvic images are obtainable. The ideal pelvic inlet image superimposes the upper sacral vertebral bodies as concentric circles. The ideal outlet image is usually obtained when the symphysis pubis is superimposed on the second sacral vertebral body (Fig. 3A and B).

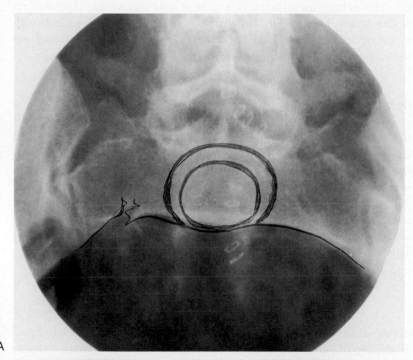

A

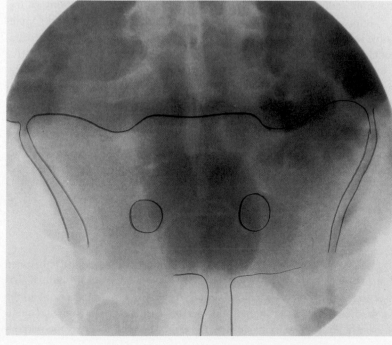

B

Figure 3. A: The pelvic-inlet (caudal) view superimposes the first and second sacral vertebral bodies, as seen on this intraoperative fluoroscopic image. **B:** The upper sacrum is best seen on the outlet (cephalad) pelvic view when the top of the symphysis pubis is located at the second sacral vertebral body as shown.

These views are essential to visualize the upper sacrum. Image enhancement and alternating negative images on the fluoroscope often improve imaging of the posterior pelvis. The arc of rotation of the fluoroscope needed to obtain these "perfect" images varies for each patient depending on the degree of lumbosacral lordosis and deformity. The amount of tilt needed to obtain perfect inlet and outlet views is marked on the fluoroscope by the technician to facilitate subsequent rapid imaging. Minor rotational changes of the fluoroscope identify the posterior pelvic disruptions tangentially and may be useful in certain sacral fractures. An "almost true" lateral sacral view is next obtained by adjusting the fluoroscope to superimpose the greater sciatic notches. On the almost true lateral sacral image, the iliac cortical densities are identified and correlated with the preoperative pelvic CT scan. The safe sacral segment for screw insertion is reconfirmed. Significant hemipelvis deformity causes this "almost true" lateral sacral view to be of little use. A "true" lateral sacral image is possible only after accurate posterior pelvic fracture reduction or in patients with minimal posterior pelvic deformities (Fig. 4). Lumbosacral osteophytes are confusing and complicate orthogonal imaging. These are best seen on the "true" lateral sacral image.

Skin Preparation/Draping

The perineum, abdomen, bilateral flanks, and lower extremities are prepared with iodine solution followed by isopropyl alcohol. The scrotum, penis, and any urinary catheter are included in the operative field when combined urologic procedures are planned. Wide preparation of the posterolateral buttock skin is important and simplifies iliosacral screw insertion. Femoral vascular catheters, enteral feeding tubes, suprapubic urinary catheters, and other essential anterior abdominal lines are prepared as skin. Chest tubes are positioned and isolated from the planned operative field. Sterile electrodes for neurodiagnostic monitoring are applied to the lower extremities when indicated.

Reduction

Accurate reduction of the posterior pelvic ring is the goal of surgery to diminish late pain and deformity. Reduction of pelvic-ring fractures can be accomplished by using a variety of techniques. Anatomic reduction and stable fixation of the *anterior* pelvic injury frequently "indirectly" improves the *posterior* pelvic displacement, especially when supplementary manipulative techniques are used. Reduction forceps are used temporarily to stabilize open reductions, whereas other techniques are used to maintain closed manipulative reductions. Early surgical treatment improves the accuracy of closed manipulative posterior pelvic reductions. An anterior pelvic external-fixation device [or a femoral distractor (Synthes, Paoli, PA, U.S.A.) attached to the external fixator pins] can be used as a "pelvic compressor or distractor" to improve the closed reduction. Distal femoral traction alone often improves posterior and cephalad deformities of the posterior pelvic ring. The fluoroscopic pelvic inlet and outlet images confirm the reduction before iliosacral screw fixation. Open reductions are performed when closed manipulative techniques fail to provide an accurate posterior-pelvic reduction.

Fixation

By using fluoroscopic control, a smooth 0.62-mm Kirschner wire (K-wire) is inserted from the lateral buttock onto the lateral ilium. This small-diameter smooth wire resists bending during insertion, which allows accurate aiming, yet causes minimal trauma to the local soft tissues. A predictable skin starting point is located in the posterior cephalad quadrant formed by intersecting lines. One line parallels the femoral shaft, whereas the perpen-

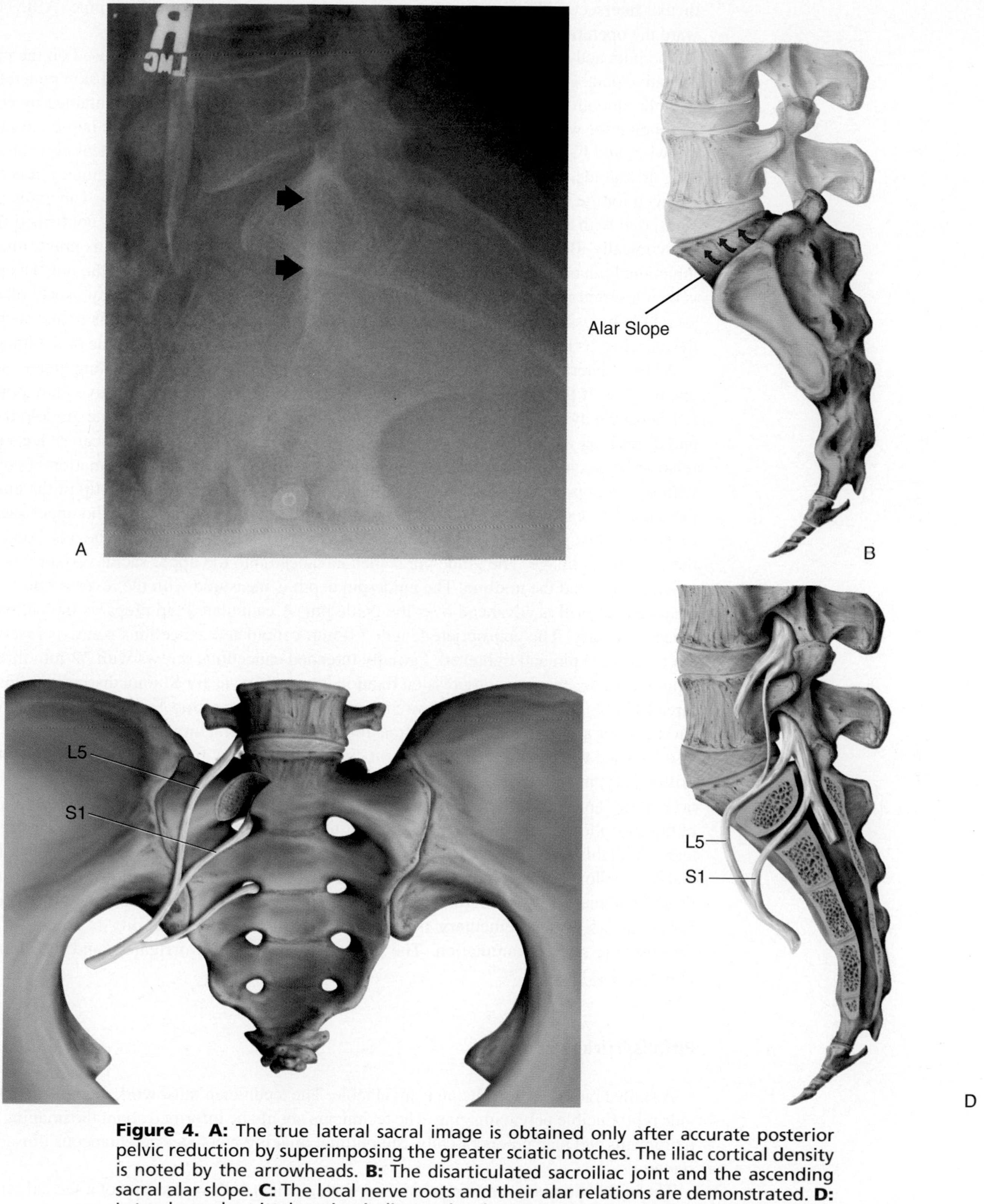

Figure 4. A: The true lateral sacral image is obtained only after accurate posterior pelvic reduction by superimposing the greater sciatic notches. The iliac cortical density is noted by the arrowheads. **B:** The disarticulated sacroiliac joint and the ascending sacral alar slope. **C:** The local nerve roots and their alar relations are demonstrated. **D:** Lateral sacral sagittal section indicates the changing structure of the alar zone and its neural relations. The fifth lumbar and first sacral nerve roots are highlighted.

dicular intersecting line is made from the palpable anterior–superior iliac spine (ASIS) toward the operating table.

The inlet and outlet pelvic images direct the orientation of the K-wire based on the preoperative plan. Perfect wire direction and starting point may require several skin punctures with the smooth wire. The perfect starting point and wire direction are maintained by gently tapping the wire to engage the lateral iliac cortical bone. The skin is then incised around the wire, and blunt deep dissection is accomplished with a narrow periosteal elevator. A long drill guide is placed over the wire, and a 2-mm terminally threaded guide pin is exchanged for the wire. The drill guide provides deep control of the guide pin. The guide pin is inserted with a power drill into the lateral iliac cortex, and its direction is confirmed fluoroscopically. Because the guide pin is only slightly engaged in bone at this point, minor directional pin corrections are still possible by using the drill guide to aim the pin. The pin is then inserted from the ilium, across the SI articulation, and into the lateral aspect of the sacral ala by using frequent inlet and outlet pelvic images. The guide pin is halted within the ala when its tip is located just cephalad to the upper sacral foramen on the outlet image.

A "true" lateral sacral image is obtained fluoroscopically by superimposing greater sciatic notches. If the posterior pelvic reduction is accurate, and the preoperative plan identifies no sacral dysmorphism, then the "true" lateral sacral image identifies the guide-pin tip and its relation with the iliac cortical density (ICD). The preoperative CT scan reflects the relation between the ICD and the sacral ala. The correlation of this information coupled with the intraoperative ICD indicates whether the pin is safely placed. The tip of the guide pin should be caudal to the ICD and cephalad to the intraosseous path of the upper sacral nerve root. The guide-pin tip should be located within the midportion of the alar bone on the true lateral image. The guide pin is then advanced into the upper sacral vertebral body to but not beyond the midline. The guide-pin depth is measured with the reverse ruler, and a cannulated drill is advanced over the guide pin. A cannulated tap prepares the pathway when necessary. The appropriate-length 7.0-mm cannulated cancellous screw is inserted over the guide pin and tightened. Partially threaded cancellous screws with 32-mm thread lengths are chosen when compression fixation is necessary, as for SI joint disruptions. Fully threaded 7.0-mm cancellous screws are used when compression fixation is not desired, such as after accurate reductions of transforaminal sacral fractures. Fully threaded screws also are used when needed to supplement compression screw fixations. During cannulated drilling, tapping, and screw insertion, frequent fluoroscopic images are obtained to assure no binding and inadvertent advancement of the guide pin. A 20- to 30-degree obturator oblique ("rollover") image visualizes the posterior ilium tangentially as the screw is tightened. With this image, the washer is noted to flatten as it contacts the ilium. Using a washer and this "rollover" image prevents screw penetration into the posterior ilium. The guide pin is removed manually. The fixation construct is stressed under fluoroscopic imaging. Additional screws or supplementary fixation are used if residual instability is noted on the fluoroscopic stress examination. The percutaneous wound is irrigated, and the skin is closed (Fig. 5).

Pitfalls/Tricks

A skilled radiology technician is invaluable. The technician must work diligently to provide reproducible pelvic imaging. The technician should be informed about the imaging requirements and plan preoperatively. Suboptimal imaging precludes percutaneous iliosacral screws.

The initial iliosacral screw is positioned strategically to allow insertion of a second screw if needed. The number of iliosacral screws necessary sufficiently to stabilize each posterior pelvic disruption depends on the degree of local instability, as well as the quality of supplementary fixation of the associated pelvic-ring injuries (Fig. 6).

Screw orientation and type are very important. The "SI joint" screw is different from the "sacral" screw in several ways. Compression lag screws are routinely used to treat SI-joint disruptions. Sacral fractures may involve the sacral neuroforamina; therefore further com-

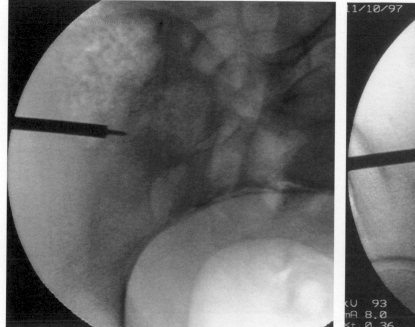

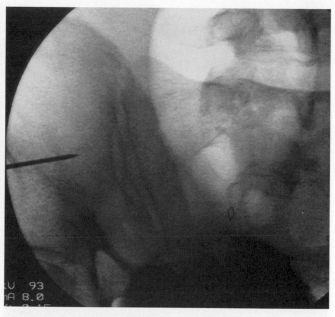

A   B

Figure 5. A, B: The technique of iliosacral screw insertion by using fluoroscopic guidance. After reduction of the right-sided sacral fracture is accomplished, the guide pin is inserted through the buttock and contacts the lateral iliac cortical bone. Pelvic inlet and outlet images are obtained to perfect the pin's starting point and aim.

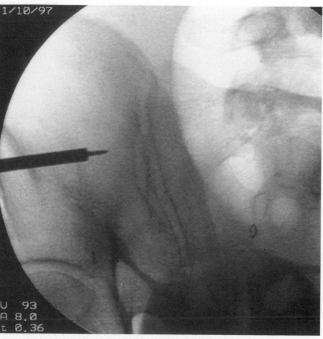

C   D

C, D: A small incision is made, and a drill sleeve is inserted over the guide pin. Final aiming adjustments are made by using the drill sleeve.

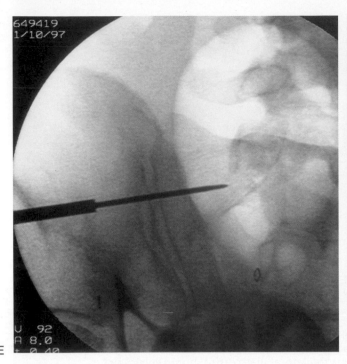
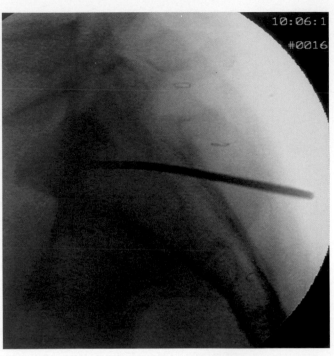

Figure 5. *(continued)* **E:** The guide pin is advanced across the sacroiliac articulation and into the sacral ala, stopping as it enters the area superior and lateral to the sacral foramen, according to the outlet image. **F:** The lateral sacral view confirms the safe location and direction of the guide pin relative to the iliac cortical density. The surgeon should understand the relations of the fifth lumbar and first sacral nerve roots with the guide pin. In this example, the guide-pin tip is directed superior to the first sacral nerve root pathway and inferior to the fifth lumbar nerve root pathway.

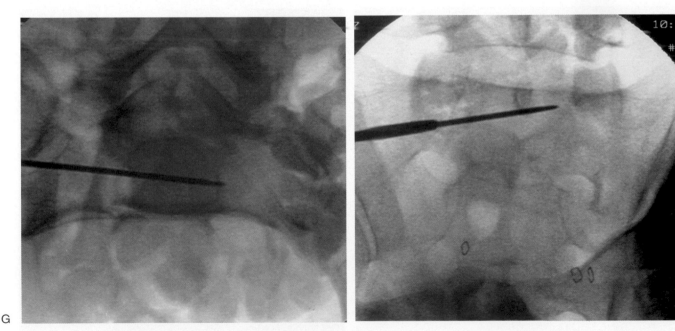

G: The guide pin is then advanced into the upper sacral vertebral body, but not beyond the boundary of the vertebral body. **H, I:** The cannulated drill prepares the pathway. Intermittent imaging avoids inadvertent guide-pin advancement due to binding.

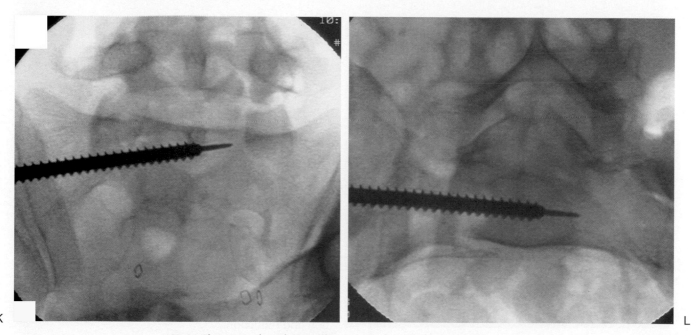

Figure 5. *(continued)* **J:** The tap is used across the sacroiliac area and removed.

K, L: The cannulated cancellous screw is inserted over the guide pin.

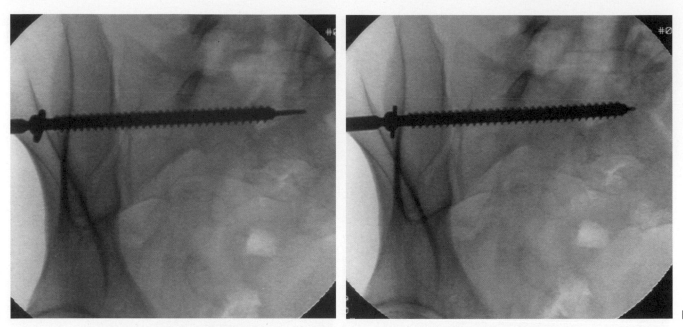

M   N

Figure 5. *(continued)* **M, N:** The fluoroscope is then positioned to visualize the posterior iliac cortical bone tangentially as the screw is tightened. The washer is observed as it contacts the cortical bone to avoid overinsertion.

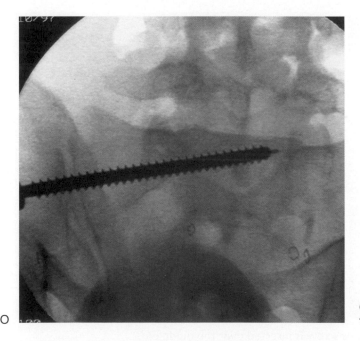

O: Final views are obtained to assure accurate screw location and reduction.

O

pression with a lag screw may produce nerve root injury. In a transforaminal sacral fracture, a fully threaded noncompression cancellous screw is required. Screws used to treat sacral fractures are usually longer than those for SI joints, because the sacral fracture is more medially located (Fig. 7). To obtain optimal stability through improved medial fixation, the sacral screw must be oriented more horizontally and tends to cross the chondral SI surfaces. To increase the screw length, the screw orientation is slightly different for "sacral" screws as opposed to "SI-joint" screws.

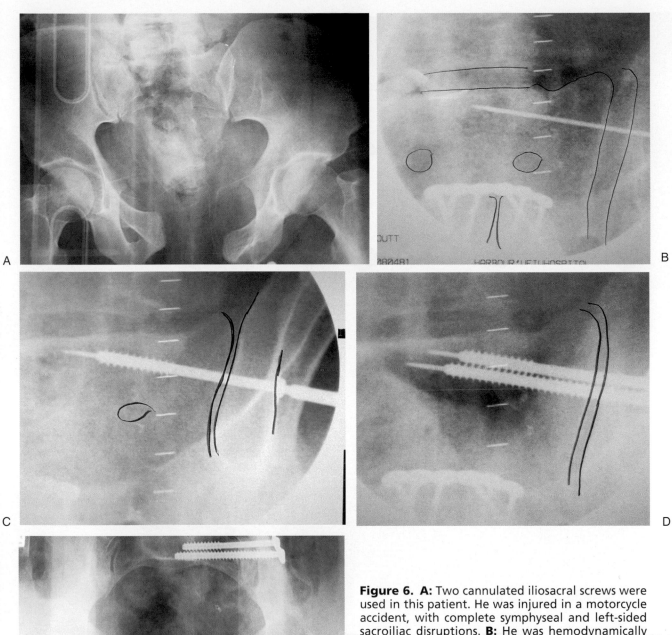

Figure 6. A: Two cannulated iliosacral screws were used in this patient. He was injured in a motorcycle accident, with complete symphyseal and left-sided sacroiliac disruptions. **B:** He was hemodynamically unstable after adequate volume resuscitation and pelvic angiography. He had urgent open reduction and internal fixation of the symphysis pubis. The sacroiliac joint remained distracted despite the anterior pelvic accurate reduction and fixation. A percutaneous iliosacral screw was chosen to stabilize the posterior pelvis. The guide pin was inserted. **C:** The iliosacral lag screw completed the compressive reduction as it was tightened. **D, E:** Because of the initial sacroiliac displacement and instability, a second fully threaded "locking" screw was inserted percutaneously further to stabilize the sacroiliac joint.

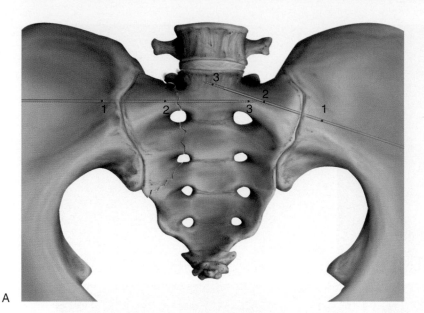

A

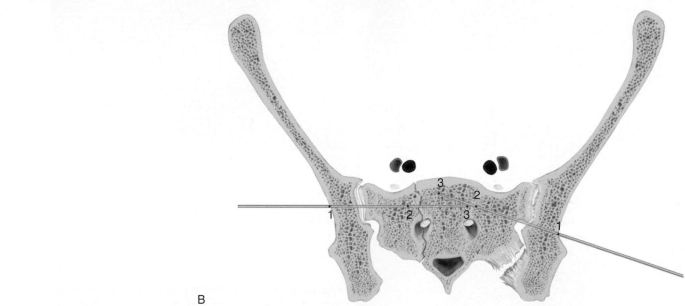

B

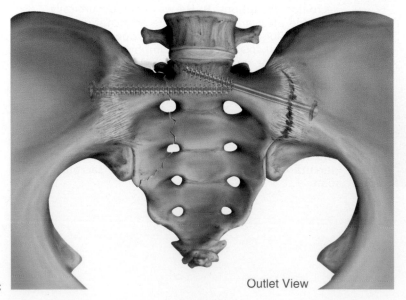

C   Outlet View

Figure 7. A, B: These illustrations demonstrate the screw orientations for sacral fractures (right side) and sacroiliac joint (SI) disruptions (left side). Critical fluoroscopic imaging intervals are numerically labeled. **C, D:** The screws are oriented according to the injury. The SI joint is anatomically oblique, whereas most sacral fractures occur in a sagittal plane. Sacral fractures are medially located relative to SI-joint injuries. For these two reasons, screw orientation and length are different for each. The screws are inserted perpendicular to the injury; therefore sacral and "SI" screws are different. "Sacral"-screw orientation is more horizontal, which orients the screw perpendicular to the fracture and allows longer screw length to balance the fixation. "SI" screws are oriented obliquely to remain perpendicular to the disrupted joint surfaces.

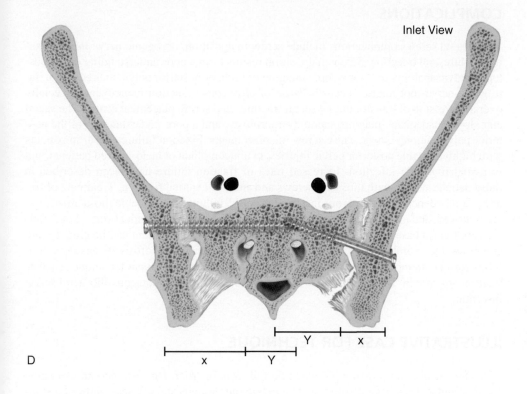

Inlet View

D

Figure 7. *(continued)* Compression screws are used for SI-joint injuries, whereas fully threaded screws stabilize transforaminal sacral fractures. "Sacral" screws are inserted through the articular surfaces of the SI joint because of their orientation, whereas "SI" screws avoid the chondral surfaces when inserted correctly.

"SI-joint" screws begin caudad/posterior on the ilium and are directed cephalad/anterior to be perpendicular to the oblique SI articulation. This screw direction usually avoids violation of the articular SI-joint cartilaginous surfaces.

The pathway of the fifth lumbar and first sacral nerve roots must be understood and respected. The nerves exit the spinal canal and are directed anteriorly/laterally and caudally.

Because of this nerve orientation, the "safe" zone for screw insertion becomes the elliptical area within the ala. A pelvic model and preoperative drawing outlining the surgical tactic are helpful.

POSTOPERATIVE MANAGEMENT

Intravenous antibiotics are administered for 24 hours after surgery when percutaneous fixation has been used alone or in combination with anterior pelvic external fixation. If open techniques are used, the antibiotics are continued until the surgical drains are removed. Sequential compression stockings are used to diminish the risk of deep venous thromboses. A licensed physical therapist supervises the rehabilitation. The rehabilitation schedule is dependent on the overall condition of the patient and associated injuries. The stabilized hemipelvis is protected by partial weight bearing with crutches or a walker for the initial 6 weeks after operation. Progressive weight bearing follows, with a goal of crutch-free ambulation 3 months after operation. Inlet/outlet pelvic radiographs are obtained in the recovery room and at the 6- and 12-week postoperative clinic visits. A postoperative pelvic CT scan assesses the reduction and implant location. Patients are seen in the clinic at 2, 6, and 12 weeks after operation. Thereafter, patients are seen annually. Most adult patients can return to work 4 to 6 months after surgery. Some patients return sooner, and others require job-site modifications. Heavy lifting and working at heights are avoided until the patient's strength and conditioning goals are achieved. Vocational reeducation is advocated for polytraumatized individuals with heavy job demands, or those patients who are unable to return to work. Nonimpact aerobic and water activities are allowed 6 weeks after operation.

COMPLICATIONS

Iliosacral screw complications include screw malposition, iatrogenic nerve injury, fixation failure, and infection. Screw malposition results from a poor understanding of the posterior pelvic anatomy or fluoroscopic imaging or both, or posterior pelvic malreduction. Iatrogenic nerve-root injuries occur because of erroneous reduction maneuvers, especially overcompression of transforaminal sacral fractures and screw-placement errors. The sacral alar slope, inadequate imaging, sacral dysmorphism, and a poor understanding of the posterior pelvis, among others, cause screw misplacements. Fixation failures occur in patients with highly unstable posterior pelvic injuries, in noncompliant or head-injured patients, and in association with infection. Increased rates of fixation failure have been described in those patients treated with iliosacral screws and anterior external fixation. Treatment of fixation failure depends on numerous factors. In "early" failures, the unstable iliosacral screws are removed, and alternative fixations are performed after repeated reductions. "Late" failures are treated based on the amounts of posterior pelvis displacement and healing. In rare situations, the overall condition of the patient or posterior pelvic soft-tissue envelope prohibits further attempts at surgical fixation, and traditional management techniques such as traction are chosen. Deep infection is rarely associated with percutaneous iliosacral screw insertion.

ILLUSTRATIVE CASE FOR TECHNIQUE

A 48-year-old man was injured when he fell from his roof. He sustained an olecranon fracture and a pelvic-ring disruption. The pelvic radiographs and CT scan showed a symphysis pubis separation, bilateral pubic ramus fractures, and bilateral sacral fractures (Fig. 8).

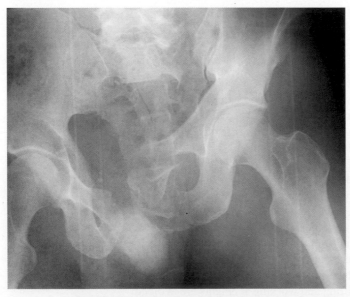

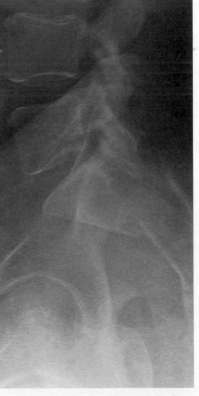

A   B

Figure 8. This patient fell from his roof, sustaining a pelvic ring disruption and olecranon fracture. **A:** The anteroposterior (AP) pelvic radiograph demonstrates the displaced transforaminal sacral and anterior pelvic fractures. **B:** The lateral sacral image identifies the displaced transverse component of the sacral injury. The lateral sacral view is helpful in patients with posterior pelvic disruptions.

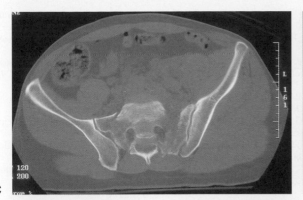

C

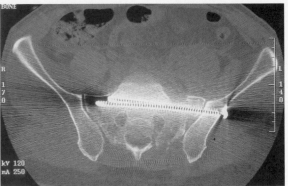

E

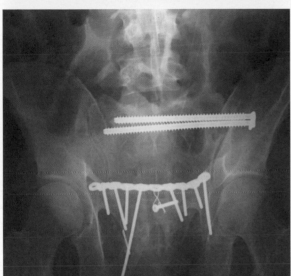

D

Figure 8. *(continued)* **C:** The pelvic computed tomography (CT) scan identifies the displacements and comminution. **D:** Distal femoral traction was used on the patient's left side. The anterior pelvic disruptions were reduced by using a Pfannenstiel exposure. A pelvic reconstruction plate and tension-band wire fixations provided anterior pelvic stability. Fluoroscopic imaging confirmed acceptable indirect reduction of the sacral fractures. Two fully threaded iliosacral screws were percutaneously inserted with the patient supine with the same anesthetic to stabilize the sacral fractures. **E:** The postoperative CT scan confirms the screw safety and reduction quality. He returned to work as a minister without problems.

The pelvis was grossly unstable to physical examination; however, the neurologic status was normal. He was brought to the operating room urgently and placed in the supine position. With a Pfannenstiel exposure, the anterior pelvic injuries were reduced and fixed with a plate and tension-band wire. The sacral fracture displacement was improved after anterior pelvic reduction and fixation along with distal femoral traction. Percutaneous iliosacral screws were used to stabilize the sacral fractures bilaterally. His recovery was uneventful. He returned to work as a minister.

RECOMMENDED READING

1. Burgess, A.R., Eastridge, B.J., Young, J.W., et al.: Pelvic ring disruptions: effective classification system and treatment protocols. *J. Trauma,* 30:848–856, 1990.
2. Goldstein, A., Phillips, T., Sclafani, S.: Early open reduction and internal fixation of the disrupted pelvic ring. *J. Trauma,* 26:325–333, 1986.
3. Gruen, G.S., Leit, M.E., Gruen, R.J. Peitzman, A.B.: The acute management of hemodynamically unstable multiple trauma patients with pelvic ring fractures. *J. Trauma,* 36:706–711; discussion 711–713, 1994.
4. Helfet, D.L., Koval, K.J., Hissa, E.A., Patterson, S., Di Pasquale, T., Sanders, R.: Intraoperative somatosensory evoked potential monitoring during acute pelvic fracture surgery. *J. Orthop. Trauma,* 9:28–34, 1995.
5. Kraemer, W., Hearn, T., Tile, M., Powell, J.: The effect of thread length and location on extraction strengths of iliosacral lag screws. *Injury,* 25:5–9, 1994.
6. Latenser, B., Gentilello, L., Tarver, A.: Improved outcome with early fixation of skeletally unstable pelvic fractures. *J. Trauma,* 31:28–31, 1991.
7. Matta, J., and Saucedo, T.: Internal fixation of pelvic ring fractures. *Clin. Orthop.,* 242:83–87, 1989.
8. Oliver, C.W., Twaddle, B., Agel, J., Routt, M.L.C., Jr.: Outcome after pelvic ring fractures: evaluation using the medical outcomes short form SF-36. *Injury,* 27:635–641, 1996.
9. Routt, M., Simonian, P., Inaba, J.: Iliosacral screw fixation of the disrupted sacroiliac joint. *Tech. Orthop,* 9:300–314, 1994.

10. Routt, M.L.C., Jr., Kregor, P.J., Simonian, P.T., Mayo, K.A.: Early results of percutaneous iliosacral screws placed with the patient in the supine position. *J. Orthop Trauma,* 9:207–214, 1995.
11. Routt, M.L.C., Jr., Meier, M., Kregor, P.: Percutaneous iliosacral screws with the patient supine-technique. *Tech. Orthop.,* 3:35–45, 1993.
12. Routt, M.L.C., Jr., Simonian, P.T., Agnew, S., Mann, F.: Radiographic recognition of the sacral alar slope facilitates optimal placement of iliosacral screws: a cadaveric and clinical study. *J. Orthop. Trauma,* 10:171–177, 1996.
13. Routt, M.L.C., Jr., Simonian, P.T., Ballmer, F.: A rational approach to pelvic trauma: resuscitation and early definitive stabilization. *Clin. Orthop.,* 318:61–74, 1995.
14. Shuler, T., Boone, D., Gruen, G., Peitzman, A.: Percutaneous iliosacral screw fixation: early treatment for unstable posterior pelvic ring disruptions. *J. Trauma,* 38:453–458, 1995.
15. Simonian, P.T., Routt, M.L.C., Jr., Harrington, R.M., Tencer, A.F.: Anterior versus posterior provisional fixation in the unstable pelvis: a biomechanical comparison. *Clin. Orthop.,* 310:245–251, 1995.
16. Simonian, P.T., Routt, M.L.C., Jr., Harrington, R.M., Tencerr, A.F.: Internal fixation for the transforaminal sacral fracture. *Clin. Orthop.,* 323:202–209, 1996.

Master Techniques in Orthopaedic Surgery,
FRACTURES, edited by D. A. Wiss,
Lippincott–Raven Publishers, Philadelphia © 1998.

38

Pelvic Fractures: Sacral Fixation

Brent L. Norris, Michael J. Bosse, James F. Kellam, and Stephen H. Sims

INDICATIONS/CONTRAINDICATIONS

Sacral fractures most commonly occur after pelvic-ring injuries but occasionally occur in isolation. Transverse, longitudinal (vertical), and dissociative H types are the most commonly identified fracture patterns. Transverse fractures usually occur after axial-load injuries and rarely require operative intervention, unless there is neurologic involvement. They are often associated with thoracolumbar compression or burst fractures. Longitudinal (vertical) and dissociative sacral fractures are invariably part of a pelvic-ring injury, and the decisions regarding treatment are based on pelvic stability and displacement. Denis classified sacral fractures according to their relation to the sacral foramina (Fig. 1). This description correlates closely with neurologic injury. Zone I injuries are lateral to the sacral foramina and are associated with L5 nerve-root injury in 24% of cases. Fractures through the sacral foramina are zone II injuries, and in 50% of patients, there is an injury to the sacral roots, including L5. If the fracture is medial to the sacral foramina, the injury is in zone III, and neurologic injury with bowel or bladder dysfunction or both occurs in up to 70% of patients.

Generally, sacral fractures associated with stable pelvic-ring injuries can be managed symptomatically with protected weight bearing until healed. On the other hand, sacral fractures associated with displaced unstable pelvic-ring injuries frequently require reduction and fixation. Relative indications for reduction and fixation of sacral fractures include posterior or vertical displacement or both (>1 cm), rotationally unstable pelvic-ring injuries and sacral fractures in patients with unstable pelvic-ring injuries who require mobilization. Displaced sacral fractures associated with neurologic injury often require decompression and stabilization to improve the chance of neurologic recovery.

A closed reduction done within the first 3 to 5 days may reduce a displaced sacral frac-

B. L. Norris, M.D., M. J. Bosse, M.D., J. F. Kellam, M.D., B.SC., and S. H. Sims, M.D.: Department of Orthopaedic Surgery, Carolinas Medical Center, Charlotte, North Carolina 28232.

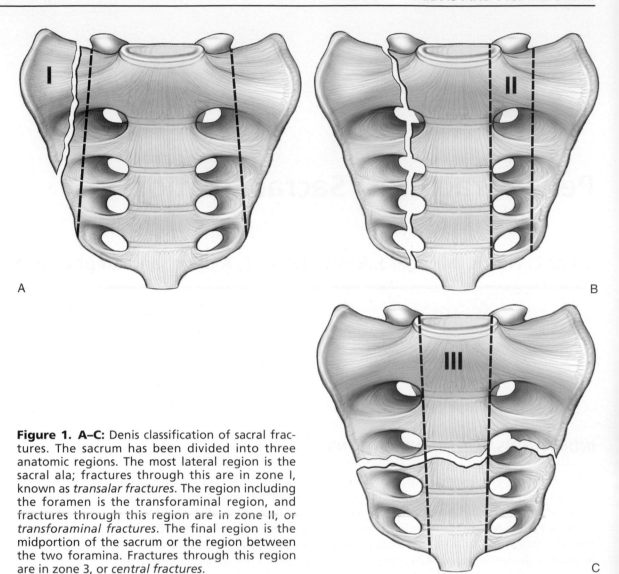

Figure 1. A–C: Denis classification of sacral fractures. The sacrum has been divided into three anatomic regions. The most lateral region is the sacral ala; fractures through this are in zone I, known as *transalar fractures*. The region including the foramen is the transforaminal region, and fractures through this region are in zone II, or *transforaminal fractures*. The final region is the midportion of the sacrum or the region between the two foramina. Fractures through this region are in zone 3, or *central fractures*.

ture, averting the need for open reduction and stabilization. Skeletal traction is recommended to maintain the reduction of these significantly displaced (usually posteriorly and vertically) sacral fractures. External fixation helps control rotational displacement.

In patients with displaced and unstable sacral fractures who require open reduction and internal fixation, the benefits of surgery must be weighed against the risks. If operative treatment is selected, the status of the posterior soft-tissue envelope must be critically assessed. If the condition of the soft tissues is not satisfactory, then open treatment of the sacral fracture should be deferred until an exposure can be made through a viable soft-tissue envelope. Age, by itself, is usually not a factor in decision making, but associated injuries and comorbidities may be considered in determining appropriate treatment.

PREOPERATIVE PLANNING

If the mechanism of injury involves direct application of force to the pelvic region (crush), the soft tissues around the pelvic region may be severely compromised. Indirect forces that disrupt the posterior pelvis usually cause less damage to the tissues. The direction of force may be predictive of the fracture pattern and its resultant stability. A laterally directed force will result in a stable or rotationally unstable pattern, whereas an anteroposterior (AP) or vertical force usually results in a more unstable fracture pattern.

A thorough evaluation and resuscitation in the emergency department is imperative, especially in the multiply injured patient. The orthopaedic surgeon assuming care or consulting on a patient with a sacral fracture must reassess the patient to assure that a life- or limb-threatening injury has not been missed. Visual examination and palpation of the back, flanks, buttocks, and groin are mandatory. Contusions and fluctuation in these regions may indicate a severe closed soft-tissue degloving injury (Morel-Lavelle lesion). Inspection of the perineum, including a rectal and vaginal examination, are appropriate to determine the presence of an occult open fracture or associated injury of the lower genitourinary system. A concise well-documented neurologic examination is essential before treatment. The common pattern of nerve injury is usually at the root level involving L5, S1, S2, and S3, and is clinically expressed as loss of bowel or bladder function and weakness or paralysis in the affected muscle group.

The diagnosis of a sacral fracture can be difficult to make based on an AP radiograph of the pelvis alone. If an injury to the posterior pelvic ring (i.e., sacral fracture) is suspected clinically or from the AP radiograph, then 40-degree cephalad and caudad (inlet and outlet views) radiographs should be obtained. These views often assist in visualizing sacral fractures, as well as give clues to the mechanism of injury. Obturator and iliac oblique views occasionally give further information of posterior pelvic injury. A sacral fracture should be suspected when there are pubic rami fractures (especially oblique patterns), interruptions of the arcuate lines of the sacrum (especially S1 and S2), fracture of the transverse process of L5, or avulsion fractures of the sacrospinous and sacrotuberous ligaments. These findings, combined with the history and results of physical examination, should increase the physician's awareness of the possibility of a sacral fracture. However, if doubt exists, a computed tomography (CT) scan of the pelvis provides definitive information about the bony anatomy of the pelvis and sacrum and is essential if a displaced fracture requires surgical stabilization.

The method of fixation is dependent on the condition of the soft tissues, the fracture pattern, and stability. If the soft tissues are viable, most techniques are suitable. Minimally invasive procedures such as percutaneous iliosacral screws are desirable but may not be possible if reduction cannot be achieved or nerve-root decompression is required. In this cases, open reduction with internal stabilization is necessary. With rotationally unstable fractures, external fixation may prevent internal and upward displacement.

For most sacral fractures, surgery is usually delayed 3 to 7 days to allow the patient's condition to stabilize, to obtain appropriate imaging studies, and to assemble the operative team. On the other hand, if the fracture is well delineated, the surgeon has all the necessary resources available, and the patient is stable clinically, surgery need not be delayed. Indications for early intervention are control of hemorrhage, debridement of open fractures, or that the patient requires emergency surgery for other reasons and all the necessary resources are available. In patients with closed soft-tissue degloving injuries, debridement may be necessary to excise devitalized tissue or drain hematomas or both. Serial debridements may be necessary, depending on the magnitude of the soft-tissue injury. Open reduction and internal fixation of the posterior pelvis requires a healthy posterior soft-tissue envelope. Significant ecchymosis, abrasion, or degloving (or a combination of these) in the posterior soft tissues are contraindications for "open" operative treatment, despite the nature of the sacral fracture/pelvic-ring injury.

SURGERY

Several surgical techniques can be used to stabilize sacral fractures and include iliosacral screws (lagged and nonlagged), posterior sacral bars, posterior iliosacral plating, and posterior sacral plating (direct).

The open reduction and internal fixation of sacral fractures is done with the patient in the

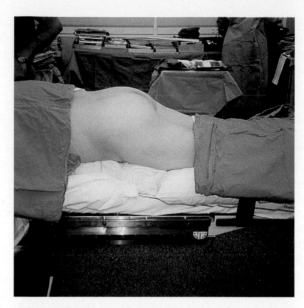

Figure 2. The most versatile position for fixing sacral fractures is with the patient in the prone position placed on bolsters. Although sacral fixation can be done in the supine position, it is limited to percutaneous techniques. The prone position allows open reduction and internal fixation if a closed reduction is unsuccessful.

prone position. Insertion of percutaneous iliosacral screws can be done with the patient in either the supine or prone position (Fig. 2). The patient is placed in the prone position with two longitudinal chest rolls. The upper and lower extremities are carefully padded and adequately supported to prevent compressive nerve injury. Depending on the need for traction or manipulation to obtain fracture reduction, one or both of the lower extremities are prepared into the surgical field. If the patient has a previously placed anterior external fixator, the patient may be suspended between two operating room tables placed in line and with the leg extensions dropped 90 degrees. The gap between the two tables allows the anterior external fixator to be placed between the tables when the patient is prone. Alternatively, if reduction/manipulation of the fracture is necessary, the anterior frame can be disassembled, leaving the pins in situ. With the patient placed prone on a single table, bolsters are positioned about the pins to support the patient. These bolsters must be radiolucent. Specialized radiolucent operating tables are mandatory. A C-arm fluoroscopy unit must be available, and adequate AP, inlet, outlet, and lateral radiographs of the sacrum/pelvis must be rehearsed before surgery is started (Fig. 3). The posterior aspect of the patient from the thoracolumbar junction to the popliteal fossa is surgically prepared and draped. The lateral extent of the surgical field should extend anteriorly to the table to allow an extensile exposure if necessary. Care must be taken to ensure that the sacrum has been adequately draped into the field and that the gluteal cleft has been excluded from the operative field. A self-adhesive biooclusive drape seals the surgically prepared field.

Percutaneous Iliosacral Screw Stabilization

Percutaneous iliosacral screws are indicated for unilateral or bilateral sacral fractures, preferably in zones I or II. Fractures in zone III are amenable to this technique, but great care must be used in placement of screws.

This technique is reserved for sacral fractures that can be adequately reduced by closed methods. A thorough understanding of the direction of fracture displacement improves the chances of reducing the fracture by closed means. Closed reduction is accomplished by

A1

A2

A

B1

B2

B

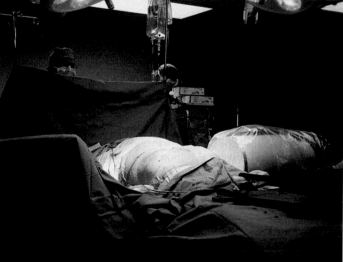

C

Figure 3. C-arm position for appropriate radiographic control of sacral fixation. **A1, A2:** This shows the position of the patient prone with the C-arm in the outlet position. The appropriate radiographic image is noted. **B1, B2:** The C-arm has been moved 90 degrees into the inlet position. The appropriate view is now seen. It should be remembered that because of the prone position, the views are reversed. What appears to be an inlet view is really an outlet position of the C-arm. **C:** This shows a lateral position of the C-arm. Note that on the image, the greater sciatic notches are aligned perfectly with no overlap. This allows an excellent position of the sacrum. The radiodense line in the superior portion of the S1 body is the ala of the sacrum.

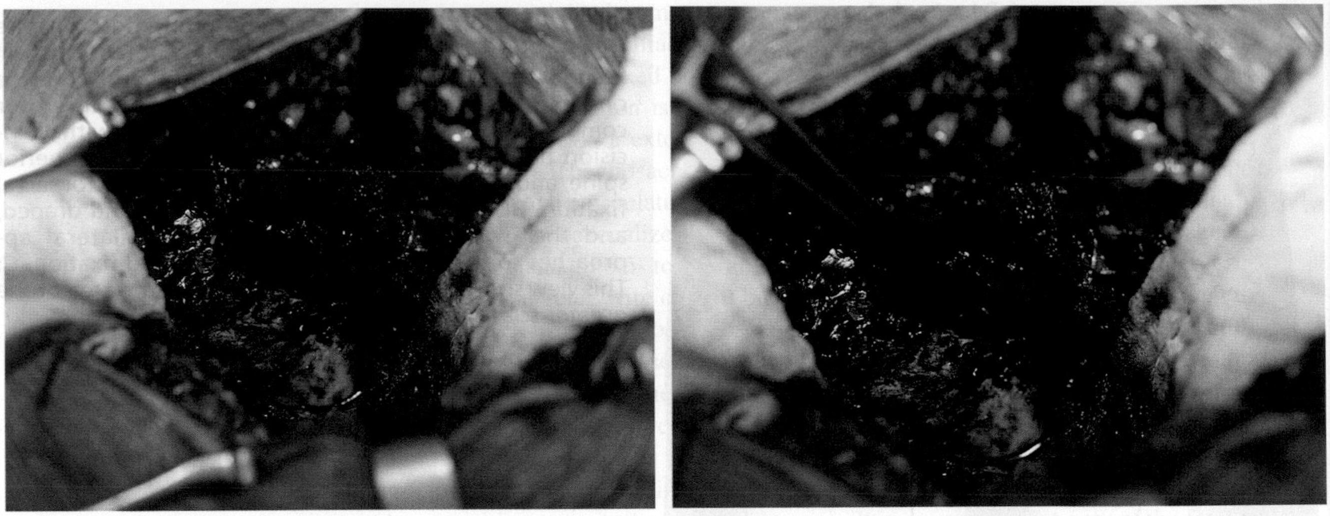

Figure 5. Deep exposure to sacral fracture. **A:** View through the longitudinal incision over the posterior–superior spine. The sacral fracture is noted to be well exposed. **B:** Retraction laterally will allow exposure of the iliac wing for placement of transiliac rods or screws. Note the fracture still is visualized.

with iliosacral screws. A straight 10- to 12-hole 4.5- or 3.5-mm reconstruction plate is used. The optimal position of the posterior sacral spanning plate is just below the posterior spine and just above the greater sciatic notch, as the best bone stock is found here. For transiliac plate placement, the plate is passed through each posterior spine by drilling two 4.5- or 3.5-mm holes 0.5 cm apart and approximately 1 cm lateral to the posterior superior iliac spine. The drill holes are connected, and a straight plate is passed through the spine and over the dorsum of the sacrum. The plate is secured to each iliac wing in the same manner as the more caudal plate with the most medial screw placed obliquely between the two tables. A long 6.5-mm cortical screw (>80 mm) between the iliac tables provides excellent purchase. The screws on each side should be left loose and then sequentially tightened. The sacral fracture is watched closely for displacement or overcompression. The reconstruction plate is contoured in situ to the outer table of the iliac crest with the use of a pointed ball pusher and mallet or screwdriver "lever." The plate is malleable enough to bend in this plane but is strong enough in tension to resist displacement of the sacral fracture. Two more screws are added on each side of the plate, further securing the plate to the ilium. Precontoured plates can be more difficult to place, and exact contouring is mandatory, or fracture displacement will occur (Fig. 7).

Direct Sacral Plating. Direct sacral plating is performed for zone II fractures and the more medial zone I fractures. Lateral zone I and zone III fractures are often difficult to plate directly because the fracture lines do not allow fixation on both sides of the fracture. For this reason, lateral zone I fractures usually require fixation crossing the sacroiliac joint, and zone III fractures usually require a bridging construct crossing the midline and obtaining fixation into the opposite ala.

The advantage of direct sacral plating is that the sacroiliac joint is spared. The sacral exposure is similar to that used for iliosacral plating, except that the incision is usually placed over the affected side and is medial to the posterior iliac spine, splitting the difference between the sacral spines and the posterior iliac spine. The multifidus and erector spinae muscles are divided distally and raised as a flap cephalad to expose the sacrum. During the subperiosteal dissection, care must be taken to avoid entering the sacral canal, especially if the lamina is fractured. Zone III fractures can be directly plated with the use of bilateral incisions or more commonly through a long midline incision. Bilateral incisions are placed more lateral than the unilateral incision to help obtain an adequate soft-tissue bridge. The same deeper dissection is performed with the addition of a subfascial dissection under the skin bridge at the S1 and S3 regions (Fig. 8).

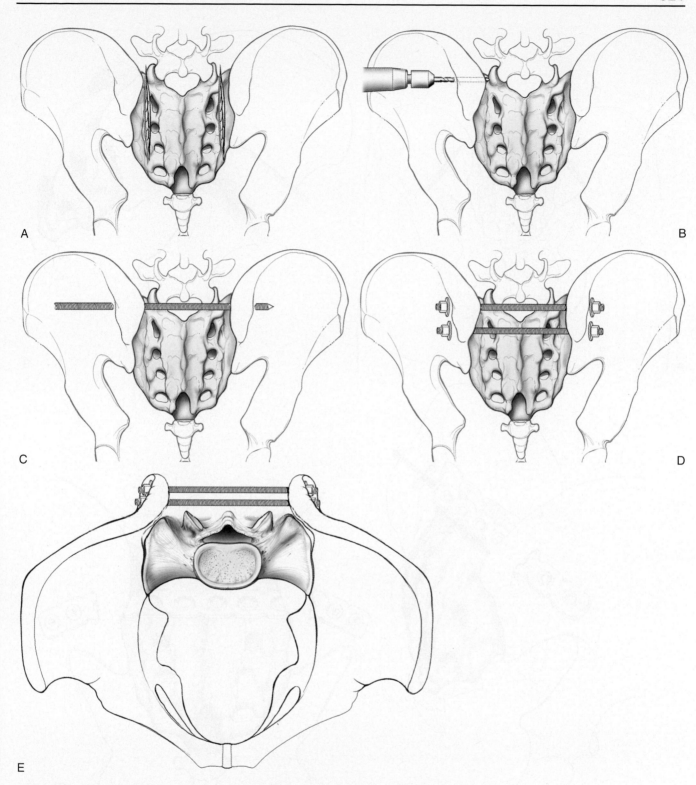

Figure 6. Transiliac bar posterior fixation. **A:** Bilateral incisions are made just lateral to posterior–superior spine. **B:** After a reduction and provisional stabilization of the sacral fracture, a 6.5-mm drill bit is used to drill a hole at the level of the L5–S1 interspace through the posterior spine. **C:** A sacral bar can then be inserted through this glide hole and, with a sharp trocar, driven through the opposite iliac crest. **D:** The sacral rods are then affixed to the bone through nuts and washers. **E:** The position of transiliac rods is noted in the inlet view to be posterior to the sacral lamina.

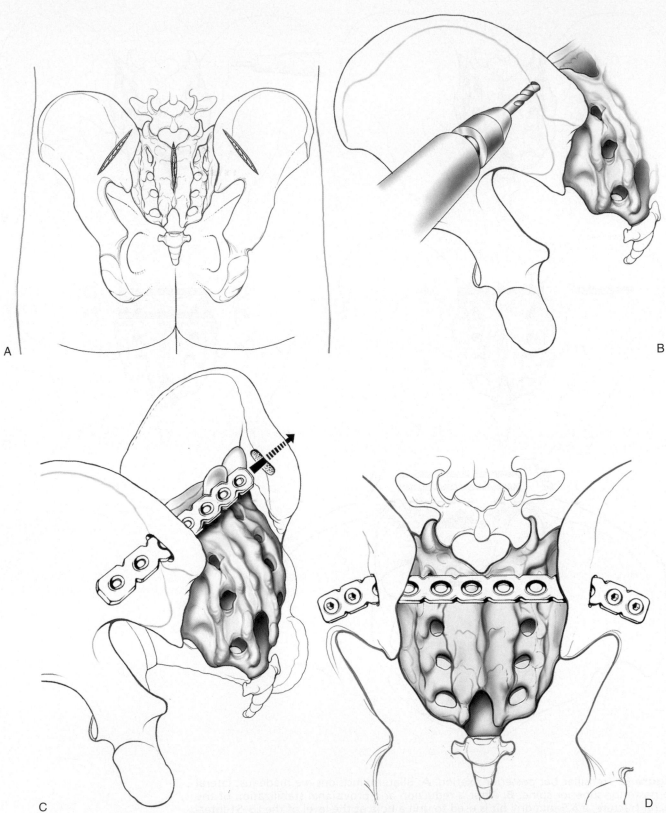

Figure 7. Posterior sacral plating. **A:** Incisions for posterior sacral plating can be as mentioned previously or as described by Albert, with oblique incisions starting at the posterior tubercle and a midline incision to allow reduction and plate passage. **B:** Drill holes are placed under the posterior tubercle just above the junction with the sacrum. **C:** The plate is chiseled through the drill holes toward the opposite crest. **D:** Final contouring is undertaken after the plate has been driven through the opposite posterior–superior spine and then fixed.

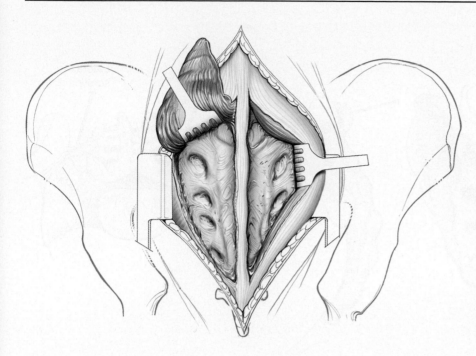

Figure 8. Deep exposure through a midline incision allows elevation of the lumbosacral musculature to expose the posterior aspect of the sacrum. This allows an extensile approach to the posterior aspect. A limited incision allows removal of the lumbosacral fascia from the medial sacral crest and lateral displacement of the muscle.

Once the sacrum has been exposed, decompression of the sacral nerve roots is performed if indicated, and the fracture reduced. Care must be taken to avoid overcompression of the sacral foramina. Exactly contoured small fragment plates, 3.5-mm reconstruction, one-third tubular, DCP, LC-DC, and H plates are then used to stabilize the fracture. The lateral plate screws are placed into the ala directly inferiorly and in a plane parallel to the sacroiliac joint.

Inferiorly directed screws avoid potential injury to the L5 nerve root, which crosses the ala superiorly. Care must be taken to avoid placement of this screw medially. The medial screws are placed between the dorsal foramen. The drill is placed perpendicular to the sacral lamina and, with transforaminal fractures, directed 20 degrees medially into the pedicle of the sacral vertebrae (Fig. 9). The medial screw can be placed perpendicular to the lamina if the transforaminal fracture line is based laterally. For the zone III fractures, direct sacral plating can be achieved by placing a "spanning" plate dorsally and obtaining purchase in each alar region. However, two plates (small fragment) are usually necessary and should be placed over the S1 and S3 regions. This construct is "distance keeping" and is commonly used for bilateral fractures, dissociated H-type fractures, and fractures with extensive comminution. Intraoperative imaging with C-arm fluoroscopy is used to avoid foraminal or central-canal hardware placement.

Regardless of the technique used to fix the sacral fractures, attention to detail and meticulous handling of the soft-tissue envelope is paramount. The wound should be copiously irrigated and complete hemostasis obtained. Anatomic closure of the deeper gluteal musculature and thoracolumbar fascia should be accomplished. The subcutaneous tissues are reapproximated, followed by closure of the skin. Drains should be placed deep to the fascia when hemostasis is questionable. Sterile dressings are applied, and the patient turned supine. If a displaced or unstable anterior pelvic injury (or both) exist, anterior stabilization should be performed. This is extremely important with direct sacral plating to neutralize the stresses on these small relatively weak plates.

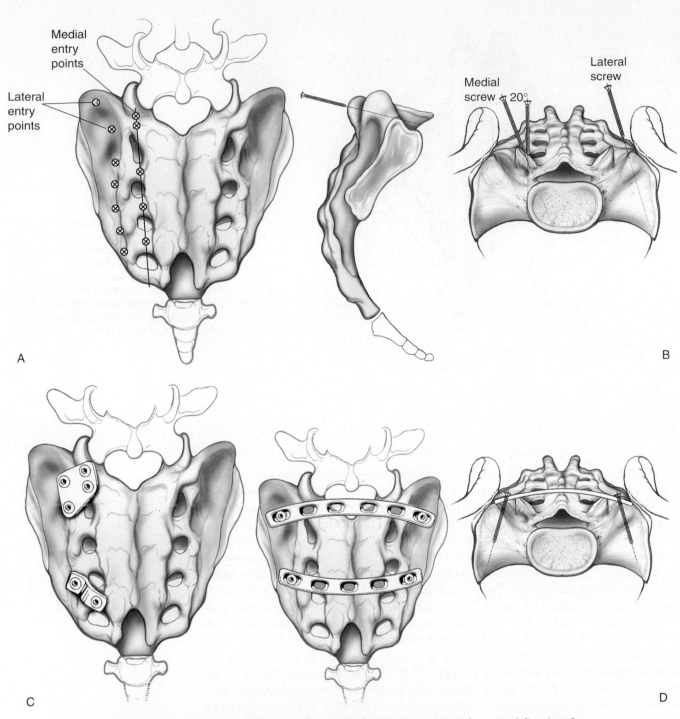

Figure 9. Insertion for direct sacral plating. **A:** Insertion points for sacral fixation for direct plating are demonstrated. Lateral entry points are shifted as far lateral as possible. The limiting factor is the attachment of the iliosacral ligaments. The medial insertion points lie along an imaginary line through the foramina. The entry point is in the middle of the distance between the two foramina along this line. In S1, the distal border of the L5–S1 facet also helps to identify the insertion point. **B:** The orientation of the lateral screw is always parallel to the plane of the sacroiliac joint. This is identified by insertion of a K-wire into the joint posteriorly. In S1, orientation must also be in the plane of the craniosacral lamina. The medial screws are oriented in the sagittal plane perpendicular to the dorsosacral lamina. In a transforaminal fracture, the direction should be inclined 20 degrees to the lateral side to be transpeduncular. **C:** Implant position for transforaminal plating. **D:** The implant for central or bilateral fractures is shown as a posterior plating expanding the whole sacrum.

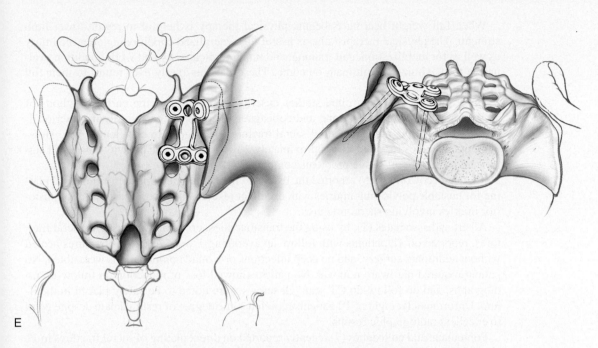

E

Figure 9. *(continued)* **E:** With comminution or difficult plate placement, a plate may be extended over into the ilium and a screw placed through the ilium, as noted.

POSTOPERATIVE MANAGEMENT

An unstable sacral fracture requires bed rest with turning until the patient is comfortable sliding to a chair. Bed-to-chair slides are done for 6 to 8 weeks postoperatively. Mobilization to partial weight bearing may occur earlier if the surgeon is confident that the fracture-fixation stability can resist the physiologic forces of these activities. Protected weight bearing is then begun on the unstable side and continued for an additional 4 to 6 weeks or until the fracture union is complete. Bilateral sacral fractures will usually require bed rest or bed-to-chair slides for a total of 10 to 12 weeks. Weight bearing can be started when the fracture has healed, but patients should be monitored closely for late displacement. If loss of reduction occurs, weight bearing is restricted.

Antibiotics are used for 24 to 48 hours. If considerable soft-tissue damage is compounded by the surgery, a longer duration may be indicated. Thromboembolic prophylaxis is a matter of surgeon preference, and we recommend it when there are specific contraindications.

At 2 weeks, the sutures are removed. If nonoperative treatment is used, radiographs at weekly intervals (for 3 weeks) are necessary to evaluate fracture position. At 6 weeks, the patient is assessed as to wound healing, pain, mobility, and general heal. Radiographs are taken only if a change in weight status is to be instituted. At 3 months, the patient is assessed for pain, mobility, sexual function, and overall general health status. The three pelvic views are obtained, and fracture union is assessed. If union is complete, weight bearing is increased; if not, further review is done in 6 weeks. It may take up to a year for union to occur. Patient review is performed at 6 months, 1 year, and yearly thereafter. It usually takes up to 2 years for maximal medical and functional recovery to occur. It is not uncommon for these patients to complain of nondisabling lumbosacral pain for many years.

When full weight bearing is begun, physical therapy is helpful to regain lower-limb strength. The physical therapist also is useful for generalized conditioning after the injury as well as for mobilization, gait training, and functional-capacity and work-condition evaluation to maximize the ultimate outcome. These patients rarely ever return to their full preinjury status.

Unfortunately, few controlled studies described outcomes of the current methods of sacral fracture treatment. DeLong and colleagues (2) reported on the use of posterior iliosacral bars for the management of sacral fractures, with good to excellent results. However, other studies reported that approximately 20% to 25% of the patients developed significant posterior soft-tissue problems/complications.

Matta and coworkers (5) reported the results of the technique of posterior iliosacral plating for unstable pelvic-ring injuries with excellent results, but few of these were for posterior injuries involving sacral fractures.

Albert and associates (1), by using the transiliac iliosacral plate for unstable sacral fractures, reported on 12 patients with follow-up averaging 1 year. All sacral fractures healed without additional surgery, and no deep infections or wound complications were noted. No patient required hardware removal. No patient showed loss of reduction on follow-up radiographs, and on follow-up CT scan, all screws were noted to be safely placed in the ilium. Unfortunately, eight of 12 patients reported some degree of residual pain despite good to excellent radiographic results.

Pohlemann and colleagues (7) recently reported on direct plating of sacral fractures in 11 patients. Anatomic reduction was obtained in nine of 11 fractures. No perioperative local complications were observed. All patients were allowed partial weight bearing within 5 days of surgery and continued for 6 weeks. In six patients with neurologic injury, four had complete recoveries after decompression and stabilization. Six patients were graded as having good to excellent functional results; however, seven of 11 patients reported some residual pain. Final radiographic analyses showed bony healing in all cases, with no implant failure. However, implant removal was performed in seven of the 11 patients at final follow-up.

COMPLICATIONS

Internal fixation of sacral fractures can lead to major or catastrophic complications. For this reason, the management of these injuries should be done by surgeons familiar with the anatomy and surgical problems of this injury.

The energy needed to disrupt the pelvic ring is substantial, and forces are transmitted not only to the bone but also to the surrounding soft tissues. Damaged posterior soft tissues are often further compromised with surgery, and a high rate of deep infection and wound dehiscence has been seen after surgical management of posterior pelvic-ring injuries, including sacral fractures.

If wound hematoma or drainage occurs, prompt assessment is necessary to avoid wound infection or necrosis. Open surgical drainage and debridement of hematomas or infections is recommended over radiologic percutaneous techniques.

Significant hemorrhage can occur from inadvertent injury of the superior gluteal vessels. If the blood or nerve supply of the gluteal musculature is disrupted, the functional result is usually compromised despite anatomic alignment of the pelvic ring. Additionally, this further compromises the soft-tissue envelope covering the posterior pelvis, leaving it more susceptible to infection and wound slough.

Nonunion of the sacrum is uncommon; however, when it occurs, it is difficult to treat because, in most cases, it occurs after operative treatment. Revision of fixation (both anterior and posterior) with bone grafting usually results in union, but not without additional morbidity. Malunion is more common than nonunion, and, fortunately, the incidence is decreasing with better reduction and stabilization techniques.

Iatrogenic nerve injury is usually permanent. Nerve-root injury and even paralysis after operative treatment of sacral fractures has been reported. However, as experience with the surgical techniques grows and as better fluoroscopic imaging of the pelvis occurs, iatrogenic nerve injury should diminish.

ILLUSTRATIVE CASE FOR TECHNIQUE

A 35-year-old woman was involved in a motor-vehicle collision in which her car was struck broadside. She was hemodynamically stable without a head injury. Assessment showed that she had several rib fractures and bilateral tibial fractures, as well as the pelvic fracture (Fig. 10).

Evaluation of the pelvic fracture led the surgeon to the conclusion that this was relatively stable and could be managed nonoperatively, especially because she would be non–weight bearing on her lower extremities because of her tibial fractures. She was mobilized from bed to chair by means of sliding transfers and discharged home at 8 days after injury.

Review at 3 weeks showed that her sacral fracture had displaced into an unacceptable position. In addition, a large fluctuant mass was evident over the dorsal aspect of her sacrum. Investigation showed that she was afebrile with a normal white count. Further studies revealed a pseudomeningocele arising from the sacral canal and exiting through the sacral fracture (Fig. 11).

Because of the displacement, instability of the fracture, and the pseudomeningocele, open reduction and internal fixation was performed. Decompression of the mass was accomplished and the dura repaired, after which an open reduction of the sacrum was performed and stabilized with a transiliac-spanning plate (Fig. 12).

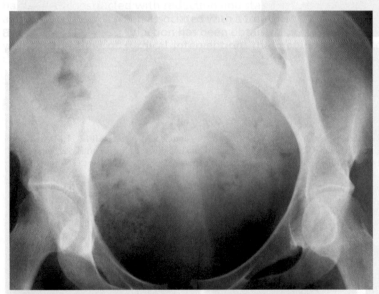

A

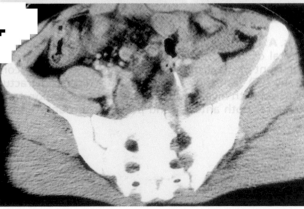

B

Figure 10. Initial radiograph. **A:** Inlet view demonstrates a fracture through the sacrum on the left transforaminal region. There is a widening of the symphysis. The sacral fracture shows a complete fracture through the foramina with a potential for instability. **B:** Computed tomography scan.

Figure 12. Postoperative fixation. **A:** Anteroposterior view of the pelvis demonstrating the postoperative stabilization. Radiographs at 5 months show that the sacrum has been reconstructed with reduction and stabilization with a dome plate. Note that a posterior sacral position associated with a transiliac lattice been used to stabilize the posterior aspect. The reduction has been obtained. The pelvic subsequent status normal well. At the time of surgical intervention, the meningomyelocele was excised and closed. **B:** Inlet view confirms anatomic reduction and satisfactory position of implants.

RECOMMENDED READING

1. Albert, M.J., Miller, M.E., MacNanahan, M. Stripet, W.A. Posterior pelvic fixation using a transiliac 4.5-mm reconstruction plate: a clinical and biomechanical study. J Orthop Trauma 7:226, 1993.

2. Browner, W.G., and Dukes, R.M. Posterior stabilization of the pelvis with sacral bars. J Int. Orthop 5:10.

3. Denis, F., Davis, S., Comfort, T. Sacral fractures: an important problem. Clin Orthop 227:67, 1988.

4. Letournel, F., and Browner, E.D. Fractures of the pelvic ring, in Browner, II. Jupiter, J. Levine, A. Trafton (Eds.), Skeletal Trauma. W.B. Saunders, Philadelphia, 1991, 1117-1180.

5. Matta, J.M., and Saucedo, T. Internal fixation of pelvic ring fractures. Clin Orthop 242:83, 1989.

6. Pohlemann, T., Angst, M., Schneider, F., Culemann, U., Techotni. Fixation at transforaminal sacral fractures: a biomechanical study. J Orthop Trauma 11:107, 1997.

7. Schildhauer, T., and Fearonte, H. Bilateral of sacral fixations. J Orthop Trauma 9:365, 1995.

8. Schnoske, H.L.C. Simonian, P.T. Routt, jr., O. Tencer, E.A. Biomechanical comparison of the sacral rod plate to iliosacral fixation of thevertical shears. J Orthop Surg. Part. Clinical Orthop. Research 10:13, 1996.

Figure 11. Radiograph at 6 days. As inlet view shows significantly more displacement posteriorly than original. **B:** Lateral of lumbosacral spine at the time of myelogram shows extravasation of the dye in front of the sacrum (arrow). **C:** Reconstruction (coronal) of the computed tomography (CT) scan shows a significantly displaced fracture paraforaminal. **D:** Axial cut of CT scan with myelogram and dye in place demonstrates the pseudomeningocele as it traverses both anterior and posterior through the fracture site.

Master Techniques in Orthopaedic Surgery,
FRACTURES, edited by D. A. Wiss,
Lippincott–Raven Publishers, Philadelphia © 1998.

39

Acetabular Fractures: The Kocher–Langenbeck Approach

Berton R. Moed

INDICATIONS/CONTRAINDICATIONS

Displaced fractures of the acetabulum resulting in joint incongruity or instability are best treated by open reduction and internal fixation. Contraindications to surgery are ill defined and not absolute. Important concerns include preexisting patient factors, such as poor general medical status and osteopenia, and factors that relate to overall patient prognosis, such as advanced age and associated injuries. All of these conditions must be considered with the knowledge that with nonoperative treatment in the face of joint incongruity or instability or both, the prognosis for hip-joint function is poor.

In choosing the appropriate surgical approach, the objective is to select the least extensive exposure that allows sufficient bony access for anatomic joint reconstruction. The Kocher–Langenbeck approach provides direct visualization of the entire lateral aspect of the posterior column of the acetabulum (Fig. 1; 7). Indirect access to the true pelvis and to the anterior column can be attained by the palpating finger or through the use of special instruments (Figs. 1–3; 7). Therefore, the Kocher–Langenbeck approach has its application in the treatment of fractures with the main displacement involving the posterior column. In the classification of Letournel and Judet (Table 1), this group consists of six fracture types: posterior wall, posterior column, posterior column and wall, transverse, transverse and posterior wall, and T-shaped. The Kocher–Langenbeck approach is the surgical exposure of choice for the first three types, in which the fracture extent is limited to the posterior wall or column or both. For the transverse, transverse and posterior wall, and T-shaped fractures, some decision making is required. All three of these fracture types have a transverse fracture line as a common component. As a general guideline, if the fracture is less than 15 days

---

B. R. Moed, M.D.: Department of Orthopaedic Surgery, Wayne State University, Detroit, Michigan 48201.

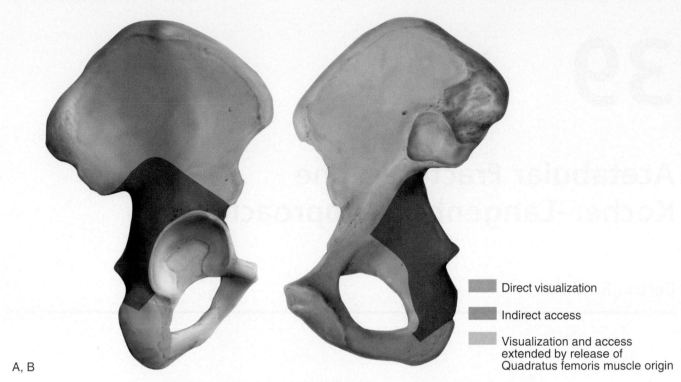

A, B

Direct visualization

Indirect access

Visualization and access extended by release of Quadratus femoris muscle origin

Figure 1. A, B: Access provided by the Kocher–Langenbeck approach.

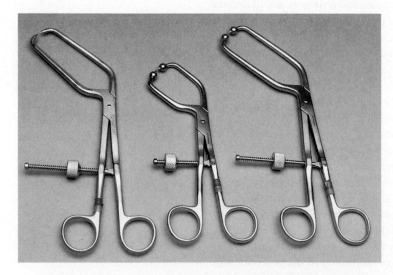

Figure 2. Examples of available special instruments (Synthes, Paoli, PA, U.S.A.) that permit intrapelvic and anterior column access.

TABLE 1. *Acetabular fracture classification*

Elementary fractures
    Posterior wall
    Posterior column
    Anterior wall
    Anterior column
    Transverse
Associated fractures
    Posterior column and wall
    Anterior column or wall and posterior hemitransverse
    Transverse and posterior wall
    T-Shaped
    Both columns

From Letournel and Judet (6,7).

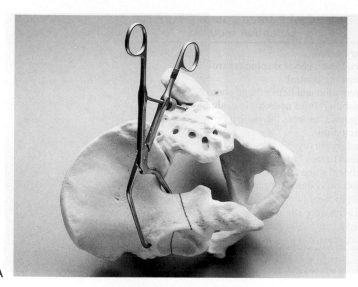
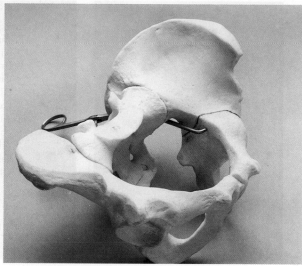

A

B

Figure 3. A, B: Example of clamp application for fracture reduction with a bone model.

old, and the transverse component is located at (juxta-) or below (infra-) the level of the roof (tectum) of the acetabulum (therefore not involving the weight-bearing area of the acetabulum), use of the Kocher–Langenbeck approach is indicated (7). Otherwise, an alternative exposure such as the extended iliofemoral approach should be used. For acute juxta- and infratectal level transverse and T-shaped fractures in which the major displacement occurs anteriorly at the pelvic brim and only minor displacement posteriorly the ilioinguinal approach is perhaps the best choice.

The status of the local soft tissues is an important additional consideration. Acetabular fracture surgery through a compromised soft-tissue envelope is ill advised because of the increased risk of infection. Closed degloving soft-tissue injuries over the trochanteric region associated with underlying hematoma formation and fat necrosis (the Morel-Lavallé lesion) or open wounds may require debridement followed by delayed wound closure (7). The fracture pattern should be reassessed to determine whether reduction and fixation can be accomplished by using an alternative surgical approach located outside of the zone of soft-tissue injury. Another treatment option is to delay surgery until wound healing. This delay, as noted previously, may preclude use of the Kocher–Langenbeck approach.

PREOPERATIVE PLANNING

In most cases, patients with an acetabulum fracture have sustained high-energy trauma. Therefore, examination of the injured limb, even in those with an apparent isolated injury, should be just one part of a comprehensive and systematic approach. Associated injuries can be life or limb threatening. The Advanced Trauma Life Support evaluation sequence should be followed (Table 2). Detailed examination of the hip and lower extremity is performed during the secondary survey. As previously noted, soft-tissue injury has important implications regarding subsequent surgery; therefore, the soft tissues should be evaluated carefully. The incidence of preoperative, posttraumatic sciatic nerve injury was reported as being as high as 31% (12). Other peripheral nerves, such as the femoral and obturator nerves, also may be injured. A complete and clearly documented neurologic examination is extremely important both for patient prognosis and for medical–legal concerns. Preoperatively, this evaluation should be repeated periodically.

The initial anteroposterior (AP) radiograph of the pelvis is obtained during the secondary survey and can provide substantial diagnostic information regarding fracture type,

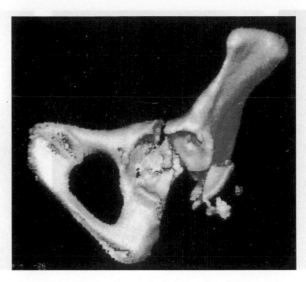

Figure 7. Three-dimensional computed tomography (CT). The fracture as deduced by evaluation of the plain radiographs and two-dimensional CT is shown fairly clearly. An overall appreciation of the fracture pattern is provided. However, there is some loss of definition, especially of the quadrilateral plate fracture involvement.

After careful physical examination and radiographic study, the appropriate surgical approach can be determined. The indications for emergency fracture fixation are uncommon (Table 3). Operative treatment is generally delayed 3 to 5 days to allow stabilization of the patient's general status and for preoperative planning. My preference is to use preoperative skeletal, femoral pin traction both to maintain an unstable hip in a located position and to prevent further femoral head articular-surface damage from abrasion by the raw acetabular bony fracture surfaces (Fig. 8). Significant intraoperative blood loss can occur. Two to four units of blood should be made available, depending on the extent of the fracture pattern. The use of an autologous blood-transfusion system, such as the cell saver, may decrease the need for intraoperative homologous banked blood transfusion.

TABLE 3. *Indications for emergency acetabular fracture fixation*

Recurrent hip dislocation after reduction despite traction
Modifier: None
Progressive sciatic nerve deficit after closed reduction
Modifier: None
Irreducible hip dislocation
Modifier: After open reduction (stable with traction), fracture fixation may be delayed because of declining medical status of the patient or limitations of the surgical team
Associated vascular injury requiring repair
Modifier: When the fracture is directly related to the vascular injury and fracture stabilization is an important adjuvant to the vascular repair, such as an anterior-column fracture associated with laceration of the femoral artery, urgent fracture fixation is required
Open fractures
Modifier: Open fracture-treatment principles require emergency irrigation, debridement, and fracture stabilization. Fracture stabilization options include traction followed by delayed open reduction and internal fixation (ORIF) or acute ORIF

From Tile (12).

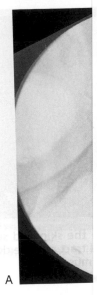

A

Figur
rior w
ducec

Surgical Procedure

With the patient in the
lar to that in hip arthropl
posterior superior iliac sp
ile field consists of the b

The skin incision (Fig
of the incision is directec
cm short of this bony lai
the midlateral aspect of t
sue and superficial fasci
thin, deep fascia overlyi

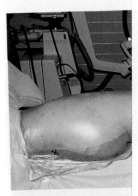

Figure 13. Patient fr
and draping. The pos
with an "X." The righ
matosensory evoked
through a sterile plas

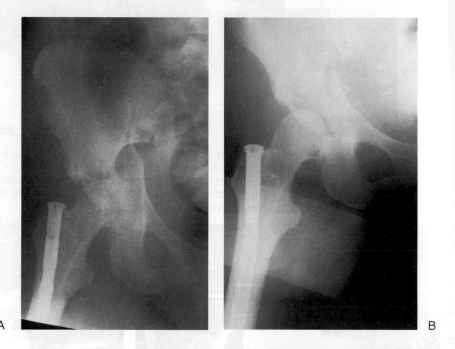

Figure 8. Anteroposterior pelvis radiograph before **(A)** and after **(B)** the application of traction. The hip joint is distracted with the application of traction, pulling the articular cartilage of the femoral head a safe distance away from the acetabular fracture surface. A defect in the femoral head from the impact of the injury is evident **(B)**. The femoral nail is from a previous injury.

SURGERY

Patient Positioning

Acetabular fracture fixation using the Kocher–Langenbeck approach can be performed with the patient in either the lateral or the prone position. Orthopaedic surgeons from North America are more familiar with and perhaps more comfortable using lateral positioning with the affected extremity draped free, as in hip arthroplasty surgery (Fig. 9). However, the Kocher–Langenbeck approach is most effective with the patient placed prone on a fracture table. The benefits of the prone position are realized by maintaining the femoral head in a reduced position. Gravity becomes a help rather than a hindrance in fracture exposure and reduction. The fracture table provides controlled traction and limb positioning, further assisting in fracture reduction. Traction is applied by using a distal femoral pin with the knee flexed to approximately 90 degrees (Fig. 10). This angle of knee flexion places the sciatic nerve in a relaxed position, minimizing the risk of intraoperative sciatic nerve injury. An unscrubbed assistant is required for intraoperative adjustment of the table.

With the patient placed prone, chest rolls should be used to elevate the head and to avoid excessive abdominal pressure. The fracture table generates the added risk of injury (i.e., pudendal nerve palsy) from pressure against the perineal post. The Judet fracture table adequately addresses these concerns (Figs. 10 and 11).

No matter what the patient position, use of a radiolucent operating table is advisable. Intraoperative C-arm fluoroscopy can then be used to assess fracture reduction and hardware location (Fig. 12). Before the sterile preparation and draping of the patient, the hip area should be quickly scanned with the C-arm to ensure adequate fluoroscopic visualization.

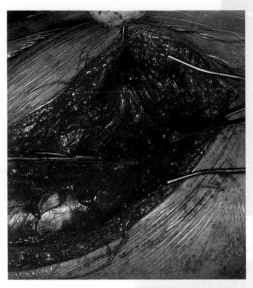

Figure 34. Muscle bellies of the gemelli have been dissected to reveal the obturator internus tendon.

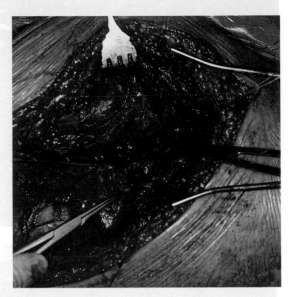

Figure 35. Obturator internus tendon is isolated and tagged with a suture. The stump of the previously released piriformis tendon can be seen just cephalad to the obturator internus tendon as it inserts into the greater trochanter.

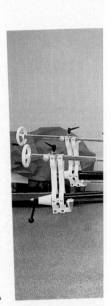

A

Figure 10. Pati[...] with a detailed [...]

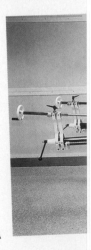

A

sciatic nerve runs deep to the piriformis muscle, appearing in the buttock at the inferior border of this muscle (Fig. 27; 5). Three variations of this "normal" anatomy have been reported, and others probably exist (5). The most common variation (12%) is for one part of the nerve (the peroneal division) to pass through the muscle and the other part (the tibial division) to appear below the muscle. The entire nerve also may pass through the muscle (1%). These two variations result in a split piriformis muscle with two tendons of insertion. The third variation is passage of the peroneal division above the piriformis and the tibial division below (3%). Given enough operative cases, one will eventually encounter one of these anatomic anomalies (Fig. 31). Knowledge of the anatomic variability of this area and the prior identification of the sciatic nerve on the posterior surface of the quadratus femoris muscle will prevent intraoperative confusion and decrease the risk of iatrogenic sciatic nerve injury. After its identification, the piriformis tendon is isolated, tagged with a suture, and released from its insertion (Fig. 32). The anastomotic branch of the inferior gluteal artery (which participates in the cruciate anastomosis of the thigh) runs in proximity to the piriformis muscle almost in parallel with the piriformis tendon (2). Failure to locate this artery may result in its unintentional laceration, followed by troublesome intraoperative bleeding. This vessel does not provide an important blood supply. Formal ligation is the easiest and best course of action.

The obturator internus tendon with the superior and inferior gemelli muscles on either side can be found just inferior and slightly deep to the piriformis (Fig. 28). The gemelli muscles insert onto the tendon of the obturator internus, and the bellies of these two muscles may actually obscure this tendon (Fig. 33). If this situation occurs, the tendon can be identified by palpation, with either a right-angle clamp or a finger placed deep to the tendon. External rotation of the hip will relax the tendon, allowing easier access to its deep surface. Internal rotation of the hip, placing the tendon under tension, will verify its position. Alternatively, the overlying gemelli muscles can be teased away to reveal the obturator internus tendon (Fig. 34). Once located, the obturator internus tendon is isolated, tagged with a suture, and released from its insertion. Both the piriformis and obturator internus tendons should be incised approximately 1.5 cm from their insertion points into the greater trochanter to avoid injury to the blood supply of the femoral head (Fig. 35). A fascial layer running from the undersurface of the gluteus maximus muscle to the posterior column of the acetabulum separates the piriformis muscle from the obturator internus and gemelli muscles. This fascia is easily visualized after the release of the piriformis

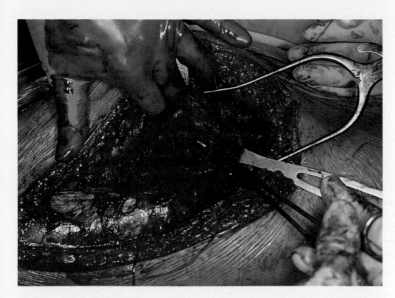

Figure 36. Delineation of the fascia separating the piriformis muscle from the superior gemellus muscle/obturator internus tendon/inferior gemellus muscle group. A right-angle clamp clearly shows the medial margin of this fascia and its proximity to the sciatic nerve. The sciatic nerve can be seen running superficial to the obturator internus tendon and gemelli muscles and then coursing deep to the piriformis muscle.

and obturator internus tendons (Fig. 36). The sciatic nerve lies directly adjacent to the medial origin of this fascia (Fig. 36). Care must be taken not to injure the sciatic nerve when this fascia is released during the clearing of the soft tissues from the posterior column (Fig. 37).

The obturator internus muscle arises from within the true pelvis from the internal circumference of the obturator foramen and the obturator membrane (2). The muscle fibers end in four or five tendinous bands that converge and pass through the lesser sciatic notch. These bands turn a right angle around the grooved external surface of the lesser sciatic notch, joining to form the single tendon of insertion. The bony surface is covered by cartilage and is separated from the tendon by a bursa. Once the obturator internus tendon is released from its insertion into the greater trochanter, it is elevated away from the hip capsule (along with the gemelli muscles) and followed medially toward the lesser sciatic

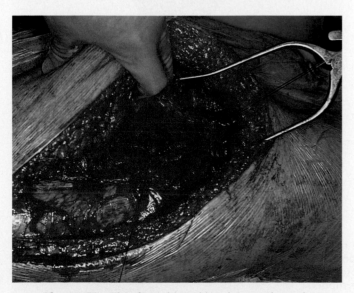

Figure 37. This fascial band has been released.

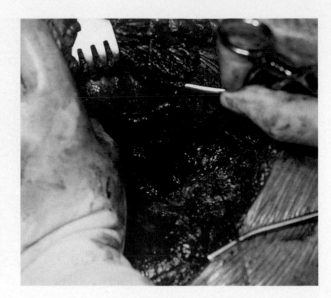

Figure 38. Obturator internus tendon has been elevated, allowing access to the lesser sciatic notch. In this photograph, the hemostat is directed toward, and its tip inserted into, the lesser sciatic notch.

notch. The underlying bursa is opened, permitting access to (and palpation through) the lesser sciatic notch (Fig. 38). A specially designed sciatic nerve retractor can now be placed with its tip anchored in the lesser sciatic notch (Fig. 39). Use of this instrument facilitates the bony exposure by permitting controlled retraction of the sciatic nerve and the posterior soft tissues. The retractor is positioned such that at the level of the lesser sciatic

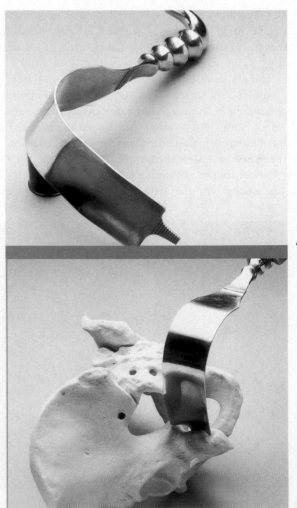

A

B

Figure 39. Sciatic nerve retractor **(A)** and its desired position in the lesser sciatic notch, as demonstrated in a bone model **(B)**.

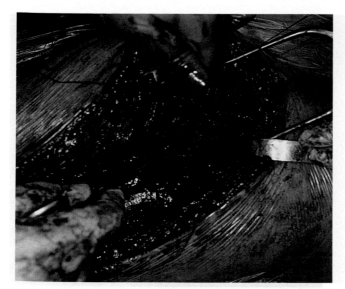

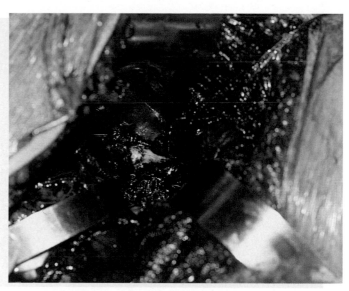

Figure 40. Sciatic nerve is unprotected both below and above (as marked by the tip of a hemostat) the obturator internus tendon and gemelli muscles.

Figure 41. Sciatic-nerve retractor is placed in the lesser sciatic notch. Just superior to this retractor, the greater sciatic notch and the overlying piriformis muscle can be seen. Two curved retractors reflect the hip abductors. The external surface of the posterior column with its overlying soft-tissue debris is well visualized.

notch, the obturator internus tendons and gemelli muscles lie between the retractor and the sciatic nerve, cushioning the nerve. However, it is very important to realize that the sciatic nerve retractor extends beyond the limits of this muscle cushion and directly contacts the nerve at the superior and inferior aspects of the retractor (Fig. 40). The relation between the sciatic nerve and the sciatic nerve retractor must be such that the edges of the retractor do not impinge or place undue pressure on the nerve. The surgical assistant in charge of maintaining position of the retractor must be cognizant of the importance of this task. The position of the retractor should be checked frequently during the operative procedure.

Once the sciatic nerve retractor has been appropriately positioned, the posterior hip capsule and retroacetabular surface of the posterior column are explored and cleared of debris. The dissection is carried from lateral to medial, progressing from the fracture site superiorly toward the greater sciatic notch and inferiorly toward the ischial tuberosity. Superiorly, the hip abductors are elevated from the external surface of the ilium and held with a curved retractor (Fig. 41). As the dissection approaches the greater notch, care must be taken to prevent injury not only to the sciatic nerve that is unprotected at this level, but also to the superior gluteal neurovascular bundle. The superior gluteal neurovascular bundle exits the greater sciatic notch above the piriformis muscle, superior to the level of the sciatic nerve. Its position can often be assessed by palpation of the superior gluteal arterial pulse at the level of the greater sciatic notch. The superior gluteal neurovascular bundle tethers the abductor muscle mass. It can be injured not only by direct laceration but also by traction from excessive retraction of the abductor muscle mass. Inferiorly, the tendon of the obturator externus muscle may be encountered (Fig. 42). Release of this tendon usually is not necessary. In cases with fracture involving the ischial tuberosity, or others requiring increased access to this area, more extensive exposure may be obtained by releasing the quadratus femoris muscle and, infrequently, the obturator externus tendon. The quadratus femoris muscle is extremely vascular. It should be released at its origin from the ischial tuberosity to avoid excessive bleeding and damage to the branches of the medial circumflex artery. The obturator externus tendon can be released in a manner similar to that described for the piriformis and obturator internus tendons.

The extent of the fracture pattern dictates the extent of the surgical approach. For fractures limited to the posterior wall that do not require access to the true pelvis, the dissec-

ments or femoral head fractures. Axial CT scans also can identify associated injuries to the posterior aspect of the pelvis such as a sacroiliac-joint disruption and sacral fractures. Advances in imaging software technology have led to the development of three-dimensional computerized tomography (3D CT), which provides an even better understanding of the spatial relation of the fracture pattern relative to the pelvis (Fig. 5B).

Trauma patients, especially those with lower extremity/pelvic injuries, are at extremely high risk for developing deep vein thrombosis (DVT), as high as 60% in some series (5,40). All acetabular fracture patients should be screened for a DVT and treated with compression boots and subcutaneous heparin if a delay in surgery is anticipated. Our preferred method of screening is magnetic resonance venography, which has proved extremely sensitive and reliable (33). Patients with an increased risk of DVT or those with documented DVT preoperatively are managed with a vena cava filter and intravenous heparin before surgery.

SURGERY

Surgical Anatomy

The physician performing an extended iliofemoral approach requires special training and a familiarity with the complex anatomy of the pelvis, particularly the many neurovascular structures that are encountered. Those structures that require identification are listed below.

Sciatic Nerve. The sciatic nerve is at risk during exposure of the posterior column and must be identified, as in the Kocher–Langenbeck approach, along the belly of the quadratus femoris muscle. Traction along the nerve should be minimized by maintaining the hip in extension with the knee flexed at all times.

Lateral Femoral Cutaneous Nerve. The lateral femoral cutaneous nerve is at risk during exposure of the anterior superior iliac spine. It is also very susceptible to a traction injury during mobilization of the soft tissues. Patients should be warned preoperatively of the significant risk of numbness, in the anterolateral thigh, after this exposure.

Superior Gluteal Neurovascular Bundle. The superior gluteal neurovascular bundle is at risk during exposure of the greater sciatic notch and must be protected from undue traction or penetration by retractors.

Femoral Neurovascular Structures. The medial margin of the extended iliofemoral approach is the iliopsoas muscle and the iliopectineal eminence. Further medial dissection without an ilioinguinal incision places the femoral neurovascular structures at risk.

Pudendal Nerve. The pudendal nerve is at risk as it exits the pelvis through the greater sciatic notch, wraps around the ischial spine, and travels back into the pelvis through the lesser sciatic notch.

Operating Room Preparation

General or spinal anesthesia is administered. We prefer the continuous epidural anesthesia as it provides improved postoperative pain relief (29). The patient is supported on a beanbag and placed in the lateral decubitus position on a radiolucent operating table or fracture table, depending on the surgeon's preference. Before surgery, a Foley catheter is placed in the patient's bladder.

Vascular access in two separate sites with large-bone catheters is important for these lengthy procedures in which significant blood loss is common. The patient's age and medical condition often dictate placement of an arterial or central line.

We routinely use an intraoperative cell saver to minimize transfusion requirements. This permits recycling of about 20% to 30% of the effective blood loss and is best used when blood loss of more than 2 L is expected (30).

The hip is kept extended and the knee flexed throughout the procedure to minimize sciatic nerve injury. In addition, intraoperative sciatic nerve monitoring with spontaneous electromyography (EMG) and somatosensory evoked potentials (SSEP) is used in all cases (9,11,14). The entire pelvis, hip, abdomen, and involved extremity is prepped free, and sterile subdermal electrodes are inserted. The sensory electrodes are inserted adjacent to the common peroneal and posterior tibial nerves and the motor adjacent to the tibialis anterior, peroneus longus, and abductor hallucis.

Surgical Approach

The incision is in the form of an inverted "J" (Fig. 6) and begins at the posterior–superior iliac spine, extending along the iliac crest toward the anterior–superior iliac spine (ASIS). From here, the distal arm of the incision proceeds along the anterolateral aspect of the thigh for a distance of 15 to 20 cm (Fig. 7). There is a tendency for the surgeon to make this arm more medial than desired. To avoid this, one should visualize a point 2 cm lateral to the superolateral pole of the patella. With the leg held in neutral rotation, this location is generally in line with the desired incision (22,29). Furthermore, a gentle curve posteriorly may be helpful in more obese patients (29).

The fascial periosteal layer at the iliac crest is identified (Fig. 8) and divided sharply along its avascular "white line," where bleeding will be minimized. Often it is easiest to start in the area of the gluteus medius tubercle where landmarks are more obvious, and to progress posteriorly and anteriorly from this point (29). Posteriorly, the strong fibrous origins of the gluteus maximus should be sharply released from the crista glutei (22). De-

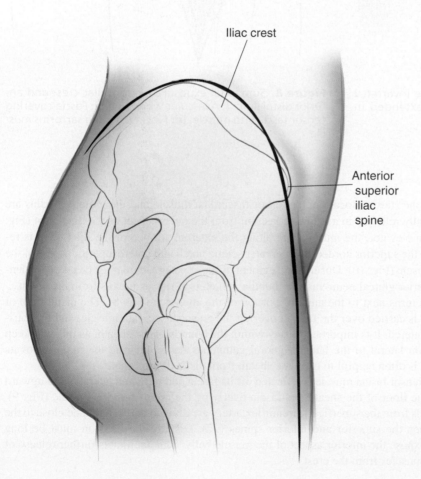

Figure 6. Inverted "J" skin incision, right side.

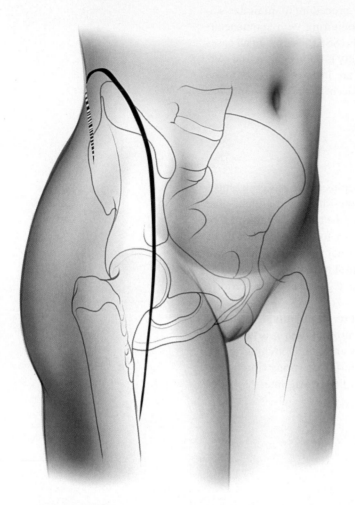

Figure 7. Anterolateral view, right side. The inverted J skin incision with distal extension for the extended iliofemoral approach.

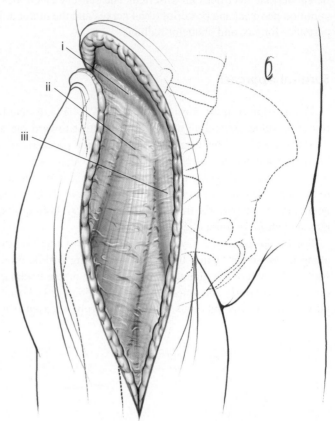

Figure 8. Subfascial exposure of right iliac crest and anterior distal limb. **i:** Avascular white line. **ii:** Fascia covering tensor fascia lata muscle. **iii:** Fascia covering sartorius muscle.

pending on the starting location, the tensor fascia lata muscle and the gluteus medius are subperiosteally released in a stepwise fashion from the outer aspect of the iliac crest (Fig. 9). Using an elevator, the musculature along the external surface of the iliac wing is released up to the superior border of the greater sciatic notch and anterosuperior aspect of the hip joint capsule (Fig. 10). During this segment of the exposure, care must be taken to identify the superior gluteal neurovascular bundle, which is at risk as it exits from the notch.

Attention turns next to the anterior portion of the approach (Fig. 8). The distal limb of the incision is carried over the fascia covering the tensor fascia lata muscle, and the muscle sheath entered. It is important to stay within the bounds of the sheath, as this will keep the dissection lateral to the lateral femoral cutaneous nerve, sparing the majority of its branches. It is often helpful to open the sheath from distal to proximal.

Next the tensor fascia muscle is reflected off its fascia and retracted laterally and upward to expose the floor of the sheath and fascia overlying the rectus femoris muscle (Fig. 9). Small vessels from the superficial circumflex artery are divided and coagulated close to the bone between the superior and inferior spines (22). Distally the incision must be long enough to expose the inferior aspect of the muscle belly. This facilitates further release of the gluteal muscles from the crest.

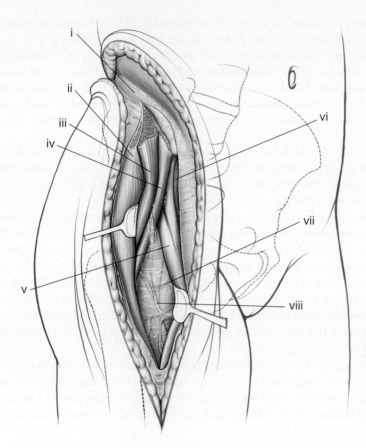

Figure 9. Subfascial reflection of tensor fascia lata and abductor muscle origins from right iliac crest. **i:** Avascular white line. **ii:** Tensor fascia lata muscle. **iii:** Gluteus medius muscle. **iv:** Gluteus minimus muscle. **v:** Rectus femoris muscle. **vi:** Sartorius muscle. **vii:** No-name fascia covering vastus lateralis. **viii:** Ascending branch of the lateral femoral circumflex artery.

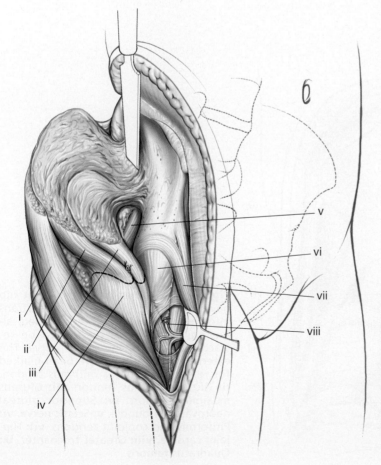

Figure 10. Proximally, the abductor and tensor fascia lata muscles have been stripped subperiosteally from the outer table of the right ileum. Distally, the ascending branch of the lateral circumflex artery has been ligated. The abductor insertions have been marked for release. **i:** Tensor fascia lata muscle **ii:** Gluteus medius muscle. **iii:** Gluteus minimus muscle. **iv:** Greater trochanter. **v:** Piriformis muscle. **vi:** Hip-joint capsule. **vii:** Two heads of the rectus muscle. **viii:** Ligated ascending branch of the lateral femoral circumflex artery.

The fascia overlying the rectus muscle is divided longitudinally and horizontally, and its reflected head and direct heads retracted downward and medially to expose a very strong aponeurosis (the "no name" fascia) over the vastus lateralis muscle (Fig. 9). When the rectus is retracted, a constant small vascular pedicle reaching the lateral border of the muscle always requires coagulation (22). The aponeurosis can be divided longitudinally to expose the ascending branches of the lateral circumflex vessels, which must be isolated and ligated (Fig. 10). Should the upper portion of this exposure be unnecessary, these vessels can occasionally be spared.

Next the thin sheath of the iliopsoas muscle is exposed and longitudinally incised. This allows the use of an elevator to strip the fibers of the psoas from the anterior and inferior aspects of the hip capsule. The exposure of the iliac wing is complete when the reflected head of the rectus femoris is sharply released from its insertion.

The gluteus minimus tendon is identified as it inserts into the anterior edge of the greater trochanter and tagged and transected, leaving a 3- to 5-mm cuff for repair (Figs. 10 and 11). The gluteus minimus muscle also has extensive attachments to the superior aspect of the hip capsule that may need to be released. Posteriorly and superiorly, the gluteus medius tendon, measuring 15 to 20 mm in length, is also isolated, tagged, and transected, leaving a 3- to 5-mm cuff (Figs. 10 and 11). It is important to transect and tag these structures sequentially and carefully for subsequent reattachment. The tensor fascia lata and gluteal muscles are held in continuity as a flap and reflected posteriorly to expose the external rotators and sciatic nerve (Fig. 11).

The tendons of the piriformis muscle, obturator internus muscle, and the inferior and superior gemelli muscles are tagged and transected as in the Kocher–Langenbeck approach (Figs. 11 and 12). The tendinous femoral insertion of the gluteus maximus is identified, tagged, and released with a cuff for repair (Fig. 12). It cannot be overemphasized that the

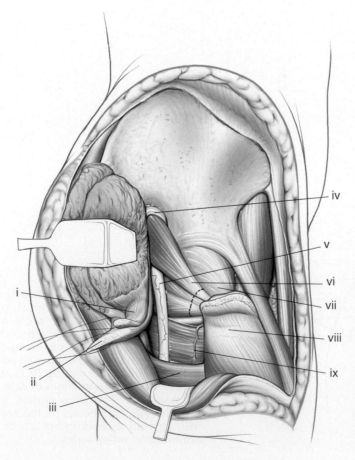

Figure 11. Abductors of the right hip have been tagged and their insertions into the greater trochanter released, allowing their muscle pedicle to be retracted to expose the sciatic nerve. The external rotators also have been marked for release. **i:** Gluteus minimus tendon. **ii:** Gluteus medius tendon. **iii:** Gluteus maximus tendon. **iv:** Superior gluteal neurovascular bundle. **v:** Sciatic nerve. **vi:** Piriformis and conjoint tendons. **vii:** Hip-joint capsule. **viii:** Greater trochanter. **ix:** Quadratus femoris.

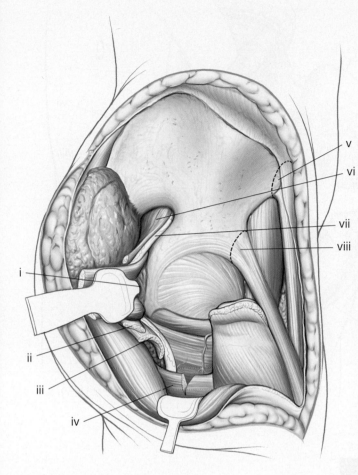

Figure 12. Retraction of right hip external rotator muscles and release of gluteus maximus insertion distally. Medially, the anterior superior and inferior iliac spines have been marked for either release or osteotomy. **i:** Blunt Hohmann in lesser sciatic notch. The conjoint tendons have been positioned between the retractor and the sciatic nerve. **ii:** Gluteus minimus tendon. **iii:** Gluteus medius tendon. **iv:** Partial release of gluteus maximus tendon. **v:** Anterior–superior iliac spine and sartorius muscle origin. **vi:** Piriformis muscle. **vii:** Sciatic nerve. **viii:** Anterior–inferior iliac spine and reflected head of rectus femoris muscle.

quadratus femoris and its blood supply to the femur via the ascending branch of the medial femoral circumflex artery must be preserved. The dissection is now complete (Fig. 1).

The piriformis muscle can be followed toward the greater sciatic notch and the obturator internus muscle to the lesser sciatic notch. A Hohmann or sciatic nerve retractor is then placed into the lesser notch, allowing complete exposure to the posterior column of the acetabulum. The surgeon must ensure that the tendon of the obturator internus maintains its position in the lesser notch between the sciatic nerve and the retractor. Should additional retraction be required, a blunt Hohmann is gently placed into the greater sciatic notch, knowing that there is no structure protecting the nerve. The distal portion of the posterior column can be visualized to the ischial tuberosity, by using sharp dissection of the origin of the hamstring muscles proximally, if necessary.

Although medial exposure of the anterior column is limited by the iliopsoas muscle and the iliopectineal fascia (Figs. 2, 8, and 12), further access to the internal iliac fossa and acetabulum is possible. This is obtained by subperiosteal dissection beneath the sartorius and direct head of the rectus or by osteotomizing the superior and inferior iliac spines, which will, respectively, release these muscles (Figs. 12 and 13). The insertion of the external oblique muscle onto the crest can also be subperiosteally released to reveal the inner table of the pelvis, which is further exposed by stripping off the iliacus muscle with a periosteal elevator. However, extensile exposure of the outer and inner tables of the iliac wing, especially in the presence of local fractures, will create a risk of iliac-bone devascularization.

Although devascularization of the iliac wing is rare, Matta (28) warned of its occurrence, especially in associated both-column fractures. To avoid devascularization of the iliac bone in this case, he suggested leaving the direct head of the rectus femoris and anterior hip capsule attached to the anterior column as a minimum. Also of concern with this exposure is the blood supply to the dome of the acetabulum, which is at risk during dissection of the anterior inferior iliac spine (4).

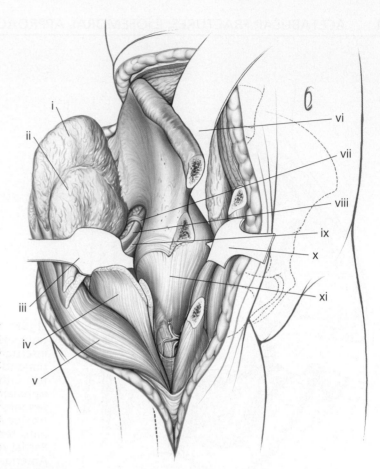

Figure 13. Maximal exposure of right acetabulum via the extended iliofemoral approach. **i:** Gluteus medius muscle. **ii:** Gluteus minimus muscle. **iii:** Blunt Hohmann in lesser sciatic notch. **iv:** Greater trochanter. **v:** Tensor fascia lata muscle. **vi:** Malleable retractor under the iliacus muscle. **vii:** Superior gluteal neurovascular bundle. **viii:** Piriformis muscle. **ix:** Sciatic nerve. **x:** Pointed Hohmann retractor over the anterior capsule of the hip. **xi:** Hip-joint capsule.

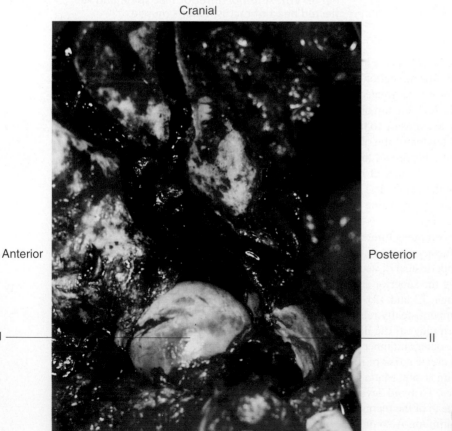

Figure 14. Close-up of acetabular-joint exposure of patient in Figure 1. **i:** Femoral head. **ii:** Loose articular fragments.

Displaced acetabular fractures often tear the hip-joint capsule. If not present, exposure of the acetabular articular surface can be obtained with a marginal capsulotomy, leaving a cuff of tissue for repair. Once the hip joint is exposed, distraction with either a Schanz screw placed into the femoral head or a femoral distractor will facilitate visualization (Figs. 1 and 14). This is important to evaluate the articular reduction, rule out any intraarticular hardware, and remove any incarcerated osteochondral fragments.

Once the exposure of the extended iliofemoral approach has been completed, the fracture can be reduced according to the preoperative plan. It is important to keep the soft-tissue flaps moist with wet sponges and periodic irrigation throughout the procedure.

Reduction Technique

Several regions of bone are optimal for screw placement. These include the iliac crest, the superogluteal ridge, the greater sciatic buttress (above the sciatic notch and to the anterior–inferior iliac spine), the anterior column, and the posterior column (30). Extra-long screws, ranging from 50 to 120 mm, should be available.

In a transverse fracture, there may be rotational malalignment of the inferior portion of the acetabulum. In the T-type fracture patterns, the anterior and posterior fragments may be separate and both columns become displaced and malrotated. Usually the anterior segment has medial displacement of its inferior portion so that the radius of curvature of the acetabulum is greater than that of the femoral head (31). In both transverse and T-type acetabular fractures, reduction is achieved with a pelvic-reduction clamp attached to 4.5-mm screws, placed proximal and distal to the posterior-column fracture. The pelvic-reduction clamp initially allows distraction to debride of the fracture surfaces, and then facilitates manipulative reduction of the fracture. A bone spreader in the fracture site can also facilitate exposure of the fracture or the joint (Fig. 15A). Additional control of rotation is provided by a Schanz screw placed into the ischium and a pelvic clamp in the greater sciatic notch.

For the reduction of the T-type and more-comminuted variants, the anterior column should be reduced first with respect to the residual acetabular "roof" portion of the ilium (31). The adequacy of reduction of the posterior column can be visualized by direct assessment of the articular surface and also with digital palpation through the greater and lesser sciatic notches.

Before definitive reduction, a gliding hole can be inserted into the proximal aspect of the posterior column from superior to inferior (Fig. 15B), assuring the position of the gliding hole in the middle of the posterior column.

A gliding hole can also be inserted from the lateral aspect of the iliac wing into the anterior column, distal and medial to the articular surface. Generally, this requires the insertion of a lag screw 6 cm proximal to the superior aspect of the articular surface, and 2 cm posterior to the gluteal ridge. The lag screw is then angled from posterosuperior to anteroinferior directly down the superior pubic ramus to secure the anterior column of the acetabulum. In large individuals, this can be accomplished with a 4.5-mm cortical screw. In women and small individuals, a 3.5-millimeter cortical screw is preferred. Care must be taken to assure that this screw remains extraarticular and also does not penetrate the anterior aspect of the superior ramus in the area of the iliopectineal eminence where the femoral vessels are in close proximity. The use of intraoperative fluoroscopy for the insertion of this screw is highly recommended.

Proper placement of pelvic-reduction forceps with respect to the plane of the fracture and geometry of the osseous surfaces is crucial for an adequate reduction (30). A variety of instruments are available to facilitate reduction. These include narrow curved osteotomes, bone hooks, ball spike pushers, "King-Tong" and "Queen-Tong" forceps, and the Farabeuf and pointed reduction clamps (Fig. 15C).

To ensure an anatomic reduction of the acetabulum, the surgeon should work from the periphery toward the acetabulum (Fig. 16), by reducing each fracture fragment sequentially. Once the iliac wing is stabilized with lag screws, by 3.5-mm laterally applied reconstruction plates, or both, the posterior column is reduced to the iliac wing with direct visualization of the acetabular articular surface.

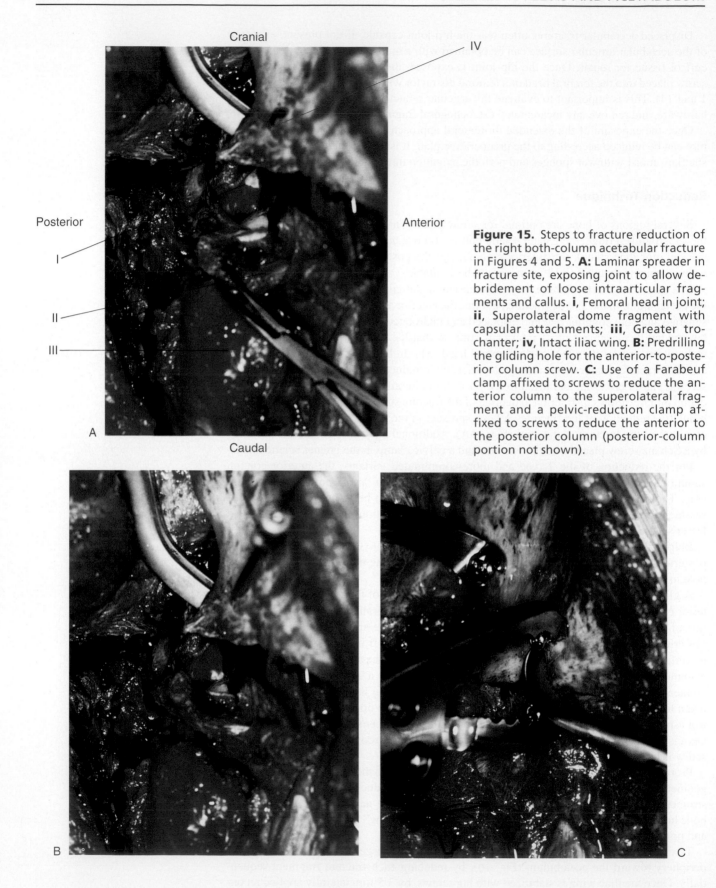

Figure 15. Steps to fracture reduction of the right both-column acetabular fracture in Figures 4 and 5. **A:** Laminar spreader in fracture site, exposing joint to allow debridement of loose intraarticular fragments and callus. **i**, Femoral head in joint; **ii**, Superolateral dome fragment with capsular attachments; **iii**, Greater trochanter; **iv**, Intact iliac wing. **B:** Predrilling the gliding hole for the anterior-to-posterior column screw. **C:** Use of a Farabeuf clamp affixed to screws to reduce the anterior column to the superolateral fragment and a pelvic-reduction clamp affixed to screws to reduce the anterior to the posterior column (posterior-column portion not shown).

Cranial

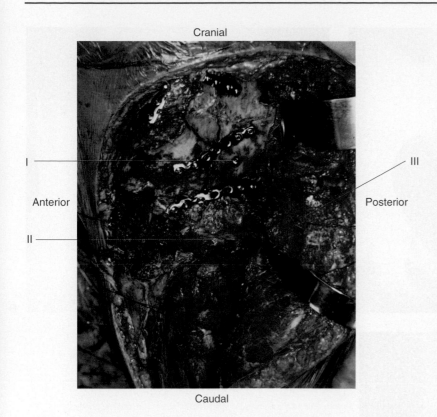

I

Anterior

II

III

Posterior

Caudal

Figure 16. Reconstruction of comminuted left both-column acetabular fracture from Figures 1 and 14. Reconstruction proceeds centripetally from the periphery. **i**: Posterior to anterior column lag screw. **ii**: Greater trochanter. **iii**: Abductor muscles and tensor fascia lata.

The posterior-column lag screw and 3.5-mm reconstruction plate fixation is utilized for transverse and T-type fractures. The anterior column is then reduced to the intact posterior column. This can be accomplished with anterior to posterior 4.5-mm lag screws inserted from the anterior–superior spine into the sciatic buttress, or anterior-column lag screws from the lateral aspect of the iliac wing as described previously, or both. The adequacy of the reduction is assessed, both by direct visualization of the acetabulum, with finger palpation of the greater and lesser sciatic notches and quadrilateral plate, and, if necessary, in the internal iliac fossa. The use of fluoroscopy is essential to assure the adequacy of reduction and the position of the fixation (Fig. 17).

Closure

Because intraarticular hardware can lead to rapid chondrolysis, it is important to confirm hardware position before closure. This is best achieved radiographically by using intraoperative fluoroscopic Judet views (especially the obturator oblique) and clinically by rotating the hip back and forth while a finger is placed along the quadrilateral surface, to feel for any crepitus.

At the completion of osteosynthesis, suction drains are placed along the external surface of the iliac wing in the vicinity of the posterior column and vastus lateralis muscle. If the internal iliac fossa has been exposed, a third drain is placed here. All drains should exit anteriorly.

The hip capsule is repaired first, followed by reattachment of the tendinous insertions of the short external rotators to the greater trochanter through drill holes, and the femoral insertions of the gluteus maximus. Next the trochanteric insertions of the gluteus medius and minimus muscles are repaired, by using five or six sutures for each tendon, as recommended by Letournel (22). Finally the tensor fascia lata and gluteal muscles are reattached to their origins on the iliac crest.

If a medial exposure has been performed, then the origins of the sartorius and direct head of the rectus femoris muscles are reattached through drill holes (or lag screws if osteotomies have been performed).

Finally the fascia overlying the tensor fascia lata muscle is repaired, followed by placement of a subcutaneous suction drain and skin closure.

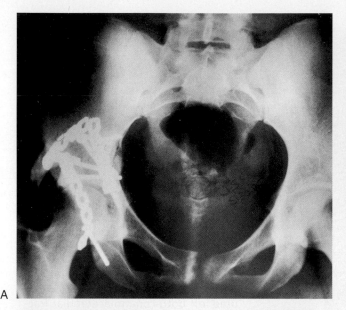

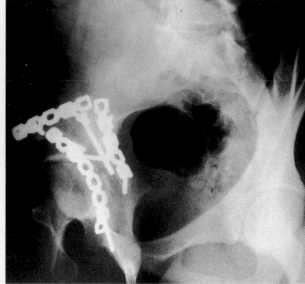

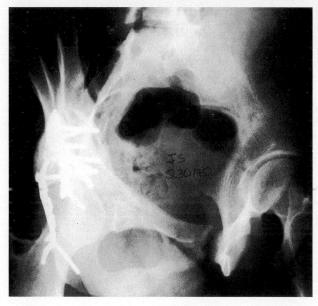

Figure 17. Patient from Figures 4 and 5 at 1-year follow-up, showing congruent reduction and maintenance of joint space. **A:** Anteroposterior pelvis. **B:** Iliac oblique view. **C:** Obturator oblique view.

POSTOPERATIVE MANAGEMENT

Postoperatively, patients are maintained on intravenous cefazolin for 48 to 72 hours. Our postoperative anticoagulation regimen includes six weeks of warfarin in conjunction with compression boots. Heterotopic ossification prophylaxis is also mandatory, preferably with indomethacin, 25 mg orally 3 times each day for 6 to 8 weeks. Drains are not removed until output has tapered to 10 to 20 ml per 8-hour shift, usually over the first 48 to 72 hours.

We stress early mobilization during the postoperative period, allowing patients to sit at the edges of their beds, and dangle their legs, and progress to chairs within the first 24 to 48 hours after surgery. We do not use continuous passive motion (CPM) as we have not had difficulty regaining hip motion in this patient population.

After the removal of drains, patients are allowed toe-touch weight bearing up to 20 pounds with crutches and strengthening exercises, along with gait training, initiated by the physical therapist. However, weight bearing is not advanced, and active abduction, any adduction, and flexion of the hip past 90 degrees are avoided for 6 to 8 weeks.

Acetabular fractures with a concomitant neurologic injury can pose a difficult rehabilitation problem because of lack of muscle activity or neurogenic pain. These frequently require consultation with a neurologist and the pain-management service.

We routinely obtain postoperative roentgenograms (anteroposterior pelvis and 45-degree oblique Judet views) and a CT scan critically to assess the fracture reduction and hardware position. The CT scan is usually obtained on postoperative day 5, just before discharge, which typically occurs on postoperative days 5 to 7. At the time of discharge, home physical therapy should be arranged.

During the first follow-up visit at 2 weeks, staples or sutures are removed. At 6-week follow-up, new roentgenograms are obtained, and generally, the abduction/adduction/fixation precautions are discontinued. The patient returns at 8 to 10 weeks, and depending on the roentgenographic findings, progression to full weight bearing is allowed, as tolerated, over the ensuing month. An aggressive outpatient rehabilitation program should be initiated at this stage.

At 3 months after surgery, the patient is reevaluated and should be weight bearing as tolerated with a cane. In the absence of any contraindications, rehabilitation becomes more aggressive, with strengthening and weights, and the patient is followed up at monthly intervals for a period of 3 more months. At 6 months, the patient should be back to all activities. From this point, there should be additional evaluation with radiographs at 1 year after surgery, and then annual follow-up visits.

Rowe and Lowell (37) reviewed 93 acetabular fractures treated nonoperatively and noted poor results for all 10 patients in whom the weight-bearing dome was not anatomically reduced. After the pioneer work of Letournel (22) and others (1,12,19,25,27), many investigators have shown that long-term clinical outcomes correlate closely with the quality of reduction achieved during surgery. In his review of 569 acetabular fractures treated within 3 weeks of injury, Letournel (22) achieved an anatomic reduction (a maximum of 1 mm of displacement on any of three views) in 74% of cases, with 82% of these patients having very good clinical outcomes at a follow-up of as much as 33 years. Of the 26% with an imperfectly reduced acetabulum, very good results were obtained in 54% of cases if the femoral head was centered under the dome, and only in 23% of cases in which there was residual subluxation of the femoral head.

Kebaish et al. (19), in a retrospective review of 90 displaced acetabular fractures, showed superior long-term results in their patients when the articular surface was restored to within 4 mm. In a similar retrospective study, Matta et al. (27) demonstrated satisfactory clinical outcome if the femoral head remained congruous within the weight-bearing dome and if articular-surface incongruity did not exceed 3 mm. However, in a recent prospective study, Matta (25) suggested that 3 mm is probably not acceptable. He reported that an anatomic reduction was achieved in 71% of 262 acetabular fractures, with 83% of these patients having good or excellent outcomes at an average follow-up of 6 years. Of the 29% with an imperfectly reduced acetabulum, good or excellent results were obtained in 68% of cases if the defect measured 2 to 3 mm, and only 50% if more than 3 mm. The most predictive initial factor for a poor result was damage to the femoral head.

Matta's (25) more recent results are in agreement with Helfet and Schmeling (12), who previously noted that an articular step-off of more than 2 mm or a gap of more than 3 mm was associated with a fourfold increase in joint-space narrowing at early follow-up. Alonso et al. (1) noted an 81% rate of good or excellent results in 21 patients treated with an extended iliofemoral approach, which in all cases achieved a reduction within 2 mm. Finally, Malkani et al. (23) and Hak et al. (6) recently used cadaver models further to support 2 mm or less as the criterion for an acceptable reduction.

COMPLICATIONS

Complications after operative treatment of acetabular fractures are best divided into three groups: intraoperative, early, and late. Intraoperative complications include neurovascular injury, malreduction, articular penetration of hardware, and death. Early postoperative complications include DVT, pulmonary embolism (PE), skin necrosis, infection, loss of reduction, arthritis, and death. The late group includes heterotopic ossification (HO), chondrolysis, avascular necrosis, and posttraumatic arthrosis.

Iatrogenic sciatic nerve injury or worsening of a preexisting deficit is a significant problem. Patients at increased risk include those with preoperative sciatic nerve compromise and those with fracture patterns that involve the posterior wall or column (11). The most significant factor in reducing the incidence of iatrogenic sciatic nerve injury appears to be the experience of the surgical team.

Letournel (22) initially reported an 18.4% incidence of postoperative iatrogenic sciatic nerve injury by using the Kocher–Langenbeck approach, which he subsequently reduced to 3.3%. However, he also noted that none of his 114 patients treated with an extensile approach developed this complication (22). Matta (27) initially reported a 9% incidence of iatrogenic nerve palsy, which he reduced to 3.5% (25) with further experience (3.4% of 59 extended iliofemoral approaches). Furthermore, only two of nine neurologic injuries involved the sciatic nerve. Alonso et al. (1) observed a postoperative sciatic nerve palsy in only one of their 21 patients treated with an extended iliofemoral approach. Importantly, the use of intraoperative sciatic nerve monitoring by using SSEPs has reduced the incidence of iatrogenic sciatic nerve injury to 2% (11,14). This risk is further lessened by the addition of intraoperative monitoring of motor pathways (9).

Superior Gluteal Neurovascular Injury

Superior gluteal vessel injury is difficult to diagnose and is caused by either the fracture or an iatrogenic insult during surgery (2,16). Letournel (22) reported an incidence of 3.5% in his series. This potentially lethal occurrence is more likely with severe displacement of the sciatic notch (e.g., high transverse fractures with marked medial rotation; 2,29). Acutely, hemodynamic instability with an arterial injury must be addressed during the initial evaluation and resuscitation, usually with arteriography and embolization. However, once the bleeding has been stopped, there may be concerns as to the viability of the muscle flap.

Because the intended iliofemoral approach completely detaches the gluteal muscles from the iliac wing (Fig. 1), the superior gluteal vessels are the only blood to supply to the flap. If this is compromised, them complete ischemic necrosis in theory is likely. Mears and Rubash (31) developed their "triradiate" approach partly in response to reports of flap necrosis following the extended iliofemoral approach; however, it has not been established whether superior gluteal injury is to blame in these cases (29). In fact, the incidence of this complication is relatively low. In over 400 acetabular fractures treated with an extended iliofemoral approach by Letournel, Matta, Mast, and Martimbeau, there have been no reports of abductor flap necrosis (22). Alonso did not observe this complication using either an extended iliofemoral or a triradiate approach in 59 cases of complex acetabular fracture (1).

Furthermore, massive abductor necrosis resulting from a superior gluteal artery injury combined with an extended iliofemoral approach was postulated based on early animal and cadaver studies alone (35,42). A recent canine study by Tabor et al. (41) showed that although necrosis of muscle and loss of mass does occur after an extended iliofemoral approach in the presence of gluteal vessel injury, this does not appear to be functionally significant. In their study, none of the gluteal muscle flaps sustained complete ischemic necrosis. Thus, some collateral flow to the abductor muscles must be present and may increase in the presence of superior gluteal vessel injury.

Letournel (22) reported a 2.3% incidence of in-hospital death after operative fixation of acetabular fractures, with the majority of the deaths occurring in patients older than 60 years. Although DVT probably plays a major role, its true incidence after an acetabular fracture is unknown. However, patients with lower extremity trauma are particularly at risk. Kudsk et al. (20) demonstrated a 60% incidence of silent DVT by venography in patients with multiple trauma immobilized 10 days or more. Geerts et al. (4) in a prospective study also demonstrated a 60% incidence of DVT in patients with primary lower extremity orthopaedic injuries. Letournel (22) reported a 3% incidence of clinically evident DVT with four fatal and eight minor pulmonary emboli in a series of 569 patients, despite the majority receiving anticoagulant prophylaxis. By using a pre- and postoperative protocol, Stickney and Helfet (40) significantly decreased their incidence of DVT. Improved detection of venous thromboembolism by using magnetic resonance venography also has led to a lower incidence of pulmonary embolism (33).

The incidence of infection has been reported to be as high as 9% but probably is between 4% and 5% (1,13,22,25,28,37). Matta (25) noted a 5% incidence of postoperative wound infection in 262 patients. Of 59 extended iliofemoral approaches, five (8.5%) developed deep infection. Letournel (22) reported 24 postoperative infections in 569 patients (4.2%) with nine superficial, ten early deep, and five delayed or late infections. Furthermore, he observed skin necrosis in 1.8% (10.2% of extended iliofemoral approached) and hematomas in 6.7% of cases (22). To minimize wound problems, he advocated the use of prophylactic antibiotics, the use of multiple suction drains in all recesses to prevent hematoma formation, surgical evacuation of hematomas, and if present, debridement of the Morel–Lavalle lesion over the greater trochanter.

The most common complication after the operative fixation of acetabular fractures is HO (Fig. 18), with an incidence ranging from 18% to 90% (3,18,22,25,32,41). However, functional limitation in patients with HO occurs in only 5% to 10% of cases (1,28,30,36). Nevertheless, heterotopic bone formation is more common and severe with the extended iliofemoral approach because of stripping of the external surface of the iliac wing (1,3,22,25,32,41). Letournel (22) reported its occurrence in 46% of his extended iliofemoral approaches performed within four months of injury, as compared with a 21% incidence in 635 other approaches. Prior to his use of prophylaxis, these rates were respectively 69% and 24%. Matta (25) noted a significant loss of motion in 20% and Letournel observed severe HO (Brooker III and IV) in 35% of patients treated with this approach within three weeks of injury. Both indomethacin (22,32) and low dose radiation therapy (single or multiple fractions; 3,22,39) have been shown to decrease the incidence of heterotopic ossification in patients with acetabular fractures. However, Alonso et al. (1) have reported a rate as high as 86% with Brooker class III or IV ossification present in 14% of their patients, even after prophylaxis with indomethacin.

The incidence of avascular necrosis (AVN) after operative treatment of acetabular fractures has generally ranged from 3% to 9% (22,25,27), with the majority of cases identified between 3 and 18 months after surgery (22). However, Letournel (22) has noted an increased incidence of AVN of the femoral head in cases presenting after three weeks, and

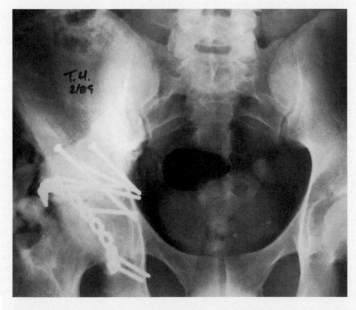

Figure 18. Anteroposterior pelvis of patient in Figure 3, at 5 months after extended iliofemoral approach. Significant (Brooker grade III) heterotopic ossification is present in the soft tissues of the right hip.

those associated with a posterior fracture/dislocation. In all probability, the fate of the femoral head is determined at the time of the injury.

The most important factor responsible for successful long-term clinical outcome after surgical fixation of acetabular fractures is the quality of the reduction. The incidence of posttraumatic osteoarthritis (OA) is greatest in patients with articular-surface incongruity or residual subluxation of the hip joint (8,19,22,27,34,37,41). After a perfect reduction within three weeks of injury, Letournel (22) noted OA in only 10.2% of his patients, as opposed to 37.5% with an imperfect reduction. Interestingly, when treatment was delayed past this time, these rates were respectively 24% and 23% (22). Loss of reduction also can occur during the postoperative period. This is more likely in elderly patients with osteopenic bone, in which it is important adequately to buttress the fractures (10).

RECOMMENDED READING

1. Alonso, J.E., Davila, R., Bradley, E.: Extended iliofemoral versus triradiate approaches in management of associated acetabular fractures. *Clin. Orthop.*, 305:81–87, 1994
2. Bosse, M.J., Poka, A., Reinert, C.M., Brumback, R.J., Bathon, H., Burgess, A.T.: Pre-operative angiographic assessment of the superior gluteal artery in acetabular fractures requiring extensive surgical exposures. *J. Orthop. Trauma*, 2:303–307, 1988.
3. Bosse, M.J., Poka, A., Reinert, C.M., Ellwanger, F., Slawson, R., McDevitt, E.R.: Heterotopic ossification as a complication of acetabular fractures. *J. Bone Joint Surg. [Am]*, 70:1231–1237, 1988.
4. Chapman, M.W.: Effect of surgical approaches on the blood supply to the acetabulum. Presented at the 1st Annual International Consensus on Surgery of the Pelvis and Acetabulum, Pittsburgh, Pennsylvania, October 11–15, 1992.
5. Geerts, W.H., Code, K.I., Jay, R.M., Chen, E., Szalai, J.P.: A prospective study of venous thromboembolism after major trauma. *N. Engl. J. Med.*, 331:1601–1606, 1994.
6. Hak, D.J., Olson, S.A., Hamel, A.J., Bay, B.K., Sharkey, N.A.: Consequences of transverse acetabular fracture malreduction on load transmission across the hip joint. Presented at the 12th Annual Meeting of the Orthopaedic Trauma Association, Boston, September 27–29, 1996.
7. Hak, D.J., Olsen, S.A., Matta, J.M.: Management of the Morel-Lavalle lesion. Presented at The Third Annual International Consensus on Surgery of the Pelvis and Acetabulum. Pittsburgh, October 5–11, 1996.
8. Heeg, M., Oostvogel, H.J.M., Klasen, H.J.: Conservative treatment of acetabular fractures: the role of the weight-bearing dome and anatomic reduction in the ultimate results. *J. Trauma*, 27(5):555–559, 1987.
9. Helfet, D.L., Anand, N., Malkani, A.L., et al.: Intra-operative monitoring of motor pathways during operative fixation of acute acetabular fractures. *J. Orthop. Trauma*, 11:2–6, 1997.
10. Helfet, D.L., Borrelli, J. Jr., Dipasquale, T., Sanders, R.: Stabilization of acetabular fractures in elderly patients. *J. Bone Joint Surg. [Am]*, 74:753–765, 1992.
11. Helfet, D.L., Hissa, E.A., Sergay, S., Mast, J.W.: Somatosensory evoked potential monitoring in the surgical management of acute acetabular fractures. *J. Orthop. Trauma*, 5:161–166, 1991.
12. Helfet, D.L., and Schmeling, G.J.: Management of acute displaced complex acetabular fractures using indirect reduction techniques and limited surgical approaches. *Orthop. Trans.*, 15:833–834, 1991.
13. Helfet, D.L., and Schmeling, G.J.: Management of complex acetabular fractures through single nonextensile exposures. *Clin. Orthop.*, 305:55–68, 1994.
14. Helfet, D.L., and Schmeling, G.J.: Somatosensory evoked potential monitoring in the surgical treatment of acute, displaced acetabular fractures: results of a prospective study. *Clin. Orthop.*, 301:213–220, 1994.
15. Johnson, E.E., Eckardt, J.J., Letournel, E.: Extrinsic femoral artery occlusion following internal fixation of an acetabular fracture: a case report. *Clin. Orthop.*, 217:209–213, 1987.
16. Johnson, E.E., Matta, J.M., Mast, J.W., Letournel, E.: Delayed reconstruction of acetabular fractures 21-120 days following injury. *Clin. Orthop.*, 305:20–30, 1994.
17. Judet, R., Judet, J., Letournel, E.: Fractures of the acetabulum: classification and surgical approaches for open reduction: preliminary report. *J. Bone Joint Surg. [Am]*, 46:1615–1675, 1964.
18. Kaempffe, F.A., Bone, L., Borden, J.R.: Open reduction and internal fixation of acetabular fractures: heterotopic ossification and other complications of treatment. *J. Orthop. Trauma*, 5(4):439–445, 1991.
19. Kebaish, A.S., Roy, A., Rennie, W.: Displaced acetabular fractures: long-term follow-up. *J. Trauma*, 31(11):1539–1542, 1991.
20. Kudsk, K.A., Fabian, T.C., Baum, S., Gold, M., Mangiante, E., Voeller, G.: Silent deep vein thrombosis in immobilized multiple trauma patients. *Am. J. Surg.*, 158(6):5151–5159, 1989.
21. Letournel, E.: Acetabular fractures: classification and management. *Clin. Orthop.*, 151:81–106, 1980.
22. Letournel, E., and Judet, R.: *Fractures of the acetabulum*. 2nd ed. Springer-Verlag, New York, 1993.
23. Malkani, A.L., Voor, M.J., Rennirt, G., Helfet, D., Pedersen, D., Brown, T.: Increased peak contact pressure following incongruent reduction of transverse acetabular fractures: a cadaveric model. Presented at the 12th Annual Meeting of the Orthopaedic Trauma Association, Boston, Massachusetts, September 27–29, 1996.
24. Martimbeau, C.L.: Effort to standardize surgical approaches in acetabular fractures. *Orthop. Rev.*, 15:39, 1986.
25. Matta, J.M.: Fractures of the acetabulum: accuracy of reduction and clinical results. *J. Bone Joint Surg. [Am]*, 78:1632–1645, 1996.
26. Matta, J.M.: Operative indications and choice of surgical approach for fractures of the acetabulum. *Tech. Orthop.*, 1:13, 1986.

27. Matta, J.M., Anderson, L.M., Epstein, H.C., Hendricks, P.: Fractures of the acetabulum: a retrospective analysis. *Clin. Orthop.*, 205:230–240, 1986.
28. Matta, J.M., and Merritt, P.O.: Displaced acetabular fractures. *Clin. Orthop.*, 230:83–97, 1988.
29. Mayo, K.A.: Surgical approaches to the acetabulum. *Tech. Orthop.*, 4(4):24–35, 1990.
30. Mears, D.C., and Gordon, R.G.: Internal fixation of acetabular fractures. *Tech. Orthop.*, 4(4):36–51, 1990.
31. Mears, D.C., and Rubash, H.E.: Extensile exposure of the pelvis. *Contemp. Orthop.*, 6:21–31, 1983.
32. Moed, B.R., and Maxey, J.: The effect of indomethacin on heterotopic ossification following acetabular fracture surgery. *J. Orthop. Trauma*, 3(2):172, 1989.
33. Montgomery, K.D., Potter, H.G., Helfet, D.L.: Magnetic resonance venography to evaluate the deep venous system of the pelvis in patients who have an acetabular fracture. *J. Bone Joint Surg. [Am]*, 77:1639-1649, 1995.
34. Pennal, G.F., Davidson, J., Garside, H., Plewes, J.: Results of treatment of acetabular fractures. *Clin. Orthop.*, 151:115-123, 1980.
35. Reilly, M.C., Matta, J.M., Olson, S., Tornetta, P.: The superior gluteal artery in the extended ilio-femoral approach. Presented at the 12th Annual Meeting of the Orthopaedic Trauma Association, Boston, Massachusetts, September 27–29, 1996.
36. Routt, M.L. Jr., and Swiontkowski, M.F.: Operative treatment of complex acetabular fractures: combined anterior and posterior exposures during the same procedure. *J. Bone Joint Surg. [Am]*, 72:897–904, 1990.
37. Rowe, C.R., and Lowell, J.D.: Prognosis of fractures of the acetabulum. *J. Bone Joint Surg. [Am]*, 43:30–59, 1961.
38. Senegas, J., Liorzou, G., Yates, M.: Complex acetabular fractures: a transtrochanteric lateral surgical approach. *Clin. Orthop.*, 151:107–114, 1980.
39. Skura, D.S., and Buchsbaum, S.: Prophylactic low-dose post-operative irradiation for the prevention of heterotopic ossification in acetabular fractures. Presented at the 59th Annual Meeting of the American Academy of Orthopaedic Surgeons, Washington DC, February 20–25, 1992.
40. Stickney, J., and Helfet, D.L.: Deep vein thrombosis prevention in orthopaedic trauma patients. Presented at the 58th Annual Meeting of the American Academy of Orthopaedic Surgeons, Anaheim, California, March 7–12, 1991.
41. Tabor, O.B., Bosse, M.J., Greene, K.G., et al.: The effects of the abductor muscles of surgical approaches for acetabular fractures associated with gluteal vascular injury. Presented at the 12th Annual Meeting of the Orthopaedic Trauma Association, Boston, Massachusetts, September 27–29, 1996.
42. Tile, M., Kellam, J.F., Joyce, M.: Fractures of the acetabulum, classification, management protocol and results of treatment. *J. Bone Joint Surg. [Br]*, 67:173, 1985.
43. Vrahas, M., Gordon, R.G., Mears, B.C., Kreiger, B., Sclahass, R.J.: Intra-operative somatosensory evoked potential monitoring of pelvic and acetabular fractures. *J. Orthop. Trauma*, 6(1):50–58, 1992.

Master Techniques in Orthopaedic Surgery,
FRACTURES, edited by D. A. Wiss,
Lippincott–Raven Publishers, Philadelphia © 1998.

42

Acetabular Fractures: Triradiate and Modified Triradiate Approaches

Dana C. Mears and Mark D. MacLeod

INDICATIONS/CONTRAINDICATIONS

The triradiate approach (TRI) allows visualization of the entire articular surface of the acetabulum, the adjacent lateral ilium to the gluteal tubercle posteriorly, the entire posterior acetabular column, the anterior column to the medial eminence, and the inner pelvic wall including the internal iliac fossa and the sacroiliac joint (Fig. 1). The TRI is indicated for selected acute acetabular fractures in which an extensile approach is necessary to adequately address significant displacement of both the anterior and posterior acetabular columns. These include transverse and T-type fractures and certain associated transverse–posterior wall, anterior column–posterior hemitransverse, and both-column fractures.

If the acetabular fracture is more than 2 weeks old, the need for an extensile approach such as TRI increases. Another indication for the TRI is a fracture of the posterior wall and column in which visualization is impaired because of obesity or muscularity of the patient. In this scenario, even a limited anterior-limb dissection and greater trochanteric osteotomy increases visualization. In cases in which an ipsilateral sacroiliac-joint injury complicates a transverse or T-type fracture, both injuries may be approached via a triradiate exposure.

Apart from acetabular fractures, the TRI is a highly effective approach for a periacetabular osteotomy. A TRI may be used as an anterolateral, direct lateral, or posterior approach to the hip for reconstructive procedures such as an arthrodesis, excisional arthroplasty, or total hip arthroplasty. In complex revision hip arthroplasty, in which extensive reconstruction of the acetabulum is necessary, the TRI provides excellent exposure.

Most single-column fractures may be satisfactorily visualized through a nonextensile ap-

---

D. C. Mears, B.M., B.CH., PH.D.: Department of Orthopaedic Surgery, Albany Medical College, Albany, New York 12208.

M. D. MacLeod, M.D., F.R.C.S.C.: Department of Surgery, Division of Orthopaedic Surgery, University of Western Ontario, London, Ontario, Canada N6C 4V3.

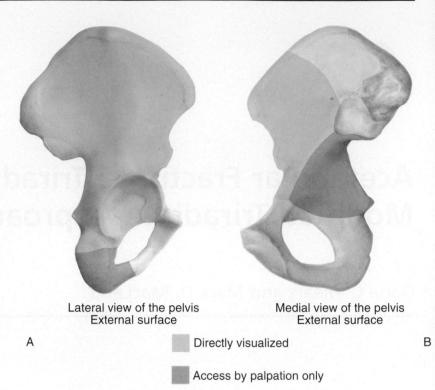

Figure 1. A, B: Classic triradiate incision allows direct visualization of the areas outlined in red and includes the entire articular surface, if a capsulotomy is performed and the femoral head is distracted. The area outlined in yellow can be palpated but not directly visualized. Division of the sacrospinous ligament from the ischial spine facilitates palpation of the lower half of the area outlined in yellow.

Lateral view of the pelvis
External surface

Medial view of the pelvis
External surface

A

B

Directly visualized

Access by palpation only

proach. Generally, the Kocher–Langenbeck is preferred for the posterior column and the ilioinguinal (IL) for the anterior column. Whenever feasible, an associated fracture pattern is visualized through an exposure that causes minimal morbidity and periacetabular devascularization. The TRI and other extensile incisions are not recommended in elderly patients, in whom a deep postoperative wound infection seems to be a frequent complication. The majority of complications associated with the TRI are a result of devascularization; a modified TRI (MTRI) reduces the amount of devascularization and the incidence of complications.

Associated disruptions of the anterior column that are medial to the medial eminence and the external iliac vessels are not accessible by either the TRI or MTRI. The use of either approach is also contraindicated where this necessitates dissection through an area of significant soft-tissue abrasion or infection. In some of these cases, an ilioinguinal or Kocher–Langenbeck approach may permit an exposure of the fracture through intact skin.

PREOPERATIVE PLANNING

A careful examination of the patient is essential. Before an acetabular exposure, the condition of the skin in the region of the incision is evaluated for features such as abrasions, contusions, or rarely an open fracture. Special attention is given to a contusion with massive ecchymosis in the lateral thigh, known as the Morel–Lavellé lesion, which results in extensive subcutaneous fat necrosis. Tenderness, extensive swelling, and ecchymosis within the buttock may represent a traumatic injury to the inferior gluteal vascular bundle. Where the inferior gluteal vessels are occluded and a TRI or an extended iliofemoral approach (EIF) is undertaken, ischemic necrosis of the abductor muscles may ensue. The necrosis occurs as a result of the combined traumatic injury to the vessels and release of the abductor muscular origins. Although a TRI does not necessitate as extensive a release of the origins of the abductor muscles as does an EIF, in patients with clinical features consistent with a traumatic injury to the gluteal vessels, preoperative angiography is recommended to determine the patency of the inferior gluteal artery. If the vessel is not patent, an alternative surgical approach is recommended.

The assessment of the presurgical neurologic status of the ipsilateral lower extremity is a crucial part of the preoperative evaluation. The integrity of the sciatic, femoral, and lateral femoral cutaneous nerves (LFCNs) is determined with documentation of any corresponding deficits. Frequently, subtle injury of the peroneal division of the sciatic nerve accompanies a posterior fracture–dislocation of the hip. Features such as minor hypoesthesia of the first web space in the foot or slight weakness of the long-toe extensors is significant. Once the sciatic nerve has been traumatized, subsequent intraoperative manipulation of or traction on the nerve may lead to further neurologic deficits.

Thorough preoperative radiographic imaging is necessary to determine the geometry of the fracture. The principal plain radiographs are an anteroposterior (AP) pelvic view and 45-degree obturator and iliac oblique views. Supplemental views of the pelvic ring, including inlet and outlet views, are indicated if there is clinical or radiographic suspicion of an associated pelvic-ring injury. A two-dimensional computed tomography (CT) scan (2D CT) with a minimum of five cuts at 2-cm intervals through the sacroiliac joints, first sacral body, acetabular dome, the center of the hip joint, and the symphysis is helpful to determine the extent of the injury, particularly to the articular surfaces of the acetabulum and the femoral head. The presence of marginal impaction of the acetabulum; impaction, abrasion, or fracture of the femoral head; an intraarticular fragment; or a minimally displaced fracture line is often better or solely seen on the CT scan.

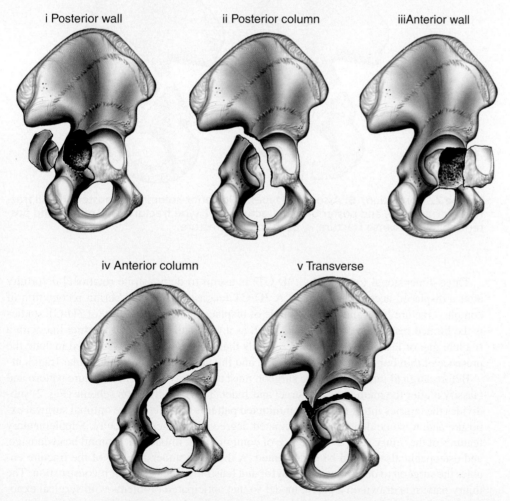

Figure 2. Classification of acetabular fractures of Letournel and Judet. **A:** Simple types: i, Posterior-wall fracture; ii, Posterior-column fracture; iii, Anterior-wall fracture; iv, Anterior-column fracture; v, Transverse fracture.

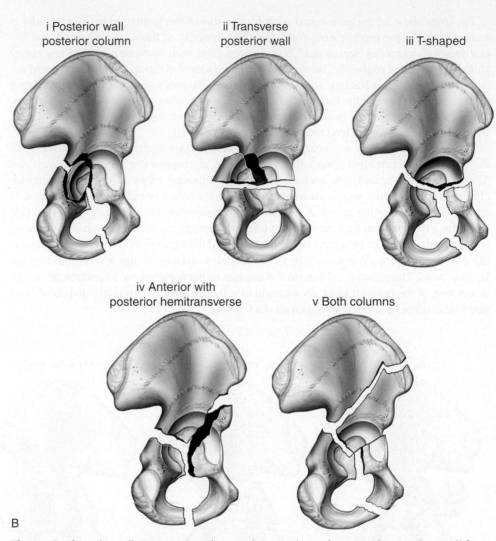

i Posterior wall
posterior column

ii Transverse
posterior wall

iii T-shaped

iv Anterior with
posterior hemitransverse

v Both columns

B

Figure 2. *(continued)* **B:** Associated types: i, Posterior-column and posterior-wall fracture; ii, Transverse and posterior-wall fracture; iii, T-type fracture; iv, Anterior and posterior hemitransverse fracture; v, Both-column fracture.

Three-dimensional tomography (3D CT) is useful to demonstrate rotational deformity after a displaced acetabular fracture. A 3D-CT reconstruction may permit recognition of complex fracture lines and the magnitude of displacement. One liability of 3D-CT studies is the limited resolution of fine details such as a minimally displaced fracture line with a fracture gap of less than 3 mm. Other details that may not be well visualized include the presence of thin bone, marginal impaction, and the presence of an intraarticular fragment.

Before surgical intervention, the surgeon must accurately define the fracture pattern and classify it after the method of Letournel and Judet. This classification scheme (Fig. 2) subdivides the injuries into simple or comminuted patterns that dictate the optimal surgical exposure and, to some degree, the anticipated degree of technical difficulty. Supplementary features of the injury such as the degree of comminution, impaction, femoral head damage, and osteopenia also should be documented. A thorough understanding of the fracture enables the surgeon to determine the need for and feasibility of acetabular reconstruction. The injury pattern is drawn on a pelvic model so that anticipated problems with surgical exposure, fracture reduction, and fixation can be defined and addressed. Fixation plates of appropriate length can be precontoured to the appropriate surfaces of the posterior and anterior columns of a life-sized pelvic model. Such preoperative preparation may decrease operating time.

SURGERY

Under general or spinal anesthesia, the patient is placed in the lateral decubitus position on a radiolucent graphite composite operating table (Fig. 3). The contralateral hip and knee are maintained in an extended position to facilitate intraoperative rotation from a semisupine to a near-prone position. This "floppy lateral" position is maintained and constrained by a suction beanbag that is evacuated initially as the patient is moved from the semisupine to the near-prone position (Fig. 4A–C). Bony prominences are padded, particularly the downside fibular head and lateral malleolus. Fixed skeletal traction is not used, as it limits movement of the limb. A Foley catheter is routinely inserted.

Preparation and draping are performed so that the surgical field includes the entire ipsilateral lower extremity and the lower trunk from the anterior to the posterior midline, extending superiorly to the level of the umbilicus. Continuous intraoperative somatosensory evoked potentials (SSEPs) and electromyogram (EMG) monitoring of the peroneal division of the sciatic nerve are used to minimize the potential for an iatrogenic nerve injury. One sterile sensory electrode is inserted subcutaneously into the popliteal fossa superior to the transverse popliteal skin crease and just lateral to the medial hamstring tendons. A second electrode is inserted 1 cm posteroinferior to the fibular head. Two motor electrodes are inserted into the anterior muscle compartment of the leg, with an interval between them of about 3 cm. Before sterile draping, similar electrodes are placed in the contralateral lower extremity. The data obtained from the operative limb is compared with data from the contralateral extremity.

A cell-saver system is used, which reduces the blood loss during the procedure up to 20% to 30%.

A high-resolution image intensifier is necessary to assess fracture reduction, concentricity of the hip joint, the presence of intraarticular fragments, the stability of the fixation, and to detect intraarticular hardware. It is essential that adequate AP, obturator, and iliac oblique views be obtained. Frequently supplementary inlet and outlet views are necessary.

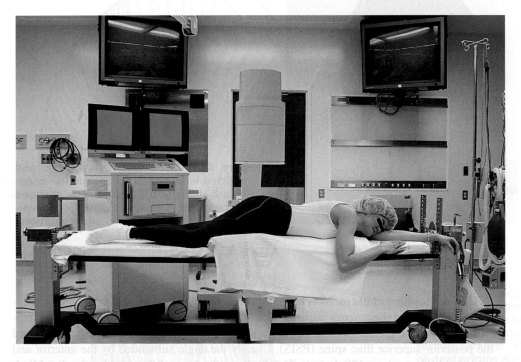

Figure 3. Surgery is performed with the patient placed on a radiolucent surgical table. High-resolution imaging with a 9-inch image intensifier is optimal.

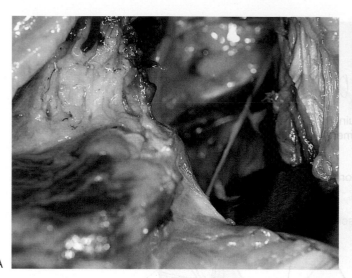
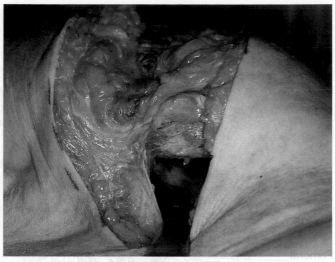

A   B

Figure 16. Exposure of the medial ilium in a cadaveric dissection. **A:** Lateral femoral cutaneous nerve is seen crossing the anterior extension of the anterior limb. The abdominal musculature, inguinal ligament, and sartorius have been released from the iliac crest. **B:** Blunt retractor inserted over the pelvic brim displaces the pelvic contents medially.

To further increase the anterior exposure, the skin incision of the anterior limb is extended toward the umbilicus 6 to 8 cm past the ASIS. The insertion of the external oblique muscle to the iliac crest is sharply incised. Division of the ilioinguinal ligament and the origin of sartorius at the ASIS permits medial retraction of the iliopsoas for exposure of the inner pelvic wall. The iliacus muscle is elevated subperiosteally from the internal iliac fossa and retracted medially (Fig. 16A and B). Blunt Hohmann retractors are placed over the brim of the true pelvis (Fig. 17). This exposure can be continued superiorly to the anterior aspect of the sacroiliac joint. If the iliopsoas is retracted laterally, the interval between

Figure 17. Development of the dissection of the medial wall of the ilium. The internal iliac fossa is exposed by the placement of a Hohmann retractor over the pelvic brim and a medial retraction of the iliopsoas. The interval between the iliopsoas and the external iliac vessels is developed by retracting the muscle laterally and identifying, and then dividing, the iliopectineal fascia. The external iliac vessels are the next most medial structures. Aberrant vessels may arise from the medial aspect of the external iliac artery such that they are relatively obscured when they are approached from the lateral aspect. Vigorous mobilization of the external iliac vessels should be avoided. The medial eminence of the acetabulum can be seen at the most anterior and medial aspect of the wound.

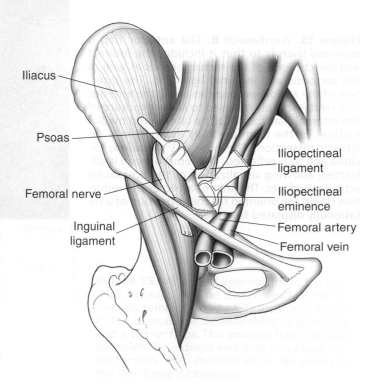

Iliacus

Psoas

Femoral nerve

Inguinal ligament

Iliopectineal ligament

Iliopectineal eminence

Femoral artery

Femoral vein

it and the external iliac vessels can be developed. The iliopectineal fascia is identified and divided down to the medial eminence, with a posterior extension to the true pelvic brim. In this way, the anterior acetabular roof is entirely exposed (Fig. 17). Attempts to achieve further medial exposure jeopardize the external iliac vessels and are unlikely to be successful.

To this point, the TRI has been described without a consideration of the specific fracture pattern or degree of comminution or osteopenia. Preservation of the soft-tissue attachments to the bone fragments for maintenance of osseous blood supply is crucial. Excessive stripping of the soft tissues from bone increases the risk of avascular necrosis (AVN) of the fragments, wound infection, and heterotopic ossification (HO). Depending on the fracture pattern, adjustments in the exposure may be necessary. For example, in a typical both-column fracture, the attachments of the rectus femoris, the sartorius, and the inguinal ligament to the anterior-column fragment that includes the anterosuperior acetabular dome are preserved. The fragment is displaced after releasing the TFL and the external oblique along the iliac crest, with subperiosteal elevation of the tensor and iliacus from the inner and outer pelvic tables, respectively. With this displacement, the quadrilateral surface and the medial eminence can be visualized for reduction and fixation. The high anterior-column fragment is then anatomically reduced and immobilized. In a similar manner, a posterior-wall fragment is preserved on its capsular attachment. In such a case, as the capsule is incised around the acetabular rim, the wall fragment is displaced in continuity with the capsule.

Modified Triradiate Incision

The principal concern with the classic TRI is the extent of soft-tissue stripping and the increased risk of devascularization of the fracture fragments, particularly those arising from the iliac wing, especially if both internal and external dissections are performed. A further concern is the high incidence of significant HO that follows this dissection, particularly where the reflected head of rectus femoris and the adjacent capsule of the hip joint are detached from bone. The MTRI was developed as a way to minimize the devascularization and HO that accompanies a classic TRI or EIF approach.

The MTRI differs from the TRI primarily by its preservation of the abductor muscle attachment to the greater trochanter, the absence of a trochanteric osteotomy, and the preservation of the anterosuperior hip-joint capsule including the contiguous origins of the indirect and direct heads of the rectus femoris.

The skin incision and fascial incisions are unchanged. The posterior limb is developed as described for the TRI. The altered development of the anterior limb begins with an identification of the interval between the TFL and the sartorius. The proximal third of the anterior-limb border of the TFL is mobilized. The origins of the TFL and the gluteus medius and minimus are preserved, along with the greater trochanter. The inguinal ligament and sartorius are incised sharply from their origins on the ASIS. The external oblique insertion on the anterior iliac crest is sharply incised. A subperiosteal elevation of the iliacus in the internal iliac fossa follows. The medial one third of the tendon of the direct head of rectus femoris is detached from the ASIS. Now the exposure of the internal wall of the ilium proceeds as described previously. The superior and anterior joint capsule are preserved along with the entire origin of the indirect head and most of the direct head of rectus femoris (Fig. 18). For a transverse or T-type fracture pattern, the accuracy of the reduction of the anterior column of the acetabulum is assessed by visualization of the extraarticular surface of the bone at the medial eminence. Image intensification is used to confirm the reduction of the corresponding portions of the articular surface. In the presence of morbid obesity or other complicating factors, the greater trochanter may be osteotomized. Because the origins of the abductors remain intact, superior reflection of the glutei is limited to the level of the upper border of the greater sciatic notch. Further reflection jeopardizes the superior gluteal neurovascular bundle resulting from excessive tension.

Wound closure begins with insertion of suction drains along the outer surface of the pelvic wall and along the inner wall when it has been exposed. The hip joint is placed in 30

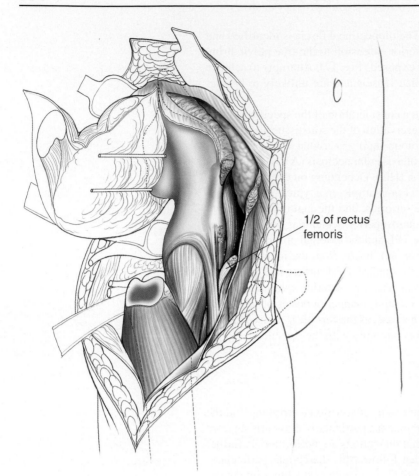

1/2 of rectus femoris

Figure 18. Modified triradiate approach (MTRI). No exposure of the articular surfaces is developed. The medial one third of the direct head of rectus femoris is released along with the sartorius and inguinal ligament. The inner wall of the ilium is exposed, whereas the capsule and the attachments of the reflected head of rectus femoris are preserved.

degrees of abduction by an elevation of the operative limb on a padded stand. This position lessens the tension in the soft tissues and further facilitates closure. The capsule of the hip joint and the origins of the indirect head of rectus femoris are reattached to the lateral ilium by the use of one or more bone anchors. The TFL and glutei, and the flap of the direct head of rectus femoris, the sartorius, and the inguinal ligament are reattached to their corresponding origins. The external oblique is reattached to the iliac crest if it was incised. The greater trochanter is accurately reduced and provisionally secured with the application of tenaculum forceps. Definitive fixation is achieved by the insertion of either two 4.5-mm cortical or two 6.5-mm long-threaded cancellous screws with ligamentous washers. In the presence of osteoporotic bone, the fixation of the greater trochanter may require the use of a supplemental heavy cerclage wire or cable-grip system. An apical stitch rejoins the three fascial edges superficial to the greater trochanter. The remainder of the fascia is repaired, and the subcutaneous and cutaneous layers are closed in a routine manner.

POSTOPERATIVE MANAGEMENT

The suction drains are maintained for up to 48 hours or until the drainage is less than 50 ml per 8-hour period. The cell-saver system is used for up to 12 hours after surgery, and when more than 250 ml of blood has been collected, it is autotransfused.

The patient is mobilized on the first postoperative day from bed to chair. When the overall condition of the patient permits, gait training begins with a walker or crutches. Patients remain partial weight bearing for 6 to 8 weeks. Active-assisted range-of-motion (ROM) exercises of the hip begin on the first postoperative day along with resisted strengthening of major muscle groups.

A second-generation cephalosporin or vancomycin is administered 1 hour before surgery and for 48 hours after surgery. Anticoagulation is initiated and maintained for approximately 6 weeks with either coumadin or low-molecular-weight heparin. After a classic TRI, prophylaxis for HO formation with indomethacin, 25 mg p.o., t.i.d., is started. The use of low-dose radiation therapy (RT) to reduce HO is not used in patients after acute acetabular reconstruction in view of the possible deleterious influences on osseous healing.

An AP view of the pelvis is obtained in the recovery room. On the second postoperative day, supplementary obturator and iliac oblique views are obtained, along with 2D-CT scans. The radiographs provide a gross assessment of the accuracy of the reduction and the congruity of the hip joint. 2D-CT scanning, although complicated by metal artifact, is the best technique to recognize intraarticular hardware and to assess postreduction joint congruity. For research purposes, we routinely additionally obtain a 3D-CT scan, including disarticulated acetabular views and reformated sagittal and coronal images. Useful 3D-CT images result only if high-quality software and experienced image collection and manipulation is available.

After discharge from the hospital, the patient continues physical therapy at home or at an outpatient facility. The sutures or skin staples are removed 10 to 14 days after surgery. The first office visit occurs about 4 weeks after the surgery. A clinical evaluation is performed, and plain radiographs are obtained. By this time, the hip should display more than 90 degrees of active flexion. Radiographic evidence of early fracture healing, such as partial obliteration of fracture lines, is anticipated. Progressive weight-bearing gait is encouraged, initially with two crutches and subsequently with a cane. Physiotherapy continues for 3 to 4 months with an emphasis on progressive-resistance exercises, including the use of weight machines. Restoration of the abductors of the hip is the primary objective. Typically, an abductor limp persists for a period of 3 to 6 months.

Repeated clinical and radiographic assessments are undertaken at 3 months, 6 months, and 1 year after surgery. Subtle clinical features of posttraumatic osteoarthritis include loss of motion, particularly internal rotation, as well as increasing pain in the groin or knee. Radiographs are carefully evaluated for congruency of the hip joint, collapse of the femoral head or the acetabulum, the formation of heterotopic bone, or the nonunion of a fracture line. The patient can expect to achieve a maximal recovery between 12 and 18 months after the time of the injury.

COMPLICATIONS

Infection

The incidence of infection after a TRI to the hip is approximately 2%. The incidence may be reduced by careful soft-tissue handling, development of full-thickness musculocutaneous flaps, and preservation of soft-tissue attachments to fracture fragments. Prophylactic antibiotics and shortened surgical times also reduce the risk of infection. If a deep wound infection is suspected, with drainage, periwound erythema or tenderness, or a persistent increase of temperature or white cell count, open exploration of the wound is warranted. Purulent fluid and hematoma are evacuated, and all necrotic tissues including bone should be excised. If the fixation is secure, it is retained; however, if it is grossly loose, it is removed. A clinical judgment regarding wound closure is based on the degree of tissue necrosis, the pathogenicity of the infecting organism, and the degree of host resistance. With minimal pus or tissue necrosis, the wound is closed in layers over suction drains. In more fulminant cases, the wound is packed open, and delayed closure is planned when the wound conditions permit. Culture-specific intravenous antibiotic therapy is administered.

Neurologic Injury

Injury to the sciatic nerve may lead to significant muscle weakness with a permanent foot drop and hypoesthesia or severe dysesthesia in the foot. The peroneal division of the sciatic nerve is more susceptible to injury than is the tibial division. The importance of an accurate preoperative clinical assessment to document any neurologic deficits cannot be overemphasized. The use of intraoperative SSEP and EMG monitoring and meticulous handling of the sciatic nerve during the dissection of the posterior column is recommended. To minimize injury to the sciatic nerve, the knee should be flexed and the hip extended throughout the case. If a postoperative neurologic deficit appear, no specific treatment is known to improve the recovery. Approximately 60% of sciatic nerve deficits will recover; however, the process may not be evident clinically for several weeks to months. Neurologic recovery may continue for 18 to 24 months after injury. During the recovery process, the painful dysesthesia in the leg and foot may be pronounced. Symptoms may be reduced with carbamazepine (Tegretol) or a tricyclic antidepressant. The clinical response to these drugs is, however, highly variable. The resources of a pain management team may be helpful. Sensory loss in the distribution of the tibial division of the sciatic nerve is particularly disabling and requires meticulous attention to footwear and foot care to diminish the risk of trophic ulceration of the plantar surface of the foot.

A foot drop or weakness of the ankle and toes extensors is managed with an ankle–foot orthosis (AFO) and passive ROM exercises of the ankle and subtalar joints. If motor function does not return within 18 months after injury and if the leg muscles are not severely atrophied, the patient may be a candidate for a posterior tibial tendon transfer. This may provide active dorsiflexion or at least a tenodesis effect, obviating the need for an AFO.

Lateral Femoral Cutaneous Nerve Injury

Despite careful identification and protection of the lateral femoral cutaneous nerve (LFCN), postoperative hypoesthesia or anesthesia in the distribution of the nerve on the anterior surface of the thigh is seen in 30% to 40% of the cases in which the dissection proceeds medial to the iliopsoas. Fortunately, loss of sensation does not lead to significant morbidity in most patients. Infrequently, dysesthesia in the distribution of the nerve may persist. In such a case, an exploration of the nerve can be undertaken in an attempt to identify a neuroma. The neuroma is resected, and the severed ends of the nerve are buried within the iliopsoas muscle.

Vascular Complications

Vascular complications are exceedingly uncommon when using a TRI to expose the acetabulum. Infrequently, persistent bleeding follows the surgical procedure, or an occlusion of the external iliac artery may occur.

Persistent bleeding of arterial or venous origin can originate from the gluteal, obturator, pudendal, or external iliac vessels, often leading to a consumptive coagulopathy. In such a case, treatment with fresh-frozen plasma and platelets may lead to cessation of the bleeding. Another effective strategy is selective arteriography and embolization. With significant bleeding or bleeding of rapid onset and progression, an open exploration of the wound is indicated. A vessel may be injured by a drill bit during open reduction and internal fixation. With impalement or laceration of the external iliac vessels, profuse bleeding results and usually requires the assistance of a vascular surgeon.

Late occlusion of the external iliac artery is a limb-threatening condition. The vessel is rendered vulnerable to occlusion if there is an intimal tear, if there is preexisting peripheral vascular disease, or if the injury resulted in significant blunt trauma to the groin. If a subsequent dissection of the vessels accompanies an exposure of the anterior column and superior pubic ramus, then even a trivial manipulation or retraction of the vessels can lead to a complete occlusion. Even in the absence of predisposing factors, a prolonged forceful retraction of the vessels can initiate an occluding thrombus. If the pulses in the limb are lost in the immediate postoperative period, an arteriogram and vascular consultation are urgently needed.

Avascular Necrosis

AVN may occur in either the femoral head or the acetabulum. AVN most commonly occurs after a posterior fracture–dislocation of the hip or disruption of the posterior wall or column. During a standard TRI, unlike the MTRI, development of the anterior limb requires division of the lateral femoral circumflex vessels. Therefore careful preservation of the medial femoral circumflex vessels is necessary, particularly during the release and subsequent retraction of the quadratus femoris from the ischium.

Progressive hip and groin pain with limitation of hip motion, particularly internal rotation, frequently occur. Radiographically, AVN is identified by an increased density of the femoral head compared with that of the other hip. Collapse of the femoral head is confirmed by loss of height and sphericity. Progressive loss of the joint space follows.

Whole-head involvement characteristic of AVN after an acetabular fracture is unlike segmental patterns of AVN attributed to other causes. Surgical interventions such as core decompression, vascularized free-fibula grafts, and osteotomies have not been successful. With AVN of the femoral head, arthrodesis of the hip is difficult to achieve and is not well accepted by most patients. Total hip arthroplasty is the treatment of choice for this problem.

AVN of the femoral head should not be confused with posttraumatic degenerative joint disease as a result of impaction or abrasion injuries to the femoral head, or traumatic loss of a portion of the femoral head. Typically in such a case, the femoral head deteriorates rapidly with a further loss of bone, resultant joint incongruity, and joint-space narrowing. This rapidly progressive joint deterioration has a similar very poor prognosis.

AVN of the acetabulum also may occur. Posterior-wall fragments or any other denuded fragments of the acetabulum and areas of marginal impaction are at risk for AVN. Patients with pain, loss of motion, and progressive radiographic deterioration of the hip joint are candidates for total hip replacement. Total hip arthroplasty to treat posttraumatic arthritis or AVN after acetabular fractures is a difficult operative procedure and is associated with high rates of component loosening.

Heterotopic Ossification

After a classic TRI for a complex acetabular fracture, the radiographic incidence of HO is between 50% and 70%. In about 7% to 13% of cases, the HO significantly or completely compromises the motion of the hip joint (1,6). With the marked decrease in the degree of soft-tissue stripping from the lateral ilium and the immediate periarticular region, the use of the MTRI has reduced the incidence and severity of HO.

If HO occurs with loss of ROM of the hip, excision of the HO and subsequent prophylactic treatment merits consideration. Excision is deferred until radiographs demonstrate no further formation of HO and maturation of the existing HO. Radiographically, if the hip has moderate to severe posttraumatic arthritis or AVN of the femoral head, then excision of the HO is unlikely to be effective unless accompanied by a total hip replacement. Excision of HO is a major procedure with the potential for profuse hemorrhage from the highly vascular bone. A variety of patterns of HO formation can be encountered. The best potential outcome occurs when the HO is discretely located between the hip muscles and the capsule. When the HO infiltrates both the hip muscles and the capsule, the prognosis is guarded. After surgery, prophylaxis with indomethacin or radiotherapy (700 to 1,000 Gy as a single dose) or both is necessary. Indomethacin is given for a period of 6 to 12 weeks. Physiotherapy begins the first postoperative day by using both active and passive motion of the hip joint.

Greater Trochanteric Complications

Nonunion of the greater trochanter occurs in approximately 6% of cases. Usually it is painful and requires open reduction and modification of the internal fixation. Most of these nonunions occur in the elderly or others with osteoporotic bone. Cable-grip fixation is particularly effective. One or two cables are passed through drill holes in the lesser trochanter, which provides a secure anchor for greater trochanteric fixation. An additional cable anchors the greater trochanter to the lateral aspect of the proximal femur, thereby functioning as a tension band. In the presence of an associated bone defect or osteoporotic bone, supplemental autologous bone graft is used.

About 20% to 30% of patients complain of pain associated with the fixation screws used to stabilize the greater trochanter. Symptoms are likely to occur in thin, active patients. Usually removal of the internal fixation relieves the discomfort.

ILLUSTRATIVE CASE FOR TECHNIQUE

This 27-year-old man was the driver of a light truck that struck a snowplow. He sustained a transverse–posterior wall acetabular fracture (Fig. 19A–C). Neurologic examination of the lower extremity was normal.

The plain radiographs and 2D-CT scans confirmed the presence of the transverse fracture line and the comminution of the posterior wall (Fig. 20A–C). The 3D-CT scan images allowed a better appreciation of the rotational displacement of the anterior column (Fig. 21A–E).

The fracture was internally fixed by using an MTRI. The anterior column was reduced and stabilized with a four-hole, one-third tubular plate. In view of the comminution of the posterior wall, a hook plate was fashioned from a second one-third tubular plate and applied to hold the comminuted fragments in position (Fig. 22A–D). Plain radiographs, 2D-CT images, and 3D-CT images demonstrated a concentric reduction (Figs. 23A–C, 24A and B, and 25A–E).

Postoperatively, the patient was gait-trained for touch-down weight bearing for 6 weeks, followed by a progressive increase in weight bearing to tolerance. In the absence of complications, the patient continued to do well for the 6-month period after the surgery.

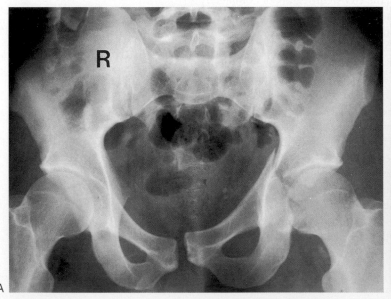
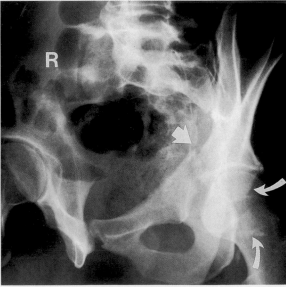

Figure 19. Preoperative radiographs. **A:** Anteroposterior (AP) radiograph documents the high transverse fracture. **B:** Obturator oblique radiograph documents the displacement of the anterior column (straight arrow) and comminution of the posterior wall (curved arrows). *(figure continues)*

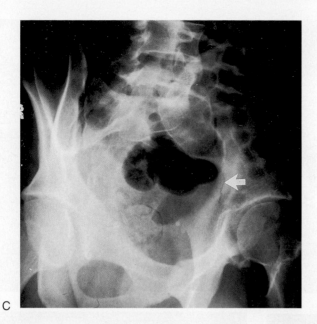

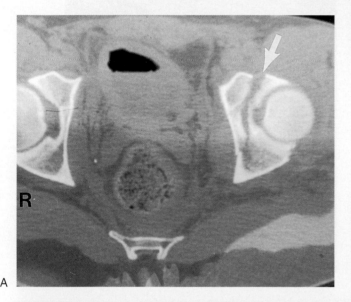

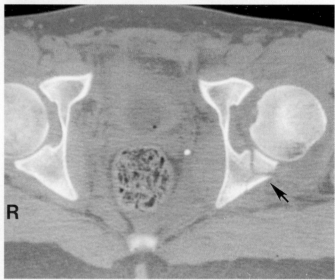

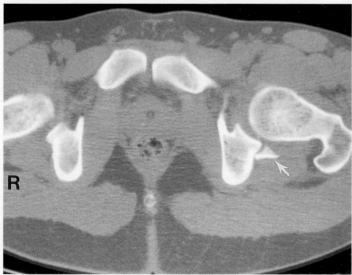

Figure 19. *(continued)* **C:** Iliac oblique radiograph documents the undisplaced fracture of the posterior column (arrow).

Figure 20. Preoperative two-dimensional computed tomography scans. **A:** Transverse fracture line. **B, C:** Comminution of the posterior wall (black arrow; **B**) and displacement of a small wall fragment (white arrow) with subluxation of the femoral head **(C).**

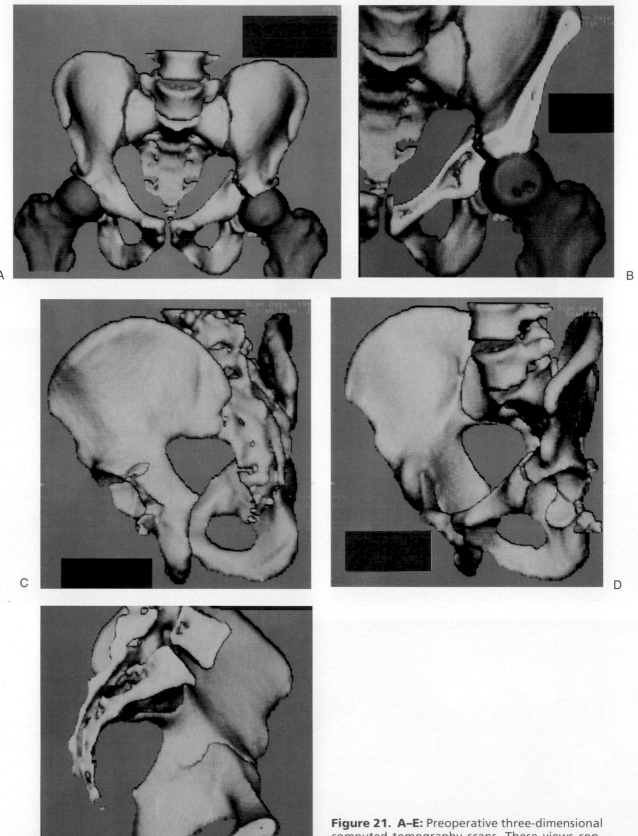

Figure 21. A–E: Preoperative three-dimensional computed tomography scans. These views confirm the findings of the plain radiographs. Rotational deformity with the displaced anterior column and the minimally displaced posterior column are emphasized in **E**.

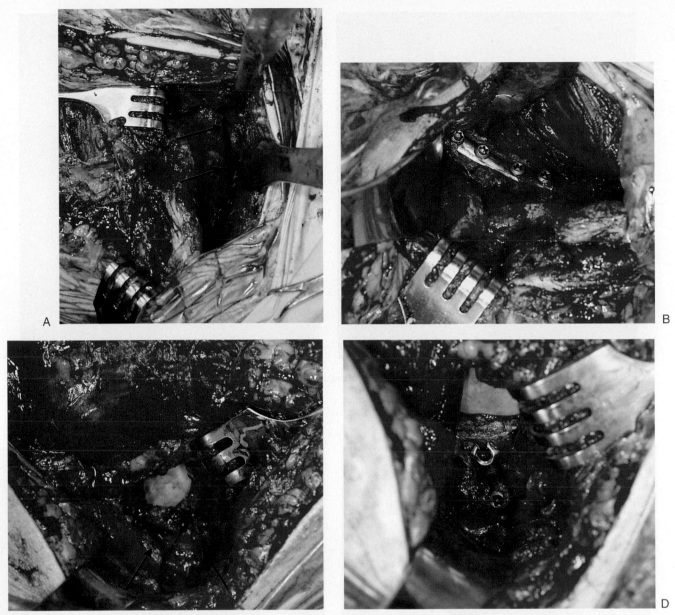

Figure 22. Intraoperative photographs. **A:** Fracture of the anterior column is marked with white arrows. The dissection has exposed the inner surface of the ilium to the fracture line at the pelvic brim. The anterior–superior iliac spine is marked with a dark arrow. **B:** A four-hole one-third tubular plate applied to the anterior column. **C:** Femoral head is exposed through the posterior limb of the incision. Comminuted fracture fragments are identified with arrows. **D:** Spring plate is applied to the largest of the comminuted fragments.

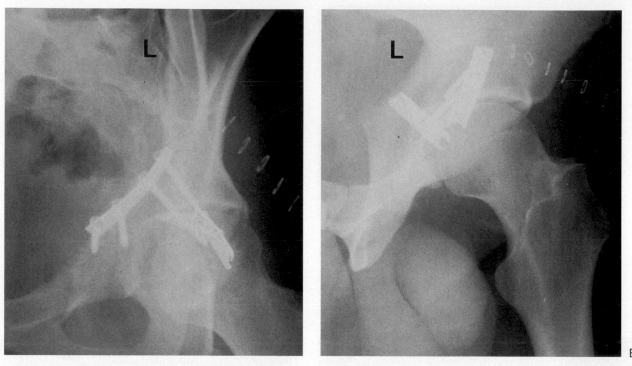

Figure 23. Postoperative obturator **(A)** and iliac oblique **(B)** views. The articular surface is concentric and congruent.

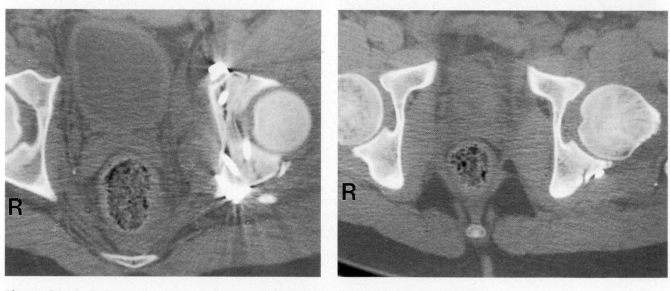

Figure 24. A, B: Postoperative two-dimensional computed tomography scans. These views confirm the accuracy of the articular reduction and the placement of the internal fixation.

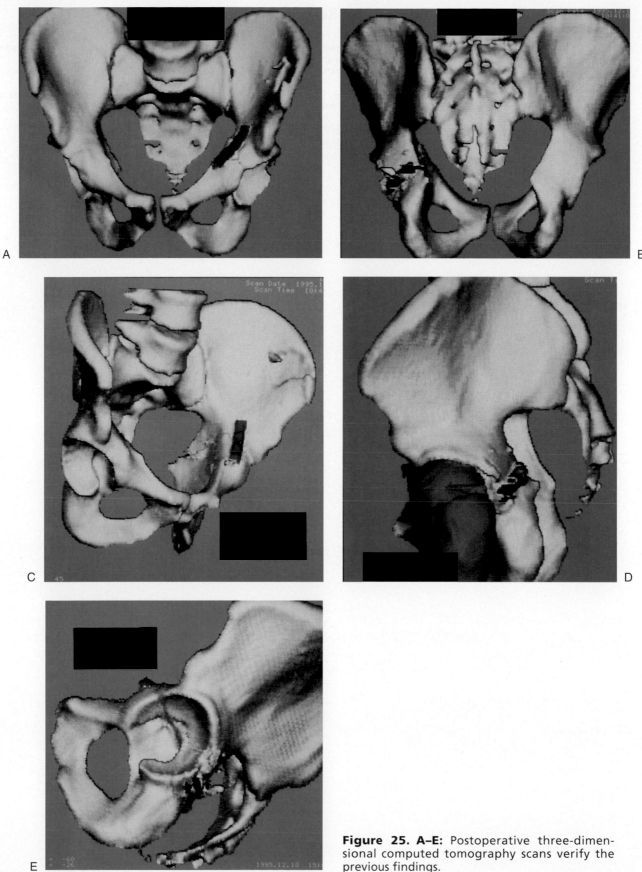

Figure 25. A–E: Postoperative three-dimensional computed tomography scans verify the previous findings.

RECOMMENDED READING

1. Alonzo, J.E., Davila, R., Bradley, E.: Extended iliofemoral versus triradiate approaches in the management of associated acetabular fractures. *Clin. Orthop.*, 305:81–87, 1994.
2. Hilde, W.J., Ferner, H., Staubesand, J. (eds.): *Sobotta Atlas of Human Anatomy,* Vol 2. Urban & Schwarzenberg, Baltimore, 1983.
3. Hoppenfeld, S., and deBoer, P.: *Surgical Exposures in Orthopaedics: The Anatomic Approach.* 2nd ed. J.B. Lippincott, Philadelphia, 1994.
4. Letournel, E., and Judet, R.: *Fractures of the Acetabulum.* 2nd ed. Springer-Verlag, New York, 1993.
5. Mears, D.C., and Rubash, H.E.: Extensile exposure of the pelvis. *Contemp. Orthop.*, 6:21,1983.
6. Mears, D.C., and Rubash, H.E.: *Pelvic and Acetabular Fractures.* Slack Inc., New Jersey, 1986.
7. Tile, M.: *Fractures of the Pelvis and Acetabulum.* 2nd ed. Williams & Wilkins, Baltimore, 1995.

Subject Index

Glenohumeral joint (*contd.*)
   dissection of, in open reduction/internal fixation of glenoid fractures, 8f
Glenoid fractures
   classification of, 4f–5f
   open reduction/internal fixation of, 3–17
      anesthesia for, 6
      bone stock for, 9, 9f
      case studies of, 15, 15f–17f
      cerclage wires in, 10f
      closure in, 12, 13f
      complications of, 14–15
      compression screws in, 9, 10f–12f
      contraindications to, 3, 4f–5f
      dissection in, 6, 7f–8f, 8
      incision for, 6, 7f
      indications for, 3, 4f–5f
      Kirschner wires in, 9, 10f–12f, 10f–13f
      positioning for, 6, 7f
      postoperative management in, 14
      preoperative planning in, 5–6
      reconstruction plates in, 9, 10f–11f
      supplemental superior approach in, 9, 12f–13f
      surgical approach to, 6
Gluteal vessels, injury to, after extended iliofemoral approach to acetabular fractures, 692
Gluteus maximus muscle, dissection of
   in extended iliofemoral approach to acetabular fractures, 684, 685f
   in Kocher–Langenbeck approach to acetabular fractures, 639, 639f–640f, 640–641
   in triradiate approach to acetabular fractures, 705, 705f–707f
Gluteus maximus tendon, release of, in Kocher–Langenbeck approach to acetabular fractures, 641f–642f, 641–642
Gluteus medius muscle, dissection of, in Kocher–Langenbeck approach to acetabular fractures, 643f–644f, 644
Guide pins
   with dynamic condylar screw, for supracondylar femoral fractures, 312f, 313
   for fixation of posterior pelvic ring disruption, 602, 603f–605f
   for reconstruction nailing of subtrochanteric femoral fractures, 259, 259f, 265, 265f–266f
Guide wires. *See also* Kirschner wires
   ball-tipped
      for reconstruction nailing of subtrochanteric femoral fractures, 259, 260f–261f, 261
   in small-diameter nailing of tibial shaft fractures, 444–445
   for fixation of talar neck fractures, 513, 514f
   for intramedullary nailing of femoral fractures, 278, 283, 283f–288f
   in intramedullary nailing of humeral shaft fractures, 85, 85f
   for open reduction/internal fixation of proximal humerus fractures, 40–41, 41f
Gustillo classification system, of tibial shaft fractures, 411, 413f

H
Hardware failure
   after reamed intramedullary nailing of tibial shaft fractures, 429
   after small-diameter nailing of tibial shaft fractures, 435, 436f, 455f–457f

Hawkins classification, of talar neck fractures, 506f
Heat necrosis, from reamed intramedullary nailing of tibial shaft fractures, 421, 422f
Hemarthrosis, after open reduction/internal fixation of patellar fractures, 344
Hematoma, evacuation of
   in open reduction/internal fixation of calcaneal fractures, 535–536
   in open reduction/internal fixation of distal humeral intraarticular fractures, 99, 101f
   in open reduction/internal fixation of distal radial fractures, 192f, 194
   in open reduction/internal fixation of patellar fractures, 340f
   in open reduction/internal fixation of radial head fractures, 132f, 133
   in open reduction/internal fixation of tibial shaft fractures, 402f
Hemorrhage, after sacral fixation of pelvic fractures, 626–627
Henry approach, to open reduction/internal fixation of forearm fractures, 145f–147f, 145–146
Herbert screws, for open reduction/internal fixation of distal humeral intraarticular fractures, 99, 103f
Heterotopic ossification
   after extended iliofemoral approach to acetabular fractures, 693, 693f
   after Kocher-Langenbeck approach to acetabular fractures, 652
   after open reduction/internal fixation of olecranon fractures, 126
   after surgical reconstruction of knee dislocation, 362
   after triradiate approach to acetabular fractures, 717
Hip, dislocation of, in acetabular fractures, 634f
Hip fractures. *See also* Acetabular fractures
   intertrochanteric, operative management of, 223 241. *See also* Intertrochanteric hip fractures
Hip-screw plates, insertion of
   in 95-degree fixed-angled blade plate stabilization of subtrochanteric femoral fractures, 251, 251f–253f
   in intertrochanteric hip fractures
      stable, 231–233, 232f–233f
      unstable, 235f, 236
Hohmann retractor, use of
   in calcaneal fractures, 533f
   in intertrochanteric hip fractures, 228f
   in open reduction/internal fixation of symphysis pubis fractures, 588f
   in supracondylar femoral fractures, 308f–309f, 308–309
Holding wires, subchondral, placement of, in ring/hybrid frame fixation of tibial plateau fractures, 386, 387f
Hook plate
   for open reduction/internal fixation of malleolar fractures, 491, 491f
   for open reduction/internal fixation of olecranon fractures, 118f
Humeral fractures
   distal, intraarticular, open reduction/internal fixation of, 95–111. *See also* Distal humeral intraarticular fractures
   proximal
      open reduction/internal fixation of, 35–44. *See also* Proximal humerus fractures
      perctunaeous fixation of, 19–33. *See also* Proximal humerus fractures
Humeral head, removal of, in proximal humeral arthroplasty, 52, 52f